TADDEO ALDEROTTI
AND HIS PUPILS

TADDEO ALDEROTTI
AND HIS PUPILS

TWO GENERATIONS OF ITALIAN
MEDICAL LEARNING

NANCY G. SIRAISI

PRINCETON UNIVERSITY PRESS

Princeton, New Jersey

Library of Congress Cataloging in Publication Data will be
found on the last printed page of this book

Publication of this book has been aided by
a grant from the Paul Mellon Fund of Princeton University Press

This book has been composed in Linotype Granjon

Clothbound editions of Princeton University Press books
are printed on acid-free paper, and binding materials are
chosen for strength and durability

Printed in the United States of America by Princeton
University Press, Princeton, New Jersey

Princeton Legacy Library edition 2019
Paperback ISBN: 978-0-691-65558-1
Hardcover ISBN: 978-0-691-65700-4

IN MEMORY OF MY FATHER

CONTENTS

ACKNOWLEDGMENTS

Numerous scholars, none of whom are responsible for any of my mistakes or omissions, have been generous with their assistance; the following are some of those to whom I am particularly indebted. Pearl Kibre, professor emeritus of Hunter College and The Graduate School of The City University of New York, knows more about medieval learned medicine in the university milieu than I can ever hope to find out. My obligation to her goes back far beyond her kindness in reading the manuscript of this book and offering suggestions for its improvement. I should like to thank Paul Oskar Kristeller, professor emeritus of Columbia University, New York, who also read the entire work in manuscript, allowing me to profit from his vast learning while saving me from many errors. I am grateful, too, to Joseph Soudek, professor emeritus of Queens College of The City University of New York, for invaluable guidance regarding the section in chapter three on Bartolomeo da Varignana's commentary on the pseudo-Aristotelian Economics; *to Professor James Etzwiler of Paterson College, Wayne, New Jersey, who read some of the philosophical material in chapter six; to Dr. Judith Neaman of The Institute for Research in History, who offered comments on the sections on psychology and mental illness in chapter seven; to Dr. Adrian Zorgniotti, M.D., Director, Department of Urology, Cabrini Medical Center, New York, who advised me on the medical content of chapter nine. I should also like to acknowledge helpful suggestions from Professor Vern Bullough of the University of California at Northridge and from Professor Michael McVaugh of the University of North Carolina. Finally, I want to express my gratitude to Professor Bert Hansen of the University of Toronto, who read most of the work in manuscript, and, in the course of innumerable conversations about Taddeo, constantly offered encouragement, informed and sympathetic criticism, and stimulating ideas.*

My thanks are also due to the staffs of the various libraries where I have worked, first and foremost the Biblioteca Apostolica Vaticana; and also the Biblioteca Marciana, Venice; the Biblioteca Medicea Laurenziana, Florence; the Biblioteca Universitaria, Padua; the Biblioteca Universitaria, Bologna; the Biblioteca Estense, Modena; the Biblioteca Am-

brosiana, Milan; the Bibliothèque Nationale and the Bibliothèque de la Sorbonne, Paris; the British Library, London; the Special Collections, Columbia University, New York; and the National Library of Medicine, Bethesda, Maryland. The Padri Redentoristi of the Church of Sta. Maria della Fava, Venice, kindly allowed me to consult and microfilm the unique manuscript (so far as is known) of Bartolomeo da Varignana's commentary on the Economics. A special debt of thanks is owed to Mrs. Alice Weaver and her staff at the Rare Book Room of the New York Academy of Medicine for their unvarying helpfulness and numerous personal kindnesses.

Earlier versions of parts of chapters three and five appeared as articles in Manuscripta and Isis, respectively: "The libri morales in the Faculty of Arts and Medicine at Bologna: Bartolomeo da Varignana and the Pseudo-Aristotelian Economica," Manuscripta 20 (1976):105-118; and "Taddeo Alderotti and Bartolomeo da Varignana on the Nature of Medical Learning," Isis 68 (1977):27-39. I am grateful to the editors of those journals for their permission to reprint.

While working on this project I have been the recipient of grants from the Faculty Research Award Program of The City University of New York, the American Philosophical Society, the Shuster Fund of Hunter College, and the National Endowment for the Humanities, to all of which am I duly grateful.

Eriko Amino assisted in the thankless task of compiling Appendix One with her usual good humor, diligence, and good grace. Lester Van Losberg typed part of the manuscript.

I wish also to thank my family, who provided moral support and necessary distraction in generous amounts. Without them, and without good friends, I might have finished the book faster; but it would have been impoverished by my own impoverishment.

December 9, 1979

ABBREVIATIONS AND
SHORT TITLES

ABBREVIATIONS

BAV   Biblioteca Apostolica Vaticana.

Comm.   Commentary on the text following.

CLM   Codex latinus monacensis (Munich, Bayerische Staatsbiblio-
         thek).

DSB   *Dictionary of Scientific Biography*, 14 vols., ed. Charles C.
         Gillispie (New York, 1970-1976).

Klebs   Arnold C. Klebs. *Incunabula scientifica et medica: Short Title
         List* (Bruges, 1938).

NLM   National Library of Medicine, Bethesda, Md.

q.   *Quaestio* or *questio*.

SF   Mauro Sarti and Mauro Fattorini, *De claris archigymnasii
         Bononiensis professoribus*, 2 vols., ed. Carlo Albicini and
         Carlo Malagola (Bologna, 1888-1896).

TK   Lynn Thorndike and Pearl Kibre, *A Catalogue of Incipits of
         Mediaeval Scientific Writings in Latin* (2d ed., Cambridge,
         Mass., 1963).

SHORT TITLES OF FREQUENTLY CITED EDITIONS

Dino, *Canon 2*   *Expositio Dini super canones generales de vir-
                           tutibus medicinarum simplicium secundi ca-
                           nonis Avicenne*, printed with Dino, *Dilucida-
                           torium* (Venice, 1514).

Dino, *Chirurgia*   *Expositio super III, IV, et parte V Fen [quarti
                           Canonis] Avicennae* (Ferrara, 1489; Klebs
                           336.1).

Dino, *De natura fetus*   *Scriptum Dini super libro de natura fetus Hy-
                           pocratis*, printed with Jacopo (Giacomo) da
                           Forli, *Expositio . . . supra capitulum Avicenne
                           De generatione embrionis . . .* (Venice, 1502).

Dino, *Dilucidatorium*   *Dyni florentini super quarta fen primi Avi-
                           cenne preclarissima commentaria: que diluci-*

xii

	datorium totius practice generalis medicinalis scientie nuncupatur . . . (Venice, 1514).
Guglielmo, *Practica*	*Excellentissimi medici Guielmi brixiensis aggregatoris dictorum illustrium medicorum ad unamquamque egritudinem a capite ad pedes practica* . . . (Venice, 1508).
Taddeo, *Aphor.*; Taddeo, *Isagoge;* Taddeo, *Pronost.*; and Taddeo, *Reg. acut.*	*Thaddei Florentini Expositiones in arduum aphorismorum Ipocratis volumen, In divinum pronosticorum Ipocratis librum, In preclarum regiminis acutorum Ipocratis opus, In subtilissimum Joannitii Isagogarum libellum* (Venice, 1527).
Turisanus, *Plusquam*	*Turisani monaci plusquam commentum in Microtegni Galieni* (Venice, 1512).

A NOTE ON NAMES AND ORTHOGRAPHY

In general, personal names of Italian origin appear in the present work in their Italian form. In a few instances, where the Latin forms are more familiar or where the Italian forms are uncertain, Latin forms have been used. I have adopted the usage Taddeo Alderotti, rather than Taddeo degli Alderotti or Taddeo Alderotto, because it appears to be sanctioned by modern Italian authors. The names of persons who are not Italian appear in whatever form seems most familiar to English-speaking readers. Wherever Latin is used, medieval orthography has been retained.

For the sake of simplicity, the author(s) of the ancient Hippocratic corpus is referred to as "Hippocrates"; works attributed to Hippocrates only in the Middle Ages are termed pseudo-Hippocratic.

A NOTE ON BANKS AND
INTEREST RATES

INTRODUCTION

Taddeo Alderotti of Florence and Bologna rose from humble origins to wealth, professional distinction, and learning. As self-made men are apt to be, he was both an innovator and a skillful adapter. Bologna was an ancient and celebrated seat of learning, especially in law, and had begun to be a center of medical education before ever Taddeo arrived there; yet Taddeo was a pioneer in establishing at Bologna what may be thought of as the "new medicine" of the late thirteenth century— a tightly organized, secular profession whose members (mostly, in Italy at any rate, married laymen like Taddeo himself) studied their discipline within a university faculty of "arts and medicine." The education of physicians in such a faculty, at Bologna as elsewhere, involved close attention not merely to medicine itself but to all the scientific and philosophical learning of the day. Taddeo himself appears to have been chiefly responsible for the introduction to the public *studium* of Bologna not only of a curriculum of Hippocratic and Galenic studies already developed at Salerno and certain schools in northern Europe, but also of Aristotelian philosophy and natural science. He and his pupils used this material to carry on the task, begun in the West only about a generation before Taddeo began to teach in the 1260s, of analyzing the differences between Aristotle's mammalian biology and Galen's physiology.

Taddeo's students, who came to him from Florence, from Padua, and perhaps from farther afield, included some of the foremost Italian physicians of the early fourteenth century—outstanding examples of successful university training for one of the two great learned professions. Subsequently they carried their learning to Florence, Siena, Paris, Avignon, and elsewhere.

Yet the learning of this group of men was neither exclusively academic nor classroom bound. Taddeo and his pupils had among their patients several popes, the Emperor Henry VII, and a doge of Venice. Furthermore, these physicians carried on an already established Bolognese tradition of surgical study and practice, and two of them, Bartolomeo da Varignana and Mondino de' Liuzzi, are famous as pioneers of autopsy and of anatomical dissection for purposes of study. Contemporary society perceived in these medical masters a highly esteemed combination of scientific learning and professional skill, and it rewarded them accordingly, with glowing eulogies, teaching positions in major *studia*, clients of high standing, and considerable wealth.

Given this range of activities by Taddeo and his fellows, it is not surprising to learn that some of their achievements have at different times attracted the attention of social historians, university historians, historians of philosophy, historians of medicine, historians of Italian language and literature, and specialists in the early Italian Renaissance, as a glance at the periodical articles in the Bibliography will show. Furthermore, the milieu in which Taddeo and his associates taught has been the focus of studies as diverse as Bullough's account of medical professionalization at Bologna and the scholarly investigations into the rise of Bolognese Averroism by Grabmann, Maier, Ermatinger, Kuksewicz, and others. (For works by scholars mentioned in the Introduction, see Bibliography.) Yet perhaps this very diversity of interest has hitherto provided a barrier to any unified study of the group as a whole. For although such aspects of Taddeo's learning as his vernacular writings, his *consilia* for individual patients, and his references to contemporary philosophical disputes at Paris have received due notice, no systematic survey of his entire output, and particularly of his Latin commentaries on authoritative medical works, has, as far as I know, ever been attempted.

This diffusion of scholarship is not peculiar to studies of Taddeo and those associated with him. In general, the content and the philosophical context of the learning of academic physicians in the medieval schools of Italy remains largely unexplored even today. Although major contributions to the study of the subject have been made—the names Thorndike, Kristeller, Kibre spring to mind—much of the enormous written output of Italian teaching physicians between the later twelfth and the fifteenth centuries remains unanalyzed and unread.

The reasons for this neglect are not difficult to find. In themselves, the main outlines of the Hippocratic, Galenic, and Arabic medical theories taught in medieval medical schools are fairly well known to historians of science and medicine. Moreover, despite a general recognition of the importance of the institutional and intellectual links between arts, philosophy, and medicine in the Italian university centers, medicine remains at best a peripheral topic for most historians of philosophy or culture. And

social historians and historians of medicine, insofar as they have concerned themselves with medicine in medieval and early Renaissance
Italy, have tended to concentrate upon its professional and practical aspects. Furthermore, although the continuing demand in the fifteenth- and
sixteenth-century universities for old, established medical textbooks ensured that a substantial number of older treatises and commentaries appeared in early printed editions, much of the output of medieval learned
physicians remains in manuscripts written in the cramped and hurried
hands of scholars more concerned with the rapid flow of their own or of
a lecturing or disputing master's ideas than with the comfort of future
readers. *Many of these works do much to justify the strictures laid upon
medical scholasticism*: lengthy, inordinately repetitive, and replete with
obscure technical terminology, they make the well-known aversion of
certain humanists for this type of learning immediately and readily
comprehensible.

Yet the major role played by learned medicine in the Italian *studia*,
the weighty social and intellectual influence in the fourteenth and fifteenth centuries of university-trained physicians, and the interactions between medicine, liberal arts, and philosophy in faculties "of arts and
medicine" all suggest that learned medicine deserves a more prominent
place in the intellectual and scientific history of the age than it usually
gets, and that the writings of scholastic physicians merit something better
than the hasty, and it must be said contemptuous, dismissal they are still
often accorded. As the reader will see, learned physicians expended much
energy in debating whether medicine was or was not a branch of natural
philosophy. Although they reached varying conclusions, it is nevertheless
plain, from our present standpoint, that their medical learning has a place
in a larger philosophical, intellectual, and scientific context. Moreover,
medical learning was itself no more static and unchanging than learning
in any other field; so our studies of its history need to be placed within
specific times and places as well as within a general intellectual context.
The vehicles of medical discussion were principally commentaries appended to lemmata from authoritative texts (such as works of Hippocrates, Galen, or Avicenna) and disputed *questiones*. Furthermore, numerous *questiones* or *dubia* were also incorporated within the commentaries
themselves. Works cast in these forms were ideally suited for the comparison of conflicting authorities and the expression of different and

changing opinions. While it is true that some arguments tended to take standard forms and became repetitive, the overall picture is one of development and debate.

It has seemed to me, therefore, that a systematic survey of the written works as well as of the careers and medical activities of Taddeo and those he trained might constitute a modestly useful adjunct to our understanding of medieval science in its intellectual and social setting. Such a survey the present work is designed to provide.

As I studied the works of Taddeo and the other authors, a number of topics especially engaged my interest. Among these were the theoretical concepts held by members of the group about the nature of medical learning and the place of medicine among the sciences (chapter five), as compared (and sometimes as contrasted) with the uses actually made in medical teaching of material drawn from natural philosophy (chapters six and seven); the extent of Taddeo's and his students' knowledge of Galen and their role in curricular development (chapter four); the relationship in their life's work and writings between medical theory and medical practice (chapters eight and nine); the use of scholastic *questiones* as tools of practical as well as abstract and speculative medical teaching (chapter eight); the place of written *consilia* for individual patients in their teaching and practice (chapter nine). Chapters one, two, and three concern the setting in which they taught, their biographies, and their contributions to moral philosophy, vernacular learning, and civic life. In an attempt to make clear their own priorities, I have compiled and arranged by subject a cumulative index of the titles of the questions discussed in their commentaries, which appears as Appendix One.

Of the problems involved in writing this work, by no means the least was that of determining which masters could legitimately be regarded as having learned from Taddeo. I have included all authors (known to me) of surviving written works who, on the basis of evidence dating from no later than the fourteenth century, can be shown to have been Taddeo's pupils, or to have had personal contact with him as younger professional colleagues, or both. Using these criteria, contemporary documentary records of the *studium* of Bologna yield Bartolomeo da Varignana and the master of arts Gentile da Cingoli; a contemporary letter by Engelbert of Admont produces Guglielmo da Brescia; a description of Taddeo as a teaching practitioner in one of the works of Mondino de' Liuzzi gives Mondino; and the collection of Florentine biographies by

Filippo Villani gives two more: Dino del Garbo and Turisanus (for references, see chapter two). All of these men (other than Mondino de' Liuzzi) were originally identified as Taddeo's pupils by external evidence, rather than by signs of response to Taddeo's intellectual influence within their written works. Yet that this group was perceived by its contemporaries and successors, as well as by myself, as constituting an intellectual as well as a professional community is interestingly suggested by a passage in one of the medical *questiones* of Gentile da Foligno (d. 1348), one of the most prolific and learned medical authors of the fourteenth century. Before proceeding to give his own views on "the reduction of medicine to act" (that is, on how medicine works in the body), Gentile summarized the views of previous authorities. He named eleven recent writers who had discussed the problem, most of them being associated with the Bologna faculty of arts and medicine; eight of the eleven are Taddeo Alderotti, all six of his pupils listed above, and a pupil of a pupil (Pancius of Lucca, follower of Guglielmo da Brescia).[1]

It should be emphasized, however, that I make no claim that the masters treated in the present study constituted a school of thought: one cannot say that either many or highly significant ideas were peculiar to them as a group. Taddeo's pupils and associates were exposed to other influences besides his; and, while some of them made their entire careers teaching at Bologna, others went far afield. In general, the very nature of medieval intellectual life—the ready interchange of both men and ideas between different centers of learning, and the widespread reliance upon a common body of authoritative texts in any given discipline—means that historians should exercise the greatest caution in attempting to demonstrate that particular concepts were the exclusive property of any one *studium* or group of masters, and that they should be aware that such efforts are often foredoomed to failure. Yet, while many of the concepts, pedagogical methods, and practices espoused by Taddeo and those exposed to his teaching might be paralleled elsewhere, it would probably not be easy to find another group of six or seven medical masters from

---

[1] Gentile da Foligno, *Questiones et tractatus extravagantes clarissimi Domini Gentilis de Fulgineo* . . . , q. 46, fols. 63r-65v. Turisanus is referred to throughout as *Plusquam commentator*, a title derived from his chief work, the *Plusquam commentum* on Galen's *Tegni* (*Microtechne*). The other recent writers named by Gentile are Antonius (probably Antonio da Parma; see next note), the Paduan professor of medicine and philosophy Peter of Abano (*Conciliator*, Petrus de Abano, Petrus Aponensis), and a master Martinus whom I have not succeeded in identifying.

the crucial period when the Italian universities of arts and medicine were taking shape whose personal contacts, common training, and institutional background are so well documented, whose reputation among their contemporaries stood so high, and whose writings survive in such quantity. These considerations, to me, more than justify the study of these men as a group.

A number of other masters who may have fallen within the orbit of Taddeo's influence have for various reasons been excluded from the present work. Although it seems highly likely that all faculty members and students in arts and medicine at Bologna in Taddeo's lifetime knew him and were to some extent influenced by him, none except those named above are included here, because specific evidence of personal association is lacking. The most important figure omitted on these grounds is probably Antonio da Parma, who seems to have taught medicine at Bologna before 1323, and who therefore may have studied under Taddeo.[2] Pupils and colleagues mentioned by name in Taddeo's own writings, but by whom no works are known to have survived, are debarred for lack of evidence concerning their thought and careers. Space and time limitations have dictated the omission of the pupils of Taddeo's pupils, several of whom were professors of medicine at Bologna in the first half of the fourteenth century (notably Giuliano, Bertruccio, teacher of Guy de Chauliac, and Alberto da Bologna, all of whose works merit further study).[3] Finally, no effort has been made to discuss the various fourteenth-century

[2] A detailed account of the philosophical contribution of Antonio da Parma, who produced a commentary on part of the *Canon* of Avicenna and a medical compendium in addition to philosophical writings, is to be found in Zdzıslaw Kuksewicz, *De Siger de Brabant à Jacques de Plaisance*, pp. 315-452. Kuksewicz denies any connection between Antonio and Bologna and unquestionably demonstrates the close dependence of his philosophical ideas on Parisian sources. Antonio's *"recollectiones"* on *Canon* 1.1 were, however, taken down "per me Albertum Bononiensem" (BAV, MS Vat. lat. 4452, 14c, fol. 47v; and similarly in a Munich manuscript—see TK 759). As far as is known, the academic career of Alberto took place entirely at Bologna. Perhaps, having studied and taught philosophy at Paris, Antonio taught medicine at Bologna.

[3] On them, see SF 1:251, n. 2, and 1:562; George Sarton, *Introduction to the History of Science*, vol. 3, pt. 1, pp. 842-845; M. Morris, *Albertus de Zancariis*; and Lynn Thorndike, "Some Medieval Medical Manuscripts at the Vatican," *Journal of the History of Medicine and Allied Sciences* 8 (1953):267. In his introduction to Mondino's *Anatomia*, Lino Sighinolfi notes (p. 16) that Alberto, then described as doctor of *physica*, and Bertruccio, described as doctor of medicine, were among the witnesses to Mondino's will in 1326. Giuliano was the *reportator*, in 1310, of Dino's commentary on the *De natura fetus* ascribed to Hippocrates (BAV, MS Vat. lat. 4464, fol. 124r); Guy de Chauliac stated that Mondino had been the teacher of Bertruccio.

physicians who are asserted to have been Taddeo's pupils by authors writing after the close of the fourteenth century. These assertions may be based on fact, even though contemporary supporting evidence cannot be found; but one suspects Taddeo's fame sometimes led to the conferment of the honor of having been his pupil on physicians who had no right to it. Thus Gentile da Foligno is excluded from consideration, despite the claim in a variety of secondary sources that he studied under Taddeo, because there appears to be no contemporary or nearly contemporary evidence to that effect, and because the chronology of their lives makes it unlikely (although not impossible).[4]

The nature of the sources presents problems of a different kind. For biographical information I have relied largely on documents already in print. Chiefly owing to the industry of the historians of Bologna and its university, there is a relatively large body of printed documentation about the six men with whom we are concerned. Doubtless, however, further search of archives of the various cities and institutions where Taddeo's pupils taught and practiced would turn up a few more documents. No such research has been attempted for this book, since its main focus is on the writings of members of the group.

[4] Taddeo probably began to teach in the 1260s and died in 1295; Gentile's birthdate is unknown, but his death in 1348 is well documented (he was the author of a *consilium* on the plague and perished during the 1348 epidemic). The last survivor among the pupils of Taddeo discussed herein was apparently Dino del Garbo, who died in 1327. The earliest documented date in Gentile's career is 1322, when he was teaching at Siena; see Carl C. Schlam, "Graduation Speeches of Gentile da Foligno," *Mediaeval Studies* 40 (1978):97, citing the Siena *Chartularium*. Furthermore, at that time Gentile was receiving a salary of 125 gold florins a year (with a supplementary payment of 60 florins a year), which rose to 180 florins in 1324. In 1321, Dino del Garbo was making a salary of 350 gold florins a year, with a 100-florin supplement for teaching at Siena; see *Chartularium Studii Senensis*, 1:169, 239-240, 243, 283-284, 313 (nos. 169, 195, 197, 228, 229, 249). Since Gentile's subsequent fame certainly came to rival that of Dino, the implication is that in the 1320s Gentile was still a young man at the beginning of his career, whereas Dino was a mature and established scholar (see Dino's biography in chapter two, below). As just noted, Gentile unquestionably knew the writings of Taddeo and his pupils well; so it seems very likely that he was a pupil of a pupil—possibly of Dino himself, whom he praised effusively in the passage cited above. Dino's son Tommaso denigrated Gentile (see note 48 to chapter eight, below), whom he may have regarded as a rival for Dino's intellectual and professional inheritance. For a discouraging glimpse of the accretion of legend around Gentile da Foligno, and the difficulties of authenticating biographical detail about him, see Fausto Bonora and George Kern, "Does Anyone Really Know the Life of Gentile da Foligno?" *Medicina ne' secoli* 9 (1972):29-53. These authors, however, appear to accept (pp. 33-34) the story of Gentile's education under Taddeo, although adducing no evidence other than assertions in earlier secondary works.

Modern editions of works by Taddeo and his pupils are few and far between. Those that have appeared in the twentieth century include Taddeo's *Consilia*, the medieval Italian version of Mondino's *Anatomia*, and a Latin commentary by Dino del Garbo on a vernacular lyric of the *dolce stil nuovo* (for details, see Bibliography). The vast bulk of their output, however, including all their medical commentaries, disputed questions, and remedy collections, remains available only in manuscript or in fifteenth- or sixteenth-century printings. To attempt to survey such a mass of material in the absence of critical editions is obviously to run grave risks of inaccuracy or imbalance.

We may note, in particular, some hazards regarding the use of *questiones* in commentaries and the use of medical recipes. As already remarked, medical commentaries by our authors normally incorporated large numbers of *questiones* on topics of traditional or current interest, or both. Obviously, such a format is extremely susceptible to interpolation; and so long as the arguments were living ones, the likelihood of subsequent emendation was no doubt fairly high. One can only admire the copyist of the commentary of Alberto da Bologna on the collection of Galen's treatises on disease known in the Middle Ages as *De accidenti et morbo* for the scruples that led him to remark, "the aforementioned doctor said many things in lecturing on this book that, saving his reverence, I do not believe to be true; and therefore what he said I have not changed, but immediately afterwards or in the margin of the book have sometimes put forward certain objections," while wondering how many other learned copyists or editors were less conscientious in the manner in which they made and acknowledged emendations.[5] Nonetheless, in the absence of specific evidence to the contrary, I have assumed that all *questiones* and arguments incorporated into a commentary bearing the name of one of the masters with whom I am concerned were in fact his work. Similarly, many collections of medical recipes and lists of herbal remedies circulated inside (and outside) the medieval *studia*. The names of famous physicians, including Taddeo Alderotti, Dino del Garbo, and Mondino, were attached to such collections, but the same

---

[5] "Et in hoc terminetur sentencia libri de accidenti et morbo recollecta sub magistro Alberto bononiensis et correpta cum scriptoque ipsemet alias scripsit propria manu. . . . Multa autem dixerat legendo hunc librum predictus doctor que salva reverentia esse vera non credo, et ideo que dixerat non mutavi sed post immediate vel in margine libri quandoque reprobavi . . . ," BAV, MS Vat. reg. lat. 2000, 14c, fol. 73r. The commentary begins on fol. 28r.

questions of authenticity of attribution and of subsequent interpolation are usually unresolved.

In consulting those works by Taddeo and members of his circle that are available only in manuscript, I have not attempted any systematic critical comparison of different manuscript traditions. (Some works, in any case, appear to survive only in a single copy.) Where early printed editions exist, I have made use of them, while referring to the manuscripts from time to time; but I have not made any systematic analysis of the transmission from script to print.

Problems of the kind indicated above are not only confined to the writings of Taddeo and the other physicians who are the subjects of this book, but also affect our knowledge of some of their own sources. These masters inherited an ancient tradition of medical learning that reached them in a variety of forms. The history, and in particular the textual history, of this process is still far from completely known, although a number of scholars are currently engaged in adding to our understanding of it. Of the proposed *Galenus latinus* we now have one volume, Richard Durling's edition of a twelfth-century translation of *De complexionibus*; a catalogue of medieval Hippocratic manuscripts and commentaries is currently being published in serial parts by Pearl Kibre; Paul Oskar Kristeller has unraveled important aspects of the formation of the collection of Hippocratic and Galenic texts known as the *ars medicine* in the late twelfth and early thirteenth century, but a number of early commentaries on works in this collection have still to be analyzed; Jerry Stannard, John Riddle, and Michael McVaugh have begun to disentangle some of the complexities of the transmission of texts and content in the medieval pharmacological tradition.

Given this situation, I can only beg the reader's indulgence for my temerity in attempting, on however small a scale, a synthesis of the kind contained in the present volume. Some of the imperfections in this book reflect lacunae in our current knowledge of medieval learned medicine; more of them, no doubt, reflect the manifold inadequacies of the author. It has nonetheless seemed worthwhile to attempt a reconstruction, even if flawed, of the thought and activities of a group of men whose lives were touched by—and who, in however small a measure, helped to shape —so many of the significant trends of their age: the growth of secular professions, the development of scientific learning, the rise of universities, and the flowering of Italian civic life.

TADDEO ALDEROTTI
AND HIS PUPILS

CHAPTER ONE

THE SETTING

This book is about a group of men who were simultaneously scholars and teachers, highly successful practitioners of a learned profession, and members of a politically and socially influential urban elite. Holders of senior professorships in the burgeoning north-Italian *studia*, medical advisers to popes and an emperor, and active members of the vigorous citizen class of the north-Italian municipalities, Taddeo Alderotti and his pupils reflected in their lives many aspects of the richly complex society in which they moved. To place them properly in their setting would require a history of the whole political, social, economic, and cultural world surrounding them. The description of this world, which was also the world of Dante, has been the task of many scholars. It will not be attempted afresh here. But of Bologna and its *studium*—the city and group of academic institutions that played the leading roles in the intellectual, cultural, and scientific formation of Taddeo and his colleagues and students—some introductory account must be given. So far as can be determined, Taddeo Alderotti (d. 1295) spent his entire academic career, as both scholar and master, at Bologna; and although some of his pupils went far afield (being variously credited with teaching or practicing in Padua, Siena, Florence, Genoa, Paris, and Avignon), they too not only developed their intellectual capacities at Bologna, but also, with a solitary exception, taught there for substantial periods of time.[1]

As is well known, the academic institutions and the delineation of fields of study that developed at Bologna served, in many respects, as a model for other medieval university centers in southern Europe, but differed sharply from arrangements usually prevailing north of the Alps. Typical of the southern European *studia* were the formation of student universities (rather than the universities of masters of arts found in the north), curricular emphasis upon law and medicine, the lay status of numerous masters and students, the tardy appearance of public teaching

[1] See the biographies in chapter two, below.

of theology, and the teaching of liberal arts and philosophy in close institutional and intellectual association with medicine. Not all these characteristics were fully developed when Taddeo Alderotti first came to
Bologna; but it seems fair to say that Bolognese education was, from an
early date, more directed toward the secular learned professions than that
provided at, say, Paris or Oxford. This secular emphasis, as much as
anything else, serves to explain the superior status and productivity
achieved in the late thirteenth and early fourteenth centuries by the faculties of medicine at Bologna and the similarly oriented *studia* of Padua
and Montpellier. It would be a mistake, however, to suppose that scholars associated with the Italian schools inhabited a different intellectual
universe or subscribed to a wholly different value system than did those
in the north. Trends in thought spread freely from one side of the Alps
to the other; so intellectual currents cannot easily be identified as peculiar
to the Italian schools, peculiar to Bologna, or peculiar to any particular
group of masters at Bologna or elsewhere. Nonetheless, Bologna was in
fact the matrix of the learning and of the professional training of Taddeo
and his pupils, and it is conditions at Bologna that will be described in
this chapter.

When Taddeo first came to Bologna from his native Florence some
time in the middle years of the thirteenth century, the former city was
already an ancient and renowned seat of learning. Schools of liberal arts
existed in Bologna in the early Middle Ages, and the city had become
a center for the teaching and study of law by the end of the eleventh
century. In the course of the twelfth century, the masters of Bologna
intensively cultivated the fields of canon and civil law, attracting students
from all over Europe and producing a great efflorescence of legal studies.
Meanwhile, the position and prestige of the jurists of Bologna steadily
advanced. Irnerius, traditionally (although probably not in fact) the
founder of legal studies at Bologna, enjoyed the protection of Matilda of
Tuscany; and from the Emperor Frederick Barbarossa came in 1158 the
celebrated *authentica habita*, an imperial decree that guaranteed a wide
range of scholarly privileges.[2]

Not only did the law schools continue to flourish, but teachers and students of other subjects, most notably of rhetoric and medicine, began to
flock to Bologna in increasing numbers. The rise of medical teaching at

[2] Gina Fasoli, *Per la storia dell'Università di Bologna nel Medio Evo*, pp. 82-91, 117-132;
Pearl Kibre, *Scholarly Privileges in the Middle Ages*, pp. 18ff.

Bologna will be considered below; here it is sufficient to say that medical teachers and students were present in the city in the first two decades of the thirteenth century. Early in the thirteenth century, too, Bologna became a notable center for the teaching of the practical rhetoric of the *ars dictaminis* (the art of letter writing) under such famous teachers as Boncompagno da Signa (d. after 1235) and his approximate contemporary, Bene of Florence.[3] But despite its importance as an adjunct or introduction to the study of law and the notarial art, thirteenth-century Bolognese rhetoric was never exclusively practical or vocational. Much evidence has been gathered that bears witness to the study of Latin poets, and Boncompagno himself cited a number of classical authors.[4] Moreover, the intimate involvement of the *ars dictaminis* with the problems of government, politics, and law in urban society meant that in Bologna, as elsewhere in northern Italy, some teachers of Latin rhetoric were much interested both in the development and use of the vernacular, and in outlining the moral attributes conducive to good government and appropriate for citizens in public life. Thus, for example, Guido Faba, or Fava, a teacher of the Latin *ars dictaminis* at Bologna from the 1220s, produced, in addition to several Latin works on rhetoric, a collection of sample letters and political discourses in the vernacular. The contribution of the schools of Bologna certainly supports the contention that the activities and interests of thirteenth-century Italian rhetoricians helped to set the scene for the early Italian Renaissance.[5]

In the middle years of the thirteenth century, then, Bologna was a major center not only for vocational training in the professional disciplines of law and medicine and in Latin grammar (the essential pre-

---

[3] A valuable account of the teaching of rhetoric and the *ars dictaminis* at Bologna in the first half of the thirteenth century is contained in Helene Wieruszowski, "Rhetoric and the Classics in Italian Education of the Thirteenth Century," in her *Politics and Culture in Medieval Spain and Italy*, pp. 589-601, where the earlier literature on the topic is also noted and discussed. See also her " 'Ars dictaminis' in the Time of Dante," ibid., pp. 359-377.

[4] Wieruszowski, "Rhetoric and the Classics," in *Politics and Culture*, pp. 596-598 and 603-604.

[5] Wieruszowski, " 'Ars dictaminis,' " in *Politics and Culture*, pp. 370, 376-377; on the general relationship of medieval Italian rhetoric to developments associated with the Renaissance, see Paul Oskar Kristeller, "Humanism and Scholasticism in the Italian Renaissance," in his *Renaissance Thought*, pp. 92-119; on the contribution of the *studium* of Bologna in this regard (not only as concerns rhetoric), see idem, "The University of Bologna and the Renaissance," *Studi e memorie per la storia dell'Università di Bologna*, n.s. 1 (1956): 313-323.

requisite for serious study in any field during the Middle Ages), but also for education in both practical and, to a lesser extent, literary rhetoric. The beginnings of a vernacular literary culture and of a concern for moral philosophy viewed in the context of civic life were also evident. Thus, the interest of Taddeo and some of his pupils in vernacular letters and in civic morality and affairs (see chapter three), like their medical learning, drew upon and carried forward existing Bolognese traditions.

It seems probable, too, that some teaching in logic was available at Bologna by around the mid-thirteenth century, since professors of logic were to be found at Arezzo in 1255 and at Padua in 1262 (and perhaps at Padua and Vercelli in 1228). The earliest public teaching in logic that can be documented at Bologna, however, appears to be that of Master Theodosius of Cremona and Master Reginaldus de Melanto in 1273. It is not known when Taddeo's own teaching of logic began, although it was before 1287; but since logic was often taught by men who were themselves still students of one of the higher disciplines, it may have been much earlier in his career.[6] No master at Bologna seems to have made any significant independent contribution to the subject before Taddeo's pupil Gentile da Cingoli (active at Bologna after about 1295); so it may perhaps be assumed that, in the thirteenth century, logic was taught only as a routine preparatory methodology.

Astronomy and astrology, too, formed part of the Bolognese learned tradition from an early date, no doubt in part because of the universal belief in the importance of astrology for medicine. The famous Michael Scot is said to have been asked by the ruling elite of Bologna to make astrological predictions in 1231; another well-known astrologer, Guido Bonatti (d. after 1282), spent much time in Bologna and almost certainly

[6] Wieruszowski, "Arezzo as a Center of Learning and Letters in the Thirteenth Century," in *Politics and Culture*, pp. 404-405; dialectic may, however, have been taught only in private schools as a preparatory course in Arezzo at this time. Master Tredecinus, "in loica providus indagator et doctor," was one of ten regent masters at Padua who attended the solemn public reading of the *Cronica* of Rolandino of Padua in 1262; see Rolandino, *Cronica in factis et circa facta Marchie Trivixane* 12.19, ed. A. Bonardi, *Rerum italicarum scriptores* (new ed. Città di Castello, 1905-1908), vol. 8, pt. 1, pp. 173-174. In 1228, seceding students from Padua made a contract with the commune of Vercelli that required the latter, among other provisions, to pay the salaries of two professors of logic; it is not known whether or not the contract was put into effect, nor to what extent it reflected the current pattern of arts teaching at Padua. See Nancy G. Siraisi, *Arts and Sciences at Padua*, pp. 17-18, and bibliography there cited. For Theodosius and Reginaldus, see SF 1:593; on Taddeo as a teacher of logic, see note 60 to this chapter.

taught there, probably beginning in the 1230s. Of the other mathematical arts, geometry and arithmetic were certainly taught in 1279, and possibly earlier. It is unlikely that music, the fourth art of the quadrivium, was wholly absent when the other three were present. In this connection, it may be noted that Bologna early became a center of the music of the *ars nova*, and that among those interested in polyphonic innovation was the learned physician Giovanni della Luna (fl. 1298-1303).[7]

In the years when Taddeo first arrived there, however, Bologna does not appear to have been particularly noted as a center for the teaching of philosophy. When and how scholars at Bologna first participated in the great intellectual revolution of the thirteenth century, namely the reception of the *libri naturales* (and *morales*) of Aristotle as basic textbooks in the schools, remains largely unknown.[8] Whether or not the Emperor Frederick II did, as claimed, send works of Aristotle to the scholars of Bologna around 1230, some natural philosophy was no doubt early studied in connection with medicine (see chapter five).[9] It is probable, however, that the *studia* of the various orders of friars played an important part in introducing the "new Aristotle" and scholastic method to the schools of Bologna. The first such *studium* to be established was that of the Dominicans, which was founded in 1218 and declared in 1248 to be

[7] Lynn Thorndike, *Michael Scot*, p. 38; idem, *History of Magic and Experimental Science*, 2:827-828; B. Boncompagni, *Della vita e delle opere di Guido Bonatti astrologo del secolo decimo terzo notizie* (Rome, 1851), pp. 21-23. Guido Bonatti disputed the assertion of Fr. Giovanni da Schio, O.P., that astrology was neither an art nor a science, which perhaps suggests that the subject was indeed treated as a learned discipline at Bologna in the 1230s, when Fr. Giovanni was present in the city (Boncompagni, *Della vita*, p. 101). For Master Johannes, who taught geometry and arithmetic in 1279, see SF 1:586-587. On Giovanni della Luna, see Nino Pirrotta, "Due sonetti musicali del secolo xiv," in *Miscélanea en homenaje a Mons. Higinio Anglès* (Barcelona, 1958-1961), 2:657.

[8] A convenient summary of the stages of the reception of Aristotle is contained in Fernand Van Steenberghen, *Aristotle in the West*. A careful study of manuscripts of Aristotle's works of Bolognese provenance or ownership, such as P. Marangon, *Alle origine dell'Aristotelismo padovano*, now provides for Padua, would probably be useful.

[9] The claim is made in a letter in the epistolary collection of Frederick's chancellor Petrus de Vinea, which contains many apocryphal items and was used as a manual of *dictamen*; furthermore it is very similar to a letter supposedly sent by Manfred to the University of Paris. The question is discussed and the authenticity of the letter of Frederick to the scholars of Bologna maintained in Roland de Vaux, "La première entrée d'Averroès chez les Latins," *Revue des sciences philosophiques et théologiques* 22 (1933):205-206. Authentic or not, the letter refers to works of Aristotle and other Greek and Arab philosophers "in sermonalibus et mathematicis disciplinis," and could therefore describe Aristotle's works on logic together with Arab treatises on astronomy and astrology, just as well as the Aristotelian *libri naturales*.

one of the six *studia generalia*, which were second only to the Parisian house in the order's hierarchy of schools.[10] According to Tommaso da Celano, an attempt to found a Franciscan house of studies in Bologna in about 1221 had drawn down the wrath of Saint Francis himself; the latter said to the founder, Johannes de Sciaca, who was "highly educated" (*"valde litteratus"*): "You want to destroy the order! I desired and wished, following the example of my Lord Jesus Christ, that my brothers should rather pray than read [or lecture—*legere*]."[11] Perhaps the saint later changed his mind, since Saint Anthony of Padua lectured on theology in the Franciscan convent at Bologna in about 1223-1224 and apparently did so with Saint Francis' approval. A Franciscan *studium* had certainly been established by 1236, when the archbishop of Ravenna gave his permission and encouragement to the Friars Minor to move closer to the center of the city so that their "schools and sermons" might be more readily accessible to "clerks and scholars." The Franciscans did not officially rank their *studia* into different categories until 1336, when Bologna was declared to be among the *studia generalia* of the order.[12] The Augustinian house in Bologna was also recognized as a *studium generale* by the general chapter of that order in 1287,[13] and a Servite house of studies had come into being before 1293.[14]

The houses of friars in Bologna were from their beginnings in close contact with the major intellectual currents of the day. For example, in the middle years of the thirteenth century, Franciscans from Bologna were regularly sent to study (and a few of them also taught) at Paris, then the chief center of theological and philosophical learning in Europe.[15] As we shall see, Taddeo Alderotti also left a bequest to finance the Parisian studies of Franciscan friars from Bologna. Although the details of the curricula offered in the *studia* of the friars of Bologna at that time cannot now be reconstructed, it is clear that the main purpose of these schools was to teach theology and the art of preaching (*ars predi-*

---

[10] Guido Zaccagnini, "Le scuole e la libreria del Convento di S. Domenico in Bologna dalle origini al secolo XVI," *Atti e memorie della R. Deputazione di storia patria per le provincie di Romagna*, 4th ser. 17 (1926-1927):230, 232.

[11] "Tu vis destruere ordinem! Desiderabam et volebam, exemplo Domini mei Iesu Christi, fratres meos magis orare quam legere," quoted in Caelestinus Piana, O.F.M., ed., *Chartularium Studii Bononiensis S. Francisci (saec. XIII-XVI)*, p. 11*.

[12] Ibid., pp. 11*-13*.   [13] Ibid., p. 9*.

[14] In that year Taddeo Alderotti bequeathed to the Servites books on philosophy.

[15] Piana, *Chartularium*, p. 38*.

candi), but that some preliminary training in arts, and perhaps also in philosophy, was also available. Thus, the Franciscan Johannes de Parma, who studied at Paris and was a *lector* at Bologna before 1247, is said to have been "a good grammarian and a master in logic" before his entry into the order; and in 1269 Friar Raymundus de Verona, *lector*, had in his possession philosophical books.[16] Logic and *natura* (presumably natural philosophy) were taught in the convent of the Friars of the Sack in 1270. The teacher, Master Lapus, seems not to have been a member of the order, and is, no doubt, to be identified with Lapus de Florentia, who was apparently teaching medicine publicly in 1268.[17] That the interests of some of the friars at Bologna included both philosophy and learned medicine in 1293 is indicated by Taddeo Alderotti's own bequests of books on those topics to the Servites and the Franciscans. (As we shall shortly see, medicine of a more practical variety flourished among the Dominicans in the shape of the surgeon Theodoric of Lucca [Teodorico Borgognoni, d. 1298].) The teaching of logic and philosophy were certainly well established among the friars by the first years of the fourteenth century; instruction in logic is recorded at the Servite convent in 1305, and a set of questions on the nature of created beings, disputed by Master Alexander de Alexandria, OFM, between 1303 and 1307, shows an extensive familiarity with the *libri naturales* of Aristotle, with philosophical topics similar to those debated in thirteenth-century Paris, and with techniques of scholastic argument. Some have also conjectured that Duns Scotus may have taught briefly at the Franciscan convent in Bologna in 1303-1304.[18]

The *studia* of the friars were open to clerics who were not members of the mendicant orders, but it is not certain whether or to what extent laymen were permitted to attend lectures and disputations in the thirteenth and early fourteenth centuries.[19] In the later Middle Ages, however,

---

[16] Ibid., p. 4, no. 3; p. 6, no. 6.

[17] Contract between Master Lapus and the syndic of the friars, printed in Francesco Cavazza, "Le scuole dell'antico studio di Bologna," *Atti e memorie della R. Deputazione di storia patria per le provincie di Romagna*, 3d ser. 11 (1894):117; the contract provides Lapus with food, drink, and a salary. Lapus was the teacher of the first scholar recorded to have received a public *laurea* in medicine at Bologna.

[18] Piana, *Chartularium*, pp. 9* and 112*-116*, where Fr. Alexander's questions are edited; for the suggestion about Duns Scotus, see p. 62*.

[19] Ibid., pp. 83*-85*; Zaccagnini, "Le scuole e la libreria del Convento di S. Domenico," p. 247.

the Franciscans of Bologna maintained close relations not only with the public college of theology (founded 1364), but also with the university of arts and medicine, many of whose members were laymen. The statutes of the university of arts and medicine compiled in 1405 reveal that the convocation of the university was regularly held in the chapter house or schools of the Franciscans; and the same statutes command scholars and masters, especially of philosophy, to attend disputations given by the *lectors* of the orders of friars.[20] In view of the career of Master Lapus, alluded to above, and Taddeo Alderotti's own personal and intellectual connection with the Franciscans of Bologna, it seems likely that close contacts between the *studia* of the friars and those who studied and taught philosophy and medicine in the secular schools of Bologna have a continuous history stretching from 1405 back to the thirteenth century.

It is, however, extremely difficult to trace the emergence of public teaching of natural and moral philosophy in the secular schools. According to John of Salisbury, one of his teachers, Master Albericus, who was outstanding *"in phisicis studiis,"* taught at Bologna, presumably in the middle years of the twelfth century. The nature of Master Albericus's exposition is unknown, however, as is that of Moneta of Cremona, who is said to have given instruction in philosophy about 1220.[21] Since Master Lapus, referred to above, taught *"natura"* in the convent of the Friars of the Sack in 1270, he may have included similar instruction along with his public medical teaching. The earliest philosophical *works* associated with Bologna appear to be Taddeo's own translation of the *Nicomachean Ethics* and a treatise on happiness by Jacopo da Pistoia written before ca. 1300 (see chapter three). In the history of secular philosophical teaching at Bologna, therefore, the generation of Taddeo takes on a particular importance.

The early institutional history of the secular academic corporations of Bologna has been extensively treated.[22] The following summary account

[20] Carlo Malagola, ed., *Statuti delle Università e dei Collegi delle Studio bolognese,* pp. 232, 260, 265-266.

[21] SF 1:586-591; John of Salisbury, *Metalogicon,* ed. Clement C. Webb (Oxford, 1929), 2.10, 867c-d.

[22] See especially SF; F. Hastings Rashdall, *The Universities of Europe in the Middle Ages,* 1:87-268, and older bibliography there cited; Albano Sorbelli, *Storia dell'Università di Bologna*; Fasoli, *Per la storia*; Kibre, *Scholarly Privileges,* pp. 18-53; Celestino Piana, *Nuove ricerche su le Università di Bologna e di Parma*; Giorgio Cencetti, *Gli archivi dello*

is designed merely to draw attention to aspects of that history that have particular significance for the careers of Taddeo and his pupils. The establishment in Bologna of formal academic organizations, namely student universities and doctoral colleges, appears to have taken place long after the city's emergence as a major center of intellectual life. As J. K. Hyde has pointed out, the development of academic societies in Bologna both paralleled and was intimately involved with the emergence of political, social, and economic associations among the citizens. The Bolognese appear to have formed a commune by 1116, and some kind of general assembly of the academic community was probably in existence by 1186. But just as more complex forms of political, economic, and social organization developed in the thirteenth century (in the shape of the *societas populi*, guilds, and military companies of Bologna), so too, from the late twelfth century, academic associations became more specialized in their functions. Thus certain foreign students of law were already joined in fraternal societies for religious and welfare purposes in the 1190's; by 1205 universities of foreign students of law had been formed and were electing their own rectors.[23]

The functions and powers of the student universities have been described many times; their members constituted a corporation that elected its own officials, made its own statutes, and claimed to regulate both curriculum and faculty. Many of the professors were, however, Bolognese citizens, and as a group enjoyed considerable political influence. Moreover, some professors were, from about 1280, salaried by the municipality, and many of them had, in any case, an independent source of income as legal consultants. Furthermore, the faculty retained control of the examination procedures leading to the doctorate. In these circumstances, the effectiveness of student regulation of the faculty, and perhaps also of the curriculum, was probably never complete, and tended to become more limited over the course of time, especially under the signorial governments of the fourteenth century. But the universities undoubtedly served

Studio bolognese; and idem, "Studium fuit Bononie," *Studi medievali* 7 (1966):781-833; G. Rossi, " 'Universitas scholarium' e commune," *Studi e memorie per la storia dell'Università di Bologna*, n.s. 1 (1956):173-266; and Manlio Bellomo, *Saggio sull'università nell'età del diritto comune*. Documents pertaining to the early history of the studium are edited in SF, vol. 2; Malagola, *Statuti*; and *Chartularium Studii Bononiensis*, cited hereafter as *Chart. Bon.*

23 J. K. Hyde, "Commune, University, and Society in Early Medieval Bologna," in *Universities in Politics*, pp. 17-46; and Fasoli, *Per la storia*, pp. 133-135.

to protect students of non-Bolognese origin and to secure them a bargaining position vis-à-vis the Bolognese municipal authorities.[24]

Relations between the universities and the commune were far from being always harmonious; as is well known, secessions of masters and scholars from Bologna, in defiance of Bolognese prohibitions, contributed to the formation of university centers at Padua, Arezzo, and elsewhere.[25] Nonetheless, various communal statutes made in the course of the thirteenth century confirmed the legal privileges of scholars and extended further protection to them, especially after the regime of the *popolo* was established.[26] Successive popes also interested themselves in the regulation of academic life at Bologna. In general, and as might be expected, given the accepted role of the church as protector of scholars and of learning, papal intervention tended to support the scholars in their disputes with the Bolognese authorities. Honorius III affirmed both the ultimate ecclesiastical authority over learning and the autonomy of the educational process in 1219, when he decreed that the right of bestowing the *licentia docendi* (license to teach) should belong to the archdeacon of Bologna, but that such license should be given only to candidates who had been diligently examined.[27] In practice, as noted, the examination of candidates was the prerogative of the teaching faculty. That the supervisory role of the archdeacon was nevertheless no mere legal fiction, at any rate in the thirteenth century, is suggested by two sample letters included in an *ars dictaminis* of that period by the Bolognese notary Matteo de' Libri. In one of these, the archdeacon is petitioned to appoint to a professorial chair the writer's relative, who is stated to have studied the arts continuously and to be worthy of the position; in the other, the archdeacon invites his correspondent to take up a professorship.[28]

Little is known of the origins of the colleges, or societies, of doctors of civil and canon law in Bologna, since the oldest surviving statutes of these bodies date, respectively, from the late fourteenth and the fifteenth

[24] Kibre, *Scholarly Privileges*, pp. 18-53; Bellomo, *Saggio sull'università*, pp. 25-52, 81-112, 149-169, 212-217. Bellomo (pp. 40-42) specifically associates the rise of student universities with the thirteenth-century rise of the *popolo* in Bologna.

[25] Rashdall, *Universities*, 1:168-171; regarding Arezzo, however, see also Wieruszowski, "Arezzo as a Center of Learning," in *Politics and Culture*, passim.

[26] Hyde, "Commune, University, and Society," pp. 43-44; Bellomo, *Saggio sull'università*, pp. 40-42, 91-93, 103.

[27] Rashdall, *Universities*, 1:221, 231.

[28] Paul Oskar Kristeller, "Matteo de' Libri, Bolognese Notary of the Thirteenth Century, and His *Artes Dictaminis*," in *Miscellanea Giovanni Galbiati*, 2:291, 316.

centuries. Whether, or to what extent, the teaching masters of law (who, unlike many of their students, were normally Bolognese citizens) felt the need to organize themselves into any kind of formal association before the end of the twelfth century is unclear. It seems likely that a doctoral college (or colleges) was already in existence by 1259, when the Bolognese citizen professors of law had to be restrained by the municipal government from preventing doctors of foreign origin from taking up professorial chairs to which they had been elected by the student universities. Subsequently, the city government intervened on at least three occasions (1295, 1299, and 1304) to prevent the doctors of civil law from reserving professorial appointments for members of their own families. These actions suggest the existence of a strongly organized legal caste, linked by ties of blood as well as by collegiate organization.[29] The jurists were of course also members of the guild of judges and notaries, which from about 1272-1274 came, for a time, to dominate the political life of the city.[30] The political importance of the professors of law is indicated by the insistence of the city government in 1295 that appointees to professorial positions be members of the dominant party of the Geremei.[31]

Thus, by the second half of the thirteenth century the jurists of Bologna, both masters and students, had achieved highly effective forms of institutional organization that added to their status, dignity, and actual political and economic power. Moreover, the *studium* of Bologna shone throughout Europe as the center par excellence of legal studies and hence of precisely those skills that were of the greatest possible practical value in the increasingly complex governmental, administrative, and juridical arrangements that characterized both ecclesiastical and secular life in that period.

It is against this background that the rise of Bologna as a prominent center of medical learning, and the institutional organization there of the teaching of medicine in association with liberal arts and philosophy, must be understood. To the physicians of Bologna, the position of the jurists stood as a continuing example of the possibilities inherent in the organization of a learned profession.[32]

[29] Rashdall, *Universities*, 1:213-214.
[30] V. Franchini, *Le arti di mestiere in Bologna nel secolo XIII*, p. 158.
[31] Rashdall, *Universities*, 1:214, n. 3.
[32] On the professionalization of medicine at Bologna, see Vern L. Bullough, "Medieval

The presence of numerous physicians and surgeons is recorded in Bologna throughout the thirteenth century. Moreover, there are a number of indications that medicine was fairly widely taught and studied as well as practiced there quite soon after 1200.[33] One of the most noteworthy of these indications is the prohibition laid by Pope Honorius III in 1219 upon the study of medicine in the schools of Bologna by certain categories of clergy.[34] Private teaching of surgery, and probably also of medicine, was certainly carried on from early in the thirteenth century. For example, the *medicus* Ugo Borgononi da Lucca, who was engaged by the Commune of Bologna as a municipal surgeon in 1214, taught the members of a small circle deliberately restricted to his own sons and perhaps a few apprentices.[35] According to his son Theodoric, author of a well-known work on surgery, Ugo usually imposed an oath of secrecy upon those to whom he imparted his methods,[36] and he left no written works.

The contrast to public teaching in a *studium generale* could hardly be sharper. Yet the relationship between Ugo and his sons and apprentices in some ways parallels the oldest and simplest form of academic association, that between an individual master and his own *socii*, that is, his pupils and assistants. A teacher and his students shared not only, ideally, a bond of mutual loyalty and common intellectual concerns, but also, like a craftsman and his apprentices, certain economic interests. An apt pupil could hope to take over his master's teaching or, if he were a physician, practice, on the latter's retirement, or at any rate to benefit from his reputation.[37] Even after the establishment of a student university and

---

Bologna and the Development of Medical Education," *Bulletin of the History of Medicine* 32 (1958):201-215, and idem, *The Development of Medicine as a Profession.*

[33] Vincenzo Busacchi, "I primordi dell'insegnamento medico a Bologna," *Rivista di storia delle scienze mediche e naturali* 39 (1948):128-144.

[34] Sorbelli, *Storia,* 1:108.

[35] His contract with the city is printed in SF 2:214-215. On his career, see Mario Tabanelli, *La chirurgia italiana nell'alto Medioevo,* 1:196-198, and bibliography there cited.

[36] *The Surgery of Theodoric,* 2 vols., trans. C. Campbell and J. Colton (New York, 1955-1960), 1:110-111.

[37] The *Rhetorica Novissima* of Boncompagno (d. after 1235), who, as noted, achieved fame by his teaching of the *ars dictaminis* at Bologna, contains a sample "*exordium* for masters who establish their disciples as their successors in teaching," in which the younger master is referred to as "fratrem et socium nostrum"; Boncompagno, *Rhetorica Novissima* 6.1, in A. Gaudenzi, *Bibliotheca Iuridica Medii Aevi: Scripta Anecdota Glossatorum* (Bologna, 1892), 2:273. The warm gratitude of a model *socius* to his master was expressed

doctoral college of arts and medicine at Bologna, therefore, masters and their *socii* continued to form groups cutting across the lines of the larger organizations. The relationship between master and *socius* was an intimate one, and its souring could lead to great bitterness, such as occurred when Taddeo Alderotti came to believe that his former *socius* and present colleague Bartolomeo da Varignana was deliberately luring away his (Taddeo's) students.[38]

To return to Ugo da Lucca, teaching was certainly no part of his official duties. The commune granted him a money fief (*feudum*) of 600 Bolognese lire per year, in exchange for which he agreed to reside in Bologna for six months of each year and throughout any periods of civil war; to treat resident Bolognese citizens gratis and inhabitants of the Bolognese countryside at a fixed scale of charges; and to accompany Bolognese military expeditions in order to treat the wounded. The fief was intended to be hereditary. However, if Ugo should have no son with appropriate medical or surgical skills, then his heir would receive only 400 lire per year and would owe the Commune of Bologna such services as "other vassals are held to owe their lords."[39]

In fact, no fewer than three of Ugo's sons became *medici*, the fief and the position of city surgeon being inherited by Franciscus.[40] As late as 1289, some twenty years after the establishment of public medical teaching and of academic associations of masters and scholars of medicine, Franciscus was engaged in private teaching of surgery by private contract.[41]

Another of Ugo's sons, Theodoric, produced one of the earliest of an important series of surgical treatises by writers associated with Bologna in the thirteenth century. His *Chirurgia*, written before 1266, has been praised by modern historians of medicine for its practicality and good sense.[42] It is a pragmatic work, emphasizing the treatment of wounds and making reference to the methods espoused by Ugo da Lucca. The

by Boncompagno's pupil Rolandino of Padua; see Rolandino, *Cronica* 10.4, ed. Bonardi, *Rerum italicarum scriptores*, new ed., vol. 8, pt. 1, p. 135.

[38] SF 2:223.   [39] SF 2:214.

[40] SF 1:544-545; Guido Zaccagnini, *La vita dei maestri e degli scolari nello Studio bolognese nei secoli XIII e XIV*, p. 111.

[41] Guido Zaccagnini, "L'insegnamento privato a Bologna e altrove nei secoli XIII e XIV," *Atti e memorie della R. Deputazione di storia patria per le provincie di Romagna*, ser. 4, 14 (1923-1924):261, 290-291, where the contract in question is printed.

[42] On Theodoric and his work, see SF 1:537-542; and Tabanelli, 1:198-207.

Bolognese tradition of surgical writing was continued by Guglielmo da Saliceto, whose *Chirurgia* appeared in two versions in 1258 and 1275,[43] and Lanfranco, author of a *Chirurgia magna* written in 1296.[44] The career of Theodoric, who was both a member of a religious order and a bishop, is also of interest as an illustration of the caution with which claims for the "secularization," or secularizing force of the medical and surgical professions in the thirteenth century, should be advanced. The growth of medicine as a learned profession was one of a cluster of factors in later medieval urban and academic society whose ultimate effect was profoundly secularizing. Nonetheless, one should beware of concluding too readily, at any rate as regards the thirteenth century, either that the clergy shunned medicine, or that learned physicians were particularly predisposed to religious heterodoxy or indifference. It is true that the prohibition of Honorius III referred to above was only one of several attempts made by the papacy in the twelfth and early thirteenth centuries to discourage priests and members of religious orders from attendance at secular medical schools.[45] And it is also true that by this time many *medici* in Italy were married laymen, some of them members of veritable medical dynasties. But the prohibitions on clerical medical studies were partial, subject to exemption, and substantially modified in the late thirteenth and early fourteenth centuries. Moreover, even in Italy (and to a much greater extent in northern Europe), some members of the clergy continued to study medicine and surgery and to engage in consultant practice of the former, and in some cases perhaps also the latter.[46] Theodoric himself joined the Dominican order as a young man. He was later elevated to the bishopric of Bitonto, near Bari, and subsequently to that of Cervia, near Ravenna. He does not appear to have resided permanently in either see, and he spent the latter years of his life in Bologna, where he died in 1298.[47] His *Chirurgia* was written while he was Bishop of Bitonto and was dedicated to a fellow bishop.[48] He practiced "his

[43] Tabanelli, *Chirurgia*, 2:499-521.   [44] Ibid., 2:803-811.

[45] Darrell W. Amundsen, "Medieval Canon Law on Medical and Surgical Practice by the Clergy," *Bulletin of the History of Medicine* 52 (1978):22-44.

[46] Kibre, *Scholarly Privileges*, p. 33, and Amundsen, "Canon Law," pp. 37-38, for the revocation of the prohibitions. For evidence of the predominance of the clergy in the medical profession in England, even in the late fourteenth century, see Huling E. Ussery, *Chaucer's Physician: Medicine and Literature in Fourteenth-Century England*, Tulane Studies in English, 19 (New Orleans, 1971), pp. 29-30, 35-38, 40.

[47] SF 1:537-539.

[48] *Surgery of Theodoric*, trans. Campbell and Colton, 1:3.

science" for monetary reward both after his entry into the Dominican order and after he became a bishop.[49] These activities, somewhat surprising for a person of his ecclesiastical status, have led some historians to suppose that the bishop, the author of the *Chirurgia*, and the son of Ugo da Lucca could not possibly have been one and the same. The question has been thoroughly canvassed and need not be gone into here.[50] Suffice it to say that not only has Theodoric's identity as a bishop, surgical author, and Ugo's son been established, but also that he had the sanction of his religious superiors for his way of life. A papal license granting Theodoric as bishop permission to retain his medical earnings for himself explains that after his entry into the Order of Preachers his income, although acquired by the exercise of his own skill, had been passed on to that order.[51]

The connections of the tradition of Bolognese surgical writing established by Theodoric and the other surgical writers with the development of Bologna as a center of learned medical teaching remain unclear. Both the well-known interest in anatomy of some of the learned physicians in Taddeo's circle and the ultimate inclusion of surgery in the academic curriculum in "arts and medicine"[52] suggest that it would be unwise to assume a sharp dichotomy between the two fields. For example, Guglielmo da Saliceto, according to the explicit in a fifteenth-century manuscript of his work, wrote his *Chirurgia* for the benefit of students, and he described surgery as a *scientia specialis* requiring intellectual as well as manual skill.[53] It is perhaps also worthy of note that in his last years the household of Theodoric included his personal *medicus*, Master Pancius of Lucca.[54] Pancius was described as a subtle and speculative medical author,[55] and as such he was associated with Taddeo and other members of

[49] According to the *curatores* of his will, Theodoric was sought out for his fame and industry "ante ingressum religionis Fratrum Praedicatorum, post ingressum dicti ordinis, ac postquam adeptus fuit episcopatum," SF 1:539, document dated January 14, 1299. A papal privilege granting Theodoric permission to retain his own earnings states: "multa perquisivit mediantibus laboribus et peritia suae scientiae et valde multa collata sibi fuerant a magnis baronibus et praelatis aliisque personis," ibid., 1:539-540.

[50] For the bibliography of this controversy, see Tabanelli, *Chirurgia*, 1:203-208.

[51] SF 1:539-540.

[52] Malagola, *Statuti*, pp. 247-248. On anatomy and surgery in Taddeo's circle, see further below, chapters four and nine.

[53] Tabanelli, *Chirurgia*, 2:517.

[54] Will of Theodoric of Lucca, printed in SF 2:233-237.

[55] SF 1:541.

his circle by the fourteenth-century scholastic physician Gentile da Foligno; and Theodoric himself was the owner of medical books.[56]

As the thirteenth century wore on, more and more of the medical men who congregated in Bologna ceased to apply to themselves the very general title *medicus*, a term that, as we have seen, could be used both for the pragmatic surgeon Ugo da Lucca and for the "subtle and speculative" medical author Pancius. They began to assume the titles of *magister*, *doctor*, and sometimes *professor*, while some of them began to describe their art as *scientia physicalis*.[57] This development suggests that the ancient tradition linking medicine with natural philosophy and with the other disciplines studied in the schools of arts (see chapter five) was increasingly coming to shape the direction of medical study and teaching at Bologna.

Up until the last four decades of the thirteenth century, however, the regulation or organization of medical teaching appears to have been haphazard. It is possible that the physicians of Bologna may have had some form of association before the 1260s, but, if so, no information concerning it is known to have survived. The barbers, who included phlebotomists, and therefore perhaps some surgeons among their number, apparently attempted to secure civic recognition as a guild in 1233, but were at that time unsuccessful. (They seem to have had better fortune in 1288, but the statutes they are known to have made in that year are lost.)[58] The relative lack of regulation and organization no doubt offered a good deal of scope for individual enterprise and for the self-definition of medical qualifications. It was in such circumstances that Taddeo Alderotti rose to fame. The creation of an institutional framework for medical study, which structured the social, intellectual, and scientific role played by his successors, was, at least in part, his work.

Those of the *medici* of thirteenth-century Bologna who chose to associate themselves with the masters of arts and to participate in the creation of academic institutions "of arts and medicine" were pursuing very real practical advantages. As an intellectual discipline, learned, theoretical medicine had a tradition of impressive antiquity and, by the thirteenth century, a substantial corpus of authoritative Latin texts available for academic study. Medicine was therefore perfectly viable as a branch of

---

[56] SF 2:233-237. For Gentile da Foligno's mention of Pancius, see Introduction, above.
[57] Busacchi, "I primordi," pp. 133-134.
[58] Franchini, *Le arti di mestiere*, pp. 32-33, 36.

higher education at the university level. In association with the masters
of arts, the medical masters could hope to achieve an institutional position
comparable, if never quite equal, to that of the jurists—a position they
were unlikely to attain as members of a nonacademic guild of *medici*,
chirurgi, or the like. In general, the degree of political and social influence exercised by any medieval craft or professional guild was pro-
portionate to the extent to which the activity in question was crucial to
the economic well-being of the community; the *studium* was not only
the glory of *Bononia docta*, it was also the city's chief economic resource.
Both the prestige attached to learning and economic factors combined
to assure that a medical professoriate would occupy a more exalted position than would practitioners who were not organized as members of a
learned profession.[59]

The institutional organization of public medical teaching and its association with the teaching of liberal arts and philosophy appears to have
taken place at Bologna during the last forty years of the thirteenth century. Taddeo himself taught logic as well as medicine.[60] A college of
doctors, made up of professors who examined candidates for a public
laurea (degree) in medicine, and no doubt also in arts, seems to have
been in existence by 1268, when a scholar contracted to give his master a
gift worth twenty-five Bolognese lire upon graduating and receiving his
"public [degree] in medicine." The agreement was signed in Taddeo
Alderotti's house and Taddeo was a witness to it.[61] In 1292 the college
of doctors (*collegium magistorum*), together with the archdeacon's
vicar, imposed penalties upon Bartolomeo da Varignana for his all-too-
successful attempt to attract the medical students of the aging and ailing
Taddeo.[62] That the membership of the college included masters of arts
as well as physicians, and that some of the latter were primarily practitioners rather than teachers, is indicated by a document of 1298. In that
year Master Boninsegno, a doctor of *physica* (that is, medicine) and as-

[59] See further the works cited in note 32, above.

[60] Ugolino Nicolini, "Documenti su Pietro Ispano (poi Giovanni XXI?) e Taddeo degli
Alderotti nei loro rapporti con Perugia," in *Filosofia e cultura in Umbria tra Medioevo e
Rinascimento, Atti del IV Convegno di Studi Umbri, Gubbio 22-26 maggio, 1966*, pp. 283-
284, document no. 5, dated April 5, 1287, in which Taddeo is described as "medico et
professore loice et medicine."

[61] Busacchi, "I primordi," pp. 135-136; "[lauream] pubblicam in medicina" (editor's
brackets), *Chart. Bon.* 8:22, document dated February 22, 1268.

[62] See note 38, above.

trology, petitioned for appointment as a municipal physician and for admission to the college of *medici*, doctors and masters "of the said arts," despite the fact that he had not yet attained the requisite age of thirty. In 1298, too, a group of four professors of *physica* swore obedience to the archdeacon while promising not to receive into the schools, either publicly or privately, any scholar who rebelled against the archdeacon's authority. It is not clear whether these four, whose number included Taddeo's associate and later rival, Bartolomeo da Varignana, constituted the entire publicly teaching medical faculty at the time, or only its senior members.[63]

The election of a "*doctor et rector in fisica*" in 1268 may indicate that some form of association of scholars in arts or medicine, or both, was then in existence. Whatever the case, by 1295 non-Bolognese scholars of arts and medicine had formed a university and had begun, greatly to the annoyance of the scholars of law, to elect their own rector; their right to do so was officially confirmed in 1316.[64]

Scholarly privileges were first formally extended to professors and scholars of medicine by the city government in a series of decrees issued some time between 1274 and 1288.[65] Apparently the civil disorders resulting from the feud between the Geremei and the Lambertazzi factions in Bologna made it necessary to offer various inducements to masters and scholars to stay in the city.[66] Among these were tax exemptions and legal protection, at first granted to Taddeo Alderotti and his pupils, and subsequently extended to all professors and scholars of medicine who were not

---

[63] SF 2:232-233. Regarding the oath of Liuzius, Maglius de Sulimanis, Bartolomeus de Varignana, and Johannes de Parma, "omnes Fixice professores," to Archdeacon Guido Baisio, see Giovanni Fantuzzi, *Notizie degli scrittori bolognesi*, 1:318.

[64] Busacchi, "I primordi," pp. 136-137; Cavazza, "Le scuole dell'antico Studio," p. 76. "*Fisica*" usually means "medicine" in a thirteenth-century Italian context; "*doctor et rector*" does not necessarily refer to the rector of a student university (on this question, see Busacchi, "I primordi," pp. 135-136). In 1289 a rector "ultramontanorum medicine" was elected; see Carlo Malagola, *Monografie storiche sullo Studio bolognese*, p. 136.

[65] A. Gaudenzi, "Gli antichi statuti del Commune di Bologna intorno allo studio," *Bullettino dell'Istituto storico italiano* 6 (1888):118, 121, 125, 130. The suggestion that the privileges may be dated in the 1270s is Gaudenzi's; Kibre, *Scholarly Privileges*, notes however that a threatened migration of scholars led the municipality to promise to uphold a variety of privileges in 1284. The scholarly privileges were incorporated, no doubt with some emendations and perhaps additions, as Book 8 of the Bolognese law code of 1287-1288; see G. Fasoli and P. Sella, eds., *Statuti di Bologna dell'anno 1288*, where the privileges accorded to Taddeo Alderotti appear at 2:102.

[66] Gaudenzi, "Gli antichi statuti," p. 118.

of Bolognese origin.[67] The municipal government soon began to pay stipends to professors in the faculty of arts and medicine. Taddeo himself was probably salaried, as well as privileged, by the commune. By 1305 the city was paying the salaries of professors of *physica* (medicine), grammar, and the notarial art.[68] In 1324 two professors of philosophy (one specializing in the *Parva naturalia, De celo,* and *Meteora* of Aristotle—that is, in natural science), a professor of practical medicine, and a professor of *astrologia* (that is astronomy and astrology), all elected by the student university of arts and medicine, were on the public payroll at annual salaries of 100 Bolognese lire each.[69] This expansion of the publicly supported arts and medical faculty reflects both the growth of the medical school under Taddeo and his pupils and the closely connected development of philosophical studies at Bologna: the professor of practical medicine was Taddeo's pupil, the anatomist Mondino de' Liuzzi; and one of the professors of philosophy was Angelo d'Arezzo, a pupil of Taddeo's pupil Gentile da Cingoli. The professor of *astrologia* in 1324 was the notorious Cecco d'Ascoli, soon to expiate his astrological determinism with his life. Ten years later, the municipality of Bologna reaffirmed its commitment to pay the salaries of professors of philosophy, practical medicine, and *astrologia,* while reducing the salary of the profes-

[67] "X. De privillegio magistri Thadei doctoris fixice et scolarium eius. Rubrica. Ordinamus, quia inveniamus sic reformatum in consciho sexcentorum et populi, quod magister Thadeus condam Aldegrotti [*sic*] de Florentia et sui heredes sint immunes et exempti ab omnibus collectis et serviciis realibus et personalibus civitatis Bononie.

"Item quod pro alique possessione quam emet ipse magister Thadeus vel alio modo vel titulo quereret, non teneatur pro ipsa solvere aliquam collectam; salvo quod non possit emere a bannitis vel confinatis communis Bononie et non possit cogi ipse magister Thadeus ire ad videndum aliquos vulneratos, vel aliquam relationem de vulneratis facere: *et sit tanquam forensis magister et scolaris in protectione communis et populi Bononie, et* eodem modo tractetur et habeatur, sed libere possit exercere artem suam prout eidem placuerit ubilibet exercere. . . ." Ibid., p. 130.

"XI. De privillegio scolarium magistri Tadei et aliorum doctorum fixice. [Rubrica] Statuimus quod scolares forenses qui audiunt vel audient in futuro fixicam a magistro Tadeo et aliis doctoribus fixice gaudeant omnibus et singulis privillegiis quibus gaudent scolares qui student vel studebant in civitate Bononie in iure civili vel canonico ex forma alicuius statuta vel reformationis vel ordinamenti communis vel populi Bononie," ibid., p. 130; and Fasoli and Sella, *Statuti di Bologna,* 2:102.

[68] Rashdall, *Universities,* 1:239.

[69] Elia Colini-Baldeschi, "Per la biografia di Cecco d'Ascoli," *Rivista delle biblioteche e degli archivi* 22 (1921):71, document no. 2, January 23, 1324. Colini-Baldeschi points out (p. 67) that this document corresponds closely to a list of professors, faculties, and salaries of the early fourteenth-century provided in Cherubino Ghirardacci, *Della historia di Bologna.*

sor of *astrologia* to 50 Bolognese lire per year.[70] Perhaps Cecco d'Ascoli's condemnation by the Inquisition had lowered the value of the teaching of the last-named discipline in the eyes of the city fathers. For comparison, the annual endowment of a chair in law was 100 lire in 1324 and 150 lire in 1334.

Those of the arts and medical faculty who were professors of medicine did not entirely have to depend either upon obtaining one of the municipal salaried chairs or upon the modest fees they were permitted to collect from individual students. The rewards of a successful consultant practice, such as Taddeo Alderotti's were many times greater than those of teaching.[71] Moreover, teachers of *astrologia* could practice their art, either by preparing predictions for private clients or by entering the service of a prince. The latter course is said, for example, to have been chosen by the famous Guido Bonatti (d. after 1282), who was probably a professor at Bologna. Later professors of *astrologia* at Bologna were obliged, by university statute, to provide individual "judgements of the year" without charge for scholars of the university of arts and medicine, a requirement that may indicate that professors normally prepared such judgments for other clients for a fee.[72]

Archival evidence regarding the internal organization of the faculty of arts and medicine at Bologna in the late thirteenth and early fourteenth centuries is almost entirely lacking. The earliest extant statutes of the College of Doctors of Arts and Medicine and of the University of Scholars of Arts and Medicine date from the late fourteenth and early fifteenth centuries.[73] It seems likely, however, that many of the arrangements reflected in the doctoral college statutes of 1378, 1395, and 1410, and in the student university statutes of 1405, may also have prevailed at an earlier date.

Judging from the content of the statutes of the college of doctors, the main function of this body, apart from jealously guarding the interests of its members and gathering for religious devotions, continued to be the conduct of the examinations leading to the degree officially conferred by the archdeacon or his vicar.[74] To this prerogative the college had by 1378

---

[70] Gaudenzi, "Gli antichi statuti," pp. 134-135; Rashdall, *Universities* 1:210-211.

[71] Taddeo left the sum of 10,000 lire Bolognese in various religious, charitable, and educational bequests; his will is printed in SF 2:223-230. See further below, chapter two.

[72] Malagola, *Statuti*, p. 264.   [73] Cencetti, *Archivi*, pp. 45, 47, 53, 68.

[74] Malagola, *Statuti*, pp. 425-522; Rashdall, *Universities*, 1:221-229.

added the licensing of all medical and surgical practice in the city.[75] Thus, its members determined and administered the process of admission to the learned profession of medicine in Bologna. In one important respect the qualifications required for membership in the college of doctors evidently became more stringent as time went on. In 1378 the members of the college were required both to be Bolognese citizens by birth themselves and to be the sons of Bolognese citizens by birth,[76] a regulation repeated with minor modifications in subsequent sets of statutes. By contrast, several of the leading professors of medicine in the first years of the college, most notably Taddeo Alderotti himself and his pupils Dino del Garbo and Turisanus, were Bolognese only by adoption.[77] The members of the college, limited in 1378 to fifteen in number, not only tried to monopolize the senior professorial positions in the faculty of arts and medicine themselves, but also legislated to oblige non-Bolognese candidates for the license to teach medicine to swear not to lecture in the morning hours, not to attempt to join the college, and not to present candidates for examination.[78] The impression that the college developed into a preserve of the Bolognese citizen class is strengthened by the existence of a provision allowing the admission of the sons or brothers of members even when all fifteen places were filled.[79] The medical profession, like other occupations open to laymen, tended to run in families. A close network of blood and marriage relationships already bound together various members of Bologna's medical elite in Taddeo's day, as a glance at the biographies in the next chapter will indicate.

No statutory description of the arts and medical curriculum at the *studium* of Bologna is known to survive from the period when Taddeo and his pupils taught there. It is clear from their works that at Bologna, as elsewhere in Europe, the arts curriculum had come chiefly to emphasize the study of philosophy and natural science found in Aristotle's works on physics, the soul, the heavens, animals, and so forth, and that this curriculum was studied not only by those pursuing a degree in arts as their final goal, but also by all those intending to proceed to the study of medicine. Of the liberal arts, logic and *astrologia* were regarded as particularly important preparatory studies for medicine and therefore continued to flourish. The survival, and indeed the fresh development, of

[75] Kibre, *Scholarly Privileges*, p. 50. [76] Malagola, *Statuti*, p. 426.
[77] See chapter two, below, for biographical details.
[78] Malagola, *Statuti*, p. 431. [79] Ibid., p. 438.

rhetorical, literary, and humanistic interests in academic circles in Bologna after the institutionalization and association of arts teaching with scholastic natural philosophy and with medical science is demonstrated by the appointment in 1321 of the celebrated classicist Giovanni del Virgilio to lecture on the major Latin poets, namely Virgil, Ovid, Statius, and Lucan.[80]

Taddeo himself probably played an important part in adapting the more or less standard thirteenth-century curriculum in Aristotelian natural philosophy to the needs of the newly established public faculty of arts and medicine at Bologna. He was the first author associated with Bologna to produce major works making extensive use of Aristotle's teachings and of scholastic method, and the growth of the now well-known school of radical Aristotelian philosophy among masters of arts at Bologna owed much to Taddeo's pupil Gentile da Cingoli. Similarly, significant innovations in medical teaching at Bologna, including the addition to the curriculum of major works of Galen and of the *Canon* of Avicenna, appear to have originated with Taddeo and younger professors who had studied under him. Detailed discussion of the probable contributions of this group of masters to the shaping of the Bolognese medical curriculum and of their conceptions of medical learning is therefore reserved for more extended treatment in chapters four and five below. Much of the significance of the men with whom we are concerned lies precisely in the fact that their careers spanned the crucial period when the institutionalization of medical learning in association with arts and philosophy was taking place at Bologna. Taddeo and his pupils helped both to shape a singularly durable form of university medical teaching and to carry it to other centers far beyond Bologna, and indeed beyond Italy. It is now time to turn to an account of their lives and work.

---

[80] Rashdall, *Universities*, 1:239-240; Paul Oskar Kristeller, "Un 'ars dictaminis' di Giovanni del Virgilio," *Italia medioevale e umanistica* 4 (1961):182, no. 5; Wieruszowski, "Rhetoric and the Classics," in *Politics and Culture*, pp. 619-626.

CHAPTER TWO

THE MEN

Like social and institutional history, biography has its own relevance to the history of thought. Moreover, the collective biographies of relatively minor figures may, more than the exceptional accomplishments of great men, serve to exemplify typical careers. The brief biographies that follow are of Taddeo Alderotti and six of his pupils, or *socii*. As far as can be determined, only these six scholars meet the dual criteria of having had an association with Taddeo that can be demonstrated on the basis of contemporary or near contemporary evidence, and of having left surviving written works from which their intellectual contribution can be evaluated.

Lest more seem to be implied by the use of collective biography than is in fact intended, it is perhaps necessary to enter a caveat here. Taddeo's was not the only intellectual influence to which his pupils were exposed; moreover, while innovative in important respects, he also frequently followed established conventions and traditions. Furthermore, the paths of some of Taddeo's students diverged widely in later life. Therefore it is not claimed, and should not be assumed, that as mature scholars they either adhered to any uniquely distinctive body of opinion or engaged in lifelong intellectual interchange. They nonetheless merit study as a group simply because they were products of a celebrated school at a crucial moment in its history and, in the case of Taddeo's students, of an almost equally celebrated master.

All six of the masters connected with Taddeo who are treated here were learned authors of some note, and most of them were men of significant practical achievement as well. The scope of their activities and influence was much more than merely local, or even merely Italian; not only are a number of manuscripts of some of their written works found in libraries in northern Europe, but also, as will be seen, some of them made their influence felt in such major intellectual centers as the *studia* of Paris and of Montpellier and the papal court at Avignon. Among them, Bartolomeo da Varignana (d. after 1321) wrote on both medicine and moral

philosophy, was responsible for some of the earliest recorded autopsies at
Bologna, and was personal physician to the Emperor Henry VII. Guglielmo de' Corvi da Brescia (d. 1326) was physician to three successive
popes, founder of one of the first residential colleges at Bologna, and
partly responsible for the medical curriculum of the *studium* of Montpellier. Mondino de' Liuzzi (d. 1326), although he may not have merited
the title he is sometimes accorded of "restorer of anatomy," nonetheless
wrote a deservedly famous textbook on the subject. Turisanus (Pietro
Torrigiano de' Torrigiani, d. ca. 1319) taught at Paris, while Dino del
Garbo (d. 1327) was in his day one of Italy's leading medical authors
and teachers. The philosopher Gentile da Cingoli (active from 1295), the
only one of the group not to pursue a medical career, was a founder of
Bolognese Averroism. The collective record is a remarkable one, of which
any teacher might be proud.

Yet it must be admitted that the very distinction of these students
makes them atypical members of Taddeo's circle, most of whose members
are no doubt lost to us. A few of his colleagues appear fleetingly in his
works and in his will: the ingenious and subtle Master Odone, who
knew the *Tegni* like his Psalter;[1] Master Clarellus, who kept Taddeo
alert;[2] and Master Bonagratia, who had his own opinion on the ages of
man.[3] Taddeo presumably had high hopes for the professional career of
his *socius* Master Johannes of Assissi, to whom he bequeathed his copy of
Serapion and a copy of Avicenna, *De naturalibus*, but Johannes seems
otherwise unknown to history, as does Master Nicholas of Faenza, to
whom Taddeo left the holograph copies of his own writings and his
Almansor.[4] Not even this much is known of most of those who were
Taddeo's students; they are nameless and faceless.

[1] "hoc dico magistro Odoni qui omnia scrutatur proprio sermone. . . . et per hoc possunt
omnia solvi ab ingenio subtili magistri Odonis facti pisis. . . . et solvitur ista questio
hoc modo a Galieno in libro de creticis diebus ibi enim legas domine Odo qui scis tegni
sicut psalterium," *Thaddei Florentini Expositiones in arduum aphorismorum Ipocratis volumen, In divinum pronosticorum Ipocratis librum, In preclarum regiminis acutorum Ipocratis
opus, In subtilissime Joannitii Isagogarum libellum*, fols. 357v, 376r, 384v. Taddeo's references to his colleagues are noted in Taddeo, *I "Consilia,"* p. xviii.

[2] "finitus est tractatus de febribus domino Clarello qui facit nos evigilare et transire per-
mentem nostram quicquid mali potest," Taddeo, *Isagoge*, fol. 389r.

[3] "hec sufficiant de etatibus: licet etas aliter sumatur apud magistrum Bonam gratiam
cuius plenam disputationem relinquo magistro Clarello," ibid., fol. 369r. For other personal
allusions of a similar kind, see ibid., fols. 367v, 390r.

[4] Will of Taddeo Alderotti, in SF 2:223-230, at p. 227. The widely circulated *Liber
Almansoris of Rhazes* (d. ca. 923) was a general encyclopedia of medicine in ten books.

Nor can one attribute all the accomplishments, intellectual and otherwise, of the most successful among Taddeo's pupils to his influence alone. Obviously other teachers and, more importantly, a general learned tradition in which Taddeo's own instruction was only one small—and wholly congruent—element also played a part in their formation. To disentangle Taddeo's personal contribution is seldom possible. Nonetheless, that Taddeo played a major role in the education of these men seems incontrovertibly established. Thus, Bartolomeo da Varignana helped Taddeo to prepare his commentary on the Hippocratic *De regimine acutorum*[5] before quarreling with him finally and irrevocably;[6] Guglielmo was stated by his own pupil, Abbot Engelbert of Admont, to have left Padua in order to study under Taddeo at Bologna;[7] Dino and Turisanus were said to have been Taddeo's students by their biographer Filippo Villani, writing ca. 1381-1382;[8] Mondino described Taddeo as a teacher and practitioner, evidently from the life;[9] and Gentile, one of whose works reflects training in medicine, submitted himself to Taddeo's authority as the arbitrator of a contract between himself and another professor.[10] But the master must take precedence over the pupils: first comes the biography of Taddeo himself.

TADDEO ALDEROTTI
(ALDEROTTO, DEGLI ALDEROTTI; TADDEO DA FIRENZE, THADDEUS FLORENTINUS)

The known contemporary sources for Taddeo's life consist of occasional allusions in his own writings, a few documents, most of them bearing upon various legal transactions to which he was a party or witness, his

[5] Taddeo, *Reg. acut.*, fol. 247r, where the assistance of "Bartolomeus veronensis" is acknowledged; in NLM, MS 492, 14c (a collection of all Taddeo's major commentaries in 3 volumes), 2, fol. 25r, the name appears in the form veronēsis. The assumption that Bartolomeo da Varignana is referred to seems highly probable.

[6] SF 2:223, document of March 22, 1292.

[7] Engelbert of Admont, letter to Master Ulrich, in B. Pez, *Thesaurus anecdotorum Novissimus*, vol. 1, pt. 1, col. 430; also cited in George Fowler, *Intellectual Interests of Engelbert of Admont* (New York, 1947), pp. 21-22.

[8] Filippo Villani, *Liber de civitatis Florentiae famosis civibus*, pp. 27-29. On the dating of Villani's work, see Hans Baron, *The Crisis of the Early Italian Renaissance* (rev. ed., Princeton, N.J., 1966), p. 95.

[9] Mondino, *Mesue cum expositione Mondini super Canones universales . . .* , fol. 38 (error for 37)r-v.

[10] SF 2:231-232.

celebrated privilege from the city of Bologna, and his lengthy, detailed, and informative will.[11] In addition, he was the subject of a brief biography included by Filippo Villani in his *Liber de civitatis Florentiae famosis civibus*, which was written about eighty-five years after Taddeo's death.[12] Villani's biography, although almost certainly heightened for the sake of drama, seems generally substantiated, in its main outlines, by the documentary evidence. There are also a few references to Taddeo by contemporary and slightly later authors, the most celebrated of whom is Dante.[13] These references attest to Taddeo's fame and throw some further light on his activities and character.

Taddeo's birthdate is not known. Villani says that he died an octogenarian, and his death date is established as 1295 by a verse epitaph contained in two manuscripts.[14] He was therefore presumably born sometime between 1206 and 1215 into a Florentine family that, if not as spectacularly deprived as Villani made out, was evidently of modest enough means. The family apparently had some medical connections or tradition before Taddeo's time, since he himself referred to an uncle of his who

[11] Several documents pertaining to Taddeo are printed in *Chart. Bon.*, 8:22; 9:203-204, 206, 220, 240-241; 10:113-114, 147, 165-166; as noted, his privileges from the Commune of Bologna appear in A. Gaudenzi, "Gli antichi statuti," p. 130; his will and a few other documents are to be found in SF 2:221-232. Recent secondary accounts of Taddeo are to be found in Vern L. Bullough, "Taddeo Alderotti," *DSB*, 1:167, and L. Belloni and L. Vergnano, "Alderotti, Taddeo (Thaddaeus Florentinus)," *Dizionario biografico degli italiani* (Rome, 1960-   ), 1:85. Still useful are the older accounts in Sarton, *Introduction to the History of Science*, 2:1086-1087; and Girolamo Tiraboschi, *Storia della letteratura italiana*, 4:218-223.

[12] F. Villani, *Liber de . . . famosis civibus*, pp. 26-27.

[13] *Paradiso* 12.82-84; *Convivio* 1.10 (where, however, Taddeo's name may be the addition of a copyist; regarding both passages, see further below). See also Giovanni Villani, *Cronica* 8.65. Taddeo's fame and skill were also briefly lauded by Benevenuto da Imola and Riccobaldo da Ferrara.

[14] The epitaph runs:

Mille nonaginta transactis quinque ducentis
Jove sero primo junii, sub nocte secunda
Migravit cunctorum Thadeus dux medicorum
Errores stravit, tenebras ut sol radiavit,
Oremus deum, pia mater, sume Thadeum

It is printed in P. Pansier, "Les maîtres de la faculté de médecine de Montpellier au Moyen Age," *Janus* 9 (1904):511, from Paris, Bibliothèque Nationale, MS lat. 6964, fol. 129, and is also to be found in Padua, Biblioteca Universitaria, MS al numero provvisorio 202, fol. 115r. The death date 1292, found in *Corpus chronicorum bononiensium*, 2, ed. Albano Sorbelli, *Rerum italicarum scriptores* (Citta di Castello, 1905), n.s., vol. 18, pt. 1, p. 238, is an error, as is 1303, frequently found in the secondary literature.

had been a surgeon.[15] Villani's claim that Taddeo sold church candles in his youth may indicate some association with medicine in the family: in thirteenth- and fourteenth-century Florence, the candlemakers were members of a subdivision of the same guild that embraced the medical practitioners and pharmacists.[16]

Nothing beyond his name is known of Alderotto, Taddeo's father. Taddeo had at least two brothers, Bonaguida and Simone, and perhaps also a sister or sisters, since some authors claim that the surgeon Bono del Garbo, father of Dino del Garbo, was his brother-in-law.[17] He may have been the youngest of the family, since his brother Bonaguida made his will in 1269, twenty-six years before Taddeo's death.[18] The family had some property before Taddeo's rise to fame, for Bonaguida sold his brother Simone a house in the parish of Santa Croce in 1251; conceivably it may have been, as Biscioni assumed, the family home.[19] The possibility is not necessarily incompatible with Villani's stress on the family's humble origins and Taddeo's poverty in his youth.

Taddeo himself demonstrated a strong concern for family and property. He married late in life, taking to wife in 1274 Adela, daughter of Guidalotto de' Regaletti of Florence. Adela brought with her a dowry of 300 lire of Pisa and 50 lire for wedding expenses, and she evidently came from a solid citizen and professional family. Both her father and her grandfather were referred to as *dominus*, an indication of at least a modest degree of social status, while her brother was later professor of canon law at Bologna.[20] She must have been much younger than her husband, who was in his late fifties or older at the time of the marriage; for she bore him a daughter, Mina, perhaps about the year 1280; and she (Adela) was still alive in 1321.[21] Moreover, Taddeo's will, drawn up in 1293, makes careful disposition for the event of his wife's pregnancy at the time of his death (with provisions varying according to whether she

[15] Taddeo, *Isagoge*, fol. 398v.

[16] Raffaello Ciasca, *L'arte dei medici e speziali nella storia e nel commercio fiorentino dal secolo XII al XV*, p. 45.

[17] For example, Francesco Puccinotti, *Storia della medicina*, vol. 2, pt. 2, p. 307.

[18] *Chart. Bon.*, 10:165-166.

[19] A. M. Biscioni, *Delle opere di Dante Alighieri* (Venice, 1741), pp. 30-33. On the basis of this document, Biscioni strongly contested Villani's statements concerning Taddeo's early poverty.

[20] SF 1:558.

[21] Mina was still unmarried when Taddeo made his will in 1293; Adela made her will in 1321 (Biscioni, *Delle opere di Dante*, p. 33).

proved to be carrying a male, a female, or twins of the same or different sex).[22]

By the mid-1280s, when his career reached its peak, Taddeo was a man of substantial property; most of the surviving documentary records of his activity concern his involvement in various business transactions. Evidently he multiplied the wealth brought by his profession through careful investment. He acquired real estate and a mortgage[23] and also, it would appear, engaged in money lending. Two curious contracts regarding excursions Taddeo made from Bologna to treat patients in Modena indicate this. The first, dated 1285, stipulates that three parties who have received the sum of 3,000 lire Bolognese from Taddeo are to escort him safely to Modena and back, paying a penalty of 1,000 lire Bolognese if any one of several provisions are violated, and repaying the 3,000 at Taddeo's pleasure. This certainly looks like a concealed loan contract, devised to avoid the ecclesiastical prohibitions on taking interest, as does a similar document of 1288, in which two other men again acknowledge the receipt of 3,000 lire from Taddeo and again promise to escort him to Modena and back with an indemnity for damage and, this time, at their own expense.[24] Wholly unambiguous is the contract of 1286 in which Taddeo undertook to lend the sum of 200 lire Bolognese to Guido, son of Recopro of Florence.[25] Guido is described as "emancipated from his father," which may imply that Taddeo, like other professors in thirteenth-century Bologna, did not disdain to lend money to students.[26] Moreover, in his will he was careful to provide that some of his charitable bequests be invested so that the beneficiaries might enjoy the "fruit and return" ("*fructus et redditus*"). The same document provides, in accordance with current convention, for the restitution of monies wrongfully acquired, that is, probably by usury.[27]

Taddeo's combination of professional success and business acumen enabled him to leave an estate valued at more than 3,000 gold florins[28] and 10,000 lire Bolognese, in addition to two parcels of real estate in Florence, gold and silver plate, and a respectable collection of philosophical, medi-

---

[22] SF 2:229-230.

[23] *Chart. Bon.*, 10:203-204, 220.

[24] SF 2:221-222.

[25] *Chart. Bon.*, 9:206.

[26] See Bellomo, *Saggio sull'università*, pp. 104-105.

[27] SF 2:228; excessive fees may also, however, have weighed upon Taddeo's conscience.

[28] Since the share of one of his three residuary heirs amounted to more than 1,000 florins; SF 2:228. At the time the value of the lire Bolognese was to the florin in about the ratio of 3:2.

cal, and devotional books. Alas, Adela bore no son to inherit this wealth. Evidently doubting her further fertility, in 1290 Taddeo petitioned Pope Nicholas III for the legitimization of Taddeolo, his natural son.[29] Once legitimized, Taddeolo could, of course, inherit; and he was accordingly named along with his half-sister Mina and Opizus, son of Taddeo's brother Bonaguida, as one of Taddeo's residuary legatees after 10,000 lire Bolognese had been distributed to various religious institutions and charities. The residual bequest must have been a substantial one, since Mina's share alone included a dowry of 1,000 gold florins (a striking contrast to her mother Adela's endowment of 300 lire of Pisa). With such a portion, it is not surprising to learn that Mina married into the noble Florentine family of Pulci before 1301.[30] The less fortunate Adela received a house in the parish of Santa Croce in Florence (the same one Bonaguida had sold to Simon in 1251?), furniture and personal possessions excluding gold and silverware, and 50 lire Bolognese. This modest bequest was left on condition that she led an honest and widowlike life and "served marital honor." If, however, "she chooses another way of life for herself," the will rather ominously continues, she is to receive her dowry back instead of the house.[31] No doubt Taddeo assumed that Adela, perhaps only in her early thirties, would remarry, and that it was therefore unnecessary to provide further for her. However, these provisions, taken in conjunction with the size of the other bequests, and with the apparent partial separation of the spouses, who seem not to have been living together continuously during Taddeo's last years,[32] may suggest that relations between them were something less than harmonious.

Taddeo's education is as obscure as the rest of his early career. Villani's story that he came late to academic life on account of slow mental development and extreme poverty is not inherently improbable, even in its picturesque detail, although there is no other evidence to support it. The earliest recorded references to Taddeo as a master date from the 1260s, when he was already in his forties or fifties, and did not produce his commentaries until he had been teaching for some time.[33] Obviously,

[29] E. Langlois, ed., *Les registres de Nicholas IV*, p. 474, no. 2873.

[30] Biscioni, *Delle opere di Dante*, p. 33; SF 1:559.

[31] SF 2:227.

[32] Ladislao Münster, "Taddeo degli Alderotti mancato medico condotto a Perugia (1287) e a Venezia (1293)," *Rivista di storia delle scienze mediche a naturali* 47 (1956):52.

[33] *Chart. Bon.*, 8:22, document of February 25, 1268; and "in nono anno mei regiminis

the most striking feature of Taddeo's learning is his extensive and apparently thorough knowledge of the standard medical authorities, especially
Hippocrates, Galen, and Avicenna. Almost unquestionably this knowledge was acquired at Bologna, which, as indicated above, was already
by the mid-thirteenth century an important center of medical activity,
and hence one in which copies of medical works were readily available
for study. Taddeo's writings also show that their author had acquired a
fairly broadly based academic grounding in the liberal arts and in philosophy. He seems to have had a reasonably thorough knowledge of the
logical and natural works of Aristotle; citations of the works on animals,
obviously of major concern to a physician for their physiological content,
and of the *Nicomachean Ethics*, in which he had a special interest, are
notably frequent in his works. Occasional citations of the *Timaeus*, of
Cicero, and of Boethius (the *Consolatio*) provide some evidence of familiarity with a broader culture.[34] Despite statements to the contrary
sometimes found in the secondary literature, there is no evidence that he
knew Greek or Arabic.[35] His frequent attempts to compare different
translations of the same work, with assertions of the superiority of one or
the other, are based entirely upon the usefulness of a particular version of
the Latin text for the argument he was considering at the moment.[36]
Nor does he seem to have been inspired with any notable interest in following current developments in sciences other than medicine; for example, he discussed the phenomena of vision with no more than the briefest
allusion to the work of Alhazen or to the various thirteenth-century writers on optics.[37] In discussing astronomy and astrology, too, his range of
reference was restricted, and rested, to a significant extent, upon medical
sources.[38]

However enterprising an autodidact Taddeo may have been, it is un-

---

incepi glossare aphorismos," Taddeo, *Aphor.*, fol. 194v. Of Taddeo's major commentaries,
only that on the *Isagoge* of Johannitius may have been begun before this time.

[34] For example, Taddeo, *Isagoge*, fol. 370v; *Pronost.*, fol. 195v.

[35] For example, in Puccinotti, *Storia della medicina*, vol. 2, pt. 2, 294.

[36] See, for example, Taddeo, *Reg. acut.*, fol. 250v.

[37] Taddeo, *Isagoge*, fols. 362r-363v.

[38] For example, in discussing astrological factors in connection with critical days in illness,
he cited Galen, *De creticis*; Alchabitius; the *Centiloquium* attributed to Ptolemy; and Albumasar (Taddeo, *Aphor.*, fols. 49v-50r). Elsewhere, in discussing the same topic, he added
citations of the *Canon* of Avicenna, Aristotle's *Physics*, and Isaac Judaeus (Taddeo, *Pronost.*,
fols. 236r-237v).

likely that he learned without any teachers at all. If we suppose Villani to be right about Taddeo's late start, the latter must have acquired the foundations of his learning either at Florence or Bologna, or both, sometime between the mid-1230s and the 1260s, when he appears as a master. There is good reason to suppose that his early studies (that is, those in arts and philosophy and perhaps a beginning in medicine) may have been fostered by the Franciscans or, less probably, the Dominicans. Whether or not there is any truth in the tale of his early occupation as a vendor of church candles, the undoubted fact of his family's association with the parish of Santa Croce makes it probable that Taddeo came to the attention of the Franciscans of Florence. As the studies of Charles Davis have shown, both the Franciscan and the Dominican houses in Florence were by the 1280s and 1290s major centers of learning from which at least some laymen were able to benefit.[39] Possibly a similar state of affairs prevailed there at an earlier date. Franciscan or Dominican teachers at Bologna may also have made themselves as available to Taddeo and other laymen.

Taddeo certainly had a particular attachment to the Franciscans of Bologna, of whom he became a very generous benefactor. The terms of his will indicate that he valued the intellectual as well as the evangelical activities of the friars. He left a bequest of 4,000 lire for the purchase of property for the Claresses of Bologna; as a condition of the bequest, the sisters were bound in perpetuity to give 50 lire each year from the fruits of the property to provide a scholarship enabling an additional Franciscan friar from the Bolognese province to study theology at Paris.[40] Except during the Great Schism, Franciscans from Bologna were regularly sent to study at Paris throughout the fourteenth and fifteenth centuries, and many of them benefited from Taddeo's bequest. As might perhaps have been expected, however, the terms of the will led to wrangling between the Claresses and the friars. A settlement between them reached in 1382 reveals that the nuns had been holding back the money, and that two of the friars designated as recipients of the scholarship and also the friar guardian of the convent had helped themselves to portable items of the

---

[39] Charles T. Davis, "Education in Dante's Florence," *Speculum* 40 (1965):415-435, especially 420-425. But in idem, "The Early Collection of Books of S. Croce in Florence," *Proceedings of the American Philosophical Society* 107 (1963):399, 401, it is pointed out that the thirteenth-century library of the convent seems to have been chiefly theological, although a collection of Aristotle's logical works was acquired in 1319.

[40] SF 2:224-225.

nuns' property (a silver chalice, a missal, a book *On The Wonders of the World*, and another, more appropriate for enclosed nuns, of *Legends of the Saints*) by way of enforced compensation.[41]

Taddeo also willed some of his medical books to the Franciscan friars of Bologna for their own use: his Avicenna in four volumes (no doubt the *Canon*), and his books of Galen. His books on natural philosophy, namely Avicenna's *Metaphysics* and Book 6 *De naturalibus*, and the *Nicomachean Ethics* (perhaps in the abbreviated Latin version he is said to have translated into Italian), he bequeathed to the Servites.[42] Taddeo's bequests reveal something of the intellectual interests of some of the friars at Bologna in the 1290s; they may also be an expression of his own gratitude to an earlier generation of teachers in one or more of the orders.

Whatever the means by which Taddeo acquired his education, his learning clearly demonstrates that medicine was studied as a learned discipline, in association with liberal arts and philosophy, during a period often characterized as one in which the main activities of Bolognese medical men were nonacademic and largely concerned with practical treatment and surgery. Neither institutionalization nor Taddeo's own enterprise created the association of arts and medicine *ex nihilo*; instead, institutionalization, as one might expect, merely gave formal existence to an informal relationship.

Taddeo's professional career engaged him as teacher, practitioner, and author; it is appropriate to examine each of these aspects in turn. There is no evidence that Taddeo ever publicly taught any subjects but medicine and logic, or at any place but Bologna.[43] With the exception of the

[41] Piana, *Chartularium*, pp. 40*-44*, where a list of friars from Bologna who studied at Paris is printed, together with the document recording the settlement of the dispute between the nuns and the friars.

[42] SF 2:227.

[43] Pansier, "Les maîtres de la faculté de médicine," p. 511, disproves the story that Taddeo taught at Montpellier, pointing out that the "Experimenta magistri thadei . . . in Montepessulano" found in Paris, Bibliothèque Nationale, MS lat. 6964, are dated 1301, whereas the same manuscript contains Taddeo's epitaph giving the death date 1295. In Paris University, Bibliothèque de la Sorbonne, MS 131, 13c, commentaries on Egidius on urines and pulses apparently written at Montpellier (fol. 96v) are attributed to "Thaddaeus" (fol. 108v; on fols. 88r, 96v, 102r, the author is said to be m[agister] T. or Th.). The attributions are, however, added in another hand. It is unlikely that these works are in fact by Taddeo Alderotti. Another manuscript in Paris, Bibliothèque Nationale, MS lat. 6964, 14 or 15c, contains authentic works of Taddeo; on fol. 129v his *Practica de febribus* (inc. "Quoniam nichil melius ad veritatis indagationem"—see TK 1288) ends with the words "Explicit practica magistri thadei bone memorie disputata," the whole sentence

vernacular compendium of the *Ethics* and of a short poem on alchemy,[44] all the works attributed to him are on medical subjects; any further indications of his attachment to philosophy or Aristotelianism must be sought in scattered passages in his commentaries on medical texts, just as the most celebrated instance of his interest in chemical or alchemical processes—his account of distilling and praise of *aqua vitae*—is found among his medical consilia.[45]

Taddeo was, obviously, an outstandingly successful teacher. But few things are more ephemeral than classroom triumphs, and it is hard to gain any clear idea of his merits in this regard. One more or less contemporary anecdote that may allow a glimpse of his method shows students free to question and contradict the master—but the one who does so makes himself ridiculous in a peculiarly humiliating way.[46] Taddeo's teaching career probably began in the mid-1260s. He described his commentary on the *Aphorisms* of Hippocrates as having been begun in the ninth year of his teaching and interrupted a few months thereafter by civil war.[47] If, as seems probable, the civil war in question was that of 1274, Taddeo may have begun to teach about 1264. He was certainly doing so by 1268, when he was referred to as a master in a document, cited in chapter one, concerning a public *laurea* in medicine.[48] He probably continued until some time after 1290, when he began arranging his

---

underlined. Another hand has added, without underlining, "parisius," which should probably be taken to mean that the work was copied at Paris after Taddeo's death. His epitaph, giving the date 1295, follows. This manuscript should not, therefore, be regarded as evidence that Taddeo disputed at Paris in 1295. Regarding Taddeo's teaching of logic, see note 60 to chapter one, above.

[44] The poem has been printed more than once, most recently in Concetto Marchesi, *L'Etica Nicomachea nella tradizione medievale*, p. 125. According to Marchesi it is known only from a fifteenth-century manuscript where it is described as "Carmina magistri Tadei de florentia super scientiam lapidis philosophorum ex Alberto Magno edita feliciter."

[45] Taddeo, I *"Consilia,"* pp. 235-242.

[46] Guido Favati, ed., *Il Novellino*, novella 35, pp. 208-209; see also Lorenzo Guerrieri, "Considerazioni sugli scolari bolognesi di Taddeo degli Alderotti in base ad una novella medioevale," in XXI *Congresso Internazionale di Storia della Medicina, Siena, 1968, Atti*, I:126-129. A student who does not accept Taddeo's assertion that the eating of *petronciani* (eggplant, according to Guerrieri) drives one mad, eats them, claims to his master that he has disproved the statement and then "alzasi i panni, e mostragli il culo." The *Novellino*, or *Cente novelle*, was written between 1281 and 1300 either at Florence or, more probably, in the Veneto or Marca Trivigiana (Favati, *Il Novellino*, pp. 59-61, 82-83).

[47] Taddeo, *Aphor.*, fol. 194v; for the political history of Bologna in this period, see Vito Vitale, *Il dominio della Parte Guelfa in Bologna (1280-1321)*.

[48] *Chart. Bon.*, 8:22.

effects.[49] By March 1292, at the latest, his pupils were slipping from his grasp, for at that time he brought a complaint to the archdeacon of Bologna that Bartolomeo da Varignana was luring them away.[50] Taddeo seems to have faced the reality of his own increasing incapacity by May of the same year, when he appointed a proctor to handle his affairs.[51] In 1293 he was lying sick at the Franciscan convent,[52] where he made his will in January, and was probably not very active thereafter. He was, however, still sufficiently involved in the affairs of the *studium* in March 1295 to agree to arbitrate an argument between Gentile da Cingoli and another master.[53]

His school was located in the parish of Saint Martin, where he owned more than one house.[54] Public recognition of his reputation as a master came in the shape of the celebrated privileges granted by the municipality of Bologna to Taddeo and his pupils.[55] By the first of these documents, Taddeo was freed from all municipal taxes, from compulsory attendance upon the wounded, and from any obligation to submit medico-legal reports on injuries; it was further stated that Taddeo, like other foreign (that is, non-Bolognese) masters and scholars, was to be under the protection of the Commune and people of Bologna and that he was to be free to exercise his art in any way he chose. The second privilege extended all the privileges enjoyed by foreign students of canon and civil law to foreign scholars who came to study medicine (*physica*) with Taddeo and the other doctors of medicine. As noted in chapter one, the dates of these privileges are uncertain; the possibilities range from 1274 to 1288. To reckon by Taddeo's own career, his reputation could hardly have been sufficient to attract large numbers of non-Bolognese students before he had been teaching for some years. A date or dates sometime in the 1280s therefore seems most likely. Taddeo appears to have received a salary as well as tax exemptions from the Commune of Bologna; this is asserted by Villani[56] and supported by the clauses in the first privilege that release him from obligatory attendance on the

---

[49] It was in that year that he secured the legitimation of his son Taddeolo, as noted above, in order to make him one of his heirs.

[50] SF 2:223.   [51] SF 1:558.

[52] Münster, "Taddeo degli Alderotti," p. 52.

[53] SF 2:231-232.

[54] Cavazza, "Le scuole dell'antico studio," pp. 413-416.

[55] Gaudenzi, "Gli antichi statuti," p. 130.

[56] F. Villani, *Liber de . . . famosis civibus*, p. 26.

wounded and from the preparation of medico-legal reports, duties that could presumably have been required in the first place only of a physician on the city payroll. Evidently the civic authorities came to think him even more valuable to the city as a professor than as a practitioner. Judging by the payments made to other municipal physicians in the thirteenth century and by the stipends on municipally endowed professorial chairs in medicine at a slightly later date, we must conclude that this salary is unlikely to have been very large.[57] For the source of Taddeo's wealth, we must turn to his practice.

Consultative practice was probably Taddeo's principal activity, and certainly his principal source of support, for much of his professional life. He himself referred to the interruption of his theoretical writing by "*lucrativa operatio*,"[58] and he appears to have taken full advantage of the clause in his privilege from the municipality of Bologna allowing him to practice *ad libitum*. Furthermore, the sums bequeathed in his will are far larger than he could have gained by teaching, even if his student fees and the customary graduation presents[59] were added to a municipal salary.

Taddeo's most famous, if not his most remunerative, patient at Bologna was King Enzo, natural son of Emperor Frederick II. That unhappy titular monarch was taken prisoner by the Bolognese in 1249, when the city had become involved in the papal struggle against the Hohenstaufen; and he spent the rest of his life in captivity in Bologna (d. 1272). Enzo's long imprisonment, his youth when he was captured, and his reputation as a poet gave rise to many romantic legends. A more prosaic side to his captivity is suggested by the clause in his will naming Taddeo as one of six physicians for whose services Enzo asked the Commune of Bologna to pay, since he had no funds to reward them. Medical attention was among the facilities provided for Enzo by the Bolognese government; so the physicians may well have been on the public payroll in any case.

[57] In 1214, Ugo da Lucca had from the Commune of Bologna a money fief (*feudum*) of 600 lire Bolognese per annum, of which, however, only 200 was direct payment for his services as municipal surgeon, since an annual payment of 400 lire was to be received by his heirs, even if they were not physicians or surgeons (SF 2:214); as noted, a professor of practical medicine was paid 100 lire per annum by the municipality of Bologna in 1324. But, as we shall see, on one occasion Taddeo himself was offered 1,000 lire per year to brave the wrath of the Bolognese and migrate to Perugia.

[58] Taddeo, *Aphor.*, fol. 194v.

[59] Rashdall, *Universities*, 1:240-241; *Chart. Bon.*, 8:22, where a graduation present to a master valued at twenty-five lire is mentioned (document of February 25, 1268).

In addition, Taddeo's fairly numerous surviving *consilia* indicate that he had an extensive and aristocratic clientele that was by no means confined to Bologna.[60]

In many instances, no doubt, requests for advice reached Taddeo from other cities by letter, either from other physicians or directly from the patients, and were answered in the same way; but on occasion he traveled to the bedside of his more distinguished patients. He appears to have made at least two trips to Modena for purposes of practice,[61] and he visited Ferrara, Rome, Milan, and Venice probably for the same reason.[62] He may also have visited Pisa and Apulia, since he was familiar with the dialects of those places.[63] Patients for whom his advice was sought included the Florentine nobleman Corso Donati for whom he wrote a regimen;[64] a doge of Venice;[65] a member of the house of Malatesta;[66] and, if Villani is to be trusted, a pope, probably Honorius IV.[67] Perhaps a yet more impressive testimony to his reputation as a practitioner is the fact that he was asked to write a *consilium* for the bishop of Cervia—that is, the celebrated surgeon Theodoric of Lucca.[68] Furthermore, the governments of Perugia and Venice unsuccessfully sought to secure his presence in 1287 and 1293. The Perugians apparently wanted Taddeo first to advise on the suitability of Perugia as a site for a *studium* and subsequently to stay in the city to practice (and perhaps teach). They offered him 100 gold florins just for the consultation, and the extraordinarily lavish salary of 1,000 lire per year. The Venetian proposal was only that he should practice there. Taddeo at first accepted the invitation to Pe-

---

[60] Enzo's will is printed in Celestino Petracchi, *Vita di Arrigo di Svevia, Re di Sardegna volgarmente Enzo chiamato*; the passage about "magistros Thaddeum, Paulum, Bartolum, Peregrinum, Amadeum et Alexium, medicos nostros" occurs on p. 125. I have been unable to secure access to a copy of Lodovico Frati's study of Enzo's imprisonment, published at Bologna in 1902. See below, chapter nine, for Taddeo's *consilia* for patients in cities other than Bologna.

[61] SF 2:221-222.

[62] His will repudiates earlier wills made in those cities; SF 2:230.

[63] Taddeo, *Aphor.*, fol. 181v.

[64] G. Spina and A. Sampalmieri, eds., "La lettera di Taddeo Alderotti a Corso Donati e l'inizio della letteratura igienica medioevale," in XXI *Congresso Internazionale di Storia della Medicina, Siena, 1968*, Atti, 1:91-99. The text is printed at pp. 94-99. See Bibliography for an earlier printing of this work and for the Latin text on which it is based.

[65] Taddeo, *I "Consilia*," p. 129.   [66] Ibid., p. 42.

[67] F. Villani, *Liber de . . . famosis civibus*, p. 27; the identification of Taddeo's patient as Honorius IV is made in Trithemius, *De scriptoribus ecclesiasticis . . . collectanea*, fol. cxr-v, and followed by Gaetano Marini, *Degli archiatri pontifici*, 1:28, and later authors.

[68] Taddeo, *I "Consilia*," p. 67.

rugia, but upon arriving in the city demanded a yet higher salary. At that point the Perugian city council decided to provide him with an honorable escort as far as Siena and to wash their hands of the arrangement.[69]

Although Taddeo's known patients were almost all members of the propertied classes, and although he acquired a notorious reputation for avarice, he also displayed, at any rate at the end of his life, concern for the health of the poor. His will includes large bequests to the infirm, sick, and aged poor, as well as a small legacy for every hospital or hospice (*hospitali*) in Bologna.[70] He was also credited with having left the poor a legacy of another kind, namely the powder known as *"testamentum Thadei"* (a mixture of cinnamon and other ingredients), which is described in a Vatican manuscript as left to the poor by Master Taddeo in his will.[71] The will contains no such recipe, but the assertion presumably testifies to Taddeo's reputation for charity as well as for learning.

As well as a teacher and a practitioner, Taddeo was a fairly copious medical author. His principal theoretical medical writings include commentaries on the *Aphorisms*, *De regimine acutorum*, and *Prognostica* of Hippocrates; the *Tegni* and *De crisi* of Galen; the medical *Isagoge* of Johannitius; and parts of the *Canon* of Avicenna (see Bibliography). He was also the author of two works on *practica* (one of them on fevers), as well as of the *consilia* and vernacular *regimen* alluded to above. A work on complexions attributed to Taddeo in some manuscripts, however, is probably not by him.[72] Furthermore, he was, in all probability, the translator of an Italian version of the *Nicomachean Ethics* (see chapter three). For some sense of the content and significance of this output, the reader is referred to the following chapters; here we will attempt only to place Taddeo's writings in the context of his life.

The evidence for the dating and sequence of Taddeo's works comes

---

[69] Münster, "Taddeo degli Alderotti," pp. 48-59; L. Tarulli, "Documenti per la storia della medicina in Perugia," *Bollettino della Deputazione di Storia Patria per l'Umbria* 25 (1922):194-195; Pietro Pizzoni, "I medici umbri lettori presso l'Università di Perugia," ibid. 47 (1950):10; and the documents cited in note 60 to chapter one, above. The terms of employment offered to Taddeo by Venice are discussed in Carlo M. Cipolla, *Public Health and the Medical Profession in the Renaissance*, p. 90

[70] SF 2:224-225.

[71] BAV, MS Vat. lat. 4425, medical miscellany, 14-15c, fol. 182v, in marg.

[72] Lynn Thorndike, "*De complexionibus*," *Isis* 49 (1958):397-408; and TK 240. To the manuscripts there listed may be added Aberystwyth, National Library of Wales, MS 2050 B (15c), fols. 126-135v, to which my attention was drawn by Professor P. O. Kristeller.

from statements made by the author himself. From these we learn that the commentary on the *Aphorisms* was begun in the ninth year of his teaching, its composition being several times interrupted before its completion in 1283 by work on other texts, by civil war, and by the exigencies of practice. Soon after beginning the work on the *Aphorisms*, Taddeo turned aside to complete the glosses on the *Tegni*, which he had begun at an earlier date.[73] His commentary on the *Isagoge* of Johannitius was also finished before the commentary on the *Aphorisms*.[74] The exposition of the *Isagoge* was probably written, at least in part, after 1277, since in it Taddeo mentions ecclesiastical censure of the doctrine of monopsychism, an apparent allusion to events at Paris in that year. The last of Taddeo's major works was probably the unfinished commentary on *De regimine acutorum*, which he described as a work of his old age and wrote in collaboration, apparently with Bartolomeo da Varignana. In its preface he stated that he had already produced commentaries on the *Isagoge*, the *Tegni*, the *Prognostica*, and the *Aphorisms*.[75] If the "Bartolomeus veronensis" whose assistance is acknowledged in the preface of Taddeo's commentary on *De regimine acutorum* is correctly identified as Bartolomeo da Varignana, the work was probably written before 1286; in that year, as we shall see, Taddeo and Bartolomeo were already on bad terms.

The main interest of the sequence thus suggested, which places Taddeo's principal activity as a medical author in the late 1270s and the 1280s, is that it shows that the commentary on the *Isagoge*, by far the most "Aristotelian" and "philosophical" of his works, is also among the earliest. Since the Italian version of the *Ethics* is probably also an early work, one may conclude that his interest in Aristotelian natural and moral philosophy was a product of his own early studies in arts, and that it perhaps ceased to be a major concern in his later years. It is worth noting in this connection that, in the eyes of Dante or his copyists and of Filippo Villani, Taddeo's reputation was primarily due to his achievements as a commentator on Hippocrates.[76]

The Hippocratic commentaries that won Taddeo his fame are all un-

[73] Taddeo, *Aphor.*, fol. 194v.　　　　[74] Ibid., fol. 1v.
[75] Taddeo, *Reg. acut.* fol. 247r; see also note 5 to this chapter.
[76] The translator of the *Ethics* is identified in *Convivio* 1.10 by the phrase "ciò fu Taddeo Ippocratista," which, although occurring in the manuscripts, may be a copyist's gloss. F. Villani called Taddeo "quasi alter Ypocras" (*Liber de civitatis*, p. 27).

finished,[77] while that on the *Isagoge* bears signs of haste.[78] This, with *Taddeo's tendency to set projects aside and return to them after a lapse of years,* suggests a career in which theoretical writing was fitted in, sometimes awkwardly, among numerous other occupations. Whatever the pretensions of medicine at the *studium* of Bologna to be the "philosophy of the body" deriving its principles from *scientia naturalis* (see chapter five), its study was not pursued in a cloistered academic calm such as contemporary masters of arts or, elsewhere, theology might have sought.

Such were the career and works of Taddeo Alderotti—all in all, a remarkable example of intellectual, professional, economic, and social self-advancement. Perhaps Filippo Villani was not altogether off the mark when he claimed that Taddeo had done as much for the study of medicine as an academic discipline as had Accursius for law.[79] The personality behind the achievement can be traced only in the dimmest and most faulty outline, however. Presumably Dante had good reason to select Taddeo as a type of worldly ambition, as contrasted to Saint Dominic, who acquired learning from purer motives.[80] Taddeo's account of his own sleepwalking may be thought to suggest a personality subjected to

[77] In the Venice edition of 1527, Taddeo's commentary on the *Aphorisms* breaks off at the end of Book 6; the commentary on the *Prognostica* ends in the middle of Book 3; and the commentary on *De regimine acutorum* also does not complete Book 3. Of the last, Taddeo's sixteenth-century editor remarked "duo tamen me movent ad existimandum Thaddeum ulterius non scripsisse, quorum unum est quia cum multa hac [*sic*] diversa exemplaria percurrerim, ipsam [*sic*] in nullo eorum terminum istum pertransire deprehendi, 2m vero est quia Thaddeus fere omnes suas expositiones incompletas nobis reliquit" (fol. 325r).

[78] "Scio tamen quod de his obscure dixi sed fessus sum et deficit charta," Taddeo, *Isagoge*, fol. 401r.

[79] "Hic quamquam adventitiis spretis lucris, glorie cupidus et honoris, commentandis auctoribus medicine operam concessit; qua in re tante auctoritatis fuisse relatum est, ut que pro glossis ordinariis haberentur, que operosis medicine voluminibus apposite fuere, tante in ea disciplina reputationis, quante in legibus civilibus Accursii," F. Villani, *Liber de civitas*, p. 27.

[80] Non per lo mondo, per cui mo s'affana
di retro ad Ostïense e a Taddeo,
ma per amor del la verace manna
in picciol tempo gran dottor si feo
(*Paradiso* 12.82-84)
The identification of the Taddeo alluded to by Dante with Taddeo Alderotti is vigorously defended in C. Calcaterra, *Alma mater studiorum* (Bologna, 1948), pp. 52-54.

considerable psychological tension.[81] Beyond this, one can say little more
than that Taddeo was conventionally devout, at any rate in his old age,
when he made his will. We may note that he maintained a lifelong
attachment to his native Florence, despite all that Bologna had to offer
him; he chose his wife from a Florentine family, owned property there
at his death, wrote a vernacular regimen for the Florentine notable Corso
Donati, and visited the city of his birth long after he was permanently
settled in Bologna.[82] He was trusted and respected by his colleagues and
more than once chosen as a guarantor or arbitrator of their disputes and
agreements.[83] It is also evident that, at least in his last years, he was
manipulative and suspicious, as his numerous wills and the secrecy of his
final will making suggest.[84] He was also jealous of his prestige, as the
unfortunate quarrel with Bartolomeo da Varignana attests. It is perhaps
a sobering thought for the historian that there are few laymen of the
thirteenth century who were not saints, kings, or nobles of whose lives as
much can be known as of Taddeo Alderotti's; but even in his case, the
materials for more than the briefest and most external biography do not
exist.

GENTILE DA CINGOLI

Gentile da Cingoli is the only one among Taddeo's known pupils who
did not follow a medical career. The studies of Martin Grabmann
brought to light the few ascertainable facts about Gentile's life: he presumably came from Cingoli, a town in the March of Ancona; his father,
Benvenuto, was sufficiently elevated in status to merit the honorific
"dominus"; Gentile himself appears to have studied at Paris around

---

[81] Taddeo, *Isagoge*, fol. 362r. Puccinotti, *Storia della medicina*, vol. 2, pt. 1, p. xxx, and
J. B. Petella "Les consultations oculistiques d'un maître italien du xiiième siècle," *Janus* 6
(1901):63-66, are in error in supposing that the Taddeus de Florentia who sent an emotional letter to the Augustinian evangelist Blessed Simone Fidati of Cascia bewailing the
damage done to the writer's eyesight by staring at an eclipse is to be identified with
Taddeo Alderotti. Simone Fidati died in 1348 after a preaching career lasting twenty-seven
years, which apparently reached its peak in the 1330s; see Nicola Mattioli, *Il beato Simone
Fidati da Cascia*, Antologia Agostiniana (Rome 1898), 2:27, and passim. As noted, Taddeo
died in 1295. The letter of Taddeo of Florence to Blessed Simone is printed by Mattioli,
pp. 436-438, as well as by Puccinotti.

[82] *Chart Bon.*, 9:240-241, document of September 14, 1286.

[83] Ibid.; SF 2:231-232.

[84] SF 2:230. Before making his final will he had made at least six others.

1290; and, from 1295 (or before) until the early part of the fourteenth
century, he was a professor of logic and philosophy in the *studium* of
Bologna.[85] Several pieces of evidence link him to Taddeo and suggest
that Gentile pursued medical studies in Taddeo's school. In 1295 Gentile
named Taddeo as the arbitrator of an agreement (signed in the house
where Taddeo was staying) between himself and Guglielmo da Dessara,
another doctor of logic. In this agreement the two doctors shared the
duties and profits of giving instruction in logic and philosophy: Gentile
promised to give supplementary lectures in philosophy in Guglielmo's
schools for three years and to turn back a quarter of the proceeds to
Guglielmo; Guglielmo promised to give the regular lectures in logic and
to hand over a third of the students' fees to Gentile.[86] Furthermore, as
already noted, the learned physician Gentile da Foligno, writing in the
1340s, placed Gentile da Cingoli among a group of recent authors who
had considered the problem of "the reduction of medicine to act" (that
is, how the powers of medication are released in the body). As already
noted, of the eleven such authors mentioned, all Italian and all, save Gentile da Cingoli, learned physicians, nine have associations with the *studium*
of Bologna, seven of them being Taddeo Alderotti and the other physicians of his school who are the subject of the present volume, along with
a pupil of Guglielmo da Brescia. Given Gentile da Cingoli's known connection with Taddeo, the presence of his name on this list seems to confirm the probability that he was once Taddeo's pupil. Finally, Gentile's
questio "Whether a sensible or intelligible species has the virtue of altering a body toward heat or cold" takes the form of a commentary on a
statement of Galen and shows extensive familiarity with medical writings
and concepts (see chapter seven).

Yet another piece of evidence indirectly suggesting Gentile's medical
interests is his *reportatio* of the *questiones* on Aristotle's *De generatione
animalium* by Johannes Vath, a master of arts at Paris. Aristotle's books
on animals were eagerly sought and studied by physicians; *De generatione animalium* was of particular interest because of the conflict between
Aristotle's views on mammalian conception and the views of Galen. The

[85] Martin Grabmann, "Gentile da Cingoli, ein italienischer Aristoteleserklärer aus der Zeit
Dantes," in *Sitzungsberichte der Bayerischen Akademie der Wissenschaften*, Philosophisch-
historische Abteilung, vol. 9, 1940. All information containing Gentile and his works in
the following paragraphs is drawn from this source, except where otherwise indicated.

[86] The document is printed in SF 2:231-232.

only known copy of Gentile's *reportatio* is found in MS Vat. lat. 4454, a miscellany of medical works, most of them by authors of the early fourteenth-century Bolognese school. Copied in a single hand are Gentile's version of Vath's *questiones*, two commentaries by Bartolomeo da Varignana on works by or attributed to Galen, and an anonymous commentary on the four Galenic tracts on diseases that in the Middle Ages collectively went under the title *De accidenti et morbo*.

Apart from the *questio* on sensible and intelligible species just noted, all of Gentile's own surviving writings are commentaries on books on logic. Since several of them were reported by Guglielmo da Varignana, son of Bartolomeo, the commentaries presumably reflect Gentile's teaching in the schools of Bologna in the early fourteenth century. The works commented on by Gentile included the *Categories* and *Prior Analytics* of Aristotle, the *Isagoge* of Porphyry, and the *Tractatus de modis significandi* of the thirteenth-century teacher Martinus of Dacia.

Gentile's academic career can therefore tentatively be reconstructed as follows. Possibly after some early studies at Bologna, Gentile proceeded to Paris, where he studied logic (with Martinus of Dacia?) and philosophy with Johannes Vath. Conceivably Taddeo—whose commentary on the medical *Isagoge* of Johannitius (completed before 1283) is by far the most "philosophical" of his medical works and shows apparent knowledge of and interest in recent trends at Paris, and who was teaching logic in the 1280s—inspired Gentile to go north for more advanced and specialized instruction in logic and philosophy than Bologna could offer. Alternatively, if Gentile's studies at Paris took place anything up to a decade earlier than 1290 (Johannes Vath was rector of the University of Paris in that year, but may well have begun teaching considerably earlier),[87] Gentile himself may have been the source of some of Taddeo's up-to-date philosophical learning. In either case, it seems likely that, upon returning to Bologna, Gentile studied medicine under Taddeo while simultaneously teaching logic and philosophy. Unlike his fellow students, he remained in the faculty of arts and may never have completed his medical studies.

Gentile's pupils in the school of arts included Master Angelo d'Arezzo (fl. 1325), an important early member of a group of Averroist (in the sense of defending the unicity and eternity of the intellect) philosophers

---

[87] Grabmann, "Gentile da Cingoli," p. 14.

who flourished at Bologna between the 1320s and the 1340s.[88] Much
scholarly discussion has centered on the origins of the ideas held by this
group. The most recent investigations have tended to stress the overriding
importance of Parisian influences, while according a lesser but nonetheless real significance to the interest in monopsychism expressed by Taddeo Alderotti and to the general tradition of medically (rather than
theologically) oriented philosophical teaching at Bologna.[89] Gentile da
Cingoli, who was characterized by Gentile da Foligno as an Averroist
in his view of the action of medicines,[90] certainly provides a link between
Taddeo's school and the later flowering of Bolognese Averroism. As far
as the content of his teaching is concerned, Gentile was only one—and
not necessarily a particularly important one—of a number of sources of
influence on Bolognese philosophers of the next generation. Yet he
plainly played a major role in building up the school of philosophy in
the *studium* of Bologna as a faculty of significance in its own right, and
not a mere adjunct to the faculty of medicine. Reciprocally, the professors
of philosophy retained a tradition of medical learning; thus, Angelo
d'Arezzo, Taddeo da Parma, and Jacopo da Piacenza, three of the leading members of the Bolognese Averroist school, all disputed *questiones*
on medical subjects,[91] although their major works concern philosophy.

Since this study is concerned primarily with the learning of physicians,
Gentile da Cingoli plays but a small part herein. Only his work on a
medical topic will receive further consideration below.

BARTOLOMEO DA VARIGNANA

Bartolomeo da Varignana is the only member of the group of Taddeo's
students or associates under consideration here whose family can be

[88] An account of this group and an analysis of their thought is provided in Kuksewicz,
De Siger de Brabant à Jacques de Plaisance, pp. 315-452; see further bibliography there
cited.

[89] Ibid., p. 317.

[90] "2ª opinio est Gentilis de Cingulo quam dicit esse Averrois in 5° colliget," Gentile
da Foligno, *Questiones et tractatus extravagantes*, fol. 63r.

[91] See Angelus de Aretio (Angelo d'Arezzo), "Utrum complexio in humano corpore et
sanitas sint due forme . . . ," Paris University, Bibliothèque de la Sorbonne, MS 128, fol.
123 (TK 1634); Thadeus de Palma (Taddeo da Parma), "Utrum mala complexio diversa
est que febris . . . ," fols. 109-111 (TK 1655); Jacobus de Placentio (Jacopo da Piacenza),
"Utrum post medicinam competat balneum . . . ," BAV, MS Vat. lat. 2418, fols. 180v-182r
(TK 1663).

shown to be of Bolognese origin. His family came from Varignana, a
small town in the Bolognese *contado*, and his father, Giovanni, was practicing medicine in Bologna in the mid-thirteenth century. Bartolomeo, a
married layman like his father, was in turn the father of three sons, one
of whom, Guglielmo, was the author of a medical *practica*. The family
continued to provide professors of medicine for the schools of Bologna
until the fifteenth century.[92] The date of Bartolomeo's birth is unknown,
but it was probably around 1260.

Bartolomeo had already become the owner of a respectable collection
of up-to-date scientific and philosophical books in 1286, when he accused
one of Taddeo's scholars of stealing parts of his library and other val-
uables.[93] The stolen books were: copies of Aristotle's *Metaphysics*, *De
anima*, and works on animals in the new translation (probably that of
William of Moerbeke made during the 1260s); a copy of Albertus Magnus' commentary on *De generatione et corruptione*; and a copy of Taddeo's own commentary on the *Aphorisms* of Hippocrates, completed only
in 1283. It may be assumed that Bartolomeo's personal association with
Taddeo was already established when the theft occurred, although
whether Bartolomeo was at the time a master or merely an advanced
(and wealthy) student is unclear. The fact that the works named are
mostly on natural philosophy may indicate that Bartolomeo was at a
stage of his career when he was teaching arts, but had not yet completed
his medical studies. He was certainly teaching medicine by 1292, the year
in which Taddeo complained to the archdeacon's vicar and the *collegio
magistrorum* that he was luring away his (Taddeo's) students. (As a
result, Bartolomeo was obliged to submit to penalties imposed by the
vicar and the college.)[94] After his old rival's death in 1295, Bartolomeo's
position was no doubt easier; by 1298, when he was one of a group of

[92] SF 1:568-572. The accounts of Sarti and Fattorini and Ladislao Münster, "Alcuni
episodi sconosciuti o poco noti sulla vita e sull'attività di Bartolomeo da Varignana,"
Castalia: Rivista di storia della medicina 10 (1954):207-215, assemble most of the available
documents and bibliography concerning Bartolomeo. Accounts of him are also in G. G.
Forni, *L'insegnamento della chirurgia nello studio di Bologna*, pp. 26-31; Sarton, *Introduction to the History of Science*, vol. 3, pt. 1, p. 841; and Fantuzzi, *Notizie degli scrittori
bolognese*, 8:152-155. The *practica* of Guglielmo da Varignana was printed at Lyons in
1533 and in other early editions.

[93] Zaccagnini, *La vita dei maestri*, pp. 36-37, citing Ottavio Mazzoni-Toselli, *Raconti
storici dall'Archivio Criminale di Bologna* (Bologna, 1870), 3:13, where, however, only an
Italian summary of the document is printed.

[94] SF 2:223.

professors of medicine who swore obedience to the archdeacon, he was presumably securely established as a senior member of the faculty.[95]

Bartolomeo's professorial career at Bologna apparently lasted until 1311, when he left the city for political reasons. There seems to be no indication that he held a teaching position after that date, although the city of Perugia tried to secure his services as a professor as late as 1321.[96] His principal theoretical works, which presumably reflect his classroom teaching, consist of commentaries on the *Aphorisms* of Hippocrates and on the *Tegni, De complexionibus, De interioribus,* and *De accidenti et morbo* by Galen; *rationes* on portions of the *Canon* of Avicenna; a commentary on the pseudo-Aristotelian *Economics*; and, possibly, a work on astrology.[97] As noted above, he appears to have assisted Taddeo in the compilation of the latter's last work, namely the unfinished commentary on Hippocrates, *De regimine acutorum.* Nonetheless, there were intellectual as well as other differences between the two men, and Bartolomeo was on occasion sharply critical of Taddeo's views (see chapter five).

Like Taddeo, Bartolomeo had a lucrative practice among an aristocratic clientele.[98] Particularly striking, however, is the extent of his professional and political involvement in the affairs of the city of Bologna. Whereas Taddeo, although salaried by the municipality, was specifically excused from practice on its behalf, Bartolomeo performed examinations and autopsies and in the years 1302-1310 produced a number of medico-legal reports for the civic authorities.[99] Moreover, he was a prominent

---

[95] See note 63 to chapter one, above. [96] Münster, "Alcuni episodi," p. 215.

[97] For manuscripts, see Bibliography; the only printing of any of Bartolomeo's works is a short excerpt from his commentary on *De complexionibus* edited by Puccinotti (*Storia della medicina,* vol. 2, pt. 1, pp. CXIII-CXXIX). Regarding the attribution of an astrological work to Bartolomeo, see SF 1:585. But see also note 60 to chapter five. The explicit of a *practica* occupying fols. 1r-172r of Naples, Biblioteca Nazionale, MS VIII D 68, attributes the work to Bartolomeus de Varignana (I am grateful to Professor Charles Henderson of Smith College for supplying me with a description of this manuscript, which I have not seen), but this may be the *Practica* of the earlier Bartholomaeus of Salerno.

[98] His patients included marchese Aldobrandino d'Este, whom he treated in 1293 for a fee of 390 lire Bolognese; see SF 1:569.

[99] Münster, "Alcuni episodi," pp. 208-214, where several of the reports are printed, and bibliography there cited. The autopsies performed or supervised by Bartolomeo are among the earliest recorded in the medieval West. The use of physicians and surgeons on the city payroll as expert witnesses in cases of assault or suspected homicide goes back to the mid-thirteenth century in Bologna and was systematized and regulated in 1288; see L. Münster, "La medicina legale in Bologna dai suoi albori fino alla fine del secolo XIV," *Bollettino dell'Accademia Medica Pistoiese Filippo Pacini* 26 (1955):258.

member of the White Guelf faction and in 1303, after the government
had fallen into the hands of that party, secured the important position of
prior of the *anziani* (supreme council) of the city.[100] Despite the fall
from power of the White Guelfs in 1306, Bartolomeo continued to serve
the commune in a medico-legal capacity until November 1310.[101] By
April 1311, however, he had joined the entourage of his best-known patient, namely the emperor Henry VII, and as a result he earned a sentence of banishment from Bologna in October of the same year.[102] Bartolomeo became a trusted number of the emperor's household, where his
responsibilities were more than merely medical. One of the tasks with
which he was charged was to deliver the iron crown of Lombardy, used
in Henry's Milanese coronation, to the monastery of Saint Ambrose in
Milan, where it was to be held in safekeeping.[103] When Henry died suddenly in 1313, Bartolomeo defended the emperor's Dominican confessor
from the charge of murdering him with a poisoned host. According to
his physician, Henry had ignored medical advice—perhaps that contained
in Bartolomeo's *consilium* for the emperor, which is still preserved in a
Munich manuscript—and had consequently died of natural causes.[104]
After the death of Henry VII, Bartolomeo seems to have spent much of
the remainder of his life at Genoa. He died sometime after 1321.[105]

Quite plainly, Bartolomeo da Varignana stands somewhat apart from
the rest of the associates of Taddeo Alderotti. Although there seems to
be little doubt that he was for a time Taddeo's student and *socius*, Bartolomeo sprang from a family that represented a Bolognese medical tradition antedating Taddeo's arrival in the city. Well before Taddeo's death,
and early in his own career, he established himself as an independent

[100] SF 1:570.

[101] Vitale, *Il dominio della Parte Guelfa*, pp. 88-92; Münster, "Alcuni episodi," p. 214.

[102] SF 1:570; and, for the month, note next following.

[103] *Monumenta Germaniae Historiae, Legum* sectio IV, *Constitutiones et acta publica
imperatorum et regum*, vol. 4, pt. 1, no. 609, document of April, 1311; also cited in
Gina Fasoli, "Bologna e la Romagna durante la spedizione di Enrico VII," *Atti e memorie
della Deputazione di storia patria per l'Emilia e la Romagna* 4 (1938-1939):29.

[104] Bartholomeus de Vagana [*sic*], ad postulationem imperatoris Henrici, inc. "Lavate
post cibum extremitates corporis . . . ," Munich, Bayerische Staatsbibliothek, CLM 23912,
a. 1394, fols. 253r-254v (TK 814); SF 1:571.

[105] Münster, "Alcuni episodi," pp. 214-215. Münster demonstrates that the death
date of 1318 or 1319 usually given for Bartolomeo in the secondary literature is incorrect;
he also documents attempts to secure his services as a practitioner by the governments of
Florence and Venice, and as a teacher by the government of Perugia, during his last years.

master. Conceivably, the intellectual differences and professional rivalry that developed between the two men may have reflected, in part, the jealousy of native Bolognese physicians of a Florentine invasion in the teaching of arts and medicine. The subsequent restriction of senior professorial positions and membership in the College of Doctors of Arts and Medicine to Bolognese citizens by birth makes such an hypothesis plausible.[106] It is also possible that political differences may have divided Taddeo and Bartolomeo; the former probably received his privileges from the municipality during the popular regime of the 1280s; whereas the latter was associated with the White Guelf faction, usually considered as representing aristocratic or magnate interests.

GUGLIELMC DE' CORVI DA BRESCIA (GUILLELMUS BRIXIENSIS)

The family of Guglielmo da Brescia originated in Canneto, a town in the *contado* of Brescia.[107] His father, Giacomo de' Corvi, who may have been a merchant, came to Brescia about the middle of the thirteenth century, and it was probably there that Guglielmo was born in 1250.[108] Nothing is known of his early education, which was presumably acquired at Brescia, but by 1274 he was already teaching logic and philosophy at the *studium* of Padua. Among his students was Engelbert, subsequently Abbot of Admont, who some fifty years later still recalled his master's teaching with admiration. (It is perhaps worth noting in passing that master and student were exact contemporaries.)[109] In 1279 or 1280, according to Engelbert, Guglielmo left Padua to study under Taddeo at

106 Malagola, *Statuti*, p. 426 (doctoral college statutes of 1378).

107 Paolo Guerrini, "Guglielmo da Brescia e il Collegio Bresciano in Bologna," *Studi e memorie per la storia dell'Università di Bologna* 7 (1922):60. Most of the available information about Guglielmo is collected in Guerrini's article and in Ernest Wickersheimer, "Guillaume de Brescia," in his *Dictionnaire biographique des médecins en France au moyen âge*, 1:230, and Danielle Jacquart's *Supplément* thereto, p. 101; see also Marini, *Archiatri pontifici*, 1:34-41.

108 Guerrini, "Guglielmo da Brescia," pp. 61, 70.

109 "Et cum celebrato Concilio praedicto [of Lyon, 1274] rumor . . . venisset . . . transtuli me circa Paduam . . . continuavi studium ibidem in Logica et Philosophia quinque annos sub Magistro Wilhelmo de Brixia tunc acto ad salarium legente ibidem, viro magnae reputationis . . . postquam a Padua recedens conventum suscepit in medicinis Bononiae sub Magistro Tatheo Medico praecipuo tunc ibidem," Engelbert, letter to Master Ulrich, in Pez, *Thesaurus*, vol. 1, pt. 1, col. 430. On Engelbert, see Fowler, *Intellectual Interests of Engelbert of Admont* (New York, 1947).

Bologna, where he acquired his medical degree.[110] He was described as
magister in physica (i.e., medicine) at Bologna in 1286.[111] Among his
pupils was, as already noted, Pancius of Lucca, personal physician to the
surgeon Theodoric.[112] To the end of his life Guglielmo looked back on
his years in Bologna with affection, but he could not have taught there
for much more than a decade.[113] Before 1298 he had become the personal
physician of Pope Boniface VIII; he subsequently served Clement V and
John XXII in the same capacity and as a chaplain; and he seems to have
spent most of the rest of his life at the papal court and in Paris, where he
died in 1326.[114]

Guglielmo's clerical status sets him apart from all but one of the other
members of the group under consideration. Although only in minor
orders (he was a subdeacon in 1314), after 1300 he accumulated an impressive array of important and lucrative benefices. He was a canon and
held prebends of the cathedrals of Brescia, Lincoln, Paris, and Constance,
and he was archdeacon of Bautois in the diocese of Constance.[115] He held
all these benefices in plurality and in absentia as recompense for his activities at the papal court as both physician and chaplain. His final prefer-
ment, in 1313, was to the archdeaconry of Bologna. The archdeacon of
Bologna was, the reader will recall, charged either in person or by his
vicar with the supervision of the *studium* and was the nominal source
of its medical and other degrees. The promotion of Guglielmo da Brescia
to this position, which he also held in absentia along with his other
benefices, was an appropriate recognition of his professional accomplishments and his early affiliation with the Bolognese academic community.

[110] The efforts of Guerrini ("Guglielmo da Brescia," p. 63) to interpret Engelbert's
words as meaning that Guglielmo was already associated with Taddeo and learned in
medicine before coming to Padua appear unconvincing.

[111] SF 1:434.

[112] Gentile da Foligno, *Questiones et tractatus extravagantes*, fol. 63r: "3ª opinio est
Guilelmi de Brixia quam sequitur Pancius de Lucha."

[113] "desiderans in civitate bononie que mihi est et fuit retroactis temporibus omni possessione precara doctrinae studium perpetuis temporibus . . . prepoleat," Guglielmo, foundation statute of the Collegio Bresciana, in Guerrini, "Guglielmo da Brescia," p. 89.

[114] Ibid., pp. 65-68; Wickersheimer, *Dictionnaire*, 1:230, and documents there cited;
P. Pansier, "Les médecins des papes d'Avignon (1308-1403)," *Janus* 14 (1909):405, 417-
418. Pansier points out (p. 407) the difference between physicians in regular attendance
on the popes, such as Guglielmo, and those called in for occasional consultation. In the
latter category appears to have been included Dino del Garbo (p. 405), as well as Taddeo
himself.

[115] For Guglielmo's preferments, see Wickersheimer, *Dictionnaire*, 1:230.

No doubt as a result of the brevity of his teaching career, Guglielmo was not a copious medical author. The best-known work ascribed to him is a *practica* designed to indicate treatment "for every kind of disease from the head to the foot." It is an encyclopedic collection of descriptions of particular ailments with suggested remedies for each, culled from some of the standard Greek and Arabic medical authorities, and combining topical and dictionary arrangement. The work is introduced by a learned, theoretically oriented preface that incorporates numerous citations of the *libri naturales* of Aristotle and of the philosophical writings of Avicenna and Averroes. The only known surviving manuscript of this *practica* dates from the fifteenth century and is anonymous and perhaps incomplete; the attribution of the work to Guglielmo by a sixteenth-century editor may, however, reflect a valid tradition. Guglielmo was more certainly the author of a brief *practica* on surgery, of scholastic *questiones* on the supposedly universal remedy theriac, of *questiones* on the *Aphorisms* of Hippocrates and on a portion of the *Canon* of Avicenna, and of a number of *consilia* offering medical advice to individuals. He may also have written a short tract on memory and a work on fevers, although a treatise on pestilence included in his printed *Opera* (1508) was in reality the work of Pietro da Tussignano and was written after 1387.[116]

Although Guglielmo's own participation in academic life was cut short by his involvement in the affairs of the papal court, his interest in schools and learning remained. Indeed, there are grounds for regarding him as a major channel for the transmission of influences between the *studia* of Paris, Bologna, and Montpellier. For example, he may have been instrumental in transmitting Italian notions regarding the nature of surgery and surgical education to the schools of the north, since two manuscripts of the *Chirurgia* of Henri de Mondeville state that he inspired that work.[117] Henri de Mondeville (d. ca. 1320), of Norman origin, was surgeon to Philip IV and Louis X of France. In the *Chirurgia*, appar-

[116] For manuscripts and editions of Guglielmo's works, see Bibliography. I have not seen the manuscript of his *Practica* (TK 364). Regarding the pest tract attributed to him, see Karl Sudhoff, "Pestschriften aus den ersten 150 Jahren nach der Epidemie des 'schwarzen Todes' 1348," *Archiv für Geschichte der Medizin* 16 (1924-1925):112-114; 17 (1925):243. Wickersheimer doubts the attribution of the tract on fevers to Guglielmo (*Dictionnaire*, 1:230). Regarding the possibility that Guglielmo wrote on memory, see Guerrini, "Guglielmo da Brescia," p. 74.

[117] E. Nicaise, trans., *Chirurgie de Maître Henri de Mondeville* (Paris, 1893), intro., p. xxv. One manuscript, however, says that the work was written at the suggestion of the Montpellier master Bernard of Gordon. The two possibilities are not mutually exclusive.

ently his only work, Henri insisted upon the desirability of literacy and
medical learning for surgeons, and he also claimed to have lectured on
surgery at Paris and on surgery and medicine in the schools of Montpellier. Of his own education he said only that he had studied and practiced
surgery at Paris and Montpellier and that his master had been Jean
Pitard, another royal surgeon.[118] Henri was certainly at Montpellier in
1304, although Wickersheimer doubts that he taught in the faculty of
medicine.[119] Henri de Mondeville was also familiar with the works of
the principal Italian writers on surgery of the thirteenth century, namely
Lanfranco and Theodoric, although there is absolutely no evidence to
suggest that he ever went to Italy and studied with the latter, as is frequently asserted.[120] Such claims are based upon Henri's own references
to these writers as "our masters," but since in the passage in question
they are grouped with Avicenna, it is plain that the allusion is to the
study of their written works.[121] It is possible that Henri de Mondeville
acquired from Guglielmo some of his knowledge of Italian surgical
books and his desire to introduce into surgical education something of
the literacy and learning on which academically trained physicians prided
themselves.[122] Incidentally, the statement sometimes found in the secondary literature—that Henri de Mondeville was himself among Taddeo's
pupils—is an example of the way in which historical legends develop.[123]
Henri's reference to Theodoric led to the mistaken supposition that he
had studied at Bologna; and *if* he studied at Bologna he "must have"
encountered Taddeo. There seems to be no other basis for the assertion.

Guglielmo da Brescia also appears to have exercised some influence
upon the shape of the medical curriculum at the *studium* of Montpellier.
He was one of three experts—the others being Johannes de Alestio and
Arnald of Villanova—called upon in 1309 by Pope Clement V to assist
in drawing up or approving regulations concerning the granting of degrees in medicine.[124]

[118] Julius L. Pagel, ed., *Die Chirurgie des Heinrich von Mondeville* (Berlin, 1892), p. 11.

[119] Nicaise, *Chirurgie*, intro., p. xxv; Wickersheimer, *Dictionnaire*, 1:282.

[120] Ibid, 1:283.   [121] Pagel, ed., *Die Chirurgie*, p. 11.

[122] It may be noted, however, that Henri's colleagues as royal surgeons included two
Italians, namely Jacobus of Siena and Giovanni of Padua (Nicaise, *Chirurgie*, intro.,
p. xxiv), who no doubt also brought him into touch with Italian trends.

[123] See, for example, Charles Singer, *The Evolution of Anatomy*, p. 72.

[124] See *Cartulaire de l'Université de Montpellier*, vol. 1, pp. 219-221, no. 25. Regarding
the medical faculty at Montpellier, see the forthcoming study by Luke Demaitre, *Doctor*

Guglielmo's undisputed writings and what is known of his career after he left Bologna suggest a concentration upon medical practice and professional training which, one might suppose, would leave little room for broader learning. Yet on the one occasion when Guglielmo directly involved himself in academic affairs during the latter part of his career, he manifested a special concern for liberal arts and philosophy, as will become evident from what follows. Perhaps his residence in Paris during his last years reawakened broader interests, dormant since his youthful teaching experience at Padua and his exposure to the circle of Taddeo Alderotti at Bologna.

In his will, made in Paris in 1326, Guglielmo provided for the foundation at Bologna of a college for poor scholars, possibly the first such house to be set up at Bologna; it seems likely that he had in mind the example of several similar colleges already established at Paris. Guglielmo died a wealthy man, with much of his property in real estate and other investments at Brescia, Bologna, and elsewhere. His college was generously endowed from the proceeds of moneys owed him by creditors—including the bishop of Bologna—in and near Bologna. The foundation statute of the *domus scholarium magistri Guillelmi de brixia archidiaconi bononsiensis*, as Guglielmo wished his college to be called, provides that a house be specially constructed to accommodate fifty poor scholars. In the meantime, immediate provision was made for the needs of eight poor scholars from Brescia who were to live in common. Various regulations were intended to ensure that the scholars should be serious students in genuine need of financial assistance. Guglielmo further specified that two of the eight should be students of canon law, two of medicine, and four of liberal arts, to be studied along with natural and moral philosophy. His interest in fostering the study of the arts, sciences, and philosophy is further demonstrated by the provision that one of the eight should be a master or a suitably qualified bachelor of arts and that he should lecture to his fellows on metaphysics and natural and moral philosophy. Thus Guglielmo stood at the very beginning of an important new trend in higher education that was to become widespread in the later Middle Ages at various university centers and to become predominant in some of them (most notably Oxford and Cambridge)—namely, the provision not only

Bernard Gordon, Professor and Practitioner (Pontifical Institute of Mediaeval Studies, Toronto), and the various articles by Michael R. McVaugh listed in the Bibliography.

of housing and moral supervision, but also of instruction within the setting of a residential college. Guglielmo also willed his books to his college, unfortunately without listing them; we may suppose that they would have been chiefly medical, but might also have included some titles pertaining to arts and philosophy.[125]

According to Francesco Malvezzi, who annotated the manuscript of the foundation statute of Guglielmo's college in 1431, Master Guglielmo showed more concern for students of the arts, especially of natural and moral philosophy, than for those of medicine or law, because he thought the former disciplines both nobler and ultimately of greater social and spiritual usefulness than a strictly professional education; medicine in particular he held to be of little use for civil life and positively damaging to the soul if pursued with too much ardor.[126] Although in the extreme form in which it is stated this opinion is no doubt Francesco's own rather than Guglielmo's, it is nonetheless probably true that Guglielmo's statutes contain an implied criticism of the attitudes and priorities of the lawyers and physicians of Bologna and of what Guglielmo perceived as an excessively vocational emphasis in the *studium*. But his conviction of the desirability of liberal and philosophical learning (even though he himself set this ideal aside for much of his busy professional career) in no way represents a rejection of medical science as such; on the contrary, it is fully congruous with the values implanted by Guglielmo's early medical training under Taddeo.

[125] The foundation statute of the college and Guglielmo's will are printed in Guerrini, "Guglielmo da Brescia," pp. 90-106; the College of Avignon, founded at Bologna in 1267, has priority in time over Guglielmo's College, but may only have provided pensions without communal living arrangements for its members (see Rashdall, *Universities*, 1:198). Guglielmo's foundation was relatively short-lived as an independent institution, being amalgamated, along with several other small colleges, in 1436-1437 with the Collegio Gregoriano founded at Bologna by Pope Gregory XI in 1371; see Berthe M. Marti, ed. and trans., *The Spanish College at Bologna in the Fourteenth Century: Edition and Translation of Its Statutes with Introduction and Notes* (Philadelphia, 1966), p. 18. Regarding colleges at Paris, see Rashdall, *Universities*, 1:498-517.

[126] "Nota hic in statuto quod magister G. plus curavit de scolaribus debentibus studere in artibus et maxime in physica [*sic* Guerrini;? philosophia (phyā)] naturali et morali quam de medicis et iuristis et causa esse quod maiorem utilitatem consideravit id sequi, et quod nobilior est illa scientia et cum maiori profectione et meliori dispositione, quod minime a civili medicina tetigisset, et quod consideravit quantum potuit quod in usu illius quam plurima delicta maxima contra committuntur, et per illam scientiam, si large sciatur, minime [*sic*] beneficium percipi animam quam per alias scientias," Guerrini, "Guglielmo da Brescia," p. 96. On Francesco Malvezzi and his annotations, see idem, "Guglielmo da Brescia," pp. 77-88.

DINO DEL GARBO (DINUS DE FLORENTIA)

The little that is authentically known of the family and background of Dino del Garbo can soon be told. His father, Bono del Garbo of Florence, was a well-known surgeon and the founder of a dynasty of physicians and surgeons that flourished in that city until the eighteenth century.[127] The two most celebrated members of the family were Dino himself and his son Tommaso.[128] There appears to be no contemporary evidence to support the frequently repeated assertion that Dino del Garbo and Taddeo Alderotti were related or that, as most versions of the tradition imply, Bono del Garbo was Taddeo's brother-in-law.[129] It is quite probable that the two families were acquainted in Florence, and it may well be that the master Bono or Giovanni Bono referred to in Taddeo's commentary on Johannitius[130] is to be identified with Dino's father, but this is not evidence of kinship. Moreover, there is some negative evidence that seems to weigh against the tradition, namely, that no such relationship is mentioned either by Filippo Villani in his biographies of Taddeo and Dino or, more significantly, by Taddeo in his will. Taddeo showed a strong sense of family obligation in his will (as when, for example, he bound his nephew Opizus to take care of the latter's mother and sister); it seems inconceivable that if he had a young relative who, at about the

---

[127] A. Corsini, "Nuovo contributo di notizie intorno alla vita di maestro Tommaso del Garbo," *Rivista di storia delle scienze mediche e naturali* 16 (1925):268-278, contains much of the available information about the family and refutes the identification sometimes made of Dino's father with the surgical author Bruno da Longoburgo of Calabria. One of the most detailed biographical accounts of Dino, although containing some errors, is still that in Tiraboschi, *Storia della letteratura Italiana*, 5:245-249; see also Wickersheimer, *Dictionnaire*, 1:119-120, with Danielle Jacquart's *Supplément* thereto, pp. 60-61; Sarton, *Introduction to the History of Science*, vol. 3, pt. 1, 837-838; and Giulio Negri, *Istoria degli scrittori fiorentini*, pp. 146-147.

[128] Regarding Tommaso, see Corsini, "Nuovo contributo," passim; and I. Cappellini, "Date importanti per la biografia di Maestro Tommaso del Garbo e per gli inizi dell'insegnamento medico nello Studio Fiorentino desunte da codici del Fondo Vaticano Latino," *Rivista di storia delle scienze mediche e naturali* 41 (1950):212-218: M. A. Mannelli, "Tommaso del Garbo ed Ugo Benzi da Siena lettori di medicina nello studium generale di Firenze," *Rivista di storia della medicina* 8 (1964):183-190; and Francesco Guido, "Cenni biografici su Dino e Tommaso del Garbo," in xxi *Congresso Internazionale di Storia della Medicina, Siena, 1968, Atti*, 1:156-163; and Sarton, *Introduction to the History of Science*, vol. 3, pt. 2, pp. 1672-1674. Tommaso was the author of a *Summa medicinalis* and was prominent as a teaching physician in both Bologna and Florence.

[129] See e.g. Puccinotti, *Storia della medicina*, vol. 2, pt. 2, pp. 358-359; and *Biographisches Lexikon der hervorragenden Ärzte aller Zeiten und Völker*, 2:682.

[130] Taddeo, *Isagoge*, fol. 390r.

time the will was made, was following in Taddeo's own footsteps by embarking on a medical career, he would not have included him among the legatees.

Although Dino's period of study under Taddeo may not have been of very long duration, the careers and interests of the two men ran nearly parallel. Indeed, Dino seems to have had more in common with his master than had any of the other physicians discussed in this chapter. Dino and Taddeo shared not only Florentine origin, prolific authorship, a pronounced leaning toward philosophy, and a lifetime of medical teaching and practice in the north Italian cities, but also, as we shall see, an interest in Tuscan vernacular literature. Moreover, it appears that only Dino of Taddeo's known students came near to achieving a reputation equal to Taddeo's own among his contemporaries and immediate posterity. Such a statement must be made with caution, since it is necessary to make allowances for the Florentine patriotism of Dino's earliest and most enthusiastic boosters, namely Giovanni and Filippo Villani. Nonetheless, their assertions must bear some relation to contemporary opinion. According to Giovanni, Dino was "the very greatest of doctors in medicine (*fisica*) and especially in natural science and philosophy who in his time was the best and sovereign physician (*medico*) in Italy"; Filippo termed him the most notable of physicians after Taddeo.[131]

Dino's birthdate is unknown. As a young man he went to Bologna to pursue his education, but was forced by civil disturbances to return home to Florence after only one year of medical study.[132] It has variously been conjectured that the disturbances in question were the internal factional struggles of the 1270s or Bologna's war against Azzo d'Este, ruler of Ferrara, in 1296-1299.[133] The later dating is more likely, since Dino's professional career did not begin until after 1300. But if so, and if the

---

[131] "grandissimo dottore in fisica et in più scienze naurali e filosofiche, il quale al suo tempo fu il migliore e sovrano medico che fosse in Italia," G. Villani, *Cronica* 10.41; "Dinus de Garbo Taddei auditor, post eum medicus fuit insignis," F. Villani, *Liber de . . . famosis civibus*, p. 28.

[132] Tiraboschi, *Storia della letteratura italiana*, vol. 5, pt. 1, pp. 246-247.

[133] The chronology of Dino's education is vigorously argued in Bruno Nardi, "Noterella polemica sull'averroismo di Guido Cavalcanti," *Rassegna di filosofia* 3 (1954):55; and Guido Favati, "Guido Cavalcanti, Dino del Garbo, e l'Averroismo di Bruno Nardi," *Filologia romanza* 2 (1955):80-81, Nardi supporting the earlier and Favati the later dating. However, these authors were engaged in controversy over the origins of the supposed Averroism of Cavalcanti or of his commentator Dino, and each was using the dating to make a polemical point.

only time Dino spent at Bologna before 1296 was a single year of medical study, the period when he was, in Filippo Villani's words, the *"auditor"* of Taddeo must have been very short, since Taddeo died in June 1295 and was probably not teaching much during the last part of his life. Perhaps, however, the year of medical study followed several years of education in arts and philosophy. Both Giovanni and Filippo Villani stressed that Dino was as learned in liberal arts and philosophy as he was in medicine, and Filippo added that Dino studied all these disciplines at Bologna.[134] Before Dino began his medical studies, Taddeo may have been his instructor in logic (which, as we have seen, Taddeo was certainly teaching along with medicine in 1287) as well as in medicine, and perhaps also in philosophy.

Upon returning to Florence from Bologna, Dino appears straightaway to have launched himself into medical practice. In 1297 both he and his father were members of the Florentine guild of physicians and pharmacists (*medici e speziali*), a membership Dino maintained for most of the rest of his life.[135] He subsequently returned to Bologna, completed his medical studies, and began to lecture there, probably in 1305, but perhaps a year or two earlier.[136] Between 1306 and 1308, studies at Bologna were interrupted by an interdict imposed on the city by Pope Clement V. Dino migrated with some of his students to Siena, which at that time had only the rudiments of a *studium*.[137] The municipality nonetheless provided Dino with a salaried chair of medicine, which he held during the academic year 1308-1309 for an emolument of 90 florins.[138] Dino was back in Bologna in 1310, however, and there, except for a brief tenure of a chair at Padua in 1311-1312, he seems to have remained for a number of

[134] See note 131, above; and "Studio vero Bononie datus est, ubi tantum liberalibus artibus philosophie, medicineque doctrinis invaluit," F. Villani, *Liber de . . . famosis civibus*, p. 28.

[135] Corsini, "Nuovo contributo," p. 268.

[136] "Expositio quarte fen primi canonis Avicenne. quam ego Dynus de Florentia incepi componere cum legi Bononie anno sexto mee lecture. MCCCXI," Dino, *Dilucidatorium*, fol. 2r. It is not clear whether Dino meant the sixth year of his lecturing, or the sixth year of his lecturing at Bologna.

[137] "scholares omnes mei amici veri existunt: maxime tamen scholares qui de Bononia et aliis partibus ad civitatem Senarum gratia reformationis studii in eadem civitate, quod Bononie tunc temporis fuit destructum, venerunt mihi," Dino, *Dilucidatorium*, fol. 2r. For the interdict, see Rashdall, *Universities*, 1:589. Regarding the *studium* of Siena, see Rashdall, *Universities*, 2:31-34.

[138] *Chartularium Studii Senensis*, 1:91-92, 95-97 (nos. 112, 114, 117, 119).

years.[139] But by 1319 he had returned to medical practice in Florence, one of his patients being the humanist poet and historian Albertino Mussato, who commemorated the occasion with verses in which he referred to Dino's brisk figure and friendly face.[140] In 1320 Dino returned to his professorship at Siena, where he lectured publicly and magisterially in the *studium* on both theoretical and practical branches of surgery.[141] This time, his annual salary was 350 gold florins, with additional payments for moving expenses and for lectures on *practica*.[142] Both Dino's reputation and the economic position of the *studium* of Siena had evidently made a dramatic advance. In 1323 the city government of Perugia invited Dino to come from Siena to conduct examinations and preside at the graduation ceremonies of doctoral candidates in medicine "for the increase and honor of the *studium* of Perugia"—yet further testimony to Dino's distinguished academic position.[143] Dino held his professorship at Siena at least until September 1323, but sometime between then and 1325 he was obliged to leave "on account of the diminution and annihilation of that *studium*."[144] Dino's career illustrates with great clarity the political and fiscal uncertainties that beset academic life in early fourteenth-century Italy.

[139] *Monumenti della Università di Padova (1222-1318)*, p. 363, establishes the dates at Padua.

[140] Adveniunt medici duo, quorum junior alter

    Dinus forma alacer, vultu quoque amabilis ipso,

    Praeterea laudes

Albertino Mussato, "Somnium in aegritudinem apud Florentiam," *Albertini Mussati Patavini Tragoedia Eccerinis et Achilleis*, ed. Niccolo Villani, col. 65, in J. G. Graevius, ed., *Thesaurus antiquitatum et historiarum Italiae*, vol. 6, pt. 2 (Leiden, 1722); Dino himself stated in the explicit of his *Dilucidatorium* that he finished that work in Florence in 1319 (*Dilucidatorium*, fol. 166r).

[141] "Hic juvenis adhuc super tertia et quarta parte seu [*sic*: fen] quinti Canonis Avicenne expositiones conscripsit utiles et subtiles tam in practica quam in theorica cyrugie, que in studiis ordinariis magistraliter perleguntur, cum jam grandevus Senis legeret," F. Villani, *Liber de . . . Famosis civibus*, p. 27; reprinted, SF 2:296. The reference to Dino's age makes it clear that these lectures were given during his second sojourn at Siena.

[142] *Chartularium Studii Senensis*, 1:164, 198, 202, 216, 224, 226, 228-229, 244-246.

[143] A. Rossi, ed., "Documenti per la storia dell'Università di Perugia," *Giornale di erudizione artistica* 4 (1875):323-325, nos. 47, 48, 50; "pro augmento et honore studii perusini," at p. 323.

[144] "Et finita est ac completa hec expositio et declaratio huius partis Avicenne anno christi 1325 die 27 mensis octobris. Quam ego Dynus de florentia minimus inter medicine doctores incepi cum viguit studium in civitate Senarum: et hanc partem Avicenne ibi in cathedra legi: sed eam complevi cum florentiam redii propter illius studii diminutionem et annihilationem," Dino, *Canon* 2, fol. 62r.

According to Filippo Villani, Dino was obliged to make his second move to Siena because his fellow professors and students at Bologna discovered that he had passed off arguments from the *Plusquam commentum*, the principal work of Turisanus, as his own. The story is told with a good deal of circumstantial detail. Supposedly, when Turisanus was on his deathbed, he dispatched his work to Bologna, hoping thus to secure himself a lasting reputation in the schools. Dino laid hands on the work, kept his possession of it a secret, but drew from it so much new material that students began to flock to him from other masters. The other professors, surprised by Dino's sudden access of wisdom, paid a student to keep a watch on him; the spy soon found out the truth, and Dino was forced to publish the *Plusquam commentum* for general consumption. His embarrassment and annoyance were such that he left Bologna forever, and went to Siena.[145]

The veracity of this picturesque anecdote has been disputed, on account of various improbabilities.[146] For one thing, Dino did not go directly from Bologna to Siena, but, as indicated above, first spent some time in practice in Florence. For another, Dino del Garbo was by 1320 already an established medical author; he scarcely needed to bolster his reputation by plagiarism from a lesser-known contemporary. Also, numerous masters and scholars migrated to Siena from Bologna in 1321;[147] so no personal problem need have been involved in Dino's decision to move at about that time. Yet Villani was well informed about Dino's works and had spoken with people who had known him; it seems unlikely that his account is wholly without basis, although its details may be fictitious. It is probable that Dino was eager to secure access to the *Plusquam commentum* as soon as he knew of its existence. Turisanus, perhaps as a result of his studies in natural philosophy at Paris, went further than almost any other medical writer of his day in incorporating material pertaining to philosophy and natural science into a commentary on a medical text. The *Plusquam commentum* derives its name from its use of a commentary on Galen's *Tegni* as a framework to support a massive weight of this kind of interpolation. Dino, a physician who, as we have seen, had the reputation of being especially interested in natural and moral philosophy, may well have wanted to be the first at Bologna to study this work. Professional

[145] F. Villani, *Liber de . . . famosis civibus*, pp. 28-29.
[146] Most notably by Tiraboschi; see *Storia della letteratura italiana*, 5:248.
[147] Rashdall, *Universities*, 2:33.

rivalry could easily lead to accusations of outright plagiarism in such circumstances.

Whatever the reasons for Dino's departure from Bologna, he seems never to have returned there after 1319. The remainder of his life after his second departure from Siena was apparently spent in Florence. There he enjoyed the patronage of King Robert of Sicily, signore of the city from 1313 to 1322, to whom Dino dedicated the final versions of two of the works he had originally composed in the course of classroom teaching.[148]

At Florence, too, the last noted episode of Dino's career took place, namely his involvement in the trial of the astrologer and poet Cecco d'Ascoli (Francesco Stabile), who was burned at the stake on September 16, 1327.[149] Cecco, perhaps the only medieval intellectual to pay the extreme penalty for ideas disseminated in the classroom, was called to account supposedly because of his refusal to renounce astrological determinism, necromancy, or both. But according to Giovanni Villani, a contemporary witness, in reality Dino del Garbo was a major cause of Cecco's death, "and many said he did it out of envy."[150] It has been claimed that hostility arose between the two men as a result of professional rivalry when both were teaching in the faculty of arts and medicine at Bologna —and that it was Cecco who spread accusations of plagiarism against Dino.[151] Cecco did indeed sharply criticize the character of a physician named Gualfridinus, by whom it has been suggested he may have meant Dino,[152] but made no specific accusations against him, at any rate in

[148] "Serenissime princeps mundi rex Roberte accipe hoc opus. . . . Quare hec opera ut rex benignus sit: et benigne recipere placeat. nam et si aliquid utile continent, erit vobis etiam ascribendum possessio, enim vera est et opus et auctor. In uno autem horum operum exponuntur canones generales de virtutibus medicinarum simplicium secundi canonis Avicenne in quibus quam grandis sit utilitas per suum prohemium indicatur. In altero vero operum exponuntur canones curative quarte fen primi canonis Avicenne . . . ," Dino, Canon 2, fol. 1r. See notes 136 and 144, above, for the classroom origin of these works.

[149] On Cecco, his teachings, and his fate, see G. Villani, Cronica 10.40; Thorndike, History of Magic, 2:948-968; idem, "More Light on Cecco d'Ascoli," The Romantic Review (1946):293-306, in addition to the works cited below.

[150] "E questo maestro Dino fu grande cagione della morte del sopradetto maestro Cecco, riprovando per falso il detto suo libello, il quale aveva letto in Bologna, et molti dissono che il fece per invidia," G. Villani, Cronica 10.41. Villani began to compile material for his chronicle in 1300, and died in 1348.

[151] See for example [Cecco d'Ascoli], L'Acerba, intro., pp. 10-11; and F. Filippini, "Cecco d'Ascoli a Bologna," Studi e memorie per la storia dell'Università di Bologna 10 (1930):26.

[152] Thorndike, History of Magic, 2:957.

writing. Moreover, Dino and Cecco could have been colleagues at Bologna only briefly, if at all. Cecco had taken up residence in Bologna by 1318, when he was living with medical students there; he had probably begun to lecture by 1322.[153] By that time, however, Dino had already left Bologna. Cecco's lectures on the *Sphere* of Sacrobosco, the source of his difficulties with the Inquisition, may not have been given until 1324, when, as already noted, he held a salaried chair in astrology. They were certainly not delivered before 1322. His commentary on Alchabitius, *De principiis astrologiae*, which contains material strongly critical of Bolognese society and individuals, dates from 1324 at the earliest and perhaps from 1325-1326.[154]

Following an inquisitorial sentence in 1324 forbidding him to teach astrology, Cecco came to Florence as astrologer to Charles of Calabria, who in 1326 succeeded his father, King Robert of Sicily, as lord of the city.[155] Perhaps Dino resented Cecco's success in obtaining the patronage of the royal house of Naples, formerly enjoyed by Dino himself. Cecco and Dino also differed in their estimate of the Florentine vernacular lyric poet Guido Cavalcanti, whom Dino greatly admired, but Cecco denigrated (see chapter three, below). It is plain from Villani's account, however, that the only action Dino took against Cecco consisted in publishing an analysis of the errors in one of Cecco's academic commentaries, a deed not necessarily inspired by malice. Yet such an analysis would provide a useful weapon for an attack on Cecco if for other reasons he had fallen

---

153 Thorndike, "More Light on Cecco d'Ascoli," pp. 296-297.

154 The dating of Cecco's commentaries has been disputed, largely because of a controversy over whether he continued to teach at Bologna after the first inquisitorial sentence in 1324, and over which work was the subject of condemnation. Thorndike (ibid., p. 301) maintained that neither commentary dates from before 1324, and that Cecco did not teach after his first condemnation; Filippini believed the commentary on the *Sphere* to date from 1322-1323 ("Cecco d'Ascoli a Bologna," p. 9); Crespi (ed. Cecco d'Ascoli, *L'Acerba*, intro.) suggested the late date of 1325-1326 for the commentary on Alchabitius, which none of the three authorities is willing to place before 1324. Cecco's commentary on the *Sphere* is edited in Lynn Thorndike, *The Sphere of Sacrobosco and Its Commentators*; that on Alchabitius is to be found in Cecco d'Ascoli, *Il commento di Cecco d'Ascoli al Alcabizzo* (ed. Giuseppi Boffito). Cecco may also have taught medicine, since he wrote a commentary on the *Aphorisms* of Hippocrates; see Filippini, "Cecco d'Ascoli a Bologna," p. 9.

155 For the sentence of 1324 see Thorndike, *History of Magic*, 2:952, where, however, it is pointed out that the available documents are late and unreliable. In 1325-1326 Cecco commented (but perhaps did not lecture on?) a work of Ptolemy and entitled the result *De excentricis* (Filippini, "Cecco d'Ascoli a Bologna," p. 9); G. Villani, *Cronica* 10.40, provides an account of Cecco's career.

out of favor with Charles of Calabria, as another version of the story has it. Whatever the case, Dino did not long survive his rival, since he died only a few days later, on September 30, 1327.[156]

According to Filippo Villani, those who had known Dino said he was so entirely wrapped up in speculation as to be almost unaware of the world about him; he was withdrawn and severe at all times except when visiting the sick, with whom he was affable and cheerful.[157]

Evidently neither the accusation of deliberate plagiarism of Turisanus nor that of murderous malice against Cecco d'Ascoli discredited Dino in the eyes of fourteenth-century Florence, if one may judge from the place of his portrait among the Just in Orcagna's Santa Croce frescoes of the Last Judgment, completed before 1368.[158] Whether the accusations were not at that time generally known, were known but not believed, or were known and believed but not thought damaging, remains obscure. Most likely, Dino's son Tommaso, who was a prominent citizen of Florence in the 1360s and who took great pride in his father's fame, played a part in securing his representation.

In any event, whatever his moral failings, Dino's reputation rested mainly on his impressive array of written works.[159] His principal achievement, which occupied him, with interruptions, from before 1311 until 1325, was in extending the range of commentary on the *Canon* of Avicenna. He concentrated his attention on the parts of the *Canon* relating

[156] G. Villani, *Cronica* 10.41 (see note 150, above), where Dino's death date is also given. The other story says that Cecco provided unfavorable horoscopes for the duke's children, surely a suicidal act for a court astrologer. One version claims that he announced that the duke's daughter would give herself over to a life of sensual pleasure; since the daughter in question grew up to be the notorious Queen Giovanna of Naples, the story seems a little too pat to be believed, although it has been traced to a late fourteenth-century source; see Thorndike, "More Light on Cecco d'Ascoli," p. 295.

[157] F. Villani, *Liber de . . . famosis civibus*, p. 28.

[158] "se ne torno Andrea a Fiorenza, dove nel mezzo della chiesa di Santa Croce . . . dipinse afresco le medesime cose che dipinse nel Camposanto di Pisa [the Last Judgment]. . . . Fra i buoni . . . fra i medesimi è maestro Dino del Garbo, medico allora eccellentissimo, vestito come allora usavano i dottori e con una berretta rossa in capo foderata di vai, e tenuto per mano da un Angelo," Giorgio Vasari, *Le Vite*, ed. Rossana Bettarini and Paolo Barocchi (Florence, [1968]), vol. 2, pt. 1, pp. 220-221. The frescoes in question are almost entirely destroyed, but are considered to have been completed as late as possible before Orcagna's death in 1368; see Richard Offner, *A Critical and Historical Corpus of Florentine Painting* (New York, 1962), section 4, vol. 1, *Andrea di Cione* [Orcagna], pp. 24, 25, 43.

[159] For manuscripts and editions of the works named in this paragraph, see Bibliography. Regarding the dating of the works, see notes 136, 141, 144, above.

to *practica,* beginning early in his teaching career with an exposition of the sections of Book 4 dealing with surgery. From 1311 to 1319 he was engaged in the composition of his *Dilucidatorium totius practice medicinalis scientie,* a commentary on *Fen* 4 of Book 1 of the *Canon,* which sets out remedies for particular diseases. Thereafter he began work on his *De virtutibus medicamentorum,* a commentary on Book 2 of the *Canon,* which concerned simples, and completed it in 1325. He also wrote on the tract on fevers in *Fen* 1 of Book 4. One is struck by Dino's omission or postponement of comment on the more theoretical parts of the *Canon*— the exposition of medical theory and regimen in the first three *fen* of Book 1, the description of anatomy and diseases in Book 3, and the section on prognostication and critical days in Book 4. He did, however, produce a set of *questiones* on the chapter on ingested substances in Book 1.[160] Dino was among the earliest Latin authors to comment systematically on large portions of the *Canon.* His expositions are said to have become standard textbooks during his lifetime.[161] A collection of remedies for surgical cases that Dino based on Galen's *De simplicibus medicinae* and on Book 2 of the *Canon* also appears to have been widely read by physicians and surgeons, for it exists in a number of manuscripts and early editions.[162] He also wrote what may be the only Latin commentary on the *De natura fetus* (or *puerorum*) attributed to Hippocrates, into which he incorporated a good deal of philosophical speculation about the origins of man, and he produced three treatises or commentaries on Galenic complexion theory. More conventionally, he also commented upon the *Aphorisms* of Hippocrates and the *Tegni* of Galen. His output also included a few *consilia* and *questiones* (on these genres of medical writing in the circle of Taddeo, see chapters eight and nine, below), and perhaps a treatise on weights and measures.[163] And, finally, he was the

[160] Inc. "Quod comeditur et bibitur. Queritur utrum aliquid operatur a qualitate . . . ," MS SG Vadian 433, a. 1465, pp. 598-618, attribution in explicit; I have not seen this work, which is on microfilm at the NLM.

[161] "in studiis ordinariis magistraliter perleguntur," F. Villani, *Liber de . . . famosis civibus,* p. 27.

[162] See TK 1027, 1348.

[163] In at least one manuscript (BAV Vat. lat. 2418, fol. 164r) this work is attributed to Mondino de' Liuzzi ("Mundinum de leuciis de bononia"); in several others what is apparently a variant of the same text appears anonymously (see TK 439; I have not seen these manuscripts). In several printed editions the work is ascribed to Dino; that consulted for this study is *Expositio Dini florentini super tertia et quarta et parte quinti canonis Avicenne . . . Tractatus Dini de ponderibus et mensuris* (Venice, 1499; Klebs 336.3). The

author of a learned Latin commentary on one of the Italian love lyrics of Guido Cavalcanti, namely, the *Canzone d'amore* beginning "Donna mi prega."

TURISANUS (PIETRO TORRIGIANO DE' TORRIGIANI)

Although, according to Filippo Villani, Turisanus excelled the other pupils of Taddeo in the power and acumen of his intelligence, his writings were few and his activities are obscure. Almost nothing is known of his life beyond the information provided in Villani's brief biography.[164] From this we learn that he was a member of a well-known Florentine family and that he began his studies at Bologna some time before Taddeo's death. (According to one of his sixteenth-century editors, he subsequently returned to Florence, but was exiled as a result of the struggle of Blacks and Whites in 1302.)[165] He then moved to Paris to continue his education; there, having learned liberal arts and all philosophy, he occupied a chair of medicine for many years. According to Villani, Turisanus practiced and publicly taught medicine at Paris about the same time Dino del Garbo was teaching at Bologna—that is, for some of the years between 1305 and 1319. The records of the *studium* of Paris, however, reveal no trace of his presence; if Villani's assertion that Turisanus was near death while Dino del Garbo was still teaching at Bologna (at latest about 1319) is correct, Turisanus cannot be identified with the Petrus de Florentia who was a professor of medicine at Paris from 1325 until 1336.[166]

Turisanus is unique among the learned physicians who were Taddeo's pupils in that no records of medical practice by him appear to survive,

---

printed text appears to be an abbreviated version of that appearing in Vat. lat. 2418, at least as far as the proem is concerned (fol. 163v in the manuscript, fol. 152r in the edition). To complicate the problem, the works cited in the text include the *Sinonima* (a medical dictionary) of Mondino Friuliano (d. ca. 1340).

[164] F. Villani, *Liber de . . . famosis civibus*, pp. 28-29; the biography of Turisanus here is drawn from Villani, except where otherwise indicated. For more recent secondary accounts, see Wickersheimer, *Dictionnaire*, 2:770; Sarton, *Introduction to the History of Science*, vol. 3, pt. 1, pp. 839-840. Still useful are Tiraboschi, *Storia della letteratura italiana*, 5:250, and Puccinotti, *Storia della medicina*, vol. 2, pt. 2, pp. 340-343.

[165] *Plusquam commentum in parvam Galeni artem Turisani Florentini . . .* (Venice, 1557), unnumbered folio facing fol. 1r.

[166] *Chartularium Universitatis Parisiensis*, ed. H. Denifle and E. Chatelain (Paris, 1891), vol. 2, pt. 1, nos. 845, 852, 919, 996, 1129.

neither as definite references in his own theoretical works, as *consilia* for individual clients, nor in any other documents that have so far been brought to light. Whether his practice was nonexistent or merely not especially extensive is not clear. Trithemius, who wrote towards the end of the fifteenth century and was Turisanus' earliest biographer after Villani, spoke of Turisanus as dogged by misfortune, a statement expanded by the sixteenth-century Florentine historian Michael Pocciantius into the assertion that Turisanus, although extremely learned, had little luck in curing patients.[167] Turisanus certainly never achieved the kind of reputation as a practitioner that attached to Taddeo, Bartolomeo da Varignana, or Guglielmo da Brescia; if indeed he was perceived by contemporaries as inferior to his colleagues in this respect, it would be interesting to know on what basis, given the relative ineffectiveness of all medieval medical treatment. To the nature of his failure, however, the sources give no clue.

The chief fruit of Turisanus' teaching, the *Plusquam commentum*, a commentary on the *Tegni* of Galen incorporating much philosophical learning and a measure of scientific originality, was not completed until his old age, when he seems to have returned to Italy (as Villani's anecdote about his sending the work to Bologna implies). He was also the author of a brief *questio* or treatise on urinary sediments (see Bibliography).

As an old man, presumably after his return to his native country, Turisanus renounced his secular studies, turned to theology, and entered a religious order. Whatever role personal misfortune may have played in this decision, it seems reasonable to suppose that his philosophical studies, begun in connection with medicine, may also have led him toward theology and toward a religious vocation. Here we have a type of ecclesiastical career very different from the efficient gathering of benefices typified by that other clerical physician, Guglielmo da Brescia. Once again, one should beware of the assumption that the development of medicine as a learned profession can always and without qualification be described as a secularizing force in the medieval world.

According to Villani, Turisanus became a Dominican, but he is not listed among Dominican authors. Trithemius and the early historians of

---

[167] Trithemius, *De scriptoribus ecclesiasticis*, fol. cxixr; Michael Pocciantius, *Catalogus scriptorum florentinorum*, p. 165.

the Carthusian order claimed that he became a Carthusian monk. He is said to have taught theology and to have written on religious subjects after entering religion, but, if so, all trace of these works has been lost.[168]

MONDINO DE' LIUZZI (LIUCCI, LUZZI; MONDINUS, OR MUNDINUS, DE BONONIA)

Today, the best-known by far of Taddeo Alderotti's pupils and associates is the anatomist Mondino de' Liuzzi.[169] Mondino had the good fortune to write a textbook of anatomy that remained standard for more than two hundred years and that consequently exists in numerous early and several modern printed editions.[170] Moreover, this work was intended to be, at least on occasion, illustrated by an accompanying dissection of a human cadaver; and Mondino himself supervised and may have performed dissections.[171] Mondino is hence deservedly recognized by historians of medicine as a pioneer in establishing the dissection of human bodies as an integral part of the systematic study of anatomy. As a result, not only does Mondino occupy a fairly prominent place in general histories of medicine,[172] but his *Anatomia* has been the subject of detailed

[168] Trithemius, *De scriptoribus ecclesiasticis*, fol. cxixr; Pierre Cousturier [d. 1537], *De vita cartusiana . . .* 2.3.7, p. 586; Theodorus Petreius, *Bibliotheca Cartusiana, sive Illustrium sacri cartusiensis ordinis scriptorum catalogus*, pp. 294-295; Benedetto Tromby, *Storia critico-cronologica diplomatica del patriarca S. Brunone e del suo ordine cartusiano* (Naples, 1777), 6:135—all of which claim Turisanus wrote religious works.

[169] The most recent secondary account of Mondino is Vern L. Bullough, "Mondino de' Luzzi," *DSB* 9 (1974):467-469; detailed accounts, based on documents relating to Mondino from the archives of the city of Bologna, are to be found both in Fantuzzi, *Notizie*, 6:41-46; and in the editor's introduction to Mondino's *Anatomia*, ed. Lino Sighinolfi, pp. 12-18. See also Sarton, *Introduction to the History of Science*, vol. 3, pt. 2, pp. 842-845; and SF 1:550-551. The works of Mondino de' Liuzzi are distinguished from those of other authors of the same forename in Eugenio dall'Osso, "Una questione dibattuta: quanti anatomici e medici di nome 'Mondino' esistevano all'inizio del '300," *Bollettino dell'Accademia Medica Pistoiese Filippo Pacini* 26 (1955):245-255.

[170] For those used in the present study, see Bibliography; others are noted by Sarton, *Introduction to the History of Science*.

[171] Bullough, "Mondino de' Luzzi," p. 468, for the controversy over whether or not Mondino performed his own dissections. To the bibliography there cited may be added Giuseppe Ongaro, "Il metodo settorio di Mondino de' Liucci," in XXI *Congresso Internazionale di Storia della Medicina, Siena, 1968, Atti*, 1:68-92. On anatomy and surgery in Bologna in the early fourteenth century, see further below, chapters four and nine.

[172] See, for example, Arturo Castiglioni, *A History of Medicine*, trans. E. B. Krumbhaar (2d ed., New York, 1947), pp. 341-344; and Singer, *The Evolution of Anatomy*, pp. 74-78.

study that has revealed, unsurprisingly, that Mondino shared most of the
medical limitations of his age: his errors in anatomy, his reliance on
Galen and the Arabs, and the possibility that he may have delegated the
actual performance of his (infrequent) dissections to an assistant have
been many times pointed out; more recently even the extent of his
knowledge of Galen has been called into question (see further chapter
four, below). It would be superfluous to repeat here the information
about the career and work of Mondino that is very generally available.
Nevertheless, it may be useful to place Mondino in the context of Taddeo's circle.

The Liuzzi family appears to have been of Florentine origin, but by
1270 Albizzo de' Liuzzi and Liuzzio, his son (the grandfather and
uncle of Mondino) had already established themselves in Bologna, where
they set up a pharmacy. No doubt the growth of the Bolognese medical
school associated with the spreading reputation of Taddeo's teaching
stimulated such ancillary trades. No doubt also, the members of the
Liuzzi family were acquainted, at Bologna if not before, with Taddeo,
a fellow Florentine in a related profession. Liuzzio de' Liuzzi seems to
have followed a career somewhat similar to Taddeo's own, moving from
a related trade into medical practice and teaching. By 1281 he was referred to as *medicus*, and by 1295 he was one of the lecturers in *physica*
in the faculty of arts and medicine. Liuzzio died in 1318; his family
commemorated his death by a handsome sepulchral relief in the church
of San Vitale depicting him in the master's cathedra lecturing to his
students. Liuzzio's career, if not as spectacularly successful as Taddeo's,
was therefore not undistinguished, although he left no written works. It
was most likely Liuzzio, rather than Taddeo, who provided the most
substantial part of his famous nephew's medical training. Mondino's
name was added to Liuzzio's on the monument just referred to; moreover, the pharmacy remained a family business and was in due course
inherited by Mondino.[173] These facts suggest a closely knit family involvement in medicine and related concerns that would have been en-
hanced, rather than disrupted or diminished, by the engagement of some
members of the family in public teaching in the schools.

That Mondino also studied under Taddeo is not, however, in doubt.

[173] *Anatomia*, ed. Sighinolfi, intro., pp. 12-13, 17-18; Fantuzzi, *Notizie*, 6:42; and
note 63 to chapter one, above.

Attention has been drawn to an anecdote about Taddeo contained in Mondino's commentary on the *Canones generales* of Mesue,[174] a work in which Taddeo is the only contemporary physician referred to; it is a story that implies a knowledge of Taddeo's methods from the point of view of a subordinate. In order to illustrate the effects of regimen upon the efficacy of medication, Mondino described a visit of Taddeo, accompanied by other physicians, to the bedside of the count of Arezzo. Seeing the patient somewhat better, Taddeo retired for the night and left the junior physicians in charge, despite their reluctance. He also left careful instructions for the administration of medication. Upon returning next morning, he found the patient near death; the other physicians protested they had given the medicine exactly as directed. Taddeo then pointed out that they had failed to close an open window and were therefore entirely responsible for the failure of the medicine to act as expected, and also for the patient's deteriorating condition.[175]

Mondino's birthdate is unknown, but could have been no later than about 1270; the date of his death has been established as 1326.[176] He was a married layman and the father of three sons.[177] He seems to have spent his entire career as a professor of medicine at Bologna. By 1316, about the time he composed the *Anatomia*,[178] Mondino was not only a regent master in the schools, but also a respected and influential citizen, who, with his uncle Liuzzio, served as the city's ambassador to Giovanni, son of Robert of Sicily.[179] In the following year, Mondino lectured on the

[174] Mary C. Wellborn, "Mondino de' Luzzi's Commentary on the *Canones Generales* of Mesue the Younger," *Isis* 22 (1934):8-11.

[175] Mondino, *Mesue*, fols. 38 (mistake for 37) r-v.

[176] He made his will in February of that year, and a posthumous inventory of his goods was drawn up in May; see his *Anatomia*, ed. Sighinolfi, intro., pp. 15-17. The will is preserved in the Archivio di Stato of Bologna. A Bolognese chronicler noted under 1326 that Mondino's internment took place "cum grande honore," *Corpus Cronicorum Bononensium*, vol. 2, ed. Albano Sorbelli, in *Rerum Italicarum Scriptores*, n.s., vol. 18, pt. 1, p. 369.

[177] According to Fantuzzi, *Notizie*, 6:42. Mondino, *Anatomia*, ed. Sighinolfi, intro., p. 17, indicates that a fourth son was born to Mondino posthumously, by his second wife.

[178] Mondino, *Anathomia Mundini*, in Charles Singer, ed., *The Fasciculo di Medicina Venice 1493*, 1:76. "A woman I anatomized last year, that is in the year of Christ, 1315, in the month of January, had a womb double as big as her that I anatomized in March of the same year" (Singer's translation).

[179] Fantuzzi, *Notizie*, 6:42; Mondino, *Anatomia*, ed. Sighinolfi, p. 13. Mondino is described as "regenti in medicina" in a property transfer of 1315-1316 printed in Umberto

Prognostica of Hippocrates, with Galen's commentary, on the first three books of his *De regimine acutorum*, and in 1319 on the chapter of the *Canon* of Avicenna on the generation of the embryo. *Reportationes* of all three sets of lectures were taken down by Mondino's student Bertruccio, or Bertuccio, who was himself to become in turn the teacher of the famous surgeon Guy de Chauliac.[180] In 1324, as already remarked, Mondino was holding a publicly salaried professorship in practical medicine. The works on which he commented and therefore probably lectured also included the *Tegni* of Galen, and, as noted, the *Canones generales* of Mesue. In addition, he produced *consilia*, which show him to have engaged in the usual type of consultant practice, disputed *questiones*, and wrote brief tracts on fevers and medicinal dosage. A *practica de accidentibus morborum* and other works are variously attributed to him and to other physicians.[181]

We have pursued at perhaps tedious length the careers of six physicians (not counting the philosopher Gentile da Cingoli) in an effort to view learned medicine in its social context. The results are in some ways instructive. We can find no division between "theoretical" and "practical" physicians; five of the six gave medical advice to individual patients,

---

Dallari, "Due documenti inediti riguardanti Liuzzo e Mondino de' Liuzzi," *Rivista di storia delle scienze mediche e naturali* 14 (1932):3-6.

[180] BAV, MS Vat. lat. 4466, fol. 55v: "Expliciunt reportationes super libro pronosticorum et primo secundo et tertio libro regiminis acutorum morborum facte sub egregio doctore Magistro Mundino per Bertuccium de bononia in anno domini M°cccxvii; MS Reg. lat. 2000, fol. 23v: "Explicit expositio capituli de generatione embrionis primi tractatus fen xxi[1] 3[1] Canonis Avicenne recollecta ab eximio medicine professore magistro Mundino de leuciis bononiensis per me Bertuccium . . . reportata ab anno domini mcccxviiii." For the relationship of Guy de Chauliac and Bertruccio, see Guy de Chauliac, *Cyrurgia* (Venice, 1498; Klebs 494.1) 1.1.1, fols. 5r-v.

[181] Mondino's commentaries on the *Prognostica*, *De regimine acutorum*, and the *Tegni* survive, as far as I know, in only two manuscripts, each containing all three commentaries. That consulted for the present study was BAV, Vat. lat. 4466, but the works are also to be found in Cesena, Biblioteca Malatestiana MS sinis. Pluteo xxvii[5], fols. 53r-226r (not in TK). The latter copy, which I have not seen, is described in Ladislao Münster and E. dall'Osso, "Mondino de' Liuzzi lettore-clinico presso lo studio di Bologna e le sue opere mediche ancora inedite," xv *Congresso italiano di storia della medicina, Torino, 1957, Atti*, pp. 212-220. These authors also note the presence in Malatestiana, MS sinis. Pluteo xxvii[4], of Mondino's brief tract on fevers at fols. 173v-174v, and of his tract on doses at fols. 161v-162r of MS destro Pluteo xxiv.[8] For the other works mentioned, see Bibliography.

lectured in the schools, and wrote both practical and theoretical works. In the cities of Italy, medicine is confirmed as a predominantly secular profession by ca. 1300—four of our six were married laymen—and its followers as involved in economic, civic, and political affairs. Thus Bartolomeo wrote on economic theory (see chapter three); Taddeo and Guglielmo were keenly interested in investment and the acquisition of property; Bartolomeo and, to a lesser extent, Mondino were politically active; Dino sought the patronage of Robert of Sicily and involved himself in the trial of Cecco d'Ascoli; and Guglielmo guided the educational policies of a pope. Only Turisanus, naturally enough, considering what was evidently an authentic monastic vocation, seems to have played no part in public affairs. If a monastic calling was exceptional, conventional piety and conservative religious views were the norm. Taddeo and Guglielmo left pious and charitable bequests; Dino attacked the unorthodoxy of Cecco; and Bartolomeo opened a medical treatise with an elaborate logical justification of the practice of prefacing all works with an invocation of the name of God.[182] None of the group acquired any contemporary reputation for unorthodoxy or skepticism. Turning to their social background, we note that medicine was often a middle-class family tradition; Taddeo, Dino, Bartolomeo, and Mondino (all the laymen) came from families where at least one older member is known to have been a physician or surgeon before them, and a medical tradition continued in the families of those (Mondino, Dino, and Bartolomeo) who had legitimate sons. Taddeo and Guglielmo seem probably to have come from a rather modest background among the trading classes—and they alone of the six can definitely be said to have died wealthy men. Three—Taddeo, Dino, Turisanus—came to Bologna from Florence; the first two maintained lifelong connections with their native city. A fourth, Mondino, came from a Florentine family established in Bologna in the generation prior to his own; Guglielmo was drawn by Taddeo's fame from the *studium* of Padua. Only Bartolomeo da Varignana can be thought of as representing an older, native Bolognese medical tradition. Guglielmo da Brescia alone seems to have attended any other *studium generale* before coming to Bologna, although, upon leaving, Turisanus went to Paris to study and teach; and Dino taught subsequently at Siena and Padua.

---

[182] BAV, MS Vat. lat. 4452, fol. 83r, proem to a commentary on Galen's *De interioribus* [*De locis affectis*]. Anonymous in this manuscript, the commentary is identified as Bartolomeo's in MS Vat. lat. 4454, 14c, fol. 55r.

On the whole it seems fair to say that the six can be characterized as a fairly homogeneous group of eminently practical, level-headed, and professionally successful men. The contributions of these men to the society in which they lived were not limited solely to medical teaching and practice, as the following chapter will show.

CHAPTER THREE

CITIZEN-PHYSICIANS AS MORAL PHILOSOPHERS AND MEN OF LETTERS

T*addeo and his pupils lived at a time and place when a vigorous urban political life and a prosperous, cultivated citizen class provided the setting both for the burgeoning of vernacular literature* and for the birth of Renaissance humanism in its moral, civic, and literary aspects. In this world, many currents flowed between academic and nonacademic milieux. Political and economic thought and poetry itself (with Dante as the prime example) drew upon and were enriched by theoretical concepts deriving from the academic learning of the day, and in particular from the reception of both the moral and the natural philosophy of Aristotle. At the same time, professors in the *studia*, whether religious or secular, responded to current political, ethical, and literary issues; thus, for example, Fra Remigio de' Girolami, OP (d. 1319), who lectured in the Dominican *studium* of Santa Maria Novella in Florence for some forty years, in his treatise *De bono communi* idealized the heroes of Roman republican history, expressed Florentine republican patriotism, and so helped to construct a Florentine historical and political mythology.[1] Members of all the learned professions, as well as some among the numbers of educated men who pursued studies in liberal arts without proceeding to any higher faculty, assisted in adapting simplified Aristotelian philosophy and other elements of school knowledge to the needs of the increasingly sophisticated and literate society outside the schools. Physicians were well equipped to take part in this interchange by their studies in liberal arts and philosophy and by their own intimate involvement in cultivated secular society.

Taddeo Alderotti and some of his associates were both among the pioneers in the study of moral philosophy at Bologna and were themselves deeply enmeshed in the *vita activa civilis*. As a result they produced sev-

---

[1] See Charles T. Davis, "An Early Florentine Political Theorist: Fra Remigio de' Girolami," *Proceedings of the American Philosophical Society* 104 (1960):662-676.

eral works indicative of an interest in social, ethical, and economic questions and in contemporary literature. In this category belong the Italian translation of an abbreviated version of the *Nicomachean Ethics* attributed (almost certainly correctly) to Taddeo;[2] Dino del Garbo's Latin commentary on the poet Cavalcanti's *Canzone d'Amore*,[3] in which Dino drew upon Aristotle's *Ethics, Politics,* and *De anima* to elucidate Cavalcanti's thought; and the commentary upon the pseudo-Aristotelian *Economics* by Bartolomeo da Varignana,[4] which incorporates much material taken from the *Politics*. Before we proceed to a closer look at each of these works, some general considerations about the study at Bologna of the subject matter they encompass are in order.

Obviously, the works just named were in large part the fruits of studies of the *libri morales* of Aristotle. The *Ethics,* the *Politics,* the *Rhetoric,*[5] and the (supposedly Aristotelian) *Economics* served as textbooks for the subject of moral philosophy (*philosophia moralis*), which had a place— albeit a minor one, in view of the concentration of attention upon logic and natural philosophy—in the curricula of the faculties of arts in the fourteenth century, and probably also the latter part of the thirteenth. Thus, for example, it has been demonstrated that lectures upon one or more of the *libri morales* were given in the early fourteenth century at Oxford, Paris, and Toulouse.[6] It is not known when these treatises, among the last works of Aristotle to be translated into Latin, were first lectured upon at Bologna. The earliest statutory reference to them dated from 1405, but they were clearly in use long before that time.[7] The two

[2] Extensive excerpts from the vernacular *Etica* attributed to Taddeo are printed in Concetto Marchesi, "Il compendio volgare dell'Etica aristotelica e le fonti del vi libro del 'Tresor,' " *Giornale storico della letteratura italiana* 42 (1903):31-63; for manuscripts and earlier editions (none of them critical), see ibid., pp. 2, 65-72. Since the work is incorporated as part of the thirteenth-century Italian translation of Brunetto Latini's *Tresor,* see also note 19, below.

[3] Otto Bird, "The Canzone d'Amore of Cavalcanti According to the Commentary of Dino del Garbo," *Mediaeval Studies* 2 (1940):150-203; 3 (1941):117-160. The text of the commentary appears at 2 (1940):160-174. But see also note 49, below.

[4] Venice, Padri Redentoristi, Chiesa della Fava, MS 3 (formerly 445), fols. 33-50; Paul Oskar Kristeller, *Iter Italicum,* 2:291; Charles H. Lohr, "Medieval Latin Aristotle Commentaries. Supplementary Authors," *Traditio* 30 (1974):126.

[5] Considered as one of the *libri morales* in the thirteenth and fourteenth centuries.

[6] James A. Weisheipl, "Curriculum of the Faculty of Arts at Oxford in the Early Fourteenth Century," *Mediaeval Studies* 26 (1964):148, 175, and literature there cited.

[7] The whole of the *Politics* was apparently translated into Latin for the first time by

pioneers in this regard appear to have been Taddeo himself, whose version of the *Ethics* dates from early in his career, and Jacopo da Pistoia, who dedicated a treatise on happiness, written at Bologna, to Cavalcanti (d. ca. 1300).[8]

Jacopo's work is a highly academic production. By means of a full array of scholastic arguments, he demonstrates that happiness, the highest good, lies in the exercise of the intellective faculty in contemplation. Relying heavily upon Aristotle's *Ethics* throughout, Jacopo asserts that such happiness is attainable in this life, that health and a measure of this world's goods are its prerequisites, and that obstacles to its achievement, such as greed, wrath, and sexual desire, should be restrained by temperance. He did, however, conform to current religious ideology to the extent of saying that perfect happiness can only be reached when the object of contemplation is God. Jacopo alludes to differences between the teachings of faith and of philosophy, while announcing his intention to investigate philosophy; so he, like Taddeo, may be classed loosely as Averroist in tendency[9] and as in some sense a precursor of the Bolognese Averroist philosophers of the 1330s and 1340s.

No direct connection between Taddeo and Jacopo da Pistoia has so far come to light. However, given that the philosophical portions of Taddeo's output (chiefly his version of the *Ethics* and parts of his commentary on the *Isagoge* of Johannitius), Jacopo's *Questio de felicitate*, and perhaps parts of the writings of Gentile da Cingoli are the only works on philosophy now considered definitely to have been produced at Bologna before 1300, one must suspect that some connection existed.[10] Moreover, the admiration for Cavalcanti shared by Jacopo and Taddeo's pupil Dino suggests a circle with common concerns embracing both Florence and

---

William of Moerbeke in the 1260s (*Aristoteles Latinus*, 1 [1957]:74-75). For the reference to the *libri morales* in the university statutes, see Malagola, *Statuti*, p. 252.

[8] Paul Oskar Kristeller, "A Philosophical Treatise from Bologna Dedicated to Guido Cavalcanti: Magister Jacobus de Pistorio and his 'Quaestio de felicitate,' " in *Medioevo e Rinascimento: Studi in onore di Bruno Nardi*, 1:425-463; the text of the *questio* appears at pp. 442-463. On the growth of Aristotelian studies at Bologna, with special reference to Taddeo, see further Martin Grabmann, "Das Aristotelesstudium in Italien zur Zeit Dantes," in his *Mittelalterliches Geistesleben*, 3:197-212; Bruno Nardi, "L'Averroismo bolognese nel secolo XIII e Taddeo Alderotto," *Rivista di storia della filosofia* 4 (1949): 11-23; and below, chapters four and five.

[9] Kristeller, "A Philosophical Treatise from Bologna," p. 437. For Taddeo's discussion of monopsychism, see chapter six, below.

[10] Ibid., pp. 438-439.

Bologna; both formal philosophy and a highly intellectual and sophisticated vernacular lyric poetry; and both academic and nonacademic
writing.

The *libri morales*, thus introduced into the curriculum of the Bologna
faculty of arts and medicine before 1300, continued to attract the attention
of the physicians of the school of Taddeo in the early fourteenth century.
Bartolomeo da Varignana's commentary on the *Economics* was, as will
become apparent, almost certainly produced at Bologna for teaching purposes, while, as already noted, Guglielmo da Brescia provided for lectures
on moral philosophy to be given within the residential college that he
founded there. Furthermore, in his commentary on Galen's *Tegni*, Turisanus (who may have acquired his moral philosophy at Paris as well as
from Taddeo or other teachers at Bologna) several times drew the subjects of good government and moral virtues into his discussion, with
appropriate citations from the *Ethics*.

For example, Turisanus remarked that the health or sickness of individuals is important to the body politic, in that it is essential for those
who rule to enjoy the best possible health, since such men ought not only
to exercise wisdom and prudence to the fullest, but also to have, in fact,
every other perfection supposedly belonging to man's nature.[11] This restricted view of public health reflects, of course, a social situation in
which the most highly esteemed form of medical attention (that of
learned teaching physicians like Turisanus himself) was probably available chiefly to the aristocracy, the higher clergy, and the property-owning
class of urban citizens. Turisanus' remark parallels the declaration of the
humanist educator Pier Paolo Vergerio (writing about 1404) that the
duty of educating their children is common to all parents but "especially
incumbent upon such as hold high station."[12]

Turisanus also drew from Aristotle's teaching on social justice, in order
to explain to his readers the refinements of the medical concept of *complexio* (that is, the balance of the qualities of hot, cold, wet, and dry).
Wishing to make the point that very different complexions might be

---

[11] "Sed maxime necessarium est optime sanum corpus ad regimen civile hominum:
quoniam talem hominem concomitatur esse sapientissimum et prudentissimum, et habere
omnem perfectionem que homini deputatur secundum naturam," Turisanus, *Plusquam*,
fol. 16r.

[12] Pier Paolo Vergerio, *De ingenuis moribus*, trans. William H. Woodward, *Vittorino
da Feltre and Other Humanist Educators* (repr. New York, 1963), p. 96. The dating is
Woodward's.

described in medical terminology as equally good (*equalem ad justi-tiam*), not in the abstract but insofar as each of them was appropriate to a particular individual, Turisanus cited and briefly expounded the definition of justice as due proportion and the mean that he found in *Ethics* 5.3-5, 1131a10-1134a15. In any city, said Turisanus (following Aristotle), honor is distributed among citizens according to their worth (some holding this to be determined by excellence—*virtus*—some by nobility of birth, and some by wealth); and such a distribution is, proportionately, just. The evaluation of variations in *complexio* should be undertaken in the light of this example.[13]

Elsewhere, Turisanus discussed the determinants of human social behavior, in what seems an early adumbration of the nature versus nurture controversy. He pointed out that although Aristotle had said in the *Ethics* (1.10, 1100b11-15) that no function of man was as constant as virtuous activity, in fact human behavior varied widely both because of variations in the innate complexions of individuals and because of differing ethnic or class mores. Thus, the custom of Jews and Moslems, of the religious and the laity, of students of liberal arts and manual workers, of writers and merchants—all were very different from one another. Moreover, variations in the laws and customs of the races and nations of men had in part a natural basis, being to some extent determined by variations in stellar influences in different regions of the globe. Within any ethnic or social group the behavior of an individual was determined by a mixture of social custom, law, and the habits of his own individual life style (*vita et conversatione*). How then was the physician (or the philosopher) to determine what elements in a person's behavior were due to his own innate complexion? Citing Haly, Turisanus declared that the natural behavior was that which appeared when an individual was sufficiently aroused emotionally to ignore social norms and his own ideals. Thus, someone whose respect for law and personal values taught him to prize religion, chastity, mercy, and justice might nonetheless be an easily enraged domestic tyrant and a ravening wolf toward the members of his own household.[14] Turisanus's concern with ethics also appears in yet another passage in which he turned aside from a discussion of pulse to mull over the distinction between courage and rashness.[15]

A similar interest in human nature is also displayed in the paean to the

---

[13] Turisanus, *Plusquam*, fol. 12r.   [14] Ibid., fols. 53v-54r.
[15] Ibid., fol. 50v.

nobility of man that opens Mondino's *Anatomia*. This description of man's nature is in sharp contrast to the rather dour views on the subject held by Turisanus: Mondino lauded man's upright stature, his partaking of qualities common also to the angels and Intelligences, his condition as a "political animal," and his manual skill. Thus Mondino united ideas about man's physical constitution, drawn at least in part from Galen, with Christian-Platonic teaching about man's spiritual nature and with Aristotelian enthusiasm for political life.[16] The mix was a potent one, and it would be used by a number of humanist writers in the fourteenth and fifteenth centuries.[17]

Finally, in the early fourteenth century, Aristotelian moral philosophy was studied at Bologna not only in the scientific and secular atmosphere of the public *studium* but also in at least one religious house. Fra Guido Vernani da Rimini, who lectured in the Dominican *studium generale* at Bologna between 1310 and 1320, was apparently the author of commentaries on all of the *libri morales*: the *Ethics*, the *Politics*, the *Rhetoric*, and the *Economics*.[18]

Against this background, the *Ethics* ascribed to Taddeo, Dino's commentary on Cavalcanti, and Bartolomeo's commentary on the *Economics* may now be examined more closely.

TADDEO ALDEROTTI AND THE NICOMACHEAN ETHICS

Although there is little doubt that Taddeo translated a version of the *Ethics* from Latin into Italian, his precise role in the preparation of the extant thirteenth-century vernacular *Etica*, after much scholarly discussion, remains unresolved. It seems unlikely that the question will ever

[16] Mondino, *Anatomia*, trans. Singer, 1:59-60. Marco Cesare Nannini, "La cultura mistico-teologica Dantesca in Mondino de' Liucci," xxi *Congresso Nazionale di Storia della Medicina, Perugia, 1965, Atti*, 1:209-215, regards the passage as "mystical" rather than, as it seems to me, humanistic.

[17] For a comprehensive account of the ancient sources and medieval and Renaissance treatment of the various themes relating to the dignity of man, see Charles Trinkaus, *In Our Image and Likeness: Humanity and Divinity in Italian Humanist Thought* (2 vols., Chicago, 1970). Enthusiastic praise of human manual skills is contained in the opening passage of Galen's *De usu partium*, of which Mondino knew, and cited here, the abbreviated twelfth-century Latin version entitled *De iuvamentis membrorum*.

[18] Charles H. Lohr, S.J., "Medieval Latin Aristotle Commentaries, Authors G-I," *Traditio* 24 (1968):191; Grabmann, "Das Aristotelesstudium," in *Mittelalterliches Geistesleben*, 3:200.

be settled definitively unless new linguistic studies are undertaken or fresh evidence turns up.[19] All that is possible at present is to summarize the state of the argument.

A free rendering into Italian of an abbreviated version of the *Ethics* (originally prepared in Arabic at Alexandria and translated into Latin by Hermann the German in 1243 or 1244)[20] is found in manuscript in two forms: as an independent treatise; and as part of the *Tesoro*, which is the Italian version of the French *Tresor* of Brunetto Latini. Despite extensive variants in the manuscripts, it is not questioned that substantially the same translation is involved.[21] Most copies of the independent version are anonymous, but in six of them Taddeo is named as translator. None of the "independent" manuscripts is older than the fourteenth century; of those naming Taddeo, two date from the fourteenth century, the rest from the fifteenth. Furthermore, at least three fourteenth-century manuscripts of the *Tesoro*, name Taddeo as the translator of a portion of the work.[22] In addition, manuscripts and early editions of the *Convivio* of Dante include a phrase identifying Taddeo as responsible for translation of the *Ethics* from Latin into Italian, a translation characterized by Dante as *laido*.[23] While the identifying remark, "cio

[19] For the bibliography, see Bianca Ceva, *Brunetto Latini, l'uomo e l'opera*, pp. 144-146, and notes here following. One of the most detailed studies of the manuscripts of the vernacular *Etica* is still Marchesi, "Il compendio volgare dell'Etica aristotelica"; but see also L. Frati, "Per due antichi volgarizzamenti. II. L' 'Etica' volgarizzata da Taddeo di Alderotto," *Giornale storico della letteratura italiana* 48 (1916):192-195; and Brunetto Latini, *Li livres dou Tresor*, intro., pp. xxviii-xxix. Detailed linguistic comparisons of the vernacular *Etica* with other vernacular writings attributed to Taddeo and Bono Giamboni might solve the problem of its ascription; however, such studies must be left to authorities on the early history of the Italian language.

[20] *Aristoteles Latinus*, 1:68, and Marchesi, *L'Etica Nicomachea*, pp. 105-129, at p. 125; the Latin compendium itself is printed at pp. xli-lxxxvi.

[21] Marchesi, "Il compendio volgare dell'Etica aristotelica," pp. 1-16; Frati, "Per due antichi volgarizzamenti, pp. 192-195.

[22] Marchesi, "Il compendio volgare dell'Etica aristotelica," pp. 65-72. The portion of the *Tresor* and the *Tesoro* devoted to a version of the *Ethics* is, according to one division of the work, followed by Marchesi, Book 6; according to a tradition in other manuscripts followed by Francis Carmody, the most recent editor of the French *Tresor*, it is Book 2, chaps. 1-49. Marchesi claimed also to have identified two manuscripts of another Italian version of the *Ethics*, separate and distinct from that attributed to Taddeo and incorporated in the *Tesoro*; excerpts from this version, are printed, side by side with the version attributed to Taddeo, in Marchesi, "Il compendio volgare dell'Etica aristotelica," pp. 30-47.

[23] "La gelosia dell'amico fa l'uomo sollecito a lunga provedenza; onde pensando che per lo desiderio d'intendere queste canzoni, alcuno illitterato avrebbe fatto lo comento

fu Taddeo ippocratista," has been held by some authorities to be a copy-ist's gloss,[24] it is accepted as Dante's in the critical edition of the *Convivio* by Busnelli and Vandelli.[25] In any case, even if a gloss, the statement is found in manuscripts dating from the fourteenth century, and thus re-flects an early tradition regarding the translator of the Italian versions of the *Ethics*.[26]

Despite this impressive evidence, there are some difficulties in the way of accepting without question the attribution to Taddeo of the extant vernacular *Etica*. The *Tresor* claims that Brunetto Latini himself trans-lated the *Ethics* "de latin en romanc."[27] It is, therefore, presumably the results of his labors that were incorporated into the French *Tresor*. But this section of the *Tresor* consists of a French translation of the same Latin compendium on which the Italian version attributed to Taddeo is based; and the French and Italian versions are so closely related as to make it virtually certain that one of them is in some way dependent upon the other.[28] Moreover, the translation of the whole of the *Tresor* from French into Italian has generally been attributed to Bono Giam-boni.[29]

Various hypotheses, none of them wholly satisfactory, have been put forward to account for this state of affairs. It has been suggested that Brunetto made use of an already existing Italian translation by Taddeo as well as of the Latin of Hermann the German in preparing his French version, and that Taddeo's translation was subsequently inserted into manuscripts of the *Tesoro* by copyists who knew of Brunetto's use of it.[30] It has even been suggested that when Brunetto claimed to have translated

---

latino transmutare in volgare, e temendo che 'l volgare non fosse stato posto per alcuno che l'avesse laido fatto parere, come fece quelli che transmutò il latino dell'Etica, ciò fu Taddeo ipocratista, providi a ponere lui, fidandomi di me di più che d'un altro," *Convivio* 1.10, ed. G. Busnelli and G. Vandelli (2d ed., Florence, 1968), 1:64.

[24] See, for example, *Convito di Dante Alighieri*, ed. Giangiacomo Trivulzio (Padua, 1827), p. 39, n. 1; and Pietro Fraticelli, *Il Convito* (Florence, 1879), p. 91.

[25] Dante Alighieri, *Convivio*, ed. Busnelli and Vandelli, 1:64.

[26] Frati, "Per due antichi volgarizzamenti," p. 193.

[27] Latini, *Tresor*, p. 175.

[28] Passages of the Italian and French versions are printed side by side by Marchesi, "Il compendio volgare dell'Etica aristotelica."

[29] On the basis of fifteenth-century editions and an attribution in one manuscript only, according to Cesare Segré and Mario Marti, eds., *La prosa del Duecento*, p. 311.

[30] Marchesi, "Il compendio volgare dell'Etica aristotelica," pp. 18-29.

the *Ethics* from "*latin*" he meant Italian and was indicating his dependence on Taddeo's work.[31] Others have claimed the reverse—that Taddeo
depended on Brunetto's preexisting French translation to prepare his
Italian text,[32] or that the text contained in the independently existing
manuscripts of the *Etica* is no more than an excerpt from the *Tesoro*,
translated from Brunetto's French by Bono Giamboni, and that Taddeo
had nothing to do with any of it.[33] The author of the most recent extensive scholarly study of Brunetto Latini and his works tends to the belief
that Taddeo and Brunetto both made translations of the Latin compendium, into Italian and French respectively, and that Taddeo's version was
later inserted into the Italian rendition of the French *Tresor*, possibly
with subsequent correction to bring it into line with the French.[34] It
should be added that so eminent an authority as Cesare Segré is of the
opinion that the attribution of the translation of the *Tresor* from French
into Italian to Bono Giambono is by no means certain and should be
carefully reexamined.[35]

In sum, there is an early and authoritative tradition that Taddeo did
indeed prepare an Italian translation of the *Ethics*. Furthermore, his
translation was from Latin,[36] a statement that by no means excludes the
possibility that he also made extensive use of an existing French version
by Brunetto Latini (the dependence of all extant Italian texts of the
Etica upon the French is strongly maintained by the most recent editor
of the *Tresor*).[37] Hermann the German's Latin translation of the compendium, completed only in 1243 or 1244, may have become known to
Brunetto in Paris some twenty years later.[38] It seems likely that Brunetto
may have introduced the Latin compendium to Italy, along with his own
French translation, when he returned to Florence from Paris in about
1267. It is probably legitimate to assume, therefore, that Taddeo played
some part in the preparation of the extant vernacular *Etica* inserted in

[31] G. B. Zannoni, ed., *Il Tesoretto e il favoletto di ser Brunetto Latini* (Florence, 1824),
p. xxxvi.

[32] Thor Sundby, *Della vita e delle opere di Brunetto Latini*, trans. Rodolfo Renier
(Florence, 1884), pp. 139-141. Sundby believed the extant texts of the *Tesoro* and of the
surviving vernacular *Etica* to be the work of Bono Giamboni as translator, but nonetheless
held that Taddeo did also translate the *Ethics*.

[33] Latini, *Tresor*, intro., p. xxviii and n. 2.

[34] Ceva, *Brunetto Latini*, pp. 146-147.

[35] Segré and Marti, *La prosa del Duecento*, p. 311.

[36] See note 23, above.   [37] Latini, *Tresor*, intro., p. xxviii.

[38] Ceva, *Brunetto Latini*, pp. 61-64, 146-147.

the *Tesoro*, and it is also legitimate to accept this as evidence of his special interest in Aristotle as a moral philosopher. Beyond that, perhaps, one should not venture. It would be hazardous, for example, to present minor variations in the Italian as against the French text as examples of Taddeo's own contribution, since it is unclear whether and to what extent his translation was subsequently corrected in the light of the original Latin version, against the French version, or otherwise amended.

As has frequently been noted, the compendium of the *Ethics* translated from the Arabic is a greatly simplified and abbreviated presentation of Aristotle's work. Several other superior Latin versions were available by the 1260s, including the complete translation directly from the Greek probably made by Robert Grosseteste and commented upon by Thomas Aquinas, and also including the older, partial translations from the Greek known as the *Ethica vetus* and the *Ethica nova*.[39] The compendium translated by Hermann the German had, however, the virtue of presenting an overview of the entire *Ethics* in small compass, and its simplicity might be thought to make it particularly appropriate for the lay audience for whom the vernacular translations were presumably intended. Some crucial Aristotelian concepts, highly relevant to the life of the Italian cities, would have been transmitted to the attentive reader of this shorter version. He would have learned that the art of governing a city is the highest of the arts, and one that should be exercised only by adults mature in character as well as years.[40] He would have been taught, too, that life in society is natural to man, or in the French and Italian versions that it is natural for man to be a citizen; and that the character of the government affects the character of the citizenry.[41] The statement in the Latin that there are three ways of life, namely, the way of concupiscence and pleasure, the way of probity and honor, and the way of learning and wisdom, is transmuted in the French and Italian into the assertion that besides the life of concupiscence, there are "the life of the citizen, which is one of probity and honor" and the contemplative life.[42] From the compendium could have been gathered also the ideas that material goods are necessary for happiness and that virtue consists in a mean between extremes.[43]

---

[39] *Aristoteles Latinus*, 1:67-71.

[40] The Latin and Italian passages are printed side by side in Marchesi, "Il compendio volgare dell'Etica aristotelica," pp. 38-39.

[41] Ibid., pp. 42, 44, 58.   [42] Ibid., p. 42.

[43] Ibid., pp. 48, 58.

To the extent that Taddeo prepared or contributed to the Italian version of the *Ethics*, he was participating in a widespread movement to disseminate the fruits of Latin learning to the growing audience for didactic as well as literary works in the vernacular. Dante's reservations about the value of translations as free and as oversimplified as the vernacular *Etica* were not characteristic of his age, which eagerly seized any fragments of classical culture that could conceivably be held to have relevance to contemporary life. In Dante's and Taddeo's time, translation and adaptation, whether from the Latin original or from a French intermediary, were often synonymous terms.[44]

DINO DEL GARBO AND GUIDO CAVALCANTI

Whatever may have been Taddeo's precise role or method in the production of the vernacular *Etica*, he clearly shared some of the interests of the circle of Brunetto Latini. In the next generation, a similar link between one of Taddeo's pupils and the group of scholarly Tuscan poets of the "*dolce stil nuovo*," poets who were themselves influenced by Brunetto, is to be found in the shape of Dino del Garbo's commentary upon the poem "Donna mi prega."[45] There is no evidence for any personal connection between the physician and the poet, although it is possible that in his youth Dino was acquainted with Guido, his older contemporary. Dino almost certainly knew another Tuscan poet, the jurist Cino da Pistoia, who was his colleague in 1322 at Siena, where the number of professors was probably small.[46]

Although he was among the earliest, Dino del Garbo was by no means the only fourteenth-century Italian author to find the learned and philosophical poetry of the *scuola stilnovistica* worthy of scholarly commentary.[47] Cavalcanti's poem is a recondite piece of work, studded with allusions to natural science, astrology, and metaphysics; the poet's declared

[44] See the valuable discussion of "La prosa del Duecento," and "I volgarizzamenti del Due e Trecento," in Cesare Segré, *Lingua, stile e società*, pp. 13-78.

[45] On Cavalcanti and his school, see Giorgio Petrocchi, "Il Dolce stil nuovo," *Storia della letteratura italiana*, 1:729-774, and especially 747-759, and bibliography there cited. For a critical text of "Donna mi prega" and discussion of the manuscript tradition, see Guido Favati, "La tradizione manoscritta di 'Donna mi prega,'" *Giornale storico della letteratura italiana* 70 (1953):417-494. The text of the poem is also printed in Bird, "The Canzone d'Amore of Cavalcanti," pp. 155-157, and in numerous other editions.

[46] *Chartularium Studii Senensis*, 1:245.

[47] The best-known example being Dante's *Convivio*; but works in this category also

intention was to explain the nature of love to men of understanding who brought to the subject not only refined emotional sensibilities, but also sophisticated and instructed intelligence:

> Et al presente conoscente chero,
> perch'io non spero ch'uom de basso core
> ad tal ragione porti conoscenza.

It is readily comprehensible why Dino, with his reputation for learning in natural philosophy, would have been attracted by such a poem. The production of a commentary in Latin presumably indicates that Dino believed at least some of his colleagues or students would share his interest and value his exposition of the poem. As already suggested, Dino's evident approval of Cavalcanti's definition of love may have been one of the grounds for dissension between him and Cecco d'Ascoli, who was highly critical of Cavalcanti's views on the subject.[48]

Since Dino's commentary has been exhaustively analyzed, no attempt will be made here to supply more than a few general remarks concerning it.[49] Dino announced at the beginning of his exposition that the intention of the poet was to explain the nature of love according to the laws of natural and moral science and of astrology. If we judge by his citations, Dino seems to have amplified Guido's explanation mainly by drawing upon Aristotle's natural works, especially *De anima* (cited five times) and the treatises on animals (cited twice). The *libri morales* are named three times, once each for the *Ethics*, the *Politics*, and the *Rhetoric*. The only other authors cited by Dino are the Arab astrological writer Haly Rodohan, who commented upon Ptolemy's *Quadripartitum*; Haly Abbas, the author of a widely used medical encyclopedia; and unnamed *medici*, the foremost of whom was probably Avicenna.[50] Dino referred to no modern authors by name, other than to Guido Cavalcanti himself.

---

include pseudo-Colonna's commentary on "Donna mi prega," Benvenuto da Imola's commentary on Dante's *Comedy*, and others.

[48] "Errando scrisse Guido Cavalcanti . . . ," *Acerba* 3.1.

[49] The edition of Otto Bird, cited in note 3 to this chapter, includes a lengthy study of the work. The commentary is also edited in Guido Favati, "La glossa latina di Dino del Garbo a 'Donna mi prega' del Cavalcanti," *Annali della Scuola Normale Superiore di Pisa* 21 (1952):72-103; this edition apparently corrects that of Bird in some respects, but is much less accessible to most North American readers.

[50] As is demonstrated by Bird, "The Canzone d'Amore of Cavalcanti," p. 194; Dino's labors as a commentator on Avicenna would in any case lead one to the same conclusion.

The nature and sources of some of the ideas that Dino expressed in this commentary have aroused vigorous controversy. The debate has centered on the issues of whether poem and commentary can be said to have an "Averroist" (or radical Aristotelian) cast and, if so, whether the Averroism is Cavalcanti's or Dino del Garbo's.[51] The controversial passage is one in which, in the course of expanding Cavalcanti's account of the process of falling in love, Dino referred to the role of the *intellectus possibilis* (the possible intellect). After pointing out that Guido, responding to a lady's request for information about love, was not writing as the servile lover of "courtly" tradition, but as a master instructing his disciples,[52] Dino went on to assert that love grows out of the impression of the *species* of the beloved object upon the memory; it requires a certain natural disposition in the individual, which is in part produced by astral influences, but also involves the exercise of free will. Like the other passions, love is caused in the soul by sense impressions, in this case by the sight of a desired object; from the exterior senses the impression reaches the internal sensitive virtues—namely, fantasy, thought (*cogitativa*), and memory—and ultimately passes to the highest, in man, of the apprehensive powers, namely, the *virtus*, or *intellectus*, *possibilis*. (For views on cognition and sense perception in the school of Taddeo, see chapter seven.) But although knowledge of the beloved object may reside in the possible intellect, love itself cannot, for it is a specific corporeal passion, whereas the intellect is wholly nonmaterial and is concerned only with abstract thought ("*pura consideratio et apprehensio spiritualis*").

Nowhere in this passage did Dino explicitly endorse the key Averroist doctrine of the unicity of the possible intellect (monopsychism), although he did refer to the possible intellect as universal and incorruptible. He seems, however, to have aligned himself with those who considered the possible intellect as one of several forms of the body.[53] Dino also addressed himself to the subject of the human soul and its faculties in one of his medical works. Fuller discussion of the latter passage is reserved for a consideration of the medical uses of philosophy (chapter six), but it

---

[51] Nardi, "Noterella polemica," passim; and Favati, "Guido Cavalcanti, Dino del Garbo, e l'Averroismo di Bruno Nardi," passim. Scholarly invective reaches remarkable heights in these articles.

[52] Bird, "The Canzone d'Amore of Cavalcanti," pp. 160, 162-165.

[53] "intellectus possibilis non est forma quae proveniat ex qualitatibus elementorum per admistionem eorum sicut proveniunt aliae formae corporeae," Dino, comm. Cavalcanti, in Bird, "The Canzone d'Amore of Cavalcanti," p. 165.

may be noted here that it appears to contain nothing obviously heterodox.[54]

Having examined the nature of love, Dino turned to its power and effect (*virtus* and *potentia*); love itself is not a virtue, but proceeds from a certain virtue of the soul. There are three senses in which the soul can be said to possess virtue—the term can be used for the soul's natural powers of intellect, will, fantasy, and so on; for its intellectual virtues such as wisdom, knowledge, or prudence; and for its moral virtues such as temperance, liberality, or fortitude—but love is not the fruit of any of these. It is rather an appetite of the sensitive soul, unregulated by reason. Dino then added a discussion, drawn from medical authors, of the physical effects of love, including its potentially lethal quality. He went on to enumerate its psychological effects, distinguishing passionate, erotic love from friendship, and noting the list of symptoms that had long since become traditional in both literary works and medical treatises.[55]

Dino's treatment of love is therefore concerned mainly with the application of Aristotelian psychology and metaphysics, and the medical tradition of the "lover's malady," to current literary conventions. Despite his use of the *Ethics*, his real concern with moral problems was minimal. His interest in actual personal relationships, social conditions, or mores is confined to two passages: in the first he carefully distinguished between a woman and a lady;[56] in the second he remarked that love is to be found more often among the wealthy and powerful than among their inferiors, possibly because the latter are chiefly preoccupied with the business of making a living, while the rich have more time on their hands. The observation, if one takes love to mean the highly ritualized cult of one's own emotions that was popularized by "courtly" lyrics and romance, is no doubt just. Dino went on to add that the noble and powerful give themselves more readily to love than do the poor, because they have the wealth and skills to attain the objects of their desires; moreover, women are more likely to return the love of someone noble than of someone of low degree. In Dino's view, poor people refrained from indulging passions that they knew would require substantial means to satisfy.[57] The remark exemplifies not so much Dino's cynicism or insensitivity, but the

---

[54] Such, at any rate was the opinion of Nardi; see his "Noterella polemica," pp. 52-54.

[55] Bird, "The Canzone d'Amore of Cavalcanti," pp. 123-136, and literature there cited.

[56] Dino, comm. Cavalcanti, in ibid., pp. 160-161.

[57] Ibid., pp. 170-171.

grip an essentially aristocratic literary cult held on the imagination of the educated classes in the Italian cities. The devotion to philosophy, which helped Dante to transform the conventions of "courtly love," evidently had no such effect upon Dino.

BARTOLOMEO DA VARIGNANA AND THE PSEUDO-ARISTOTELIAN ECONOMICS

Bartolomeo's Latin commentary on a text attributed to Aristotle is, obviously, a much more conventional production for a medieval university teacher than either a popularization of the *Ethics* to benefit the growing public for serious, didactic prose works in the vernacular, or the treatment of a vernacular love lyric as worthy of formal study by the learned. Yet here also is to be found evidence of interest in matters of current social concern.

The commentary appears to survive in a single manuscript, now the property of the Padri Redentoristi of the Chiesa della Fava in Venice.[58] The attribution to Bartolomeo is contained in the explicit, and it is implicitly supported by references to florins and ducats, indicating that the author was writing for an Italian audience, and by citations of medical authorities, which are sufficiently frequent to identify him as probably a physician.[59] This commentary is definitely not the work of Bartholomaeus de Brugis, another and better-known learned medical commentator on the *Economics* who flourished at Paris (and probably Montpellier) and who was approximately contemporary with Bartolomeo da Varignana.[60]

Bartolomeo da Varignana's work, unlike the productions of Taddeo and Dino considered in this chapter, is most likely a written redaction of

[58] See note 4 to this chapter. For a description of this manuscript, see my article "The *libri morales* in the Faculty of Arts and Medicine at Bologna: Bartolomeo da Varignana and the pseudo-Aristotelian *Economics*," in *Science, Medicine, and the University, 1200-1550: Essays in Honor of Pearl Kibre, Manuscripta* 20 (1976):105-118, where some of the following discussion also appeared.

[59] Ducats and florins: Venice, Padri Redentoristi, MS 3 (445), 14-15c, fols. 44v, 45v; citations of *Mesue, De appropriatis*, and of *De iuvamentis* [*membrorum*], ibid., fol. 33r; of Galen's *Tegni*, ibid., fol. 39r; of Isaac, *De dietis*, ibid., fol. 41r.

[60] Lohr, "Medieval Aristotle Commentaries," *Traditio* 23 (1967):375-376, where incipits and manuscript listings are given. I have compared the commentary attributed to Bartolomeo da Varignana with the questions and commentary of Bartholomaeus de Brugis as contained in Venice, Biblioteca Marciana, MS lat. VI, 82 (3019), fols. 105-154r.

lectures he gave in the faculty of arts and medicine at Bologna. Its pedagogical purpose is shown by the large amount of literal explication of Aristotle's text that it contains, especially in Books 1 and 3. It does not necessarily follow that the study of the *Economics* was, in Bartolomeo's day or thereafter, an essential part of the curriculum in arts and medicine. It seems more likely that individual masters enjoyed some liberty to introduce occasional courses upon works of particular interest to themselves or their students, whether or not these works were among those required for examination. Thus, the statutes of the student University of Arts and Medicine of Bologna, drawn up in 1405, provide for additional payments to masters who lectured *"extraordinarie"* upon certain books.[61] Most of the books named are listed elsewhere in the same set of statutes as required for the study of *"philosophia."*[62] Some, including the *Politics*, the *Ethics*, and the *Economics*, were not required. (A set of lectures on the brief *Economics* brought the master five Bolognese lire; one on the lengthy *Politics*, twenty.) A similar situation may well have prevailed a century earlier, during Bartolomeo's teaching career.

Several reasons can be suggested for this learned physician's interest in the *Economics*, a work chiefly concerned with *res familiaris*, the art of household management. Bartolomeo seems to have desired to limit the role of "philosophy" in general, and of Aristotle in particular, in advanced and specialized medical education (see chapter five, below); but this does not necessarily imply his rejection of the commonly accepted belief that the physician should undergo preliminary training in all the liberal arts and in philosophy. The existence of his commentary upon the *Economics* may signify Bartolomeo's preference for Aristotle as a philosopher in the broad sense rather than as a physiologist. And the *Economics* has a number of features that might have recommended it to any learned physician. It contains material on marriage, which would provide opportunity for discussion of the nature of love and human sexuality, topics that, as Dino del Garbo pointed out,[63] related both to natural and to moral philosophy, and that, as part of natural philosophy, were frequently treated by medical authors. Aristotle's supposed treatment of the relations of parents and children could be enriched by discussion of theories concerning generation and conception. And in a more practical

---

[61] Malagola, *Statuti*, p. 252, also cited in Rashdall, *Universities*, 1:241.

[62] Malagola, *Statuti*, pp. 274-277.

[63] Dino, comm. Cavalcanti, in Bird, "The Canzone d'Amore of Cavalcanti," p. 180.

vein, the art of household management might be thought to pertain to considerations of health. That the subject of *res familiaris* concerned physicians at the turn of the fourteenth century is demonstrated not only by the existence of the commentaries of Bartolomeo da Varignana and Bartholomaeus de Brugis on the Aristotelian *Economics*, but also by the translation into Latin in about 1300 of the pseudo-Galenic *Economics* by the physician Armengaudus Blasius of Montpellier.[64] In the latter work much attention is given to the health and care of children, as well as to the management of household affairs.

In addition to the foregoing, Bartolomeo da Varignana seems to have had interests less directly related to his medical background. In particular, he expatiated at some length upon questions of political thought and economic analysis, as will become apparent from the following brief summary.

The commentary opens with a proem in which the author asserts that moral philosophy is superior to every other *scientia philosophie*. The specific value of the study of *yconomica* is that it provides immediate guidance in the management of one's household and, indirectly, knowledge of politics and civic affairs (*"eorum que in politice seu civili tractantur"*). The commentary was written to instruct others and to aid the author's own understanding, as well as to bring him fame after death—the last perhaps a somewhat overoptimistic assertion. The main object of the commentary on the first book seems to be to point up the relationship of the *Economics* to the *Politics*, a work the author appears to have known thoroughly. From the *Politics* is introduced, for example, the idea that the government of the household is naturally and always monarchical, unlike that of the state. Since Book 1 of the *Economics*, although not the work of Aristotle, is believed to be an early Peripatetic compilation and is obviously based in large part on Book 1 of the *Politics*,[65] Bartolomeo easily found parallel or related passages. So frequent, indeed, are such passages that he was led to inquire whether it was superfluous to treat of *yconomica* as a separate discipline, since its parts were adequately covered in Book 1 of the *Politics*.[66] His conclusion was that a household could be

---

[64] The Latin text is edited in M. Plessner, *Der Oikonomikos des Neupythagoreers 'Bryson' und sein Einfluss auf die islamische Wissenschaft* (Heidelberg, 1928), pp. 205-213. I am grateful to Professor Josef Soudek for drawing my attention to this.

[65] Aristotle, *Oeconomica*, ed. F. Susemihl (Leipzig, 1887), intro., pp. v-ix.

[66] Venice, Padri Redentoristi, MS 3 (445), fol. 34r: "Queritur an hec scientia superflua."

considered either as an entity in its own right or as part of a state; if considered as the former, it is legitimate to speak of *yconomica* as distinct from *politica*. He added that *yconomica*, *politica*, and *ethica* are arts, not sciences, since they are directed to action rather than to understanding alone.

Despite his acceptance of a distinction between *yconomica* and *politica*, Bartolomeo continued to address political and social questions with implications extending well beyond the household. For example, he vigorously defended the natural basis of property rights, on the grounds that nature provides nutriment for imperfect animals and must therefore do the same for perfect ones; but the natural foods of man are bread, flesh, and wine, which are acquired through the ownership of land. In this passage no distinction is made between communal and private property, though it is clear from what follows that the author had private property in mind. His views may be contrasted to the well-known opinion of Thomas Aquinas, who maintained that the institution of private property is a human supplement to the natural right of all men to enjoy the fruits of the earth in common.[67] Also natural, according to Bartolomeo, is "secondary" possession, that is, ownership of precious metals with which can be purchased goods to supply natural needs. Since the ownership of the means of acquiring supplies has thus been shown to be natural, the ownership of animals for food and work is also justified.[68] Bartolomeo also accepted Aristotle's justification of slavery, which rested, first, on the assumed natural inferiority of some men, and second, on the legal disabilities imposed upon prisoners of war.[69] It may further be noted that for Bartolomeo the term *servus* comprised not only Aristotle's two categories of the naturally inferior and the legally enslaved, but also those who voluntarily proffer their services to great men and those who work for a daily wage.[70] Bartolomeo went on to claim, with Aristotle, that

[67] "si natura providet animalibus imperfectis de nutrimento multo magis et perfectis . . . sed alimentum hominis sunt panis, caro et vinum et tallia et homo naturaliter fruitur illis ad suum nutrimentum . . . sic ergo possessio secundum naturam naturaliter inest homini . . . agricultura immediate est homini naturalis possessio," ibid., fol. 36r. For the views of Thomas, *Summa theologiae* II-II, q. 66, a.2, ad primum.

[68] "ex quo aparet quod, cum ex animalibus supleatur maxime indigencie humane, quod [*sic*] possessio animalium inest homini secundum naturam," Venice, Padri Redentoristi, MS 3(445), fol. 36r.

[69] *Politics* 1.4-6.

[70] "quattuor species sunt servi secundum naturam, servi secundum leges, servi merce-

wars for the acquisition of slaves and cattle, and perhaps all wars for gain, are "perfectly natural and just."[71] Moreover, in a later passage he maintained that Aristotle's statements about the injustice of acquiring property by force should be understood only in reference to wars defined as unjust.[72]

Discussion of Aristotle's belief in the moral superiority of agriculture as a way of life led Bartolomeo to expatiate upon the advantages of recruiting peasants in time of war. He repeated the ancient truism that farm laborers, inured to rough living, meagre diet, and strenuous exercise, make much better soldiers than do urban artisans.[73]

The commentary on Book 1 also contains some fairly conventional prescriptions regarding the treatment of servants, which should be humane, and regarding the division of labor between husbands and wives. Of more interest are several folios devoted to a consideration of the relationship between husband and wife in terms of natural philosophy— namely, as a means whereby the perpetuation of the human race is ensured. After casually remarking that according to Aristotle the world is eternal[74] (apparently without feeling the need to provide a counterbalancing statement of his own orthodoxy), Bartolomeo proceeded to explain that, in the case of animals, the eternity is of the species, not the individual. The union of husband and wife is thus wholly natural and of the first importance; whence it follows that all men desire marriage, with the exception of some few who prefer to contemplate the divine. Moreover, man alone among the animals engages in sexual activity not out of blind instinct, but out of a conscious desire to produce offspring who will assist their parents in old age; and man alone regulates his sexual conduct according to principles of morality and discretion (however, Bartolomeo held the belief that domestic animals to some extent imitate man in this). There follows a lengthy discussion along medical

---

narii, et servi dillecti . . . sunt et dillecti, et hii maxime inveniuntur in curiis magnatum. sunt autem hii qui sponte serviunt alicui domino propter amorem," Venice, Padrı Redentoristi, MS 3 (445), fol. 40v.

[71] "Bella ergo et pugne que fuerint in acquisitione erunt maxime secundum naturam et iusta," ibid., fol. 36r, with a citation of *Politics* 1.8. The scribe has added "horum" in the *margin.*

[72] "non acquiruntur impie nec violenter sicut illa que belice acquiruntur et intelligendum est de bello iniusto," ibid.

[73] Ibid., fol. 36v.

[74] "secundum philosophum . . . mundus videtur esse perpetuus," ibid., fol. 37r.

lines of the influence of the seasons upon conception, the best ages for parenthood in men and women, and other physiological matters. It is, of course, in this section of the work that the author's medical learning is most fully displayed.[75] Further discussion of the relations between husband and wife occupies his commentary on Book 3, where the subject is taken up from a psychological and moral standpoint. In this last book the commentator hews fairly closely to the supposedly Aristotelian text.

The main interest of the commentary lies in Bartolomeo's treatment of Book 2, not only on account of the apparent absence of other Latin expositions of this portion of the work,[76] but also because the commentator here engages in fairly free discussion of economic concepts. The dearth of commentaries on the genuine Book 2 of the *Economics*, of which there exists a Greek text, may be due not only to the restricted circulation of this part of the work,[77] but also to the subject matter of Book 2 itself. Whereas Books 1 and 3 both relate to the art of household management and to family life, the text of Book 2 consists almost entirely of an unrelated series of anecdotes about ways in which various rulers of antiquity managed public finance. This series of examples would be difficult or impossible to make into the subject of a detailed scholastic commentary, and it is, in any case, as Bartolomeo remarked, "not very useful for those [individuals in private life] who are looking for a lot of money."[78] He therefore resolved the problem of providing an appropriate

---

[75] Ibid., fols. 38v-39v.

[76] Siraisi, "The *libri morales* in the Faculty of Arts and Medicine at Bologna," p. 109.

[77] The two principal Latin versions of the *Economics* are the so-called *translatio vetus*, perhaps dating from the mid-thirteenth century, and that of Durandus, produced in 1295. The former, on which Bartolomeo da Varignana based his commentary, includes all three books of the work, the latter only the first and third, which in medieval manuscripts of and commentaries upon the *recensio Durandi* are frequently numbered *primus* and *secundus*. No Greek manuscript is extant of Book 3 (*liber secundus*, according to the tradition of the *recensio Durandi*). See further, *Aristoteles Latinus*, 1:75-77; Josef Soudek, "The Genesis and Tradition of Leonardo Bruni's Annotated Latin Version of the (Pseudo-) Aristotelian *Economics*," *Scriptorium* 12 (1958):260-68; the same author's "Leonardo Bruni and His Public: A Statistical and Interpretative Study of his Annotated Latin Version of the (Pseudo-)Aristotelian *Economics*," *Studies in Medieval and Renaissance History* 5 (1958):51-136; and Hermann Goldbrunner, "Durandus de Alvernia, Nicolaus von Oresme und Leonardo Bruni: Zu den Übersetzungen der pseudo-aristotelischen Ökonomik," *Archiv für Kulturgeschichte* 50 (1968):200-239. According to Soudek, "Leonardo Bruni and His Public," p. 64, the *recensio Durandi* was more widely known than the *translatio vetus*.

[78] "non esse multum utilles hiis qui volunt multam pecuniam," Venice, Padri Redentoristi, MS 3 (445), fol. 44r. See also Soudek, "Genesis and Tradition," pp. 267-268.

exposition of Book 2 by announcing his intention not to comment on
each of the Philosopher's examples, but instead to supply his readers
with more useful information concerning types of trading operations;
different monetary transactions and their licitness or illicitness; and ways
of making money.[79] In fact, after briefly explaining that trade can consist
of exchange of goods for goods, or of goods for money, or of money of
one currency for that of another, he proceeded to devote most of his
attention to the legitimacy of various types of monetary transactions and,
in particular, to usury.

Although he relied upon standard conceptions drawn from Aristotelian and Roman legal sources,[80] and although his conclusions were cau-
tiously phrased, Bartolomeo's treatment of usury seems relatively advanced. Having begun by stating that usury is always unnatural and
therefore unjust (on the Aristotelian grounds that money does not breed
as animals do), he then raised the answered two objections to this for-
mula. The first of these inquired how any voluntary action, such as the
willing payment of interest for a loan, could be inherently unjust, since
Aristotle had associated injustice with constraint and force.[81] To this the
reply was that free will can be conditioned, and that the borrower's will
to pay usurious charges is conditioned by his need for money. The other
objection pointed out the apparent inconsistency of allowing the taking
of a premium for the use of gold and silver as bullion or as objets d'art
(making it, for example, permissible to rent out a silver vase) while
forbidding a similar premium for the use of the same metals coined into
money. In reply to this, Bartolomeo produced a series of standard formulations.[82] He distinguished between loans for use and loans for exchange,
stating that, in the latter, ownership of goods passes to the borrower (a
concept deriving from Roman law), and that it is therefore illegitimate
to charge him a rental for the use of his own property. He also attempted

---

[79] "oportet providere quomodo commutationes fiant [?] . . . quot sint species pecunie
et que sunt licite et que non . . . quot sint modi lucrandi particulares," Venice, Padri
Redentoristi, MS 3 (445), fol. 44r.

[80] See John T. Noonan, *The Scholastic Analysis of Usury* (Cambridge, Mass., 1957),
pp. 38-81, for discussion of the development of these concepts by canonists and theologians
from the late twelfth century.

[81] "videtur quod uxura sit iusta et licita. quia quod voluntarie fit etiam ipso petente,
hoc videtur esse iustum . . . maior patet ex hoc. quia violentum secundum philosophum
primo politice est iniustum. ergo per oppositum voluntarium est iustum," Venice, Padri
Redentoristi, MS 3 (445), fol. 45r.

[82] See Noonan, *Scholastic Analysis of Usury*, pp. 38ff.

to develop a reply based on metaphysics, pointing out that being in the form of coins is accidental for silver, but of the essence of money; so the same regulations should not necessarily be expected to apply to silver and to silver coin. But the most striking feature of this author's treatment of the subject of usury is not his theoretical analysis, but his pragmatic conclusion that without interest-bearing loans many of the indigent would perish and that cities and kingdoms would fare badly indeed if they could not get money on loan, "as is self-evident"; thus it is that the "legislator" tolerates the lesser evil in the state in order to avoid the greater.[83]

It appears likely that the immediate source of Bartolomeo's ideas about usury was the teaching of contemporary Bolognese professors of canon and civil law, a supposition borne out by Bartolomeo's own references to the views of the "*juriste*."[84] Among these Joannes Andreae,[85] in particular, has been shown to have given considerable thought to the problem of usury in society and to have moved tentatively toward some justification of interest-bearing loans.[86] For our purposes, it is interesting to note the implied existence of common intellectual concerns in the faculties of law and of arts and medicine at Bologna. The same social problems, discussed in legal terms by the jurists, could be treated in the faculty of arts and medicine in terms of moral philosophy. Moreover, in each case these discussions represented an academic response to current social realities.

The commentary on Book 2 of the *Economics* concludes with a list of five ways of getting a profitable livelihood. These are: *possessorius*, or as a landowner, from the revenues of agricultural property; *mercatorius*, from long-distance commerce, either by land or sea, whether engaged in as a principal or an employee; *mercenarius*, from local trade in foodstuffs raised by oneself; *experimentalis*, by which Bartolomeo apparently meant the use of special knowledge acquired from experience to corner a market, a process he described as highly lucrative and perfectly just; and *artificialis*, through the exercise of an art, such as that of a physician.[87]

---

[83] "multi indigentes possent sine pecunia periclitari ymo civitates et regna quoniam se male haberent nisi pecuniam mutuo invenirent, ut de se patet. hinc quod legislator ad minus malum consentit in civitate," Venice, Padri Redentoristi, MS 3 (445), fol. 45v.

[84] Ibid.

[85] He had begun to teach canon law at Bologna by 1302, and died in 1348. See J. F. von Schulte, *Die Geschichte der Quellen und Literatur des canonischen Rechts* (repr. Graz, 1956), 2:205-229, for his career and writings.

[86] Noonan, *Scholastic Analysis of Usury*, pp. 65-67.

[87] Venice, Padri Redentoristi, MS 3 (445), fol. 46r.

The first four of these categories are loosely based on *Politics* 1.8-11, 1256a1-1259a35, although Bartolomeo seems far from sharing Aristotle's disdain for commerce. He refers approvingly to Aristotle's anecdote about the philosopher Thales, who supposedly used his meteorological knowledge to fiscal advantage by securing a monopoly of oil presses at harvest time, a story Aristotle may have intended as a warning rather than as a good example. The fifth category perhaps reflects the development of medical and legal professionalism in the university centers of northern Italy in the thirteenth and early fourteenth centuries. Also listed are the qualities necessary for the successful conduct of business and professional affairs, namely, ingenuity, hard work, honesty, sophistication regarding the wiles of merchants, and good physical condition.[88]

In the hands of a professor of medicine, a commentary on the *Economics* might be expected to become largely a vehicle for a physiological or psychological discussion of human nature and for advice on family regimen. These elements are of course present in Bartolomeo's commentary; but, as the foregoing account indicates, they were by no means the writer's only, or necessarily even his principal, concerns. His announced intention to provide practical guidance as well as academic analysis, and his pragmatic and businesslike approach to socioeconomic and ethical problems, indicate that he also valued the *Economics* and the art of *yconomica* as a source of guidance concerning problems that he or his readers might encounter outside the classroom in their roles as citizens, property owners, and professional men. The academic culture of the faculties of arts and medicine was, after all, rooted in the economic and social life of the north Italian cities; in this environment, the professors of medicine and learned medical authors were at the same time members of a propertied citizen oligarchy, professional practitioners with a living to get, and, often, married laymen with households to manage. For the student of arts and medicine, who might hope to follow a similar career, the study of the *Economics* with the aid of this commentary was doubtless a worthwhile project.

Revealing though the works discussed in this chapter may be when considered as examples of the thought and activity of members of a learned profession in the earliest years of the Italian Renaissance, they

---

[88] Ibid., fol. 43v.

do not, of course, represent the chief intellectual preoccupations of Taddeo and his fellow authors. These masters were primarily concerned not with civic life, or with literature, or with moral (or even with natural) philosophy, but with medicine considered as a branch of higher learning. The vast bulk of their works concern medicine, and it is to these works and to the scope of their medical teaching that we must now turn if we wish to identify the ideas that were central to their thought.

CHAPTER FOUR

THE DEVELOPMENT OF A
MEDICAL CURRICULUM

I*n the span of about sixty years in which Taddeo and some of his pupils were teaching at Bologna, the scope of academic medical instruction expanded in important ways. Some of the changes may* have originated with Taddeo or his successors and subsequently spread to other centers of medical learning; others Taddeo and his disciples, who participated fully in current intellectual trends, adopted from elsewhere. There are, however, two ways in which Taddeo and those he taught may be credited with having a significant influence upon the development of medical education in the schools of western Europe. The first of these particularly concerns the *studium* of Bologna. At Bologna, some members of this group of masters unquestionably helped to give the medical curriculum the shape that it retained, with modifications, through the sixteenth century. There is little doubt that they introduced the study of particular books, that they developed new forms of practical demonstration, and that they played a part in developing regulations governing medical study. After Taddeo himself, those most influential in this regard were probably Bartolomeo and Mondino, who both taught at Bologna for substantial periods of time and held positions of political importance in the city, and perhaps Guglielmo, who is known to have been interested in curricular development and who held (in absentia, it is true) the position of archdeacon of Bologna, which gave him some responsibility for the schools. The high repute of Bologna as a center of medical learning no doubt ensured the imitation of the content and organization of its curriculum elsewhere.

The second kind of influence was exerted when works written by members of the group were studied in other schools. As an example, one may cite Dino del Garbo's commentaries on portions of the *Canon* of Avicenna. If we judge by the number and distribution of extant manuscripts,[1] these were among the most widely read works produced by Taddeo or

---

[1] Based on a survey of entries in TK.

any of his known pupils. The full reception of Avicenna in the medical schools, an enormously important event in late medieval medical education, was certainly fostered by Dino's efforts, but cannot be linked in any specific way with curricular development at Bologna. As we shall see, however, it is quite likely that Dino's interest in interpreting Avicenna was inspired by Taddeo's own early and fragmentary efforts in that direction.

In what follows, therefore, we shall attempt to trace the sources and nature of the medical curriculum from which Taddeo and his associates taught, and we shall attempt to determine the extent of their own contribution to curricular development.

In large part, the medical learning of the members of Taddeo's circle was, like the learning of their contemporaries in other fields, a body of knowledge transmitted through the study of authoritative texts. By the time the student university and the doctoral college of the Bolognese faculty of arts and medicine were formally established, a substantial corpus of Latin texts suitable for the handing down of medical learning in an academic setting, with the aid of lecture and commentary, had long been available and in use in the major schools of western Europe. As is well known, the few Hippocratic, Galenic, and other ancient medical treatises existing in Latin versions in the early Middle Ages were supplemented during the late eleventh and twelfth centuries by new translations of material from Arabic sources, through the efforts of Constantinus Africanus and others.[2] Not all of these works were, however, equally suitable for teaching purposes, at any rate in the eyes of twelfth-century medical masters. They preferred treatises long known in the West in one version or another that were short, somewhat simplified in medical content, and aphoristic in presentation. Recently, much evidence has been brought to light concerning the formation during the twelfth century of

[2] For the Hippocratic tradition in the Middle Ages, see Pearl Kibre, "Hippocratic Writings in the Middle Ages," *Bulletin of the History of Medicine* 18 (1945):371-412, and her "Hippocrates Latinus: Repertorium of Hippocratic Writings in the Latin Middle Ages," *Traditio* 31 (1975):99-126; 32 (1976):257-292; 33 (1977):253-295; 34 (1978):193-226, and subsequent issues. For early medieval Galenism, Augusto Beccaria, "Sulle tracce di un antico canone latino di Ippocrate e di Galeno," *Italia medioevale e umanistica* 4 (1961): 1-75, and 14 (1971):1-23; Owsei Temkin, *Galenism*; Richard J. Durling, "Corrigenda and Addenda to Diels' Galenica," *Traditio* 23 (1967):463-476. On the reception of Arabic medicine, Heinrich Schipperges, *Die Assimilation der arabischen Medizin durch das lateinische Mittelalter.*

a core curriculum in medicine and, in particular, the forging of that renowned teaching tool the *ars medicine*, or *articella*.[3] The *articella*, a collection of short treatises, underwent some variations in content and sequence in different times and places. It appears to have been formed
around the medical *Isagoge* of Johannitius, to which were subsequently
added the *Aphorisms* and *Prognostica* of Hippocrates and short works
on urine and pulse; later still, the *Tegni* (*Microtechne, Ars parva*) of
Galen, and, in the thirteenth century, the *De regimine acutorum* of
Hippocrates were also added. The early versions of the collection may
have been formed at Salerno, but the latest version, which incorporates
material translated by the Toledan school and not known in Italy before
the thirteenth century, is probably of transalpine origin. Versions of the
articella were early used at Chartres, Paris, and Montpellier, as well as at
Salerno, and the treatises of the collection have been shown to have become standard subjects of commentary in the later twelfth and thirteenth
centuries.[4]

The *articella* was probably introduced into northern Italy by Petrus
Hispanus (Pope John XXI, d. 1277). Petrus studied both in southern
Italy or Sicily under Master Theodore, astrologer to Emperor Frederick
II, and in Paris, and was teaching medicine at Siena in 1246. Petrus
commented on every work in the complete *articella* collection.[5] However,

[3] See P. O. Kristeller, "The School of Salerno: Its Development and Its Contribution to
the History of Learning," in his *Studies in Renaissance Thought and Letters*, pp. 495-551;
idem, "Nuove fonte par la medicina salernitana del secolo XII," *Rassegna storica salernitana*
18 (1957):61-75; idem, "Beiträge der Schule von Salerno zur Entwicklung der scholastischen Wissenschaft im 12 Jahrhundert," in *Artes Liberales, von der antiken Bildung zur
Wissenschaften des Mittelalters*, ed. Josef Koch (Leiden, 1959), pp. 84-90; and, most
recently, idem, "Bartholomaeus, Musandinus, and Maurus of Salerno and Other Early
Commentators of the 'Articella,' with a Tentative List of Texts and Manuscripts," *Italia
medioevale e umanistica* 19 (1976):57-87. See also Morris H. Saffron, ed. and trans.,
*Maurus of Salerno Twelfth-Century "Optimus Physicus," with His Commentary on the
Prognostics of Hippocrates*, pp. 8-9, and bibliography there cited; also Kibre, "Hippocratic
Writings in the Middle Ages."

[4] Kristeller, "Bartholomaeus, Musandinus, and Maurus of Salerno," passim; Saffron,
Maurus of Salerno and Maurus' commentary on the *Aphorisms*, in S. de Renzi et al., eds.,
Collectio Salernitana, vol. 4 (1856); and Rudolf Creutz, ed. and trans., *Die medizinisch-
naturphilosophischen Aphorismen und Kommentare des Magister Urso Salernitanus*, Quellen
und Studien zur Geschichte der Naturwissenschaften und der Medizin (Berlin, 1936), text
of commentary at 5:18-130.

[5] See Sybil D. Wingate, *The Mediaeval Latin Versions of the Aristotelian Scientific Corpus, with Special Reference to the Biological Works*, p. 79; and Kristeller, "Bartholomaeus,
Musandinus, and Maurus of Salerno," pp. 80-81.

the introduction of the *articella* to Bologna may have been the work of Taddeo himself; Taddeo commented on five of the seven treatises and was apparently the only thirteenth-century author associated with a north Italian school, other than Petrus, to expound the collection extensively. The version of the texts used by Taddeo seem to have included Galen's commentaries on the Hippocratic works.[6] All of the five younger physicians in Taddeo's circle also commented on one or more of the *articella* works.[7] Although the lack of early statutory lists prescribing the books required of medical students at Bologna in the late thirteenth and early fourteenth centuries makes it impossible to say precisely which works then constituted the official medical curriculum, it seems highly probable that all the works commented on by the masters here discussed served as textbooks at one time or another, but that the texts of the *articella* were of the first importance. Furthermore, in the hands of the Salerno masters the commentaries on the *articella* had quite frequently served as vehicles for the introduction of a good deal of natural philosophy and scholastic methodology into medical teaching;[8] so their suitability as texts in a faculty "of arts and medicine" was established.

The name of Hippocrates was held in the highest respect, although Taddeo's pupils were less prolific than their master in the output of Hippocratic commentary. Taddeo was, as we have just seen, the author of three lengthy commentaries on works attributed to Hippocrates, and his scholarly reputation was based primarily on his interpretation of that

---

[6] On the translations and influence of these Galenic commentaries, see Kristeller, "Bartholomaeus, Musandinus, and Maurus of Salerno," pp. 67-68.

[7] Mondino on the *Tegni*, *Prognostica*, and *De regimine acutorum*; Turisanus on the *Tegni*; Dino on the *Tegni*; Bartolomeo on the *Tegni*; and Guglielmo on part of the *Aphorisms*. See Bibliography for manuscripts and editions.

[8] Kristeller, "The School of Salerno," pp. 515-518. Saffron (*Maurus of Salerno*, p. 92) notes that Maurus (d. 1214) was familiar with (probably from the Aristotelian translations of Boethius) and made use of the terms *universalis, particularis, accidentalis, potentialis, actualis, opifex, substantia, forma*; see also Saffron's introduction, pp. 12-13, for discussion of the natural scientific and philosophical interests of the Salernitan masters. See also Aleksander Birkenmajer, "Le rôle joué par les médecins et les naturalistes dans la reception d'Aristote au xiie et xiiie siècles," in his *Études d'histoire des sciences et de la philosophie au moyen âge*, Studia Copernicana, 1:73-87. Particularly striking is the philosophical tone of Urso of Salerno, who dominated the medical school there from ca. 1200; for example, "Perspicuae rationi patet fidelium, quod universum rerum et invariable manet principium effectivum, cuius admirabili potentia visibilia et invisibilia sunt condita universa, eius que inscrutabili sapientia conditas formas et virtutes varias inseruit prout voluit," Creutz, *Urso Salernitanus*, p. 19 (see note 4, above).

author. Of his pupils and associates, Guglielmo, Bartolomeo, Mondino, and Dino appear to have written Hippocratic commentaries. As noted, Guglielmo and Bartolomeo wrote on the *Aphorisms*; Mondino on the *Prognostica* and *De regimine acutorum*. In the opening of the former he listed nine works of Hippocrates, explained their relevance to different aspects of medical learning, and recommended diligent study of their content.[9] He noted, for example, that among these nine treatises both *De natura humana* and *De natura fetus* provided information about the origins of the human body, the former being concerned with its remote origins (that is, the elements) and the latter with its immediate origins— namely, semen and menstrual blood. *De natura fetus* was itself the subject of commentary by Dino del Garbo, who also left a fragment of commentary on the *Aphorisms*. His exposition, the only known Latin commentary on this particular Hippocratic work, is also the only Hippocratic commentary produced by one of the masters under discussion that is not based on one of the treatises normally included in the *articella*. Moreover, only the works of Hippocrates found in the *articella*—the *Aphorisms*, the *Prognostica*, and *De regimine acutorum*—made their way into the mandatory curriculum at Bologna as it was recorded in the university statutes of 1405.[10]

In the work of Taddeo and his associates, one can also detect signs of less traditional interests, most notably a desire to study more of the works of Galen. As just noted, Galenic teaching in some form was always central to the medieval medical tradition. But although the short summaries of Galen's doctrine contained in the *Tegni* and the *Isagoge* of Johannitius were by the twelfth century standard textbooks in European medical schools and although many Galenic concepts were transmitted via the writings of Arabic physicians, a number of Galen's longer, more detailed, and more complex treatises on physiology and disease, translated into Latin during the twelfth century, were not at first the subject of much scholarly commentary. The assimilation of such works as *De locis affectis*, of the treatises on diseases known to the Middle Ages as *De accidenti et morbo*, and of *De virtutibus* (or *facultatibus*) *naturalibus* into the regular medical curriculum appears to have begun in the second half of the

[9] BAV, MS Vat. lat. 4466, fol. 1r. For the works named, see Appendix Two, below. Mondino's list may be compared with earlier listings of the works of Hippocrates and the order in which they should be studied; see Beccaria, "Sulle tracce," pp. 73-74.

[10] Malagola, *Statuti*, pp. 274-276.

thirteenth century and to owe much to the activities of the physicians of Bologna.[11]

In the circle of Taddeo, this new Galenism involved not only close study and commentary upon some of the longer Galenic treatises that had been translated into Latin in the preceding century, but also listing and collecting such works of the Galenic corpus as were available and noting titles attributed to Galen (by himself or others), but not accessible for study. These achievements, like those of Peter of Abano in translating a few more of Galen's minor works,[12] may seem slight when compared with the great monument of early fourteenth-century Galenism, namely, Niccolò da Reggio's translation of *De usu partium* (not known, as far as I can determine, to any of Taddeo's pupils).[13] They are nonetheless far from negligible, and they may have given rise to innovations of lasting significance in the Bologna medical curriculum.

Thus, for example, Taddeo himself compared two Latin translations of Galen's *De interioribus* (as *De locis affectis* was known in the Middle Ages), a book that provides a detailed account of Galen's system of internal medicine, along with much information about Galenic physiology in general. Taddeo went through the entire work, adding marginalia indicating where the translations differed and which was to be preferred. The results of his labors are found in a collection of twenty-one treatises by Galen copied in the fourteenth century; translators' names are indi-

[11] A survey of index entries in TK reveals the existence of few or no medieval Latin commentaries on any of these works antedating those produced by Taddeo and his pupils. While no commentary on *De virtutibus naturalibus* can definitely be ascribed to any of the physicians who are the subject of this book, a fragment of an anonymous commentary is included in BAV, MS Vat. lat. 4452, fols. 129-131, where it is found with medical works of Bartolomeo da Varignana and Albertus, that is, probably Alberto da Bologna (Albertus de Zancharus). The only other known commentary is that of Nicholas of Bologna (TK 1626, 1687), who is probably to be identified with Mondino's pupil Niccolò Bertruccio (see Introduction, above).

[12] Lynn Thorndike, "Translations of the Works of Galen from the Greek by Peter of Abano," *Isis* 33 (1942):649-653.

[13] Niccolò's version of *De usu partium* was finished in 1317 and apparently put into circulation in 1322, when he dedicated it to King Robert; see Galen, *On the Usefulness of the Parts of the Body*, trans. Margaret T. May (Ithaca, 1968), 1:6 (intro.). On Niccolò as a translator, see also Lynn Thorndike, "Translations of Works of Galen from the Greek by Niccolò da Reggio (ca. 1308-1345)," *Byzantina Metabyzantina* 1 (1946):213-235. The translations of Niccolò da Reggio, including *De usu partium*, were apparently known to the author of a commentary on Avicenna's chapter in the *Canon* "de generatione embrionis" ascribed to Dino del Garbo in an edition printed at Venice in 1502—but this work is not in reality Dino's; see note 142 to chapter six, below, and Bibliography.

cated in several instances—William of Moerbeke, Mark of Toledo, and Burgundio of Pisa.[14] It is probable that not only Taddeo's version of *De interioribus*, but also the whole codex, is evidence of a growing concern in the schools of Bologna for the firsthand study of authentic works of Galen.

One of the two known Latin commentaries on *De interioribus* (and the only one of Italian provenance) was written by Bartolomeo da Varignana.[15] It does not seem farfetched to suggest that the incorporation of this work into the Bologna curriculum, in which it was a statutory text by 1405,[16] in fact occurred much earlier as a result of the interest of Taddeo and Bartolomeo.

The case may be similar with *De accidenti et morbo*. Only four Latin expositions of this set of works appear to survive: the commentary by Bartolomeo da Varignana; a commentary and questions (dated 1319) by Antonio da Parma, a philosopher and physician who probably taught medicine at Bologna; a commentary by Alberto da Bologna (Albertus de Zanchariis), who was the *socius* of Antonio da Parma and an associate of Mondino de' Liuzzi, and who was himself a professor of medicine at Bologna;[17] and an anonymous commentary.[18] The possibility that the

[14] BAV, MS Urb. lat. 247. The codex is described in Cosimo Stornaiolo, *Codices urbinates latini* (Rome, 1902), 1:236-238. At fol. 281v: "Explicit liber de interioribus G correptus per magistrum Tadeum." Regarding the two translations used by Taddeo, see Durling, "Corrigenda and Addenda to Diels' Galenica," pp. 466-467, no. 60a.

[15] The other was by Johannes de Sancto Amando. See TK 760.

[16] Malagola, *Statuti*, p. 275.

[17] Questions by Antonio da Parma on *De accidenti et morbo* are contained in BAV, MS Vat. lat. 4450, 14c, beginning at fol. 73r. Antonio was probably also the author of the immediately preceding commentary on the same work, inc. (fol. 57r) "In principio huius libri sicut in principio aliorum nos oportet inquirere quatuor causas eius." The same commentary is also found anonymously in BAV, MS Vat. lat. 4466, 14c, inc. (fol. 157r) "In initio huius libri morbum diffiniri oportet. In principio istius libri sicut in principio aliorum nos oportet inquirere quatuor causas eius"; and in Munich, Bayerische Staatsbibliothek, CLM 13020, a. 1319, fols. 88v-94r (I have compared the opening sections). In the *Catalogus codicum manu scriptorum Bibliothecae Regiae Monacensis* (Munich, 1876, repr. Wiesbaden, 1968), vol. 4, pt. 2, p. 93, the work in CLM 13020 is ascribed to Mondino, but this appears to be the result of a misreading of the explicit of the previous work in the codex, Mondino's *Anatomia*. For the possible connections of Antonio da Parma with Bologna, see note 2 to the Introduction of this work; see also Anneliese Maier, *An der Grenze von Scholastik und Naturwissenschaft*, p. 81. For the relationship of Alberto da Bologna (Albertus de Zanchariis) with Antonio da Parma, see note 2 to the Introduction. Albertus' commentary on *De accidenti et morbo* is contained in BAV, MS Reg. lat. 2000, 14c, fols. 28r-73r.

[18] BAV, MS Vat. lat. 4454, fols. 3-54r, inc. "Intencio huius libri, etc. iste liber primo

last-named work originated in the circle of Taddeo is quite strong, since it occurs in a fourteenth-century codex also containing works of Dino del Garbo and Bartolomeo da Varignana, as well as Gentile da Cingoli's *reportatio* of his Parisian master's lectures on *De animalibus. De accidenti et morbo*, therefore, seems to have been the subject of a good deal of attention at Bologna in the early fourteenth century and probably entered the formal curriculum at that time; it, too, appears in 1405 as a statutory text.[19]

The foregoing does not exhaust the Galenic commentary produced in Taddeo's circle. In addition to the treatments of *De interioribus* and *De accidenti et morbo* just mentioned, and to the commentaries on the *Tegni* produced by every physician in the group except Guglielmo da Brescia, Taddeo commented on *De crisi* and *De differentiis febrium*; Bartolomeo on *De complexionibus*[20] (again, his is one of the earliest Latin commentaries); Dino, apparently three times, on *De malicia complexionis diverse* (attributed to Galen) and on *De differentiis febrium* (see Bibliography). Dino also complained about the lack of Galen's authentic *De semine* and *De spermate* (see chapter six).

In the context of the Galenic interests of Taddeo's circle, a bibliography of works from which theoretical medicine might be studied, which was drawn up by Bartolomeo da Varignana, acquires a special significance.[21] It is a list that must be approached with caution, since it may represent no more than a record of the learning that Bartolomeo wished to be thought to possess. Nonetheless, it merits attention. Bartolomeo listed forty-seven medical books, eight of them being general works on the whole of medicine, and the remainder treatises on its specific aspects. The eight general works are, predictably enough: the *Aphorisms* of Hippocrates; the *Tegni* of Galen; and the *Isagoge* of Johannitius (the three treatises that formed the core of the *articella*); together with the major Arabic encyclopedias of particulars—the *Continens* of Rasis; the *Teisir* of Avenzoar; the *Liber regalis* (or *al-Maleki*) of Haly Abbas; the *Canon* of Avicenna; and the

---

dividitur in prohemium et tractatum secundum ibi *dico*. Ergo in prohemium dat intencionem suum."

[19] Malagola, *Statuti*, p. 275.

[20] One of the two twelfth-century Latin versions of this work is edited in *Galenus Latinus I: Burgundio of Pisa's Translation of Galen's "De complexionibus,"* ed. Richard J. Durling (Berlin-New York, 1976).

[21] BAV, MS Vat. lat. 4452, fols. 83v-84r. For the identification of this work as Bartolomeo's, see note 14 to chapter five.

Colliget of Averroes. Presumably, the highly compressed treatises of the *articella* were valued as works for general orientation, and the Arabic encyclopedias as works of reference. The most remarkable feature of the rest of the list is the heavy emphasis on works of Galen, which make up thirty of the thirty-nine treatises named. Bartolomeo indicated that five of these books were known to him by name only, presumably implying that he knew the rest at first hand. He also displayed some ability to distinguish between genuine and spurious works of Galen, noting the absence of Latin versions of authentic Galenic treatises on anatomy.[22] Also striking is Bartolomeo's knowledge of major treatises by Galen that appear not to have circulated very widely, although available in Latin— for example, *De interionibus* (on which, of course, he himself commented); and *De virtutibus naturalibus*, that is, *De facultatibus naturalibus*, which a recent writer has characterized as "a very important review of Galen's physiological principles."[23] It seems likely that the list was compiled while its author was still teaching at Bologna (that is, by 1311 at latest) and that his Galenism was not, therefore, inspired by the new wave of translations that began with the work of Peter of Abano (d. ca. 1316) and Niccolò da Reggio (active ca. 1308-1345).[24]

An even longer list of Galen's works than that compiled by Bartolomeo was written down, apparently also at Bologna and a few years after Bartolomeo wrote. It occurs on the last folio of the commentary of Alberto da Bologna ("Albertus Bononiensis," that is, Albertus de Zanchariis) on *De accidenti et morbo*. According to this author or his annotator, "the complete works of Galen are seventy-one in number."[25] Of the seventy-one titles listed, however, some twenty-two bear notations indi-

---

[22] For the list of Galenic works named by Bartolomeo, see Appendix Two, below. The titles that he listed while disclaiming direct knowledge were *De medicatione per anothomiam*, *De anatomia vivorum*, *De anatomia mortuorum*, *Antidotarius*, and *De plenitudine sive multitudine*; of the first three he remarked "Et nullum horum trium habemus . . . reffert tamen G. in fine tegni se ipsos fecisse." Regarding three short Latin treatises on anatomy which in the Middle Ages passed under Galen's name, see note 3 to Appendix Two, below.

[23] Rudolph E. Siegel, *Galen's System of Physiology and Medicine*, p. 22.

[24] Regarding the Galenic translations of Peter of Abano and Niccolò da Reggio, see Thorndike, "Translations of the Works of Galen from the Greek by Peter of Abano," and "Translations of Works of Galen from the Greek by Niccolò da Reggio" (notes 12 and 13, above).

[25] "sunt numero omnes libri G.71," BAV, MS Reg. lat. 2000, fol. 73r. The list is written as a marginal notation in an extremely cramped hand, and many of the titles are hard to read.

cating that the work in question was known only at second hand and stating where, in the works of Galen or other medical authors, reference to it could be found.

Thus, while Galen's major works on anatomy were still untranslated; and while knowledge of his thought was frequently obtained from highly compressed treatises such as the *Tegni* and from such compendia as the *Isagoge*, which sometimes distorted his meaning, or via the writings of Avicenna and other Arabic writers; nonetheless, when Taddeo and his pupils taught in Bologna, serious attention was given to determining the scope of Galen's output and to studying some of his longer works in their entirety.

Taddeo and his colleagues also played a part in the final stages of the two-hundred-year assimilation of Arabic medicine in the Latin West. In particular, Taddeo, Mondino, Guglielmo, and perhaps Bartolomeo, and above all Dino del Garbo were among the pioneers in the enormous task of commenting on the encyclopedic *Canon* of Avicenna (see Bibliography).[26] Taddeo, Mondino, and Guglielmo commented only on short sections of the *Canon*, but, as already noted, Dino has the distinction of apparently being the first Latin commentator to attempt a systematic analysis of substantial portions of that monumental work. The *Canon*, translated into Latin by Gerard of Cremona (d. 1187), was assimilated by learned physicians during the course of the thirteenth century; however, its use as a fundamental textbook for formal instruction within the university milieu presumably dates from the appearance of the earliest academic commentaries. Hence Dino and, to a lesser extent, the others mentioned were instrumental in securing for the *Canon* the dominant place in western European medical education that it retained until the

---

[26] Taddeo was not, however, the earliest Latin writer to attempt an analysis and exposition of parts of the work. According to an ascription in a fifteenth-century manuscript, Urso (of Salerno?) compiled an index to Book 2; and ca. 1280 Johannes de Sancto Amando commented on Avicenna's chapter on fevers (see TK 492, 361). That the contribution of Taddeo and some of his students to the reception of the *Canon* was recognized as significant by their successors in the Italian medical schools is suggested by the fact that Taddeo and Dino, along with Dino's younger contemporary Mondino da Cividale del Friuli, are the earliest authors named in an early fifteenth-century list of eight commentators on Book 1 of the Canon. The list also attributes a commentary on this part of the *Canon* to Bartolomeo da Varignana, but I have not succeeded in locating or finding any other reference to such a work. See Ernest Wickersheimer, "Une liste dressée au xv⁰ siècle des commentateurs du 1ᵉʳ livre du Canon d'Avicenne et du livre des Aphorismes d'Hippocrate," *Janus* 34 (1930):33-37.

seventeenth century. It is perhaps worth noting in this connection that the books of the *Canon* on which Dino did not comment, even in part— namely, Books 3 and 5—had not found their way into the Bolognese medical curriculum by 1405.

The works commented on by Taddeo and his students, show that the chief sources of their medical teaching were the aphoristic writings of Hippocrates, accompanied by Galenic commentary, the *Tegni*, several authentic and major works of Galen, and the *Canon* of Avicenna. Hippocrates, Galen, and Avicenna were regarded as preeminent authorities of equal weight; but in sheer bulk, Galen and Avicenna must have dominated the curriculum; and Avicenna, of course, incorporated much Galenic material into the *Canon*. It seems, therefore, that the claim that is now sometimes made that the Bolognese medical school of the early years of the fourteenth century knew relatively little of the authentic Galen holds good only for Galen's major treatises on anatomy.[27]

Furthermore, within the fairly short time span under consideration, sixty or so years, a progressive broadening of knowledge and interest can be detected. Whereas Taddeo chiefly produced lengthy commentaries on the *articella*, commented only upon fragments of the *Canon*, and studied but did not comment upon one of Galen's longer treatises (*De interioribus*), his pupils were a good deal more adventurous. All of them commented upon at least one *articella* work (they could scarcely escape doing so, given the already established position of the collection in medical education), but only Mondino on more than one. Instead, Dino tackled substantial portions of the *Canon*, Bartolomeo explored lesser-known works of Galen, and Guglielmo was apparently partially responsible for the introduction of a modern Galenic and Avicennan curriculum at the *studium* of Montpellier. That these activities filled a perceived need is indicated by Villani's remark, already noted, to the effect that Dino's commentaries on Avicenna became standard academic medical textbooks

[27] A very negative evaluation of the state of knowledge of authentic Galenic teaching in the medical schools of Bologna in the late thirteenth and early fourteenth centuries is to be found in Fridolf Kudlien, "Mondinos Standort innerhalb der Entwicklung der Anatomie," in Robert Herrlinger and Fridolf Kudlien, eds., *Frühe Anatomie: Eine Anthologie*, pp. 1-14; Markwart Michler holds that "true Galenism" in medieval medicine is not to be found before Guy de Chauliac, who completed his work on surgery in 1363 ("Guy de Chauliac als Anatom," in ibid., pp. 15-32). It is no doubt true, however, that anatomy was the weakest part of the Galenism of Taddeo's school. Owsei Temkin, while recognizing that "much of medieval Galenism rested on spurious works, excerpts and over simplifications," takes a somewhat more positive view than Kudlien and Michler (*Galenism*, p. 116).

in his lifetime; that they met with some resistance among conservatives is perhaps suggested by a clause in the papal bull, supposedly influenced by Guglielmo da Brescia, establishing the Montpellier medical curriculum.[28] This bull prescribes the study of various treatises of Galen, namely *De complexionibus, De malicia complexionis, De simplici medicine, De morbo et accidenti, De crisi et criticis diebus,* and *De ingenio sanitatis,* together with Avicenna (no doubt the *Canon*); but it permits the substitution for Avicenna of works of Rasis, Constantinus Africanus, and Isaac, thus allowing continued study of works widely used in the schools of the Latin West after the end of the eleventh or the beginning of the twelfth century.[29] (According to the same bull, students at Montpellier had also to prepare themselves for examination on selected works from another list of books including three of the treatises of the *articella*: the *Aphorisms,* the *Prognostica,* and the *Isagoge.*)

The emphases given to the Bolognese medical curriculum in the two generations centering on 1300 are reflected in lists of prescribed books found in the statutes of the university of arts and medicine drawn up in 1405. The statutes list texts for medicine, subdivided into theoretical and practical branches, for philosophy, and for *astrologia* (in a single section). The curriculum in theoretical medicine required the student, over a four-year period, to master four treatises of Hippocrates, all or part of fifteen works of Galen,[30] and portions of the *Canon* of Avicenna and the *Colliget* of Averroes. Prescribed reading for practical medicine consisted solely of selections from the *Canon*. The assigned Hippocratic and Galenic texts included four of the treatises of the *articella* (*Aphorisms, Prognostica, De regimine acutorum, Tegni*). The other Hippocratic work was *De natura fetus,* on which Dino commented. Of the remaining Galenic treatises, at least seven are known to have been the subject of commentary or detailed study by Taddeo or one of his students.[31]

[28] *Cartulaire de l'Université de Montpellier,* 1:219-221, no. 25.

[29] On Constantine and Isaac, see Kristeller, "The School of Salerno," pp. 509-510.

[30] *De differentiis febrium, De complexionibus, De malicia complexionis* (attributed to Galen), *De simplici medicina* [*sic*], *De creticis, De interioribus, De regimine* (or *ingenio*) *sanitatis, Tegni, De accidenti et morbo, De crisi, De febribus ad Glauconem, De tabe, De utilitate respirationis, Liber terapeutice* (*De methodo medendum*), *De virtutibus naturalibus.*

[31] Namely, *De differentiis febrium, De complexionibus, De malicia complexionis, De simplici medicina, De interioribus, De accidenti et morbo,* and *De crisi* (for authors, manuscripts, and editions in the case of Dino's *Compilatio emplastorum et unguentorum,* which is in part based on *De simplici medicina,* see Bibliography). Regarding *De virtutibus naturalibus* in the circle of Taddeo, see note 11, above.

It seems likely that formal public instruction in surgery was also introduced into the curriculum of the faculty of arts and medicine at Bologna
in the age of Taddeo and his pupils, although the earliest statutory evidence for the existence of the subject as an academic discipline comes
from a later period. The tradition of surgical teaching, writing, and practice was strongly established at Bologna, as at other Italian centers of
learning, before the organization of formal academic corporations in arts
and medicine. It was impossible for learned physicians wholly to ignore
the considerable achievements of the surgeons or to dismiss the substantial corpus of their Latin works; so the subject was never excluded from
university curricula, as it was north of the Alps.[32] Thus, the textbooks
prescribed for surgery in the 1405 statutes referred to above included one
of the works of the mid-thirteenth-century surgeon Bruno da Longoburgo of Calabria, as well as portions of the *Canon*, and a work attributed to Galen.[33] Even at Bologna, obviously, not all surgeons acquired
formal training from the public faculties of art and medicine. No doubt,
as in the period before the existence of that faculty, many continued to
enter practice by way of private instruction or apprenticeship.[34] Moreover, a formal distinction between fully qualified learned physicians and
surgeons was maintained.[35] Nonetheless, it is clear that in the period with
which this study is concerned, as in the later fourteenth and the fifteenth
centuries, when statutory evidence becomes available, surgery was cer-

[32] See Pearl Kibre, "The Faculty of Medicine at Paris, Charlatanism and Unlicensed
Medical Practice in the Later Middle Ages, "*Bulletin of the History of Medicine* 27 (1953):
1-20, and especially p. 16, for examples of the attitude to surgery of learned physicians in
northern Europe.

[33] Malagola, *Statuti*, pp. 247-248. Bruno was the author of two works on surgery,
namely, the *Chirurgia magna* and the *Chirurgia parva*; in the edition of Venice, 1498 (Klebs
494.1, one of several early printings), they are bound with the *Chirurgia magna* of Guy
de Chauliac and occur at fols. 83-102 and 103-105 respectively. The explicit of Bruno's
Chirurgia magna states that it was completed at Padua in 1252.

[34] See Zaccagnini, "L'insegnamento privato a Bologna," especially pp. 261-262; Busacchi,
"I primordi," and literature there cited.

[35] See, for example, the report on the wounds of Azzolino di Domenico submitted by
Bartolomeo da Varignana and his assistants on March 1, 1302. In it, Bartolomeo and
Pace di Angelo are each identified as *doctor physice*; another doctor present is termed
medicus physicus; and two others *medici in cyrurgia*. The document is preserved in the
Archivio di Stato di Bologna, sezione del Commune, Carte di corredo agli atti della Curia
del Podestà, and reproduced as fig. 5 in *Catalogo della Mostra tenutasi nella Regia Biblioteca Universitaria di Bologna in occasione del II° Congresso della Società per la Storia delle*

tainly taught and perhaps practiced by some of the learned physicians of the faculty of arts and medicine. Among Taddeo's pupils, Dino del Garbo and Guglielmo da Brescia wrote on surgery[36] (Dino commented on the same portions of Avicenna as were subsequently made mandatory texts for the study of surgery at Bologna by the university statutes of 1405), while Mondino's *Anatomia* proclaims its author's concern with the "chirurgical usage of the subject."[37] For a definition of surgery and its relation to the rest of medicine, we may turn to Dino del Garbo.[38]

According to Dino, medicine was divided into two parts, theory and practice; and surgery pertained entirely to practice. Practice was in turn divided into the science of regulating healthy bodies and that of regulating sick bodies. With the former, surgery had little to do, except insofar as the regimen for a healthy client might include phlebotomy. But surgery was, most importantly, one of the three ways of treating a sick body (the others were diet and medication). Surgery itself could be defined in either of two ways. According to the first of these, it was any manual operation designed to restore health to a sick body. Thus defined, however, surgery was not a science and not part of the science of medicine (since neither the theory nor the practice of medicine consists of *operatio*, as Taddeo had taught—see chapter five—and as Dino repeated), although it was an instrument of medicine. Considered as a science, on the other hand, surgery was the science of teaching how to perform manual operations, or, more broadly conceived, of treating any disease in which manual operation may finally be required. The manual operations referred to included mixing and administering medicines as well as making incisions—in short, any activity involving physical manipulation of the patient. Understood in the broader sense, Dino added, the science of surgery also included teaching how to cure by diet and medication. Following the text of Avicenna on which he was commenting, Dino declared his intention of interpreting the science of surgery in the widest

---

Scienze Mediche e Naturali, Settembre 1922, to which my attention was drawn by Professor P. O. Kristeller.

[36] Dino, *Chirurgia* (Ferrara, 1489; Klebs 336.1); Guglielmo, *Practica in cyrurgia,* the preface and table of contents of which are printed in Karl Sudhoff, *Beiträge zur Geschichte der Chirurgie im Mittelalter,* 2:419-421.

[37] Mondino, *Anatomia,* trans. Singer, 1:59.

[38] Dino, *Chirurgia,* sig. A2r.

possible sense, and he observed that, thus understood, surgery involves theory as well as practice.

The education of a surgeon, Dino held, should include both general instruction in the principles of medicine and practice under an expert *medicus* whom the student should see operate and who should supervise the beginner's own efforts at operating. Yet if the surgeon must be deficient in one or the other branch of knowledge, it is better that he should lack practical experience than book learning. If he has adequate academic training, he can always pick up the practical skills with minimal trouble, though the contrary is not the case. However, he who has not seen enough of anatomy falls easily into errors whereby men are killed.[39] One may note that the thrust of the passage as a whole is to integrate surgery into the rest of medical learning, to emphasize its "scientific" and "theoretical" aspects, and to minimize the specialized and technical features of surgical practice. At least some of this emphasis was probably the result of a desire to raise the dignity of the science of surgery. A pragmatic concern with the realities of surgical practice is suggested, however, by Dino's concluding prescription that the surgeon should be bold, dexterous, not readily deflected from his purpose by cries of pain, and equipped with properly sharpened instruments.

The best-known innovation in medical teaching at Bologna to be associated with the circle of Taddeo lies in the realm of practical demonstration rather than study from books. As already noted, the *Anatomia* of Mondino de' Liuzzi was written in 1316 or 1317 to accompany dissection of a human cadaver for purposes of instruction. This is, of course, quite different from the dissection of animals for purposes of study, whether performed by Galen or by the twelfth- and thirteenth-century doctors of Salerno; it is different from the acquisition of anatomical knowledge in the course of surgical practice, which was characteristic of the thirteenth-century Bolognese tradition; and it is even different from post-mortem examinations and autopsies in cases of unexplained death of the kind

---

[39] "quia ille qui quod est in libris novit atque imaginatur cum pauca operationis noticia perveniet ad illud ad quod multi eorum qui ea que continentur in libris non noverunt nullo modo potuerunt pervenire. Et propter hoc dicit etiam Albucasis. Nos vero iam diximus in introitu huius libri, quoniam qui non est sufficiens videre anathomiam non evadit quin cadit in errorem quo interficiuntur homines," ibid.

performed or supervised by Bartolomeo da Varignana—although all of the foregoing no doubt contributed to Mondino's achievement.

It is clear from a statement of Guy de Chauliac that Mondino devised a regular course of formal academic instruction based on dissection of the cadaver, although it is not known how frequently he was able to do this (Guy says "many times"), or whether attendance at his demonstrations was mandatory for medical or surgical students or both (subsequently, of course, Mondino's textbook of anatomy had a long career as a manual to accompany the dissections mandated at Padua and other universities during the later Middle Ages). In pointing out that surgery could be learned both from books, which in this subject were useful but not sufficient, and from various forms of demonstration, Guy described the type of demonstration adopted by his own master, Bertruccio, and by Bertruccio's master, Mondino. Four successive lectures were given with a fresh cadaver, the first being on the digestive system, liver, and veins ("because these parts putrefy more quickly"), the second on the heart and arterial system, the third on the brain and nervous system, and the fourth on the extremities. At each lecture the student would be taught to recognize a set of nine characteristics of the parts in question (including such items as shape, function, and the special diseases to which the organ was liable). Guy remarked that in this way one could learn a good deal about visceral anatomy and about the blood vessels, the nervous system, and the anatomy of muscles and skin.[40] Mondino, like other four-

[40] "Experimur autem in corporibus noviter mortuis per decollationem vel suspensionem: anatomia ad minus membrorum officialium interiorum carnis musculorum et cutis et multarum venarum atque nervorum; precipue quantum ad originem secundum quod tractat Mundinus Bononiensis qui super hoc scripsit et ipsam fecit multoties: et magister meus Bertucius per hunc modum. situato corpore mortuo in banco faciebat de ipso quatuor lectiones. In prima tractabatur membra nutritiva: quia citius putribilia. In 2ᵃ membra spiritualia. In 3ᵃ membra animalia. In 4ᵃ extremitates tractabantur. Et secundum concordationem sectarum in quolibet membra videnda erat 9, scilicet compositio, substantia, complexio, quantitas, numerus, figura, colligantia, actus, atque utilitates: et que sunt egritudines que in ipso possunt contingere quibus per anothomiam in dignoscendo pronsticando: ac etiam curando medicus possit auxiliari." Guy de Chauliac, *Cyrurgia* (Venice, 1498; see note 33, above), fols. 5r-v. Regarding the development of the concept of the nine categories of anatomical knowledge, see Roger French, "A Note on the Anatomical Accessus of the Middle Ages," *Medical History* (forthcoming, 1979). On the introduction of human dissection in general, and on medieval legal and ethical attitudes thereto, see, *inter alia*, Singer, *The Evolution of Anatomy*, pp. 71-87; Mary N. Alston, "The Attitude of the Church Toward Dissection Before 1500," *Bulletin of the History of Medicine* 16 (1944-45):221-238; Corner, *Anatomical Texts*; Premuda and Ongaro, "I primordi della

teenth-century anatomists, tended to avoid skeletal anatomy because of the possible sin involved in the preparation of the bones.[41] Guy's description of the method of Mondino and Bertruccio ends by contrasting their methods to those of other professors of the subject who used dried human bodies, animals, or pictures as aids to their instruction.

Guy made no mention of any particular form of anatomical preparation used by Mondino or Bertruccio. The claim that Mondino's female assistant used to "cleanse most skillfully the smallest vein, the arteries, all the ramifications of the vessels, without lacerating or dividing them; and to prepare them for demonstration she would fill them with various colored liquids, which, after having been driven into the vessels, would harden without destroying the vessels" is presumably apocryphal.[42] Whether or not such a person as Alessandra Giliani, the supposed assistant in question, actually worked for Mondino, the technique of anatomical injection with wax, which appears to be referred to, was developed in the seventeenth century.[43] Since the same passage praises Alessandra for her ability to depict the blood vessels naturalistically (scarcely a possibility or even a value in early fourteenth-century medical illustration), the whole story is probably a reflection of post-Vesalian interest in anatomical preparation and illustration.

Mondino was not necessarily the originator of the practice of anatomical demonstration with the cadaver at Bologna. There is at least a possibility that a casual remark of Taddeo's, in his commentary on the *Aphorisms*, to the effect that he could not solve a question about the process of fetal nourishment because he had neither been able to find an

---

dissezione anatomica in Padova"; Forni, *L'insegnamento della chirurgia*, and, on Mondino as dissector, note 171 to chapter two, above.

[41] The preparation of bones by boiling was forbidden by a bull of Pope Boniface VIII. See Alston, "The Attitude of the Church," passim; and G. Martinotti, "Prospero Lambertini (Benedetto XIV) e lo studio dell'anatomia in Bologna," *Studi e memorie per la storia dell'Università di Bologna*, 1st ser. 2 (1911):147-178, to which my attention was drawn by Professor Elizabeth Brown of Brooklyn College.

[42] The passage is quoted at third hand in Muriel J. Hughes, *Women Healers in Medieval Life and Literature* (Freeport, N.Y., 1968; repr. of 1943 ed.), p. 87. The original source is said to be a chronicle of S. Giovanni in Persiceto (a small commune near Bologna), which I have not, so far, traced. Alessandra's existence and her work for Mondino are said to be attested by her tombstone. Professor Joan Ferrante of Columbia University drew my attention to Hughes's work.

[43] Henry A. Skinner, *The Origin of Medical Terms* (2d ed., Baltimore, 1961), p. 227.

authoritative discussion of the matter, nor seen the anatomy of a pregnant woman, alludes to academic demonstration rather than autopsy.[44]

In any case, the introduction of human dissection into medical education seems to be very closely tied to the appearance of a formally organized student university and doctoral college of arts and medicine at Bologna. It is likely that the practice emerged as a possibility when an organized, privileged faculty of arts and medicine felt the need of it; presumably individual physicians, however learned, or a craft guild, however practically oriented and skillful, would have been unlikely to secure legitimate access to the bodies of executed criminals, an access that appears to be taken for granted in the opening words of the text of Mondino's work. It is probable, nonetheless, that given the practice of carrying on instruction in the home of the teacher, which was common at Bologna both before and after the organization of universities and doctoral colleges, a good deal of whatever demonstration with the cadaver was available in Mondino's day took place in private. This certainly continued to be the case long after public anatomies were instituted by university statute. Public anatomies in the medieval *studia* were always infrequent, with the privilege of attendance carefully rotated among the students. Thus, even if some measure of authorized access to cadavers supplied by the municipal authorities had been attained when Mondino's *Anatomia* was written, it is unlikely to have been sufficient to satisfy the needs of medical students. Hence, presumably, occurred the prosecution in 1319 of four scholars of Master Alberto da Bologna, himself a pupil of Mondino, for grave robbing.[45]

The intimate association of the practice of dissecting cadavers with

---

[44] "neque anothomiam vidi in muliere pregnante," Taddeo, *Aphor.*, fol. 140r.

[45] See Giovanni Martinotti, "L'insegnamento dell'anatomia in Bologna prima del secolo XIX," *Studi e memorie per la storia dell'Università di Bologna*, 1st ser. 2 (1911):1-146, where both the general practice of teaching privately in the homes of professors in the medieval *studium* and the continuance of private anatomies until the seventeenth or eighteenth century are stressed. The statutes of the student university of arts and medicine drawn up in 1405 provide for public dissection; see Malagola, *Statuti*, pp. 289-290. For the prosecution of the scholars of Alberto da Bologna, see the document printed in Salvatore de Renzi, *Storia della medicina in Italia*, 2:249-250 (excerpts also in Martinotti, "L'insegnamento"). The scholars were prosecuted by the civil authorities for sacrilege in profaning a cemetery, not for dissection as such. The cadaver was that of a man who had been hanged. The chief witness for the prosecution, a servant of Master Alberto, indicated that the scholars as well as the master actually participated in the dissection.

"scholastic" medicine and the university milieu becomes yet clearer when one considers the whole range of Mondino's own written output and professional activity. As the reader has no doubt already noted, from the list of his works in chapter two, Mondino's interests fit a general pattern common to the other learned physicians discussed in this study. In no sense can his orientation be considered more "practical" than theirs, or bound by any unique links to the pre-university tradition of Bolognese medicine and surgery. Like most of his fellow students under Taddeo, he combined theory and practice both in his teaching and in advising patients. Thus, like all the other members of the group, he commented on one or more of the treatises of the *articella*; like all the others, he used the methodology of the scholastic question to discuss medical topics whenever it seemed to him appropriate to do so; like all the others except Turisanus, he wrote *consilia* for individual patients; like Taddeo, Dino, and Guglielmo, he expounded part of the *Canon* of Avicenna; with Dino he shared a particular interest in human generation; like Bartolomeo he performed or supervised autopsies. Moreover, it would be difficult to establish that his interest in *practica* or *chirurgia* was any greater or much different in kind than that of, say, Dino del Garbo. Like the *Sphere* of Sacrobosco[46] and the *Perspectiva communis* of John Pecham,[47] the *Anatomia* of Mondino is deservedly a famous and genuinely a significant work. But, like them, it owes its success largely to its author's intelligence in perceiving where in the curriculum a suitable textbook was lacking and to his skill in simplifying and abbreviating the standard teaching of his day into a handy introductory manual. It is not the product of a scholar who was isolated, original, or "in advance of his time," but part of the continuing effort of the first two generations of physicians and professors of medicine in the institutionalized faculty of arts and medicine at Bologna to establish a solidly based and comprehensive curriculum.

Many aspects of the organization of arts and medical teaching in the *studium* of Bologna seem also to have taken lasting shape in the years when Taddeo and some of his disciples taught there. One of these was

---

[46] Edited in Thorndike, *The Sphere of Sacrobosco.*

[47] Edited in David C. Lindberg, *John Pecham and the Science of Optics* (Madison, Wis., 1970).

the frequency with which the same master would teach some of the liberal arts (usually logic or astronomy), Aristotelian natural philosophy, and medicine during the course of his career. Thus, of fourteen doctors involved in drawing up a set of statutes for the medical branch of the Bolognese College of Doctors of Arts and Medicine in 1378, seven are recorded as having degrees in philosophy as well as in medicine, and five are known to have taught logic and Aristotelian natural philosophy as well as medicine.[48] Two generations earlier, among Taddeo and his pupils, the situation was very similar. Taddeo taught logic as well as medicine, Guglielmo taught logic and philosophy at Padua before studying medicine with Taddeo, Bartolomeo probably lectured on moral philosophy as well as on medicine, and Gentile da Cingoli, who spent his career teaching logic and philosophy, had also received medical training (for documentation, see chapter two). Of course, in Taddeo's day, as in the later period, not every master who taught logic, *astrologia*, or philosophy also taught and wrote on medicine, or vice versa, as the surviving output of the masters makes clear. In particular, after Taddeo's death, philosophical trends among the masters of arts at Bologna were not necessarily either reflected in or inspired by the current teaching and writing of the professors of medicine. Nonetheless, the only inviolable personnel division within the faculty of arts and medicine was apparently between the teachers of grammar and rhetoric on the one hand, and those of logic, the quadrivial arts, philosophy (including natural science), and medicine on the other. It would be interesting to know whether those portions of the statutes of the university of arts and medicine drawn up in 1405 that evince a desire to prevent a dilution of the curriculum through blurring the lines between disciplines and admitting unqualified students to the more advanced subjects represent a reaction against this state of affairs, or merely a healthy caution that was not necessarily new. In these statutes, the various areas of study are arranged in a hierarchy in which medicine holds the highest place. Only scholars who had studied and only masters who had taught a particular discipline might take part in public disputations pertaining thereto; and, at the elections to the professorial chairs, only students who had studied medicine might vote for a professor of medicine, and so on.[49]

At least some of the academic exercises that were later required by

---

[48] Malagola, *Statuti*, pp. 425, 448.   [49] Ibid., pp. 305-306.

statute of masters and scholars in arts and medicine at Bologna were instituted during the lifetimes of Taddeo and his disciples. Thus, for example,
the output of our group of masters makes it clear that they were accustomed to engage in formal disputations on medical subjects (see further,
chapter eight, below).

Less clear is the extent to which, if at all, they were responsible for
laying down regulations governing the length of study in arts and medicine and for establishing appropriate qualifying examinations. Later, a
degree in arts seems to have called for four years' study, and a degree in
medicine for four or five.[50] This resembles fairly closely the demand, contained in the papal bull regulating the curriculum for Montpellier (supposedly influenced by Guglielmo da Brescia), that students who were already proficient in arts should study medicine for five years; others
should study for six.[51] No medieval academic statute at Bologna seems,
however, to have formalized the admirable requirement contained in the
Montpellier bull that students should spend two summers "*in medicine
practicam . . . exercendam.*" The story told by Mondino de' Liuzzi of
Taddeo's presence at a patient's bedside, accompanied by junior physicians, suggests, nonetheless, that some form of supervised practice was
required as part of the curriculum.

By 1378, students at Bologna were permitted to specialize by concentrating on particular disciplines within the general category of arts and
natural philosophy. For example, by 1378 a student could choose to be
examined either in all the arts and philosophy; in logic and philosophy
alone; in grammar and rhetoric alone; in philosophy and *astrologia*
alone; or in medicine and one or more of the arts. For a general arts
degree a two-day examination was required, as was also the case for a
degree in logic and philosophy. Grammar with rhetoric and philosophy
with *astrologia* each required only a single examination. If any three
subjects were combined, two examinations were required, while a degree
in medicine combined with all the arts was granted only after three examinations. As for medicine itself, "if anyone wants to pass with distinction, then he is to take two examinations"—perhaps one in theory and another in practice. Again, these requirements are laxer, as far as medicine
is concerned, than those prescribed by the papal bull of 1309 for Montpellier. At Montpellier, possibly under Guglielmo's influence, students

[50] Ibid., pp. 274-277, 432; Rashdall, *Universities,* 1:248.
[51] See note 28, above.

were obliged to offer themselves for examination in both theoretical and practical medicine if they wished to be graduated at all in that subject.[52]

How soon after the establishment of the academic institutions of the faculty of arts and medicine at Bologna the arrangements just described were made formal is, unfortunately, impossible to say. But if no such examinations were ever taken by Taddeo, it seems only too likely that he imposed them, or similar requirements, on his pupils. Contemporaries certainly recognized Taddeo as an expert on academic organization; thus it was that in 1287 the civic government of Perugia sought his services as a consultant "to see and examine if the said city of Perugia is a suitable site for a *studium*."[53]

Because they had at their disposal the resources of formally organized corporations for the teaching and study of medicine in conjunction with arts and philosophy, and the financial and legal support of the government of Bologna, and were nonetheless untrammeled by anything much in the way of earlier institutional tradition, Taddeo and those of his pupils who taught at Bologna were in an excellent position to develop the medical curriculum as they chose. There seems every reason to suppose that they took full advantage of the opportunity and that their decisions had lasting influence. They were, of course, in the mainstream of the medical (and to some extent the philosophical) learning of their day; so few of their choices were idiosyncratic. But their actions helped to bring together and to put into a durable institutional framework some of the most characteristic features of the learned medicine of the Italian university centers in the later Middle Ages and Renaissance: the preservation of the *articella* tradition side by side with the expansion of interest in Galen; the central place given to the *Canon* of Avicenna; the retention of surgery in the formal academic curriculum; the demonstration of anatomy with the cadaver; the use of scholastic tools of inquiry (commentary and disputation) in medical teaching; and the insistence that medicine be studied in conjunction with Aristotelian natural philosophy. We may now turn to inquire what kind of learning they believed that the study of these texts and disciplines should produce.

[52] Malagola, *Statuti*, p. 489, and note 28, above.

[53] ". . . causa videndi et examinandi si prefata civitas Perusii apta sit studio et utilitati studentium." The document is that referred to in note 60 to chapter one, above. In the end, Taddeo declined the invitation; see Münster, "Taddeo degli Alderotti mancato medico condotto."

CHAPTER FIVE

THE NATURE OF MEDICAL
LEARNING

T*addeo and his pupils were self-conscious and articulate about the nature of their own discipline. They provided their readers with definitions of medicine and its various branches, expressed* opinions about the proper content of a medical education, discussed the relationship of medicine to other disciplines, and investigated the relative roles of theoretical and practical learning. What they had to say was of course often conventional and traditional, since there was at their disposal an extensive body of medical literature in which these topics were discussed. For example, fairly elaborate definitions and discussions of the nature of medicine preface early medieval commentaries on works of Hippocrates and Galen,[1] works of Salernitan masters of the eleventh through the thirteenth centuries,[2] as well as some of the major medical encyclopedias of Arab origin such as the *Pantegni*, based on the work of Haly Abbas, and the *Canon* of Avicenna.[3] Moreover, a very ancient tra-

[1] See Beccaria, "Sulle tracce," *Italia medioevale e umanistica*, 4:1-75, especially pp. 35-37, where the preface to a Latin commentary on the *Aphorisms* dated by Beccaria to the seventh century A.D. (p. 59) is printed; and Owsei Temkin, "Studies in Late Alexandrian Medicine. I. Alexandrian Commentaries on Galen's *De sectis ad introducendos*," *Bulletin of the History of Medicine* 3 (1935):405-430, especially pp. 426-427, where part of the introduction to a Latin commentary attributed to Agnellus the Iatrosophist and probably written in the sixth century is printed. I am grateful to the Frank M. Folsom Ambrosiana Microfilm and Photographic Collection of the University of Notre Dame for supplying a photocopy of the latter commentary, preserved in Milan, Biblioteca Ambrosiana, MS G 108 Inf., 9c, fols. 22r-48v. Regarding this commentary, see also Beccaria, "Sulle tracce," *Italia medioevale e umanistica*, 14:1-23.

[2] For example, Maurus of Salerno, commentary on the *Aphorisms* of Hippocrates, in *Collectio Salernitana*, 4:513-514 (see note 4 to chapter four, above); Bartholomaeus of Salerno in the prefaces of his commentaries on the *Isagoge* of Johannitius and the *Tegni* of Galen, printed in Paul Oskar Kristeller, "Bartholomaeus, Musandinus, and Maurus of Salerno," pp. 85-87. On the analytical and academic treatment of medicine by twelfth-century Salernitan masters, and on their philosophical interests, see idem, "The School of Salerno," passim. References to the "Salernitani" occur from time to time in the writings of Taddeo's circle.

[3] The *Pantegni* was the work of Constantinus Africanus.

dition, ultimately deriving from the medical schools of Alexandria, emphasized links between medicine and philosophy;[4] and brief discussions of the place of medicine among the sciences are included in the classifications of knowledge provided by such influential nonmedical writers as Hugh of Saint Victor and Thomas Aquinas.[5] From works in all these categories our group of medical masters could, and from all except perhaps the last they did, draw ideas about the nature of medical learning. But as they adapted, changed, and contradicted their sources, the better to express their own views, they revealed the preoccupations of their own time and place. In the recently institutionalized Bolognese faculty of arts and medicine, the nature of medical learning and of an appropriate medical curriculum and the links between medicine and other branches of knowledge must necessarily have been topics of living significance for learned physicians. From their expressed views on these subjects one may hope to gain some further understanding of the ways in which medicine functioned in their milieu as a "scientific" discipline and activity. This is so even though the extent to which their statements reflected the actual teaching situation in the Bolognese *studium* remains largely a matter of conjecture.

As we have just seen, well-established convention called for some sort of discussion of the nature of medical science to be placed at the beginning of general works on medical theory; somewhat similar but usually shorter and, naturally, more specific discussions frequently (but by no means always) opened specialized treatises on particular aspects of medicine. Thus, among the works of the masters here considered, elaborate analyses of the whole nature and scope of medical science occur at the beginning of Taddeo's commentary on the *Isagoge* of Johannitius and in Turisanus's commentary on the *Tegni* of Galen. Almost equally sweeping is the preface by Bartolomeo da Varignana to his commentary

[4] On the association of medicine and philosophy in Galen's own teaching and among those influenced by him in the late antiquity and the earlier Middle Ages, see Temkin, *Galenism*, pp. 1-94; regarding the transmission of this tradition to the Latin West, see also the works of Beccaria and Temkin cited in note 1, above. Another important channel for the transmission of the concept was Isidore of Seville, who declared that medicine is a second philosophy and that all the liberal arts are necessary to medicine (*Etym.* 4.13.1-5).

[5] Hugh of St. Victor, *Didascalicon de studio legendi*, ed. C. H. Buttimer (Washington, D.C., 1939), pp. 37-39, 43-44; Thomas Aquinas, *Expositio super librum Boethii de Trinitate*, ed. Bruno Decker (Leiden, 1955), pp. 168-171. On the history of the classification of knowledge, see James A. Weisheipl, "The Classification of the Sciences in Mediaeval Thought," *Mediaeval Studies* 27 (1964):54-90.

on Galen's comprehensive work on internal medicine, *De interioribus.* But, as we have seen, the preface to Dino del Garbo's lengthy commentary on the surgical portions of the *Canon* of Avicenna merely contains a brief investigation of the nature of surgery and a description of the skills required by a surgeon, and the well-known opening chapter of Mondino's *Anatomia* is devoted to a strikingly humanistic essay on the qualities that mark off man from the beasts. Elsewhere, in his commentary on the *Prognostica* of Hippocrates, Mondino began with a sober evaluation of the usefulness of this particular branch of knowledge in medical science and its relationship to astrological prediction. Taddeo introduced his commentary on the *Aphorisms* with an evaluation of the sense in which medicine could be said to be an art. In contrast, the general work on practical medicine attributed to Guglielmo da Brescia, which actually consists of an alphabetical listing of diseases and remedies, is introduced by a highly academic discussion of the value of theoretical learning in medicine as a foundation for practical skill.

Although the various passages exploring the proper definition and scope of medicine make no direct reference to the circumstances of contemporary university teaching or professional practice, they can be related to those circumstances. In practical terms, the problem that faced Italian medical masters at the turn of the fourteenth century was broadly and approximately as follows. On the one hand, the relatively recent institutional association of medicine with liberal arts and natural philosophy in the *studium* of Bologna and other university centers must surely have reinforced not only the venerable tradition linking the disciplines named, but also the concept of medicine as a fully learned discipline. Medical men could now reassert, with renewed confidence, their claims to *scientia,* to *ars* (of a kind comparable to the liberal arts in dignity), and *philosophia*—claims that had not always been respected by scholars in other fields.[6] On the other hand, medicine had a well-established tradition as an autonomous discipline, with its own authorities and its own methods. Too much insistence on the association with philosophy and the arts

---

[6] Hugh of St. Victor categorized medicine as one of the mechanical or adulterine arts that have no relation to theoretical or speculative philosophy, and provide suitable occupation for manually skilled members of the lower classes (*Didascalicon,* ed. Buttimer, pp. 38-39). Thomas Aquinas held the more moderate view that medicine, although wholly practical in purpose and excluded from among the liberal arts on account of its association with the human body, the part of man that is not free, could be held to be subalternated to *physica,* that is, natural science (*In Boethium de Trinitate,* ed. Decker, pp. 168-171).

might bring with it the risk of subordinating medicine to the Aristotelian natural philosophy that had become the mainstay of university teaching in the arts faculty. Discussion revolved around the issue of the appropriate balance to be maintained.

Thus Taddeo himself, in the introduction to his commentary on the *Isagoge*, emphasized the links between medicine and natural philosophy and the characteristics that entitled medicine to be defined as a science in the Aristotelian meaning of the term.[7] Among the various definitions of medicine provided by authorities, he indicated his preference for that of Avicenna, according to whom medicine was "the science by which the dispositions of the human body are known . . . so that health may be maintained or, if lost, recovered."[8] In the passage cited, Avicenna himself had not particularly emphasized methodological links and overlapping content between medicine and other sciences. He had admitted the necessity that physicians have some *sapientia physicalis* (for example, of the elements), but had pointed out the strictly limited medical value of such knowledge and had criticized physicians who taught natural science. Taddeo, however, introduced a different emphasis. He began by defining *scientia*, citing the *Ethics* and *Posterior Analytics*. *Scientia* is knowledge strictly demonstrable from premises. The subject of medical science is the human body; this distinguishes it from such sciences as astronomy and music, which deal with the dispositions of the heavenly bodies and with harmony, respectively; medicine is also distinct from *scientia naturalis*, which does include the study of the human body as a mobile physical object, but not its health or sickness. Medicine is divided into theory and practice, and the end of theory is practice. Yet although practice serves to exemplify the antecedent theory and direct it to its ordained end, it cannot be said to prove theory, since that which comes after does not prove that which goes before. Theory is defined by Aristotle and Avicenna as knowledge for its own sake; by Constantinus Africanus as certain information about things that are grasped by the intellect alone. Although *practica* is not grasped exclusively by the intellect, *practica*, as Avicenna says, is itself a *scientia intellectualis*. Taddeo firmly denied that *practica* was to be identified with *operatio*, despite the assertions of Johan-

---

[7] Taddeo, *Isagoge*, fols. 343r-v.

[8] "Dico quod medicina est scientia, qua humani corporis dispositiones noscuntur, ex parte, qua sanatur, vel ab ea removetur; ut habita sanitas conservetur et amissa recuperetur," *Canon* 1.1.1, proem.

nitius and Constantinus Africanus to the contrary. No science, according to Taddeo, consists of *operatio*, and *practica* is undoubtedly a science. *Practica* is properly defined as a *scientia operativa*, which teaches how and why theory should be put into operation manually and sensibly. For example, a physician knows from theory that fever is caused by heat; *practica* teaches him to cure by opposites, and he therefore prescribes that the patient be given cold water, which is a manual operation. This kind of medical practice, which is a science involving theoretical knowledge, is to be sharply distinguished "from the usual practice that old women carry on."[9] It is true, however, that medical practice is different from the practical parts of the other sciences, since the latter involve intellectual, not manual, *operatio*. The practice of grammar, for example, consists in teaching how to construe, and the practice of dialectic in teaching how to reason by syllogisms.

Taddeo then went on to defend the inclusion of material relating to *physica* (in the general sense of natural science) in a medical work, despite the definition of the subject of medicine as the human body. He also took up the question of the position of medicine in regard to the three philosophies (rational, moral and natural), which were commonly held to divide speculative science. Obviously, medicine could not be regarded as part of moral philosophy, and despite the use of logic in medical argumentation, its subject matter was not the same as that of rational philosophy, that is, dialectic. Taddeo rejected, "saving the reverence due to a monk," the contention of Constantinus Africanus that, because logic was used in medical discussions, medicine was partly subordinated to dialectic and partly to natural philosophy. Instead, he maintained strongly that it should be placed entirely under natural philosophy. Many of the received principles of medicine were drawn from natural philosophy, as Avicenna himself had admitted; as a result, medicine was subalternated to natural philosophy and therefore subjected to its principles.

Taddeo's exposition demonstrates certain definite intentions. He defined medicine as a science and indicated also that it is comparable in scope to the quadrivial arts of astronomy and music; he showed that, although medicine is distinct from *philosophia naturalis*, it is properly regarded as subalternated to it; and he demonstrated that medical practice as well as medical theory is included in the foregoing categories.

---

[9] "propter hec separatur practica que est scientia a practica usuali quam faciunt vetule," Taddeo, *Isagoge*, fol. 343v.

Effectively, this amounts to a justification of the alliance of medicine with the subjects normally studied in the arts schools, of the study of those subjects by physicians, and of the place of medicine—even practical medicine—in a university curriculum. It also constitutes an effective defense of the dignity and social prestige claimed by learned physicians.

In his commentary on the *Aphorisms*, written, as we have seen, later in his career, and possibly at a time when the influence of his own studies in arts and philosophy, so prominent in the commentary on the *Isagoge*, had somewhat faded, Taddeo Alderotti explained how it was that Hippocrates had defined medicine as an art, rather than as a science.[10] He noted that art and science differ as do "to be made" and "to be." Art is a skill in the soul of the artificer through which he works on things capable of being made; for example, the art that is in the soul of a carpenter is the skill with which he builds a home, whereas an understanding of the house as such and of wood and stone is acquired by science. As authority for this statement he again cited *Ethics*, Book 6, and *Posterior Analytics*, Book 2 (whence, as already noted, he drew his definition of science in the passage discussed above). Taddeo observed that when Hippocrates termed medicine an art, he was speaking of medicine in the way that he, Hippocrates, had discovered it, namely, by reasoning upon and experience with *factibilia*; in this sense it was more appropriate to call medicine an art than a science. The down-to-earth example of the carpenter adopted by Taddeo provides a parallel with a mechanical, not a liberal, art; it suggests that the rational, abstract, and "philosophical" view of medicine so well described by Taddeo in his introduction to the commentary on the *Isagoge* never, even in the minds of its warmest advocates, entirely succeeded in driving out more craftsmanlike notions of medical activity. Nor indeed was there any reason why the two conceptions should not exist side by side; as both Turisanus and Peter of Abano, another younger contemporary of Taddeo, were to state, medicine was both *scientia* and *ars*, just as it was both theory and practice.[11]

[10] Taddeo, *Aphor.*, fol. 2v.

[11] Turisanus, *Plusquam*, fols. 7r-v; Peter of Abano, *Conciliator differentiarum philosophorum et precipue medicorum* (Venice, 1496; Klebs 773.5), fols. 4r-8v. There are, of course, earlier antecedents: while stressing the relationship of medicine and philosophy, the commentary on Galen's *De sectis* contained in Milan, Biblioteca Ambrosiana, MS G 108 Inf. (see note 1, above) also compares the art of medicine with both liberal and mechanical arts, carpentry being named among the latter (fols. 22r-24r; see also Beccaria, "Sulle tracce," *Italia medieovale e umanistica* 14:11-12.

In his last work, the commentary on *De regimine acutorum*, Taddeo grew bold enough, or weary enough, to tackle the question of the fundamental worth of the medical science known to him.[12] He inquired whether common knowledge or folk wisdom had anything to contribute to medical science and whether, if so, information of this kind could possibly be considered a legitimate part of an art known to the wise. He asked whether a physician needed to have prior familiarity with a disease in general in order to prescribe helpful treatment in an individual case. If a physician engaged in the practice of questioning his patients about their symptoms and incorporating the results in a treatise or an individual *consilium* (as Taddeo and, later, some of his pupils were in the habit of doing), was he descending to an "unscientific" involvement with the common knowledge of the vulgar? And could anyone who had not been initiated into the mysteries of learned medicine tell the difference between a good physician and a bad one, when the treatment prescribed by the "bad" physician who did not know the appropriate measures called for by medical science might be just as effective as that of the good one, owing to the vagaries of chance or the resilience of the patient's constitution?

Taddeo defended (and exercised in practice) the right of a learned medical author to include in his writings information gained from the interrogation of his patients, even though he believed this to involve the rejection of Hippocrates' own opinion on the point. The Latin text of the passage of *De regimine acutorum* in question is somewhat obscure, but appears to mean that certain information or suggestions from patients have no part in the art of medicine. Galen's commentary on the passage, incorporated in the version of Hippocrates used by Taddeo, adds that not everything written in medical treatises is relevant to the art. Taddeo's interpretation of the passage was that Hippocrates here expressed his disapproval of those practitioners who relied solely on information gathered from their patients rather than on his, or their own, findings (*suis inventionibus*); whereas Galen, in his commentary, had taken to task physicians who incorporated information acquired by interviewing patients in

---

12 Taddeo, *Reg. acut.*, fols. 247v, 248v, 250v. The questions raised and answered in these folios are indexed in the question register of the work (fol. 342v) as follows: Utrum medicus debeat interrogare infirmum de omnibus accidentibus et de eis facere librum; Utrum aliqua nota vulgo, arti medicinali addenda sint; Utrum medicus curaturus aliquam egritudinem debeat prius eam cognoscere; Utrum iudicium vulgare sit verum; Utrum vulgus cognoscat tantum ea in quibus medicus bonus cum malo communicat.

medical treatises, on the grounds that nothing known by the vulgar could be essential to the medical art, and that such material was therefore an irrelevant excrescence in a medical work. Taddeo remarked that the symptoms reported by a patient were, on the contrary, a legitimate part of the description of the disease, although the physician must exercise discrimination in weeding out the irrelevancies that would probably be embedded in a layman's narrative.[13] Moreover, Taddeo went on to maintain explicitly that Galen was wrong to suppose that facts known to the vulgar had no place in the art of medicine; something could not be excluded from medicine just because it was a matter of common knowledge. For example, everyone knew that the cure for stone in the bladder was to remove the stone—but only the skilled physician knew what treatment would remove it. Similarly, he held that the populace are able and entitled to judge in a general way the qualifications of a competent physician and the nature of good medical treatment, although in particular cases they are incapable of estimating the physician's skill or of evaluating the element of chance in the successes of the incompetent.

Perhaps the fairly pragmatic approach to medical science that can be detected in Taddeo's commentary on *De regimine acutorum* owed something to the influence of his collaborator, "Bartolomeus Veronensis," who, as suggested earlier, is probably Bartolomeo da Varignana. Certainly Bartolomeo da Varignana elsewhere displayed considerable hesitation over the kind of association between medicine and natural philosophy emphasized by Taddeo in his early commentary on the *Isagoge*. For example, Bartolomeo chose to introduce his commentary on *De interioribus*, Galen's work on the manifestations of disease and injuries of the internal organs, with a critical exposition of the definition of medicine as "*philosophia corporis.*"[14] He drew the phrase from the proem of a com-

---

[13] "Sed hic videtur Hip[pocrates] iniuste reprehendere illos quia signum quod sumitur ab inditio patientis est unum de veridicis signis et artificialibus . . . quare videtur quod medicus debeat de omnibus accidentibus interrogare infirmum. Ad quod dicendum est quod de omnibus inquirendum est a medico in collocutionibus ad investigandum essentiam morbi, sed non sunt omnia scribenda in libris tanquam artis principia," Taddeo, *Reg. acut.*, fol. 247v.

[14] BAV, MS Vat. lat. 4452, 14c, fol. 83r. The anonymous commentary on *De interioribus* that occupies fols. 83r-102r in this manuscript (TK 857) is the same as that ascribed to Bartolomeo da Varignana in another fourteenth-century manuscript, namely, Vat. lat. 4454. The commentary in Vat. lat. 4454 occupies fols. 55r-75v (modern numbering of folios) and is identified in the explicit as "recollectiones libri de interioribus secundum M. Bartolomeum de Varignana." See TK 531, where, however, another set of folio numbers, also

mentary on the *De sectis* of Galen, probably from that ascribed to Johannes Alexandrinus, which has been shown to be familiar to another member of the circle of Taddeo Alderotti, but perhaps from the closely related work attributed in a ninth-century manuscript in the Biblioteca Ambrosiana to Agnellus the Iatrosophist.[15] These commentaries, one of which became available in Latin as early as the sixth century A.D., appear to have been an important channel whereby the ideas of Alexandrian physicians about the close relationship of medicine to philosophy reached the Latin West. In the commentary attributed to Johannes Alexandrinus, it is stated that philosophy is the medicine of the soul and medicine the philosophy of the body, and that, according to Aristotle, philosophy and medicine are sisters. In the commentary said to be by Agnellus, the remark "medicine is the philosophy of the body" is specifically attributed to Aristotle. These definitions are not, of course, Aristotelian, as Owsei Temkin long ago pointed out.[16]

According to Bartolomeo, the definition of medicine as the philosophy of the body is not entirely valid. Not only does such a definition ignore the purpose of medicine, namely, in Avicenna's words, to maintain health and recover it when lost,[17] but it is not generally true even of medicine considered as a descriptive science. Knowledge about bodies, Bartolomeo pointed out, can be either mathematical or natural; and medicine is certainly in no way connected with mathematics. Nor can medicine be equated with natural philosophy of the body in general, because in that instance it would simply be a branch of *scientia naturalis*, which is not the case. It is true that the subject matter of medicine can be described

---

found on the manuscript, is used. The principal differences between the two versions appear to be the omission of the proem and of a final chapter, *De priapismo*, in Vat. lat. 4454; but see also note 78 to chapter seven, below. On the proem, found only in Vat. lat. 4452, see further my article "Taddeo Alderotti and Bartolomeo da Varignana on the Nature of Medical Learning," *Isis* 68 (1977):27-39, where an earlier version of some of the following discussion appeared.

[15] "asumpsi diffinitionem huius scientie quam ponit commentator libri sectarum in prohemio," BAV, MS Vat. lat. 4452, fol. 83r. The commentary ascribed to Johannes Alexandrinus is printed with works of Galen in some early editions. For the commentary of Agnellus, see note 1, above. The relationship of the two commentaries and their contents is discussed in Temkin, "Studies in Late Alexandrian Medicine," pp. 403-430, and Beccaria, "Sulle tracce," *Italia medioevale e umanistica*, 14:1-23. Temkin points out that the commentary ascribed to Johannes Alexandrinus is cited in the preface to Mondino's *Anatomia*.

[16] Temkin, "Studies in Late Alexandrian Medicine," pp. 408-409, 418.

[17] "diffinitio medicine asignata est incompleta quoniam solum datur per subiectum non autem per finem," BAV, MS Vat. lat. 4452, fol. 83r.

as a type of *philosophia naturalis* of the body specifically pertaining to the human body, its properties and passions. Unlike knowledge acquired by the study of *philosophia naturalis*, however, medical knowledge always serves an ultimately practical purpose. The whole of medicine is directed toward *opus*, and therefore medicine is to be categorized as a practical-intellectual skill. Its object is hence quite different from that of *scientia* (or *philosophia*) *naturalis*, which seeks the truth for its own sake. Because sciences with different ends cannot be subalternated one to another, medicine cannot properly be regarded as in any way subalternated to *scientia naturalis*,[18] even though the latter discipline does provide theoretical knowledge of such aspects of the human body as generation, health, sickness, and so on, and even though the method of demonstration is the same in both sciences. The passage concludes with some fairly conventional remarks about the nobility and usefulness of medicine as a science and with a further emphatic statement of the practical purpose of medical knowledge. Thus Bartolomeo provided his readers with a firm defense of the autonomy of medical science, somewhat unusual in its insistence on the divorce of even theoretical medicine from *philosophia*, or *scientia, naturalis*. The contrast to Taddeo's own views could scarcely be more striking.

It should be made clear, however, that Bartolomeo did not advocate the omission of the study of Aristotelian logic or Aristotelian natural science from the training of physicians. On the contrary, immediately before discussing the definition of medicine, he took pains to demonstrate his own Aristotelian learning by means of an elaborate logical justification of the practice of beginning every work with the invocation of a deity: God is prior to everything and therefore should be at the beginning of everything. This rather commonplace assertion Bartolomeo buttressed with a formidable array of citations from the *Physics*, the *Metaphysics*, *De anima*, and the pseudo-Aristotelian *De causis*. Later in the same work he was to refer to the usefulness of a knowledge of logic for the study of medicine.[19]

The discussions of the nature of medical learning produced by Taddeo and Bartolomeo are excelled in sophistication by that produced by Turi-

[18] "inde tamen quod si [medicina] sit considerans tales passiones [corporis humani] non considerat illas propter verum sed propter opus. scientia autem naturalis illas considerat propter verum. et quia ille scientie que fine differunt una non subalternatur alteri, ideo ex dictis apparet quod medicina non subalternetur scientie naturali," ibid.

[19] Ibid., fol. 90r.

sanus. The latter author seems to be the one, of the masters under consideration, who was most fully aware of the type of analysis of scientific methodology that interested a series of natural philosophers from the thirteenth century until the fifteenth. Turisanus's introduction to his *Plusquam commentum* on Galen's *Tegni* fits into a sequence of expositions of scientific method that apparently began with Grosseteste, continued in the writings of Albertus Magnus, Saint Thomas, and other thirteenth-century scholastics, and was subsequently taken up by Peter of Abano, and afterwards by members of the Paduan "Averroist" school.[20] Like the writers just named, Turisanus attempted to analyze and reconcile the conceptions of scientific activity and scientific methodology of Aristotle on the one hand and Galen and other medical authors on the other; and, like Grosseteste and his successors, too, Turisanus wrote a lengthy disquisition on how the processes of resolution and composition lead to scientific understanding.[21]

It is difficult, however, to see just where Turisanus should be placed in this sequence, and, in particular, to understand the relationship between his discussion and that by Peter of Abano. Turisanus's *Plusquam commentum* was completed, as already noted, shortly before 1319 and was therefore presumably written in the same decade as the *Conciliator* of Peter of Abano, completed after 1310.[22] Although in discussing resolution and composition neither Peter nor Turisanus cited the other by name, there are signs that they were aware of each other's opinions on the subject. A central feature of Turisanus's exposition is his identification of the type of demonstration termed *"propter quid"* (knowledge of the reasoned fact) in the Latin version of Aristotle's *Posterior Analytics* with resolution, and of Aristotle's demonstration termed *"quia"* (knowledge of the fact) with composition. Peter of Abano and most subsequent Latin medical authors who discussed the issue followed Haly Rodohan, an eleventh-century Muslim commentator on the *Tegni*, in identifying demonstration

---

[20] See Alistair Cameron Crombie, *Robert Grosseteste and the Origins of Experimental Science* (2d ed., Oxford, 1961); John Herman Randall, Jr., *The School of Padua and the Emergence of Modern Science*; and William A. Wallace, *Causality and Scientific Explanation*, 1:28-47, 65-86, 117-127.

[21] Turisanus, *Plusquam*, fols. 3r-6r.

[22] The *explicit* of the *Conciliator* gives the completion date of 1303, but the work includes references to Peter's *Lucidator*, which, according to its author, was finished in 1310. No doubt Peter continued to add material to the *Conciliator* after his return to Italy from Paris in about 1306. See Thorndike, *History of Magic*, 2:880, and Siraisi, *Arts and Sciences at Padua*, p. 121. Peter died ca. 1316.

"*propter quid*" with composition, and demonstration "*quia*" with resolution. Peter's criticism of those who disagreed with Haly over this point may have been aimed, therefore, at Turisanus. Another sign of mutual familiarity is that both Turisanus and Peter offered a very similar example of the process of resolution and composition; Turisanus rather pointedly described his version as his own work.[23]

Turisanus was probably also familiar with other recent discussions—those of Robert Grosseteste and Albertus Magnus in particular—since he used standard examples relating to eclipses of the moon and to the supposedly purgative effect of scammony on red bile, which had been developed by those writers from the text of Aristotle and, most likely, from the writings of Galen and Avicenna.[24] The only authorities named by Turisanus in the course of his discussion of scientific method were, however, Aristotle, Galen, Boethius, Haly, Avicenna, and Averroes.

Conceivably, the discussions by Turisanus and Peter of Abano of scientific method as a process of resolution and composition may have derived from their studies at Paris.[25] This cannot be conclusively demonstrated, however, since manuscripts of earlier writings in which a similar analysis is found may also have circulated in Italy. Perhaps, though, Villani's story of Dino del Garbo's avid (even unethical) acquisition of the *Plusquam commentum*, mentioned above, is but a faint echo of the interest aroused in scholarly Italian medical circles by the introduction of this kind of sophisticated analysis of scientific method.

Turisanus began his exposition of scientific method with a consideration of the proper order of teaching any science, which, he explained, was nothing else than the dependence of posterior on prior.[26] He then asserted that the *Tegni*, at any rate in the version translated into Latin from the Arabic, endorses the use of the method of resolution, which is

---

[23] "et est demonstratio propter quid, et hec est doctrina compositiva . . . et est demonstratio quia, et hec doctrina dicitur resolutiva," Peter of Abano, *Conciliator*, fol. 10v. Compare this with the passages of the *Plusquam commentum* in notes 28 and 31, below. Jacopo da Forlì (d. 1414) noted the difference between Turisanus on the one hand and Peter of Abano and most of the "moderns" on the other over this issue; see the remarks from Jacopo's commentary on the *Tegni* translated in E. Grant, ed., *A Source Book in Medieval Science*, pp. 721-722. For the examples of resolution and composition, compare *Conciliator*, fol. 10v, and *Plusquam*, fol. 3v.

[24] See Bruce Eastwood, "Medieval Empiricism: The Case of Grosseteste's Optics," *Speculum* 43 (1968):306-321; Wallace, *Causality and Scientific Explanation*, 1:42-43, 73-75.

[25] For Peter's career, see Thorndike, *History of Magic*, vol. 2, chap. 70, passim.

[26] Turisanus, *Plusquam*, fols. 2r-3r.

described as proceeding from the nearer to the more remote—that is, beginning with an immediately evident phenomenon and reasoning back from it to "the first principle and cause of it."[27] There follows an explanation of Aristotle's teaching on scientific method in Book 2 of the *Posterior Analytics*; it is at this point that resolution is identified with demonstration *propter quid*, or absolute demonstration from the reasoned cause.[28] Turisanus then put forward as an example of resolution his own "question whether putrid fever or accidental heat is found in the body or why it is found." To demonstrate the cause of a putrid fever, it is sufficient to say that a putrid humor is produced inside the body and heats its container. But if one then inquires why the putrid humor is produced, the answer is because the prohibition of transpiration corrupts the natural heat; the reason for the prohibition of transpiration is the presence of obstruction in the passages of the body. One of the causes of obstruction must therefore be present; and these are either too many humors, or their grossness or viscosity, or excess of coldness or dryness or of dry heat. Whichever of these conditions predominates in any given instance will be the cause in that instance. Suppose that the cause in the case in question is an excess of humors; the cause of this in turn is over-eating and the resultant indigestion. This may be due to excessive appetite, which is the result of a faulty constitution (*malicia complexionis*); and the last named has, in turn, its own cause. The method of composi-

[27] "Translatio autem ex arabico [of the *Tegni*] in certificatione huius doctrine plus continet de textu, scilicet, cum dicit est ut statuas rem ad quam intendis et cuius scientiam inquiris secundum finem complementi eius: deinde consideres in propinquiori et propinquiori fine quo non stat res illa neque completur usque quo pervenias ad principia eius et est textus iste quasi expositio translationis ex greco. Sicut autem doctrina resolutiva fit [BAV, MS Urb. lat. 244, fol. 3v: fuit] ut accipiat quesitum et consideretur [Urb. lat. 244: componatur] in causa propinquiori et resolvatur usque ad primum principium et causam eius [Urb. lat. 244: ultimum quesitum ipsius]," ibid., fol. 3r.

[28] "dicit Aristotelis demonstratio que dat causam inventionis est alia a demonstratione que dat inventionem tantum: nam ea que dat causam inventionis dicitur demonstratio propter quid: que competit in quesito de quare [BAV, MS Urb. lat. 244, fol. 3v: in questione propter quid]: et est ista demonstratio per priora natura . . . Ea autem que dat inventionem tantum dicitur [Urb. lat. 244: alia est] demonstratio quia . . . Ad unum ergo istorum quesitorum quod est quesitum de quare respondetur per demonstrationem que absolute demonstratio dicitur: et [Urb. lat. 244: que] est demonstratio propter quid: et hec est doctrina resolutiva. Ad alia autem duo respondetur per demonstrationem que dicitur demonstratio non absolute sicut vult Aristotelis et est demonstratio quia: et hec dicitur doctrina compositiva [Urb. lat. 244: compositoria]," ibid., fol. 3v. See also *Posterior Analytics* 2.1-2, and Wallace, *Causality and Scientific Explanation*, 1:11-18, 213-214, regarding the translations of the key passages available in the Middle Ages.

tion, however, requires one to begin with the first principles and argue from them to the final manifestation of their activity. To provide an example, he listed the same chain of causes regarding fever in the reverse order.

Turisanus' examples of resolution and composition should perhaps warn us against attaching too much significance to early discussions of scientific method and against laying too much stress on the role of observation in medieval medicine. Most of the links in his chain of reasoning, which purports to explain the causes of a case of fever, have no basis in observable bodily processes. When he does come to an observable sequence of events (indigestion following overeating), Turisanus links it with other suppositions in what appears to us now to be a perfectly arbitrary way. Thus handled, the *doctrina resolutiva* and *doctrina compositiva* do not yield explanations any more rigorously verified than those of casual, random observation or learned or popular tradition. Turisanus should perhaps have heeded the implicit warning about the application of cause-and-effect analyses in medicine that Taddeo inserted into his commentary on an aphorism of Hippocrates (6.32), who suggested a relationship between stammering and diarrhea.[29] Taddeo pointed out that when physicians note an apparent relationship between two conditions, this should not be taken to mean that the two are necessarily linked in a one-to-one, cause-and-effect relationship, although such might be the case. Taddeo made copious use of examples to explain that, in physiology and medicine, observable "effects" do not always have a single cause, and vice versa. One cause could produce several effects that might or might not be related to one another, or several causes, related or unrelated, could produce the same effect. Thus two related conditions may both be effects of a cause distinct from either of them, or may be joint causes of yet another effect. Returning to the case of stammering and diarrhea, Taddeo asserted that these were two separate effects of excessive humidity in the brain, but that it was not inevitable that they should occur together; stammerers should watch their diet because they have a *tendency* to diarrhea.

Yet Turisanus, even if less clinically oriented than Taddeo, was himself fully aware of the limited usefulness of the *doctrina resolutiva* and *doctrina compositiva* to the medical science of his own day. He noted that the *doctrina resolutiva* was much used in geometry and other

[29] Taddeo, *Aphor.*, fols. 180v-181r.

branches of mathematics, because in mathematics the prior causes (*priora*) are well known to us; so those sciences allow certitude. But when it comes to natural sciences (*physica*), the prior causes are often hidden from us and only resultant accidents can be observed. Hence the physical sciences are less certain than mathematics.[30]

Nonetheless, Turisanus expressed his dissatisfaction with definitions of medical science provided by older authorities that did not take sufficient account of the method of resolution as the key to the acquisition of scientific knowledge. In particular, he was critical of Haly and the many who followed him on this score, noting that although Haly mentioned "*processus*" he did not really understand the distinction between resolution and composition.[31] Haly had stated that medicine was divided into curative and conservative branches, and that by ceaseless consideration of diet, regimen, and medication, and their effects, one would arrive at an understanding of first principles. Haly, in Turisanus's view, was doubly in error, both because he did not understand *resolutio* correctly and because he did not sufficiently stress that no single method of investigation could bring one to an adequate understanding of medical science. That Haly's belief in the sufficiency of general *summae*, in which the particulars of medicine were expounded one by one "by definition," was inadequate could be demonstrated by Galen's own methodology. Galen himself, Turisanus claimed, had used the method of resolution.[32] Despite his scorn

[30] "Usus autem huius doctrine apud mathematicos: ideo est maxime: quia in omnibus mathematicis ea que sunt natura priora sunt etiam notiora nobis: et ex illis declarantur posteriora: unde et illas scientias certissimas convenit esse [BAV, MS Urb. lat. 244, fol. 4r: scientias esse contingit]. In physicis autem frequenter non est sic quoniam sunt nobis occulta que priora sunt secundum naturam . . . ex quo accidit physicas scientias in quibusdam non habere tantam certitudinem quantam habent mathematice," Turisanus, *Plusquam*, fol. 4r.

[31] "Dicit Hali super isto loco quod in hac doctrina fuit inceptio ex principiis medicine, et componitur et extrahitur per compositionem totum quod est necessarium in medicina. Sed iste sermo non est verus, nam intentio eius est quod ex principiis medicine demonstretur in hac scientia quicquid posterius est principiis. et hoc appellat compositionem, cum ista sit resolutio sicut premonstravimus, et signum quod hec fuerit sua intentio est quia dixit in compositiva doctrina fieri demonstrationem propter quid cum Aristotelis in analeticis dixit ea fieri in resolutiva. . . . Et declaratur error eius ex hoc quod multi in tradendo scientias similibus doctrinis utuntur," ibid., fol. 5v.

[32] "Inquit enim Gal[enus] in fine huius libri in numeratione suorum librorum volentem artem medicine secundum rationem extrahere exerceri oportet in libro suo, quem demonstratione constituit: ex quo manifeste innuit resolutivam doctrinam nihil aliud quam demonstrationem eam esse, scilicet, que absolute demonstratio dicitur, unde et verificatur nostra

for the inadequacy of Haly's understanding of scientific method, Turisanus did not on that account reject the usefulness of encyclopedias of particulars in medicine. The proper view, he maintained, was that transmission and expansion of medical science called for the use of various types of scientific methodology, various modes of teaching, and accordingly various types of works in which the different branches of the subject were transmitted in the appropriate way. There was room both for encyclopedias and for specialized and analytical treatises such as those of Galen. Nor was Galen's own method wholly acceptable. Turisanus implied that Galen, too, had not fully understood the method of resolution; in fact, none of the ancient authorities in medicine had taught the proper use of this type of investigation, although Aristotle and other philosophers had earlier applied it in other disciplines. Medicine, like all branches of knowledge, had been crude and immature in its beginnings; and ancient medical writers, "*quasi rudes et primi*" as they were, wrote only of those external manifestations of disease apprehensible by the senses. Moreover, Turisanus asserted, medicine normally makes much more use of demonstration *quia* than of demonstration *propter quid*.[33] This, he believed, was because it is after all easier to see that a man has a fever because (*quia*) he has the symptoms of fever—headache, thirst, racing pulse—than it is to discern that he has a fever because (*propter quid*) of the presence of putrid heat in his body.

Thus, while Turisanus, like Grosseteste,[34] was apparently prepared to consider that *propter quid* demonstration was theoretically possible in physical as well as mathematical science, he was decidedly hesitant about its actual applications in medicine. He concluded his discussion by remarking that the ultimate causes of disease are often hidden, and that

---

expositio quam superius induximus in doctrinis. Sed hanc doctrinam dicit Gal[enus] se exercuisse alibi sicut in variis libris suis sicut est scrutantem videre," ibid.

[33] "Causa vero propter quam antiquorum nullus in medicina tradenda usus fuerit ista doctrina: quia in aliis scientiis non dubitamus philosophos que precesserunt G[alenum] sicut Ari[stotelem] et alios ipsa [*sic*] usos fuisse: est quia hec doctrina valde difficilior est, compositiva facilius [*sic*]. . . . Et licet Gal[enus] ea que in medicina queruntur visus fuerit ex causa demonstrare . . . scientia tamen medicine et universaliter scientia naturalis: et quecunque sub illa plus utitur in suis quesitis demonstratione quia quam demonstratione propter quid propter debilitatem nostre cognitionis," ibid.

[34] Wallace, *Causality and Scientific Explanation*, 1:39: "Rightly or wrongly, Grosseteste was apparently convinced that physical science . . . can arrive at true and appropriate causal explanations of physical phenomena, and in this sense can be a *propter quid* science."

demonstration that a disease is present because its symptoms are present (by demonstration *quia*, composition in his system) is more natural to medicine than demonstration *propter quid*, or resolution—a comment that reflects a perfectly realistic evaluation of the relative merits of the ability of medieval physicians to identify clusters of symptoms, and of their understanding of etiology. In the same passage, Turisanus used the well-worn example of the supposed purgative effects of scammony on red bile as an example of the type of medical knowledge that is purely "experimental" (that is, derived from experience) and is "as it were extraneous to any kind of (methodical and scientific) teaching."[35] From this point of departure, Turisanus went on to give his opinion on the already time-honored question whether medicine should more properly be classified as a science or an art. After explaining the principle of subalternation, according to which one science might be grouped with or subordinated to another, he declared that medicine is indeed in one sense a science, for it undoubtedly involves intellectual speculation about eternal verities.[36] However, it is also a practical activity, whose object, like that of the other mechanical arts, is to produce physical change.[37] When a physician orders treatment and the patient recovers, the result is produced partly by the physician's art and partly by the natural disposition of the human body, knowledge of which is undoubtedly a science. Yet the physician's study of man is limited to those aspects of the human body that affect health and sickness—for example, he does not consider man as the possessor of a soul or as a risible being. Moreover, the understanding of those who believe Galen to have described the division of medicine into theory and practice is vain and forever false, since such a division is not to be found in any of the works of Galen that are extant

[35] "scamoneam colere rubee evulsivam esse solo experimento convincitur, talia ergo particularia quesita extranea sunt ab omnibus speciebus doctrine," Turisanus, *Plusquam*, fol. 6r.

[36] "licet speciale subiectum alicuius scientie sit sub speciali subiecto alterius scientie ad modum quod eius suspicat [*sic*] predicationem: non propterea de necessitate scientia erit sub scientia, ita quod eius suscipiat predicationem, licet sit sub ea ad modum quod sua principia recipit ab ipsa: que est alter modus subalternandi. . . . medicina est scientia secundum quod ea de quibus est considerantur ab intellectu speculativo, id est, secundum quod ex aliquibus principiis speculatur aliquas conclusiones que sunt necessarie et eterne, sed ab hac scientia que quidem est habitus intellectus speculativi, resultat in intellectum practicum factivum quidam habitus que est ars medendi, que magis proprie dicitur medicativa quam medicina," ibid., fols. 7r-v.

[37] "hoc ergo modo secundum quod medicina est ars est una ex mechanicis," ibid., fol. 7v.

in Latin.[88] The currently recognized division between theory and practice should not, Turisanus held, be thought of as a division between knowing and doing, or paralleled with the distinction between mathematics and ethics. On the contrary, theory and practice are both integral parts of medicine: practice requires knowledge and study, just as does theory; and the purpose of theory is to direct practice. Medicine, therefore, is best categorized as an active science. Those who hold it to be a speculative science because it is subalternated to a speculative science—namely, natural philosophy—are wrong; similarly, ethics is subalternated to metaphysics, which is certainly speculative, but ethics, like medicine, is nonetheless itself an active, not a speculative, science.[39]

Thus Turisanus too, despite his obvious familiarity with and interest in current discussions of the methodology of investigative science, showed himself to be a vigorous defender of the view that the goal of all medical learning is the essentially practical one of restoring or conserving health. He found it necessary to reject explicitly the notion, which he claimed was held by some of his contemporaries, that medicine could be considered a purely speculative science. Moreover, he indicated his belief that, whatever the application in mathematics or in natural philosophy of the kind of analysis discussed by Grosseteste and others, its value for medicine was quite limited. His views were realistic, given the actual state of medical knowledge. The goal of medicine considered as a speculative science would be, presumably, improved understanding

---

[88] "Iam autem intellexerunt quidam ex antiquis magistris de Salerno quod Gal. per hoc dictum suum innueret divisionem medicine in theoricam et practicam quam nequaquam invenimus haberi in aliquo librorum suorum qui usque hodie ad latinam linguam exiverint: licet hec divisio non effugiat rationem propter habere medicinam non solum speculari passiones de subiecto: sed de conservatione et amotione earum in illo et ab illo, quorum primum videtur theorice, secundum practice, et intendunt illi quod Galie[nus] dicit secundum primam quidem rationem, id est theoricam, quod vero dicit in actionibus etiam intendunt practicam. Quorum intellectus vanus est et continuo falsus; nam ea pars medicine que theorica est numquam est de causis efficientibus et conservantibus sanitatem: sed practica," ibid., fol. 9r.

[39] "Dico ergo quod hanc scientiam quidam ascribunt esse speculativam ex eo quod subalternatur speculative, scilicet, naturali philosophie et ex eo etiam quod nulla videtur activarum, scilicet, nec monastica nec hyconomica nec politica, nec enim videtur scientia activa in plures divisa. Sed ostendemus proprio [sic] ipsam esse activam. . . . aliqui dicunt eam esse speculativam, quia subalternatur speculative. Dictum est quod medicina non subalternatur vere ad modum quo subalternatur species generi, scilicet, suscipiendo predicationem, sed secundum quod sua principia recipit ab illa qui est alter modus subalternandi. Ethica nam que est activa scientia subalternatur metaphysice que omnibus speculativior est," ibid., fol. 9v.

of human physiology and the etiology of disease, per se; to the extent that Turisanus, like Bartolomeo da Varignana, de-emphasized these goals, his views may be regarded as likely to impede scientific progress. But he was of course perfectly correct in perceiving that the existing tools of investigation in natural philosophy were unlikely to produce much further elucidation in physiological matters. Yet his perceptions in this regard did not prevent him from engaging in much speculation and ratiocination concerning humors, elements, complexion, and so on throughout the rest of the *Plusquam commentum*.

Turisanus's insistence that both structured, rational investigation and data randomly acquired from experience were integral parts of a unified medical science prefaced a work that was very general and largely theoretical in its approach. The same point was made, with equal emphasis, in the introduction to the *Practica* attributed to Guglielmo da Brescia.[40] This alphabetically arranged collection of particulars about diseases and remedies, beginning prosaically enough with baldness, is preceded by a brief commentary on the statement "He who wishes to be a master and perfect practitioner of the active arts should have no less knowledge of universals than particulars."[41] The author began by explaining that the difference between speculative and active is the same as that between theory and practice; medicine is an active art or science, even though it involves speculation, because its purpose is practical. He alluded in passing to the existence of two methods of investigation: the *via cognitionis*, which begins with general principles and proceeds to details; and the *via inventionis*, which begins with particulars acquired from experience and proceeds to general principles. Then, with a wealth of learned, mainly Aristotelian, citation (from the *Posterior Analytics*, the *Physics*, the *Metaphysics*, the works on animals, the *Ethics*), he set out to demonstrate that, although knowledge of general principles is indispensable for the physician, "he is a better practitioner who better knows how to descend to particulars."[42]

From the foregoing it will have become obvious that, whatever the variant shades of their individual opinions, the masters whose views

[40] Guglielmo, *Practica*, fol. 2r.

[41] "Illum qui vult esse magister et artifex perfectus in artibus activis oportet ut non minus habeat scientiam rei universalis quam rei particularis," ibid. The phrase is attributed to Aristotle "in xi moralis philosophie."

[42] "Et ille est melior artifex qui melius ad particularia condescendere novit," Guglielmo, *Practica*, fol. 2r.

have so far been analyzed were one in their desire to stress the interdependence of generalized "scientific" medical theory and the multi-
farious (and often apparently irrational) details of medical practice.

Within the overall scheme of an integrated medical science divided
into theory and practice, various programs of subdivision were adopted.
The ancient division of theoretical medicine into physiology, etiology,
and semiotics seems generally to have been abandoned.[43] Bartolomeo da
Varignana explicitly outlined one such program when he included a list
of the branches of medical theory in the introduction to his commentary
on Galen's *De interioribus*.[44] According to Bartolomeo, medical theory is
divided into the study of parts, passions, and causes of the human body.
Mondino de' Liuzzi, in the opening chapter of the *Anatomia*, adopted
the same scheme, remarking that "in Medicine a knowledge of the parts
of the subject—that is the human body—and the naming and relations of
those parts form a division of the science,"[45] and citing the *Colliget* of
Averroes as the source of this terminology. By "parts" Bartolomeo, too,
seems to have meant chiefly anatomy. Under the heading of "passions"
Bartolomeo included not only the all-embracing and much-discussed concept of *malicia complexionis* (the nearest English equivalent of which is
perhaps "disordered constitution"), the whole of internal medicine, such
specific conditions as fever, and particular diseases such as phthisis, but
also such controlling accidents or external factors as critical days, and
signs or diagnostic tools such as variations in pulse. By "causes" Bartolomeo meant the Aristotelian four causes; in applying them to the human
body he was following Avicenna. He thus avoided the scheme of division
into naturals (the body and its parts), nonnaturals (external factors),
and things against nature (diseases) adumbrated by Galen in the *Tegni*
and explicitly developed by Johannitius and numerous subsequent writers.[46] For Bartolomeo, material causes in medicine were the elements and

[43] Adopted, for example, in both the early medieval or late antique commentaries
referred to in note 1, above.

[44] BAV, MS Vat. lat. 4452, fol. 83v.

[45] The translation is that found in Mondino, *Anatomia*, ed. Singer, 1:59.

[46] See L. J. Rather, "The 'Six Things Non-Natural': A Note on the Origins and Fate of
a Doctrine and a Phrase," *Clio Medica* 3 (1968): 337-347; Saul Jarcho, "Galen's Six Non-
Naturals: A Bibliographic Note and Translation," *Bulletin of the History of Medicine* 44
(1970):370-377; and Peter H. Niebyl, "The Non-Naturals," ibid., 45 (1971):486-492;
Jerome J. Bylebyl, "Galen on the Non-Natural Causes of Variation in the Pulse," ibid., 45
(1971):482-485. The last-named article refers, in part, to Turisanus's use of the concept.

humors; the formal cause was *complexio*; the efficient causes were air, diet, and medication (the last two categories suggesting that the boundary between theoretical and practical medicine was in some areas rather indeterminate); and the final causes were "virtues and operations," that is to say, primarily respiration and pulsation.

Unlike Bartolomeo, neither Turisanus in the *Plusquam commentum* nor Taddeo in the commentary on the *Isagoge* included in his introductory description of medical science any single passage setting out all the subdivisions of medical theory, practice, or both. Instead, both authors, as might be expected, considering that they were commenting, respectively, upon the *Tegni* and upon Johannitius's introduction to that work, implicitly accepted the division of medicine into naturals, nonnaturals, and things contrary to nature. It is worth noting that both also found it desirable to include some special justification of the concept of nonnaturals, or external conditions inevitably affecting human health.[47] Turisanus, in particular, devoted some space to considering whether geographical location (*terra*), altitude, the stars, and human occupations and customs (*artes et mores*) should not also be included among them, since these conditions unavoidably affect the environment in which the human body flourishes or fails to flourish. He concluded, however, by deciding that the traditional six categories (air, food and drink, sleeping and waking, motion and quiet, evacuation and repletion, and the emotions) in fact provide an adequate scheme of division that should properly be understood to include the additional environmental conditions named above.

The descriptions of or allusions to the subdivisions of medical science provided by the members of Taddeo's circle do not, of course, concern medical specialization and specialties in anything like the modern sense. The masters of this group paid little or no attention in their writings to the possibility that a practicing learned physician might concentrate his attention exclusively upon particular parts of the body, diseases, or types of treatment. It is clear, for example, that the list of the various branches of theory set down by Bartolomeo da Varignana simply represented, in its author's mind, a convenient schema of the subjects of medi-

---

[47] Taddeo, *Isagoge*, fol. 372v. The questions discussed are included in the question register (fol. 401r) under the titles: Utrum diffinitio rei naturalis et non naturalis posita ab autore sit bona; Utrum res non naturalis sit de substantia nostri corporis; Utrum res non naturales sint plures quam sex. Turisanus, *Plusquam*, fol. 81r, question entitled in question register (fol. 137v): "Utrum res non naturales sint sex."

cal education. The absence of discussions of specialization is, in the main, simply a reflection of the state of medical science at the time; the practical possibilities of any would-be specialist were limited by the amount and actual usefulness of the information available to the physician about particular diseases, injuries, or bodily functions. But it is no doubt also true that the general emphasis upon the overall unity of medical science and the general respect for philosophical breadth of learning contributed to a climate of opinion that was not very hospitable to the concept of specialization as such. Even "*chirurgia*," which, as we have seen, embraced a much wider area than the modern "surgery," does not seem to have received the exclusive attention of any learned physicians. Practitioners who confined themselves to surgery alone did so because they lacked broader learning, not because, after having acquired it, they had chosen to specialize.

Taddeo and those he trained, like other learned physicians of the period, considered that the study of medicine in all its branches required knowledge not only of scientific medical theory and of the accumulated details of medical practice, but also of certain ancillary sciences. As Peter of Abano, a contemporary professor of philosophy, *astrologia*, and medicine at Padua, put it, all the arts and sciences are necessary to medicine, but logic, *astrologia*, and natural science (*scientia naturalis*) are "more necessary."[48]

Among the ancillary sciences, natural philosophy, or natural science, had pride of place. Not only were the principles of natural philosophy usually regarded as fundamental to medicine (as has been demonstrated above), but the details of natural science provided a mass of relevant information. All the members of Taddeo's circle displayed extensive knowledge of the *libri naturales* of Aristotle. Much of the discussion of the particulars of human anatomy, physiology, and psychology by Taddeo and those associated with him drew upon Aristotle and other natural philosophical writers, and compared their conclusions with those of medical authorities. In addition, certain other topics traditionally expounded by physicians lent themselves especially well to the introduction of material drawn from natural philosophy. For example, accounts of the "things natural" in the scheme of naturals, nonnaturals, and things contrary to

[48] "Ille [scientie] tamen que medicine sunt necessariores existunt iste: Logica . . . , naturalis eius principiorum ostensiva, et astrologia," *Conciliator*, fol. 3r.

nature, or of the material causes of the human body in the scheme of parts, passions, and causes, called for discussion of the elements; under the nonnaturals, discussion of the category "air" might be expanded to include material on meteorology, climate, and physical geography; optical theory could be introduced into descriptions of the eye and the sense of sight. The uses Taddeo and his pupils made of natural philosophy are, indeed, sufficiently various and of sufficiently wide-ranging import to merit separate treatment; for this the reader is referred to the following two chapters.

Of the seven liberal arts, all of them traditionally thought necessary to medicine,[49] only logic and astronomy played any significant part in the medical writings of Taddeo and his associates. Bartolomeo da Varignana, as already noted, declared that logic was indispensable in medical learning, a statement that was scarcely necessary since his own theoretical writings, like those of his colleagues and contemporaries, constituted a prolix tribute to the thoroughness of their author's dialectical training.

Astrology, along with a certain amount of introductory astronomy, undoubtedly played an important part in medical training at Bologna in the early fourteenth century, and probably before. This is sufficiently demonstrated by the teaching career of Cecco d'Ascoli and by the existence of a commentary on the *Theorica planetarum* completed by Taddeo da Parma in 1318 and written especially for the benefit of medical students.[50] Cecco prefaced his commentary on Sacrobosco's *Sphere* with an elaborate justification of the importance of astrology for medical studies, and Taddeo da Parma introduced his commentary on another standard introductory textbook in astronomy with "a long exposition and bibliography—chiefly from Arabic authors—of judicial astrology itself and a list and classification of various other occult arts."[51]

Both the *Theorica planetarum* and the *Sphere* were among the works prescribed for the study of astronomy at Bologna by the university statutes of 1405. At that time, and no doubt also in the early fourteenth century, "*astrologia*" was a basic course in arithmetic, geometry, and astronomy (including the use of instruments), as well as astrology in the modern

---

[49] See for example Haly Abbas, *Liber totius medicine* . . . (Lyon, 1523), fol. 83; Roger Bacon, *Opus tertium*, chap. 59, and other authors.

[50] Thorndike, *History of Magic*, 3:12 and appendix 2.

[51] Cecco d'Ascoli, *In spheram mundi enarratio*, ed. Lynn Thorndike, in *The Sphere of Sacrobosco*, pp. 344-346 (proem); Thorndike, *History of Magic*, 3:12.

sense. The required texts included an algorism, or arithmetic, the first three books of Euclid's *Elements*, part of Ptolemy's *Almagest*, as well as the astrological *Centiloquium* attributed to him, and a treatise on the astrolabe.[52]

The importance attached to the study of the stars in medieval medical education[53] derived from a general and widely held belief that the heavenly bodies play an intermediary role in the creation of things here below and continue to influence them throughout their existence. The actual uses of astrology in medical diagnosis and treatment by learned physicians were many and various. "Astrological medicine" is a vague and unsatisfactory term that can embrace any or all of the following: first, to pay attention to the supposed effect of astrological birth signs or signs at conception on the constitution and character of one's patients;[54] second, to vary treatment according to various celestial conditions (the well-known treatise on astrological medicine generally attributed in the Middle Ages to Hippocrates suggests general changes in medical treatment as the moon moves through the different signs of the zodiac,[55] and, of course, the physician might also vary his prescriptions according to the patient's individual horoscope); third, to connect the doctrine of critical days in illness with astrological features, usually phases of the moon;[56]

[52] Malagola, *Statuti*, p. 276. These works were all available in Latin in the thirteenth century and before; also prescribed in 1405, however, were the *Alfonsine Tables* of planetary motions with canons for their use, the latter being apparently those compiled by John of Saxony, which reached Bologna in 1344; see L. Frati et al., "Indici dei codici latini conservati nella R. Biblioteca Universitaria di Bologna," *Studi italiani di filologia classica* 17 (1909):1-171, no. 1369 (2614), *explicit*.

[53] For the teaching of astronomy/astrology in connection with medicine at other medieval university centers, see Richard Lemay, "The Teaching of Astronomy in Medieval Universities, Principally at Paris in the Fourteenth Century," in *Science, Medicine, and the University, 1200-1550: Studies in Honor of Pearl Kibre, Manuscripta* 20 (1976):197-217.

[54] For example, a set of tables to find the ascendant at the time of nativity drawn up by the Paduan professor of medicine Jacopo Dondi (Oxford, Bodleian Library, MS Canon. misc. 436, fols. 48-50; I have examined the photocopy bequeathed to Columbia University by Lynn Thorndike) were intended to assist in medical astrology of this kind.

[55] There are numerous manuscripts and early printed editions (see TK). I have consulted *Astronomia Hippocratis* in J. Ganivet, *Amicus medicorum* (Frankfurt, 1614), pp. 582-617; three Latin versions circulated in the thirteenth and fourteenth centuries (see note 66, below).

[56] For example, Taddeo, *Pronost.*, fols. 236r-v, questions listed in register (fol. 246r) as: Utrum aspectus lune et corporis supercelestis sit causa crisis; Utrum corpus superceleste sit causa mala crisis; Utrum natura creticans recipiat adiutorium a constellatione; Utrum motus celestis sit causa dierum creticorum intercidentium.

and fourth, to predict or explain epidemics with reference to planetary conjunctions, the appearance of comets, or weather conditions.[57]

There is no question that physicians in Taddeo's circle, like their colleagues elsewhere, shared the general belief in the influence of the heavenly bodies. Thus Taddeo reiterated that "specific form" was a quality given to everything on earth by the heavens or constellations, and Dino discussed the role in human generation of the Intelligences acting through the heavenly bodies (see chapter six). Furthermore, they also made specific applications of astrology to medicine: Taddeo wrote of the relationship of the aspects of the moon to crisis in illness; Turisanus explained that astrology aided medicine by indicating how dosage and strength of medication should be varied under different planetary aspects;[58] and Mondino, as we shall see, discussed the connection between changes in the weather and epidemic disease. Yet there is singularly little evidence in their writings of any special interest in, or particularly wide knowledge of astronomy or astrology. Compared with such fourteenth-century Italian physicians as Peter of Abano and Jacopo and Giovanni de' Dondi, all of whom were noted for their astronomical learning, the circle of Taddeo is markedly deficient in this regard.[59] None of its members (with the possible exception of Bartolomeo da Varignana)[60] produced any work devoted to astronomy or astrology, while the astrological excursuses in their medical works are neither very lengthy nor very numerous.

There are, indeed, a few signs that some of the members of our group of authors may have wanted to set limits to the interest in astrology among Bologna's medical students. Thus, Gentile da Cingoli declared his opposition to astrological determinism, asserting that the stars may predispose, but they do not determine[61] (elsewhere, however, Gentile

[57] A practice very widespread in the Middle Ages. A famous—and learned—example is the report produced by the physicians of the University of Paris, at the request of the king of France, on bubonic plague; see Anna M. Campbell, *The Black Death and Men of Learning* (New York, 1931), pp. 39-42.

[58] See note 56, above, and Turisanus, *Plusquam*, fol. 100r (misprint for 84r).

[59] For a summary account of the astronomical (and in the case of Peter and Jacopo astrological) interests of these Paduan professors of medicine, and citations of the literature, see Siraisi, *Arts and Sciences at Padua*, pp. 81-94.

[60] SF 1:585, referring to a manuscript formerly in the library of Santa Croce; but I have been unable to locate any manuscript answering to this description in Angelo Maria Bandini, *Catalogus Bibliothecae Mediceae laurentianae* (4 vols., Florence, 1774-1777), vol. 4, which lists manuscripts formerly in the library of Santa Croce in Florence.

[61] Grabmann, "Gentile da Cingoli," pp. 26-28, where the passage is printed.

appeared to accept at least some of the claims of astrologers and magicians—see chapter seven). Dino del Garbo is said, as already noted, to have prepared an analysis of the errors in one of Cecco d'Ascoli's commentaries, in which he presumably attacked Cecco's astrological determinism. Moreover, in his *Dilucidatorium* "of the whole of practical medicine," Dino considers a wide range of forces that might conceivably affect the effectiveness of phlebotomy; but the stars, traditionally associated with bloodletting, are the topic of only one question (although seasons and weather are discussed in several).[62]

Mondino de' Liuzzi used the first section of his commentary on the *Prognostica* of Hippocrates[63] to expound what he believed to be the true meaning of certain Hippocratic sayings pressed into service by some authors to justify medical astrology. The passages in question—namely, the statement in *Airs Waters Places* that the physician ought to be able to forecast from celestial signs, and the remark in the *Prognostica* that some diseases appear to have something of the celestial or divine about them—were, for example, soon to be used in this astrological sense by Cecco in the preface to his commentary on the *Sphere*.[64] Mondino, by contrast, labored to point out the limited, relatively pragmatic nature of the Hippocratic author's actual meaning in the passages in question. He began by inquiring whether prognosis had any place in medicine, since foretelling the future from signs was the function of astrology. His conclusion was that the usefulness of medical prognosis and the admiration that prognostic skill brought the physician more than justified its inclu-

[62] "Utrum melius sit flobothomare et ventosare in prima quadra lune quam in secunda: et in tertia quam in quarta," Dino, *Dilucidatorium*, chap. 21, q. 5. Regarding the stars and bloodletting see, for example, Robert Herrlinger, *History of Medical Illustration* (New York, 1970), pp. 25-28.

[63] Mondino, comm. *Pronost.*, BAV, MS Vat. lat. 4466, fol. 1v.

[64] *Airs Waters Places* 2; *Prognostica* 4. The passage in *Airs Waters Places* is an unambiguous justification of the study by physicians of weather and climate, and hence of the heavens. Two medieval Latin versions of the *Prognostica* respectively qualified some diseases as having about them something "celeste" or "divinum." Galen, in his commentary on the *Prognostica* (Galen, *Opera*, ed. Kühn, 18:21), had striven to repudiate the notion that Hippocrates could ever have stated disease to be a divine affliction, and had interpreted the statement as alluding to the effect on health of the atmosphere and winds. Cecco, however, placed both *Airs Waters Places* and the *Prognostica* on a list of authoritative works endorsing astrological medicine that also included the pseudo-Hippocratic tract on astrological medicine, the *Centiloquium* attributed to Ptolemy, and works of Hermes Trimegistus, Albumasar, and Messahalah (Cecco, *In Spheram*, in Thorndike, ed., *Sphere of Sacrobosco*, pp. 344-345).

sion as part of the science of medicine. Nonetheless, when Hippocrates wrote that physicians should know celestial signs, he had not meant, as some supposed, that doctors should be able, from the aspect of the stars, to know about a divine virtue that caused diseases. Hippocrates repudiated such ideas as fatuous and did not include them in medical science. Furthermore, primary causation (*primum principium*) is the province of theology, and celestial aspects, as such, that of astrology. What Hippocrates had recommended physicians to study was not celestial aspects themselves, but the influence on human health of changing atmospheric conditions caused by the passage of the sun through the signs of the zodiac— that is, the seasons and the general character of the year's weather (*constitutio anni*).[65] Obviously, the effect of the weather (*dispositio aeris*) is not something peculiar to prognostication for any individual, but is common to many men and to other creatures as well.

Replying to the objection that the knowledge of weather conditions he was recommending would not redound greatly to the physician's credit, since any countryman knew as much, Mondino pointed out that the ability to presage the impact of future weather conditions on the health of large numbers of people was far from commonplace and would indeed bring the physician credit. If people marvel at the physician's ability to say that one patient will die and another recover, should they not be the more amazed if he can correctly predict the general implications for public health of a warm winter and a cold spring? And prognostications of this sort the physician can make. He may, for example, announce that putrid and mortal diseases will be prevalent in late spring and early summer, on the basis of his knowledge that the preceding summer was unusually hot and dry and that the heat and drought continued into the middle of the autumn, when the weather suddenly turned wet and remained so for a long time. This hypothetical case demonstrates, Mondino concluded, that Hippocrates was not merely talking about knowledge of present weather conditions, such as any peasant might have, but about genuine, medical prediction.

Thus, Mondino took a conservative, not to say cautious, position toward the medical uses of astrology. Naturally enough, in a commentary

---

[65] [Y]pocratis per signum celeste non intellexit aspectum corporis celestis immediate sed dispositionem quod causatur in aere a corpore celesti et quia hec est dispositio que causatur in aere per cursum solis in celesti zodiaco per alias constellationes hec autem dispositio est tempus anni et constitutio anni," Mondino, comm. *Pronost.*, BAV, MS Vat. lat. 4466, fol. 1v.

on the *Prognostica*, he sought to maintain as strongly as he could the possibility of authentic, factually based medical predictions quite distinct from the forecasts of astrologers, especially from those involved in the forbidden and dangerous branches of judicial astrology. For him, the astrology necessary for a physician came down to not much more than the ability to take note of weather conditions. Moreover, it is noteworthy that Mondino discussed the views of Hippocrates on astrology without mentioning the pseudo-Hippocratic tract on astrological medicine, which was widely disseminated in three separate translations, at least two of which were probably of north Italian provenance.[66] In this work, the vital necessity of a knowledge of astrology for successful medical treatment is several times stressed.

Like the remarks of Gentile da Cingoli, the preface to Mondino's commentary on the *Prognostica*, written in 1317, conceivably reflects a growing uneasiness among some of Bologna's medical masters about the enthusiasm for astrological medicine among some of their colleagues and students in the faculty of arts and medicine. Their enthusiasm was soon to reach its peak in the lectures of Taddeo da Parma and Cecco d'Ascoli. Plainly, some medical masters were already anxious to disassociate themselves from possibly heterodox opinions of any kind by 1311, when Dino del Garbo's *socius*, Master Giuliano da Bologna (Julianus Bononiensis), denounced a colleague to the Inquisition on grounds so flimsy that the inquisitor subsequently reversed the sentence and fined the accuser.[67] Thus, Dino's own hostility to the astrological beliefs of Cecco d'Ascoli, even if fully developed only after Dino ended his teaching career at Bologna, may after all represent the culmination of a long-standing conflict within the arts and medical faculty there.

The foregoing sketch has outlined how the discipline of learned medicine was conceived by our group of masters, and what kind of studies it involved for them and for those they taught. From the evidence that has been assembled, it is plain that, despite the institutional union of arts

[66] See Lynn Thorndike, "The Three Latin Translations of the Pseudo-Hippocratic Tract on Astrological Medicine," *Janus* 49 (1960):104-129. Two of the translations were by William of Moerbeke and Peter of Abano respectively, both of them active in Italy for part of their careers. Turisanus appears to allude to this treatise; see the passage cited in note 58 to this chapter.

[67] Girolamo Biscaro, "Inquisitori ed ereteci lombardi (1292-1318)," *Miscellanea di storia italiana*, 3d ser. 19 (1922):492-493. Giuliano was the *reportator* of Dino's commentary on Hippocrates, *De natura fetus* (see BAV, MS Vat. lat. 4464, fol. 124r). Regarding the possible presence of some unorthodox beliefs within the circle of Taddeo, see below, chapter six.

and medicine, despite the intellectual allurements and prestige of natural philosophy, and despite the prevalence of Aristotelian logical and philosophical learning among medical faculty, the medicine of those trained in the schools of Bologna in the years circa 1265-1325 retained its autonomy as a science, its practical side, and its own distinct, learned tradition. The following chapters will show how Taddeo and his pupils and associates interpreted, developed, and used some of the content of the learning in natural philosophy, arts, and medicine that was their heritage.

CHAPTER SIX

THE USES OF PHILOSOPHY: RECONCILING THE PHILOSOPHERS AND PHYSICIANS

*A*s we have seen, the earliest writings on Aristotelian philosophy known to have been produced at Bologna are those of Taddeo: his vernacular Etica, and the philosophical passages in his commentary on the medical *Isagoge* of Johannitius. And, together with his contemporary and probable colleague Jacopo da Pistoia, who expounded the nature of true happiness in scholastic mode and with abundant Aristotelian citation, Taddeo may be regarded as the progenitor of subsequent philosophical endeavors by the masters of Bologna. Furthermore, works on philosophy were produced by Taddeo's pupils; not only by Gentile da Cingoli, who remained in the faculty of arts, but also by the physicians Bartolomeo da Varignana and Dino del Garbo. Nor was philosophy a peripheral or sparetime activity of these physicians. Taddeo and his colleagues and pupils taught and wrote within an intellectual tradition that claimed philosophy and medicine to be in some way akin and that consequently regarded knowledge of philosophy as an essential part of the learned physician's professional equipment. They would have endorsed, and the writings of some of them may have helped to inspire, the decision, mentioned above, of the compilers of the 1405 statutes of the Bologna University of Arts and Medicine to list Aristotle's *libri naturales* and the required texts in medicine under a common rubric.

Yet the information so far assembled here about their writings on moral and natural philosophy, their attempts to define the relationship of the disciplines of philosophy and medicine, and their descriptions of an essentially Aristotelian scientific method tell little or nothing about the ways they actually used in medicine knowledge that they thought of as philosophical. Two questions remain unanswered: Where, how, and on what subjects is information drawn from philosophical authors incorporated into the medical writings of Taddeo and his pupils? and What level of awareness of current philosophical trends and disputes is shown in their medical works?

So far as I am aware, the kind of systematic survey of the works of Taddeo and the others that is necessary to answer the first of these questions has not hitherto been àttempted. Yet that question is of considerable importance for the history of medieval learned medicine. The traditional assertions about the importance of philosophy for medicine might be expected to take on a new meaning in a period in which the teachings of Aristotle and his Arab commentators, with their revolutionary implications for almost every branch of Latin learning, had but recently been absorbed. Further, it seems reasonable to assume that "philosophy" (understood as material obtained from the works of philosophers) was not randomly incorporated into thirteenth- and fourteenth-century medical writings, but served specific functions. What these functions were, scholars have only recently begun to determine.[1] Clearly, however, for medicine one of the most significant aspects of the reception of Aristotle was the recognition of contradictions between Aristotelian teaching and the medieval Galenic tradition. The impact of this recognition has indeed general significance for the history of science in the Middle Ages as well as for the history of medicine, since the discrepancies between Aristotle and Galen constituted one of the principal known examples of conflict between leading scientific authorities. The way in which medical and other writers handled these discrepancies is an important key to the changing patterns of scientific thought. The medieval ideal was harmonization and reconciliation, but this proved no easier to achieve in the case of Aristotle and Galen than in that of Aristotle and Plato.[2] Discussion and attempted reconciliation of the differences between the two presentations of anatomy and physiology became a major theme in Latin medical (and some

[1] See, for example, the analysis of the development of pharmaceutical theory contained in the editor's introduction to Arnald of Villanova, *Aphorismi de gradibus*, ed. Michael R. McVaugh, in Arnald of Villanova, *Opera Medica Omnia*, ed. L. Garcia-Ballester, J. A. Paniagua, and Michael R. McVaugh, vol. 2 (Granada-Barcelona, 1975); Richard P. McKeon, "Medicine and Philosophy in the Eleventh and Twelfth Centuries: The Problem of the Elements," *The Thomist* 24 (1961):75-120; and E. Seidler, "Die Heilkunde des ausgehenden Mittelalters in Paris," *Sudhoffs Archiv für Geschichte der Medizin und der Naturwissenschaften*, Beiheft 8 (1968), pp. 91-106.

[2] On the ancient and medieval history of attempts to compare and sometimes reconcile the teachings of Plato and Aristotle, see Frederick Purnell, "Jacopo Mazzoni and His Comparison of Plato and Aristotle" (Ph.D. diss., Columbia Univ., 1971). I owe this reference to the courtesy of Professor Edward Mahoney.

philosophical) writing in the thirteenth century and remained a preoccupation of physicians until the seventeenth century.[3] The importance attached to the reconciliation of Aristotle and Galen in medical schools around 1300 is well illustrated by the title given by Peter of Abano, who taught at Paris and Padua, to his best-known work: *The Reconciler of Differences and Especially of the Philosophers and Physicians.* The manner in which Taddeo and his pupils confronted discrepancies between the most revered authorities in philosophy and in medicine reveals not only the extent of their philosophical knowledge and the way in which they used it, but also their attitudes to authority, their notions of scientific proof, and the state of development of their critical faculties.

The second question—that of the medical authors' awareness of contemporary philosophy—has attracted some attention from historians of medieval philosophy, at least as far as Taddeo Alderotti and Dino del Garbo are concerned. The belief that Taddeo may not only have inspired the study of Aristotle at Bologna, but may also have given Bolognese Aristotelianism its characteristically radical and occasionally heterodox direction, has led to careful examination of his views.[4] There is no doubt that Taddeo was familiar with the notorious Averroist thesis of the unicity of the intellect, and his exposition of it has convinced some scholars that he shared the view he was describing. As we have seen, similar opinions have been ascribed, on less firm grounds, to Dino.[5] Yet it remains to be seen whether these particular philosophical ideas attributed to Taddeo and Dino played any considerable or consistent part in the medical teaching of Taddeo's school.

Rather than simply being assumed, the role of these ideas must be demonstrated. It is no doubt true that at Bologna, as at Padua, the secular

[3] See Edwin Clarke and C. D. O'Malley, *The Human Brain and Spinal Cord: A Historical Study Illustrated by Writings from Antiquity to the Twentieth Century* (Berkeley, Calif., 1968), pp. 25-26, and Siegel, *Galen's System of Physiology and Medicine*, p. 225.

[4] See Nardi, "L'Averroismo bolognese nel secolo XIII e Taddeo Alderotto," and Martin Grabmann, *Mittelalterliches Geistesleben,* 3:197-212; this portion of the work earlier appeared, in Italian, as "L'Aristotelismo italiano al tempo di Dante con particolare riguardo all'Università di Bologna," *Rivista di filosofia neo-scolastica* 38 (1946):260-277. Regarding Dino, see the works cited in note 133 to chapter two, above. According to B. Nardi, "L'Averroismo bolognese," p. 22, Taddeo "made himself a preacher of Averroism among his numerous pupils."

[5] "Taddeo Alderotto era, nell'interpretazione del pensiero di Aristotele, averroista," B. Nardi, "L'Averroismo bolognese," p. 19; but see also the more cautious statement in Grabmann, "L'Aristotelismo italiano," p. 270.

status and the professional goals of teachers and students of medicine, especially in the absence of the restraining influence of a public faculty of theology, helped shape an approach to Aristotle in which theological considerations played little part. It is also true that, in an institutionally integrated faculty of arts and medicine, contacts between philosophers and physicians remained close; learned physicians had quite often taught philosophy at an early stage of their careers, as Guglielmo da Brescia had done, and perhaps also Bartolomeo da Varignana. Yet the philosophical output of the 1320s-1340s, on which the current reputation of the Bolognese Aristotelian school rests, does not appear for the most part to have been the work of men who produced any substantial medical writings, although some of them were undoubtedly trained as physicians.[6] Moreover, to the extent that the antecedents of their philosophical views have been traced, their ideas appear to have been influenced by Jean de Jandun and other philosophers at Paris, rather than by any tradition developed in Bolognese medical teaching.[7] It also seems likely that, as the faculty of arts and medicine developed and grew larger in the generation after Taddeo, the distinction between those who were primarily teachers of medicine, on the one hand, and those who were primarily teachers of philosophy, on the other, became clearer than it had been in Taddeo's own lifetime. There is no good reason to assume therefore, that medical teaching as such necessarily stressed philosophical controversy for its own sake or included significant contributions to contemporary philosophical debate. On the contrary, there are good grounds for supposing that their very professionalism led Taddeo's pupils, if not Taddeo himself, to limit the time devoted to philosophical studies; to treat philosophy and science in their medical works as adjuncts to medicine; and (again with the exception of Taddeo himself) to be extremely cautious about giving the slightest ground for suspicions of unorthodoxy. Nor should it be assumed that the philosophical views of those trained by Taddeo were the ideas of a close-knit coterie of thinkers, identified either

[6] The philosophers of this school whose works have so far been studied are Anselmo da Como, Angelo d'Arezzo, Taddeo da Parma, Matteo da Gubbio, and Jacopo da Piacenza; on them, see Kuksewicz, *De Siger de Brabant à Jacques de Plaisance*, pp. 315-452, and bibliography there cited. Kuksewicz (p. 342) identifies Anselmo da Como as a physician; and see note 91 to chapter two, above, for medical questions by Angelo d'Arezzo and Jacopo da Piacenza (Jacobus de Placentia). On the rise of the school, see further the studies named in note 63, below.

[7] Kuksewicz, *De Siger de Brabant à Jacques de Plaisance*, pp. 316, 399-406.

by themselves or by others as the holders of certain characteristic views. As already remarked, several of Taddeo's pupils appear to have studied under him only for relatively brief periods of time, and their later careers, in some cases, carried them far from the schools of Bologna. In their works, unambiguous references either to opinions of Taddeo or to those of another member of the group are extremely infrequent. Nonetheless, to consider their treatment, as a group, of philosophical issues is to explore an important aspect of the medical learning of their time, as it was handed down by Taddeo at Bologna and by his successors at Bologna and elsewhere.

Taddeo and those he taught were versed in both moral and natural philosophy, but natural philosophy played by far the greater part in their medical writings. A few citations of the *libri morales* can be found in the medical works; and, to the extent, admittedly fairly slight, that traditional medical teaching dealt with professional ethics, it paralleled the concerns of moral philosophy.[8] One could argue too, as Turisanus did, for parallels between Aristotle's concept of justice and Galen's complexion theory, both of which are based on the idea of balance, due proportion, and the mean; and physicians as well as moral philosophers occasionally made humanistic declarations about the nobility of man's nature. Nonetheless, in their medical writings, "philosophy" almost always meant Aristotelian natural philosophy to our authors; as the reader will have become aware, the various statements about the relationship of medicine and philosophy that were quoted or summarized in the preceding chapter all refer to natural philosophy. It is worth pausing briefly to recall what this discipline, along with metaphysics (with which physicians also sometimes concerned themselves), encompassed.

Natural philosophy, in the later thirteenth and early fourteenth centuries, was based primarily on the study of all the *libri naturales* attributed to Aristotle. Its subject matter therefore ranged over the fundamental principles of matter and motion (the *Physics*); motion in the heavens and the nature of heavenly bodies (*De celo et mundo*); principles of change in terrestrial bodies and the role of the elements (*De generatione et corruptione*); psychology and sense perception (*De anima* and some of the *Parva naturalia*); atmospheric conditions, including climate and

---

[8] See Mary C. Wellborn, "The Long Tradition: A Study in Fourteenth-Century Medical Deontology," *Medieval and Historiographical Essays in Honor of James Westfall Thompson*, ed. J. L. Cate and E. N. Anderson (Chicago, 1938), pp. 344-357.

weather (the *Meteorologica*); botany (the pseudo-Aristotelian *De plantis*); and zoology; animal and human anatomy, and physiology (parts of the *Parva naturalia* and, above all, the books on animals). In addition, those Aristotelian concepts that endeavor to explain the nature of being itself—substance, form, potency, act, the first mover, and so forth—were studied in the *Metaphysics*; while, as we have seen, the *Posterior Analytics* provided the basis for a method in natural science. As far as medieval medicine is concerned, the material contained in the *libri naturales* may be thought of as falling into two categories: accounts of basic principles that were held to underlie medicine as they underlay all physical sciences; and material directly relating to the subject of medical science, that is, to the human body. Certain works that appear decidedly non-medical to a modern reader fell into the latter of these categories for medieval learned physicians. *De celo* and the *Meteorologica* were certainly relevant to medicine in an age that held the heavenly bodies (whether directly, or indirectly via their effect on climate and weather) and "airs waters places" to be major influences upon human health or sickness; the discussion of the elements and qualities in *De generatione et corruptione* was highly pertinent to medical theories about the balance of "complexion" in each individual; and the information about plants contained in *De plantis* would have been valued by physicians trained in the use of herbal medicines.[9] Of even more obvious medical relevance, of course, were the various accounts of psychology and sense perception provided by Aristotle. But, evidently, the Aristotelian material that was likely to be of most interest to learned physicians was the Philosopher's extensive treatment of mammalian anatomy and physiology and, more specifically, of the anatomy and physiology of man. Human anatomy occupies a prominent place in Book 1 of the *Historia animalium*, while substantial portions of that work and of *De generatione animalium* are devoted to the subject of human reproduction. Further discussions of topics in or related to human anatomy and physiology are scattered throughout the biological works.

Learned physicians in the Latin West appear to have arrived at some understanding of the full range of applications of the contents of all of

---

[9] As may be seen from the fact that Albertus Magnus appended a herbal describing individual plant species and frequently indicating their medicinal uses to his version of this work; see Albertus Magnus, *De vegetabilibus et plantis*, Book 6, in his *Opera omnia*, ed. Auguste Borgnet (Paris, 1890), 10:159-268.

the *libri naturales* to medicine only during the middle years of the thirteenth century—that is, shortly before Taddeo began to teach at Bologna in the 1260s. The process had begun long before; as noted in the preceding chapter, the physicians of Salerno in the twelfth century showed some knowledge, probably mainly indirect, of Aristotelian doctrines; they also preserved a tradition of discussing questions relating to general science as well as to medicine.[10] Moreover, the most influential precedent in the handling of Aristotelian material in a medical book was probably set by the *Canon* of Avicenna, which, as already noted, was translated from Arabic into Latin before 1187. Yet the first Latin medical work to show signs of its author's extensive familiarity with the *Canon* is apparently the *Anatomia vivorum*, formerly ascribed to Ricardus Anglicus, which has been dated between 1210 and 1240, with the greatest likelihood attached to some time about the year 1225.[11] Taddeo himself was, as has already been mentioned, among the earliest Latin commentators on parts of the *Canon*. Moreover, Aristotle's works on animals and discussions of these works by the great Arab philosopher-physicians Avicenna and Averroes reached the west only between 1210 and about 1230.[12] Latin commentaries on Aristotle's works on animals began to appear in the middle years of the century, the most notable and influential no doubt being those by the theologian and natural philosopher Albertus Magnus, and by the physician and logician Peter of Spain (Pope John XXI).[13]

Given the availability of this range of philosophical material and this array of precedents for its treatment in connection with medical topics, it is not surprising to find that, while the philosophical content of the medical works of Taddeo Alderotti and his associates is almost exclusively Aristotelian, it takes a number of different forms and serves a variety of purposes.[14] In addition to the expositions of the relationship between medicine and philosophy and of scientific method referred to in the last chapter, we may distinguish: first, the explication of fundamental Aristotelian doctrines in a medical context and the discussion of related

[10] On this tradition, see Brian Lawn, *The Salernitan Questions.*

[11] See Corner, *Anatomical Texts,* pp. 38-44.

[12] *Aristoteles Latinus,* 1:80-81, 107-108; Vaux, "La première entrée d'Averroès," pp. 193-245; Wingate, *The Mediaeval Latin Versions of the Aristotelian Scientific Corpus,* pp. 72-77.

[13] Wingate, *The Mediaeval Latin Versions of the Aristotelian Scientific Corpus,* pp. 79-82.

[14] There are a few traces of the survival of earlier medieval Platonic influences; thus, for example, Taddeo cited both the *Timaeus* of Plato and the *Consolation of Philosophy* of Boethius; see Taddeo, *Isagoge,* fols. 363r and 360r.

questions of current philosophical interest; second, the introduction of supplementary information concerning the particulars of natural science in such fields as cosmology, zoology, climatology, and others; and third, the direct enrichment of medical learning by the inclusion of material on human psychology, anatomy, and physiology drawn from Aristotle's works, and the discussion of contradictions between the teaching of Aristotle and the Galenic medical tradition. While this division is excessively schematic, in that given passages in the medical writings of members of the group may include material in more than one of the foregoing categories, it will nonetheless provide a framework for analysis.

FUNDAMENTAL ARISTOTELIAN DOCTRINES AND QUESTIONS OF CURRENT PHILOSOPHICAL INTEREST

Although Taddeo and his colleagues and pupils, like all their contemporaries, were firmly grounded in Aristotelian physical science, they did not devote much space in their medical works to general expositions of such concepts as form and matter, the elements, the four causes, and the varieties of motion, with their implications for the human body in health and sickness. The chief reasons for this restraint were no doubt their own sense of themselves as specialists in medicine, not philosophy, and their discrimination between the contents appropriate to different kinds of medical work. On the whole, they were mindful of Avicenna's dictum that the physician should be familiar with natural philosophy, but should not himself attempt to expound it.[15] Their few broad expositions of the principles of natural philosophy are, for the most part, in the theoretical sections of general or introductory books such as Taddeo's commentary on the *Isagoge* of Johannitius, and Turisanus's *Plusquam commentum* on the *Tegni*; they are almost completely absent from more specialized works of practical import, such as Taddeo's commentaries on the *Aphorisms* and *Prognostica*, Dino del Garbo's *Chirurgia*, and the commentary on Galen's *De interioribus* by Bartolomeo da Varignana. A notable "philosophical" interpretation of a work on a specialized physiological topic was, however, created by Dino in his commentary on the *De natura fetus* of Hippocrates.

Furthermore, levels of philosophical concern and competence varied among the members of the group. No doubt as a result of his Parisian

---

[15] Avicenna, *Canon* 1.1.1.2.

experience, Turisanus stands out both in breadth of philosophical interest and in relative philosophical sophistication; for example, he was able to cite such important and (then) recently translated works as the commentaries of Themistius on *De anima*, and Simplicius on *De celo et mundo*.[16] Close behind Turisanus come Taddeo (in his commentary on the *Isagoge*), and Dino (in his work on the fetus); but Guglielmo, Bartolomeo, and Mondino apparently found philosophy less useful as an adjunct to medicine. For instance, Mondino's commentary on the *Tegni* appears singularly free of the philosophical subject matter in which Turisanus's exposition of the same work is rich.

Where expositions of natural philosophical or metaphysical theory do occur, they are frequently accompanied by indications of the author's familiarity with more or less recent philosophical debate. Among the questions touched upon by Taddeo and his pupils and colleagues were, as we shall see, those of the multiplicity of forms in an individual, the principle of individuation, the elements in a mixture, monopsychism, and the origin of the soul in each individual—all of them subjects of controversy among natural philosophers and theologians of the thirteenth century. Yet, although some of these topics were vigorously argued in Taddeo's own lifetime, by the early fourteenth century, when most of his pupils were mature scholars, they represented fairly traditional fields of interest. If anything, the medical masters of the next generation seem to have been less concerned than was Taddeo to keep up with the latest philosophical innovations. Thus, at Paris, apparently in the years Turisanus taught there, Franciscus de Marchia pioneered the discussions of projectile motion that were to provide the context for some of the most fruitful developments in fourteenth-century thought. But Turisanus, when he had occasion to refer, in passing, to projectile motion, did so without showing any special interest in the subject or any awareness of Franciscus's work.[17] The following brief account of the treatment by

[16] Turisanus, *Plusquam*, fols. 37r, 40r. The commentary of Simplicius was translated by William of Moerbeke in 1271 (TK 764). The commentary of Themistius, also translated by William of Moerbeke, was an important resource for leading thirteenth-century philosophers in discussions of the nature of the intellective soul; see Edward P. Mahoney, "Themistius and the Agent Intellect in James of Viterbo and Other Thirteenth-Century Philosophers (Saint-Thomas, Siger of Brabant and Henry Bate)," *Augustiniana* 23 (1973):422-467. Turisanus, however, cited Themistius in connection with sense perception. It is not clear whether or not he knew the works at first hand.

[17] See the passage from the *Plusquam commentum* quoted in note 29 to chapter seven, below. On Franciscus de Marchia, O.F.M., and his supposition that the moving force in

Taddeo and Turisanus of the elements, of form and matter, and of the nature of life may give some idea of the approach and the range of philosophical reference among these two generations of learned physicians.

The subject of the elements and of the elements and elemental qualities in a mixture, to which Taddeo devoted two chapters in his commentary on the *Isagoge*, and Turisanus several folios of the *Plusquam commentum*,[18] was, of course, a central concern of thirteenth-century Latin philosophy.[19] It was also a topic with which physicians had concerned themselves since antiquity. Whereas discussions of form and matter, the four causes, and the varieties of motion (all of which, including local motion, Taddeo pointed out as inhering in various involuntary physiological processes)[20] appear to have entered medical writing relatively late, Galen himself had devoted an entire treatise to the subject of the elements.[21] Although the Latin version of Galen's *De elementis* that was available in the thirteenth century may not have achieved very wide circulation, the *Isagoge* of Johannitius, which was enormously influential in transmitting simplified Galenic teaching to the medieval West, numbered the elements among the "things natural" that constitute the human body.[22] Constantinus Africanus gave the elements a prominent position at the beginning of his widely read *Pantegni*; some scholars also associate teaching about the elements with the twelfth-century medical schools of Salerno;[23] in addition, a tract on the same subject by the Jewish physician Isaac was twice translated into Latin, once by Constantinus Africanus

sending a projectile was impressed in the projectile itself, a theory he had developed by about 1319, see Graziella Federici Vescovini, "Francis of Marchia," *DSB*, 5:113-115; Marshall Clagett, *The Science of Mechanics in the Middle Ages* (Madison, Wis., 1959), pp. 526-531, where a translation of an excerpt from Franciscus' exposition is printed; and A. Maier, *Zwei Grundprobleme der scholastischen Naturphilosophie* (Rome, 1968), pp. 161-200, where some of the texts are printed.

[18] Taddeo, *Isagoge*, fols. 344v-347r; Turisanus, *Plusquam*, fols. 11v-12r.

[19] Maier, *An der Grenze von Scholastik und Naturwissenschaft*, pp. 1-88.

[20] Taddeo, *Isagoge*, fol. 366v.   [21] *De elementis*, ed. Kühn, 1:413-491.

[22] Regarding the medieval versions of Galen's *De elementis*, see Durling, "Corrigenda and Addenda to Diels' Galenica," pp. 465-466. For the passage in the text of the *Isagoge*, see Taddeo, *Isagoge*, fol. 344r.

[23] Richard C. Dales, "Marius 'On the Elements' and the Twelfth-Century Science of Matter," *Viator: Medieval and Renaissance Studies* 3 (1972):191-218; Rodney M. Thomson, " 'Liber Marii de Elementis': The Work of a Hitherto Unknown Salernitan Master?" ibid., pp. 179-189. See also McKeon, "Medicine and Philosophy in the Eleventh and Twelfth Centuries." I am informed by Professor Paul Kristeller that the association of Marius with Salerno has been questioned.

and once by Gerard of Cremona;[24] the elements and the mixture of elemental qualities in human "complexio" and in food and medicine also received quite extensive treatment in Avicenna's *Canon*.[25] Thus, precedents among medical writers for Taddeo's and Turisanus's treatment of the elements extended even to their special interest in the properties of elemental qualities in a mixture as exemplified in human *complexio* and in compound medicines. Their work was distinguished from that of their Latin predecessors chiefly by a much wider and more direct knowledge of Aristotelian and Galenic element theory and by the influence of Avicenna and Averroes.

Taddeo began his discussion of the elements by distinguishing between the Aristotelian definitions of "element," "principle," and "cause"; and he went on to observe that the term "element" is defined differently by philosophical and by medical authorities, since the latter include organs and humors among the elements. He then reviewed the definitions provided by Aristotle,[26] Galen (from *De elementis*), Avicenna, and Isaac. Taddeo himself adopted a definition combining those of Aristotle and Avicenna, according to which the elements are indivisible, permanent, and corporeal; he noted that thus defined they do not include either prime matter (which, according to Averroes, is not *corpus in actu*)[27] or such incorporeal entities as complexion, operations, and virtues. On the question of whether or not heat and cold are the substantial forms of elements, Taddeo concluded that there is a sense in which this is so, although in another sense the elementary qualities are accidents—just as snow appears to the eye as a white substantial form (*sic*), although if snow is considered as a substance, its whiteness is an accident.[28] Taddeo was also familiar with the terminology developed by some of the twelfth-century cosmologists that distinguished between the elements as such and the *elementata*, the composite bodies in which the elements are always found in the present world;[29] and he denied that any element could

---

[24] TK 1045.   [25] Avicenna, *Canon* 1.1.2-3; 1.2.2.1.5.

[26] Taddeo, *Isagoge*, fol. 344v. Taddeo cited *Metaphysics* 3.5, which contains a concise definition of "element." Aristotle's main discussion of the elements is, however, to be found in *De generatione et corruptione* 2.1-8.

[27] "hoc dicit [Avicenna] ut excludat materiam primam, nam ipsa non est corpus in actu, sicut dicit Averroes super primo phisicorum," Taddeo, *Isagoge*, fol. 344v.

[28] "dico quod nivis in eo quod visum disgregat est substantialis forma albedo, in eo quod est substantia quidem, est ei accidentalis," ibid., fol. 345r.

[29] See Theodore Silverstein, "*Elementatum*: Its Appearance Among the Twelfth-Century Cosmogonists," *Mediaeval Studies* 16 (1954):156-162.

have more than one quality "to the highest degree," dismissing as idiots those who maintained that it could.[30]

Taddeo's chapter on mixtures explains that these can be either natural, as in human complexion, or artificial, as in an electuary. Natural complexion, in turn, can be either primary or secondary; an example of secondary complexion is that of milk, which is composed of liquid and curds and butterfat, each of which has its own primary complexion made up from elemental qualities. Turning to the causes of mixtures, he declared their material cause to be the miscible condition of the ingredients (in physical contact with one another, not too viscous, and not too disparate in quantity—one drop of wine cannot be said to be mixed with a million jars of water); their formal cause, the tenacity of the miscible parts; their efficient cause, the heavenly bodies that Aristotle stated in *De celo et mundo* to be the cause of all terrestrial motion; and their final cause, the perpetuation of the universe by generation (for mixture produces generation) and the operation of the mixture itself.

Turisanus, too, was chiefly interested in the elements in connection with the medical concept of *complexio*. He defined the latter as a mixture of the qualities found in the prime elements, drawing his definitions of elements and mixture from *De generatione et corruptione* and the *Metaphysics*. Hence, the problem he addressed was a special case of a more general problem that had long preoccupied philosophers; namely, how the elements combine to form the compounds that constitute all existing bodies.[31] His treatment took the form of a disquisition on whether the substantial forms of the elements persist in a mixture, given that mixing somewhat changes but does not destroy the effects of the components. He stated the problems as follows: the persistence of the effect of the components suggests that their forms also persist, but this involves supposing that the mixture as an entity has more than one substantial form; moreover, it is impossible to suppose that the forms of contrary elements, such as fire and water, could persist together—if they did the resultant compound could not be regarded as a true mixture. And if it were accepted that the forms of the elements persist in every mixture that comes into being, then no "corruption" of the elements would be involved in

---

[30] "dicunt quidam idiote quod ellementa habent duas qualitates in summo," Taddeo, *Isagoge*, fols. 345r-v. Taddeo here appears to contradict Aristotle, although he himself maintained that his own view was the same as that of the Philosopher in this matter.

[31] Aristotle posed the problem in *De generatione et corruptione* 1.10, 327a29-328b25.

the formation of such natural substances as wood and flesh; yet a fundamental tenet of Aristotelian natural philosophy was that the generation of one thing involves the corruption of another. Turisanus allowed that Averroes had clarified the problem by stating that *mixtio* and *corruptio* are not interchangeable terms, but rejected as unsatisfactory his view that the forms of the elements survive in a mixture by undergoing changes.[32] According to Turisanus, Averroes had maintained that the forms of the elements are very imperfect, being close to prime matter and somewhere between substantial and accidental forms, and therefore able to increase and diminish. This Turisanus pronounced to be impossible, since a mean between substance and accident is no more conceivable than a mean between affirmation and negation; moreover, if the substantial forms of the elements were capable of augmentation and diminution, then species and mixtures would be constantly in flux. Instead, he offered a solution similar to and possibly derived from that of Aquinas, namely, that it is the virtues or qualities rather than the forms of the elements that survive in a mixture; in this way, both the existence of a mixture as a separate entity and the continued existence of the elements are assured.[33]

A problem to which Taddeo several times returned was that of reconciling two concepts widely relied upon by physicians, namely those of *complexio* and specific form, with the philosophical concept of substantial form. *Complexio* was a term applied to the controlling balance of elemental qualities in any body or its parts; specific form was a supposed quality responsible for properties peculiar to any species that were otherwise inexplicable in cause and apparently arbitrary in effect—the notion was frequently used to explain the medicinal action of certain herbs.[34] Taddeo raised the issue of the relation between *complexio*, specific form, and substantial form both in his chapter on mixtures at the beginning of the commentary on the *Isagoge*[35] and in a set of questions on specific form incorporated into his commentary on Avicenna's chapter on ingested substances. The questions on specific form were evidently a source

[32] For a summary of the teaching of Averroes on this point, see Maier, *An der Grenze von Scholastik und Naturwissenschaft*, pp. 28-29.

[33] Cf. ibid., pp. 32-35, especially p. 34.

[34] *Complexio* is, of course, Galen's *crasis*, usually rendered into modern English as "temperament." Since *complexio* was the translation universally used by the Latin physicians of Taddeo's day, I have chosen to preserve their terminology.

[35] Taddeo, *Isagoge*, fols. 346r-v; the question is "an complexio sit forma substantialis membri."

of pride to their author, since he also incorporated them in an abbreviated version into the latter part of the commentary on the *Isagoge*.[36]

In the first of the passages referred to, Taddeo inquired whether or not *complexio* is itself the substantial form of any bodily part (*membrum*). His solution was, as usual, effected by distinction: insofar as an organ (*membrum*) is a substance, complexion is not its form; but if the organ is regarded as the instrument of a bodily process (*instrumentum operationis*), then complexion may be said to be its substantial form. He also inquired whether *complexio* or substantial form comes first, given, on the one hand, Avicenna's claim that its *complexio* prepares a thing for the reception of its *specific* form, and, on the other, his assertion that *complexio* is an accident. Taddeo's conclusion is that a form of some kind already exists when a part (*membrum*) receives its *complexio*, but that complete form (*forma que est complementum et totum*) follows *complexio*.[37] His ideas on this point become clearer when we turn to his analysis of specific form.

As examples of the functioning of specific form, Taddeo proffered the effect of scammony upon choler—the supposed fact that "we see red things are moved by blood, no matter in what species the redness is found, whether in stone, or in wood, or in a liquid"[38]—and the action of a magnet. He asserted that specific form is an "added form" given by celestial virtue to an entire species and existing in individuals only by reason of their species;[39] although he denied that specific form is caused by *complexio*, he held, following Avicenna, that the *complexio* of a spe-

[36] Taddeo's commentary is contained in BAV, MS Palat. lat. 1246, 15c, fols. 78v-97v (TK 1251). The questions on specific form begin on fol. 83v. Avicenna's chapter "Quod comeditur et bibitur," the subject of the commentary, is to be found in *Canon* 1.2.2.1.15. According to McVaugh, ed., Arnald of Villanova, *Aphorismi de gradibus*—vol. 2 in Arnald, *Opera Medica Omnia*—this chapter was "cited by western pharmacists more frequently than any Galenic passage" touching on similar topics (intro., 2:17-19). For the parallel passage in the commentary on the *Isagoge*, see Taddeo, *Isagoge*, fols. 378r-v.

[37] "An complexio vel substantialis forma antecedat in subjecto," Taddeo, *Isagoge*, fol. 346r.

[38] "videmus res rubeas movetur sanguine in quacunque rerum specie existat rubedo, sive in lapide, sive in ligno, vel in liquore," Taddeo, comm. *Quod comeditur*, BAV, MS Palat. lat. 1246, fol. 83r.

[39] "dator autem huius forme est virtus exterior, scilicet, alicuius corporis celestis seu alicuius constellationis que quidem virtus influit super totam speciem et ratione speciei est postea diffusa super individua. et propter hoc vocata fuit forma specifica: quia ipsa est in individuo ratione sue speciei . . . ista forma non est tota ab elementis, sed dispositio sue receptionis, et neque est tota a corpore celesti: sed eius datio vel eductio de potentia ad actum," Taddeo, *Isagoge*, fol. 378r.

cies prepares that species to receive its specific form.[40] He believed specific form to be present in all species, and hence in all individuals, although in some things its operations are weak and occult, and in others (presumably scammony, the magnet, and so on), strong and manifest.[41] Unlike some other medical writers, he identified specific form with at any rate some aspect of substantial form;[42] and he presumably thought that it is specific form that is added after an earlier form, and after *complexio*, to produce "complete form." We may assume that Taddeo accepted the idea of multiplicity of substantial forms (although he made no direct reference to the vigorous debate on this topic, which engaged such leading thirteenth-century philosophers and theologians as Bonaventura and Thomas Aquinas),[43] since he did not identify specific form in man with the human soul, which he also held to be a substantial form. He distinguished between the soul and specific form by pointing out that, unlike the rational soul, specific form is given by the stars and is corruptible.[44] Taddeo did, however, draw a parallel between the nature of specific form and that of the soul; in the course of demonstrating that specific form

[40] "Modus autem acquirendi [talis est—deleted in MS] istam formam talis est corpori. Corpora simplicia adinvicem commiscentur ex commixtione quorum resultat complexio que preparat illam speciem ad recipiendum formam additam quam vocamus formam specificam. . . . Ista species [?] et forma addita est ipsa forma specifica quam precessit complexio . . . In hoc notatur quod ipsa complexio non est causa que ipsam formam specificam in materia fecerit. Sed habilitat eam ad recipiendum." Taddeo, comm. *Quod comeditur*, BAV, MS Palat. lat. 1246, fol. 82v.

[41] "omnis res habet formam specificam sed sunt quedam res que habent eam debilem valde . . . ," ibid., fol. 86v. Taddeo added that some things might act through their specific form only in certain circumstances: "Verbi gratia panis in humano corpore agat [*sic*] a materia et non a forma specifica tamen forte in aliis corporibus efficit operationem aliquam per formam specificam," ibid.

[42] "sed hec [forma specifica] est forma substantialis sicut dicit Avi[cenna]" Taddeo, *Isagoge*, fol. 378r. Taddeo's readiness to identify *forma specifica* with, in one sense, substantial form appears to be somewhat unusual; see Arnald of Villanova, *Aphorismi de gradibus*, intro., p. 19.

[43] On the controversy over the unicity or multiplicity of form, see Daniel A. Callus, O.P., "The Origins of the Problem of the Unity of Form," *The Thomist* 24 (1961):257-285, and Theodore Schneider, *Die Einheit des Menschen*, in *Beiträge zur Geschichte der Philosophie des Mittelalters*, n.s. 8 (Munster, 1973). The controversy that developed during the thirteenth century as to whether or not the rational soul is the single substantial form of man subsequently became involved with the dispute over the Averroist idea of the unicity of the possible intellect. In 1311 the Council of Vienne attempted to solve the question and end debate by declaring it to be an article of faith that the intellectual soul is the one substantial form of the human body.

[44] "non intelligas quod ista forma sic infundatur corpori sicut anima rationalis, nam sic esset incorruptibilis," Taddeo, *Isagoge*, fol. 378r.

can simultaneously be both a substantial form and an active principle, he remarked:

> Nor is it impossible for one form to have both properties, for the soul, when it is the substance of the animate body, has these two properties, for it is the substance of the body in which it is the form, for it prevents the body from withering away; but it is also the power and active virtue from which all the operations of the body proceed.[45]

Although Taddeo's attempt to harmonize the concepts of *complexio*, specific form, and substantial form may have taken him somewhat out of his philosophical depth, subsequent writers, including his pupil Guglielmo da Brescia, further developed the notion of specific form as an explanation of certain otherwise inexplicable actions or forces, including that of the magnet, which became a standard illustration of this idea.[46]

The material that has just been outlined shows something of the way in which the principles of natural philosophy provided the foundations of medical science. Taddeo and his students also called these principles into service in connection with specific physiological phenomena. For example, both Taddeo and Turisanus discussed nutrition and the action of medicines in terms of the theory of form and matter, and their decision to do so was neither arbitrary nor unreasonable. Although in antiquity and the Middle Ages simple observation could convey a certain amount of information about the intake and digestion of food, the biochemical processes remained obscure until the nineteenth century. Similarly, while it was plain that the absorption of drugs could affect the body in various ways, there was no possibility of knowing exactly how they worked. One way to provide a scientific explanation for these phenomena was by the application of generally accepted basic principles—that is, by reducing the

---

[45] "dico quod substantia que tenet rem in esse habet duplicem considerationem: nam consideratur in eo quod tenet rem cuius ipsa est forma in suo esse, et hoc modo proprie vocatur forma substantialis et ab ea non est actio vel passio . . . alio vero modo consideratur in quantum ipsa forma est sicut principium agens; tunc dicitur potentia sive virtus, et ab illa proprietate agit et patitur. Neque est impossibile aliquam formam istas duas proprietates habere, nam anima cum sit substantia corporis animati habet has duas proprietates, nam ipsa est substantia corporis in eo quod forma, nam tenet corpus ne marescat. Item potentia est et virtus agens a qua procedunt omnes operationes corporis," ibid.

[46] Michael R. McVaugh, "Theriac at Montpellier, 1285-1325 (with an edition of the 'Questiones de tyriaca' of William of Brescia)," *Sudhoffs Archiv für Geschichte der Medizin und der Naturwissenschaften* 56 (1972):114, 126-27.

problem to a general proposition and, in effect, inquiring: How does one thing become another? In an Aristotelian philosophical context, such an inquiry inevitably led to the consideration of form and matter. In a sense, indeed, the treatment of nutrition and the effect of medicines—that is, the absorption of one corporeal and therefore compound substance by another—may be regarded as the next stage of the discussion, which has been traced above, of the way in which natural and artificial compounds are made up from the elements and elemental qualities.

Thus, Taddeo's commentary on the chapter in the *Canon* of Avicenna "on things eaten and drunk" opens with an examination, in terms of the doctrines contained in Aristotle's *Physics*, of the principles by which and the ways in which ingested substances act in the body. Taddeo questioned Avicenna's assertion that there are three ways in which one thing can act upon another—namely, by its quality (medicine), by the matter (food), or by its whole substance—on the Aristotelian grounds that the form of any mover must always be involved in its action.[47] He went on to inquire into the fate of the form of ingested food,[48] concluding that "some quality by which it acts" is retained until the food is completely assimilated. Taddeo also briefly summarized other prevailing ideas about the difference between the action of food and that of medicine: food was held to be assimilated to the body, whereas medicine was thought to assimilate the body to itself. Assimilation of one or the other kind was apparently thought of as happening with various degrees of completeness, according to whether the ingested substance was absolute food, medicinal food, absolute medicine, tempered medicine, poisonous medicine, or poison.[49] Taddeo, however, followed Avicenna in declaring that some

[47] "hic ponit Avicenna tres modos operacionis scilicet tota [in margin: sola] qualitate, materia et tota substantia. Contra quod sic obiicitur et primo contra primum. Non enim videtur quod sola qualitas possit operari in humano corpore ista conclusione que concludebat quod omnis agens est compositum. . . . Pro tercia ponit quod aliquid operatur sola materia. Sed contra omnis actio est a forma sicut scribitur 3° phisicorum . . . Ad hoc ita respondeo dico quod cibus ab hora qua iungitur corpori usque ad horam ni qua assimilatur perfecte semper retinet aliquid qualitatis qua agit et patiur . . . Cum vero membro assimilatur tunc cibus nullam retinet qualitatem extrinsecam a membro," Taddeo, *Quod comeditur*, BAV, MS Palat. lat. 1246, fols. 78v-79v.

[48] Theologians also interested themselves in this question, although from a different standpoint; see Thomas Aquinas, ST 1, q. 119, and Thomas S. Hall, "Life, Death, and the Radical Moisture," *Clio Medica* 6 (1971):11.

[49] "cibum absolute, cibum medicinalem, medicinam absolute, medicinam temperatam, medicinam venenosam, et venenum," Taddeo, *Quod comeditur*, BAV, MS Palat. lat. 1246,

types of medicament, which neither assimilate nor are assimilated, act neither through matter nor through a quality, but through their total substance by means of their specific form (this assertion provided the jumping-off point for his questions on specific form already alluded to).

The problem of how food is transformed into the substance of the nourished animal led Turisanus into a discussion of form and matter, distinguished from that of Taddeo by its author's greater boldness in engaging in philosophical debate.[50] Turisanus began by remarking that the process of nourishment seems to be a kind of generation, similar to that of fire, which continuously generates itself from fuel. The food retains its matter, but not its form; whereas the animal that is nourished always retains its form, although its matter is continually diminished and renewed like flowing water. But this concept gives rise to the difficulty that if it were supposed that all the matter in an individual can flow away and be replaced in this way, then it would follow that the same form can successively be attached to completely different matter; yet fundamental to the concept of form and matter is the idea that form and matter are inseparable in any individual thing. According to Turisanus, the "more famous" (*famosior*) solution to this problem is that of philosophers (whom he did not name, but among whom he probably included Avicenna and Albertus Magnus), who solved the difficulty by asserting that a substance termed seminal moisture (*humidum seminale*), although requiring constant augmentation from accidental moisture (*humidum accidentale*) acquired from food, is never completely consumed during life; in a metaphor employed by Avicenna and Albertus and repeated by Turisanus, the using up of seminal, or radical, moisture over the course of life is compared to the consumption of the oil in a lamp.[51] Turisanus's own opinion was that the proponents of this explanation do not correctly understand Aristotle's meaning; a better interpretation of Aristotle's views is that nourishment takes place by means of form, not by means of matter, and that the entire matter of an individual is indeed changed over the course of a lifetime. This solution,

---

fol. 78v. Guglielmo da Brescia also discussed this concept; see his *Questiones de tyriaca* in McVaugh, "Theriac at Montpellier," pp. 141-142.

[50] Turisanus, *Plusquam*, fols. 56r-57r.

[51] Ibid., fol. 56v; see Michael R. McVaugh, "The '*Humidum Radicale*' in Thirteenth-Century Medicine," *Traditio* 30 (1974), 259-283; Peter H. Niebyl, "Old Age, Fever, and the Lamp Metaphor," *Journal of the History of Medicine* 26 (1971):351-368; and Hall, "Life, Death, and the Radical Moisture."

Turisanus noted, is not generally regarded as valid, because of the common acceptance of the doctrine that matter is the principle of individuation. Yet perhaps, suggested Turisanus, this explanation of individuation is incorrect. After all, Avicenna, in Book 6 of his *De naturalibus*, had said that the complexion of an animate being determines its matter; and Averroes, in his commentary on Book 2 of *De anima*, had declared diversity of forms to be the cause of diversity of matter. Turisanus clinched the argument, to his own satisfaction, by declaring that if matter were the principle of individuation, it would follow that: first, individuals of the same species would differ only in their matter, and therefore, all men would have one soul, which is absurd; and second, all individuals would necessarily have matter, which is not true of the separated substances (angels, for example). Thus, he seems to have been concerned to repudiate both the Averroist idea of the unicity of the human intellect, on the one hand, and the views on individuation held, for example, by Aquinas, on the other.[52]

If much of the philosophizing of the members of Taddeo's circle appears to have been designed to explain physiological processes that were otherwise obscure to them and to be remarkable chiefly for its demonstration of familiarity with the more arcane technicalities of thirteenth-century Aristotelianism, these masters were nonetheless capable, on occasion, of addressing issues that even today are recognized as simultaneously biological and philosophical. As an example, we may take the reflections of Turisanus on the question "What is life, and where does it come from?"[53]

Notwithstanding the absence of a separate tradition of biological science, distinct from natural philosophy, the sources from which an author of the early fourteenth century could draw an answer to this perennial question were several, since it was equally the concern of theology, natural philosophy, and medicine. Despite his familiarity with the philosophical works of Albertus Magnus, whom he cited by name,[54] and probably with Thomas Aquinas, Turisanus excluded overt reference to theo-

[52] Cf. Thomas Aquinas, ST 1, q. 76, a. 2, ad 1. Thomas solved the problem regarding the angels by asserting that each spiritual being constituted a separate species. Turisanus did not cite Thomas by name, and was here countering a school of thought rather than the views of any individual.

[53] Turisanus, *Plusquam*, fols. 29v-31r. The questions discussed include "Utrum virtus spiritualis det vitam" and "Utrum anima sit actus corporis habentis vitam."

[54] Ibid., fol. 30v.

logical and religious considerations and examined solely the teachings of philosophy and medicine.

He was primarily concerned with reconciling the Aristotelian concept of the soul as the principle of life, or the life-giving force, with the Galenic doctrine of the existence of a distinct *virtus vitalis*, or *spiritualis*, whose presence is manifested in the beating of the heart and the pulsation of the arteries. Taddeo had considered this problem before Turisanus and had come to the conclusion that *virtus vitalis* is not to be identified with the functioning of any of the Aristotelian faculties of soul (which he termed *virtutes* or *potentiae*)—that is, not with vegetative, sensitive, or rational faculties—but is rather an essential precondition of the activity of all of them.[55] Turisanus, as Taddeo had done, inquired whether, and how, *virtus vitalis* can be considered a virtue of the soul. He pointed out that since Aristotle had stated that the faculties of the soul are intellective, sensitive, and vegetative, or pertaining to local motion; and since the last of these refers to *appetitus*, which leads to voluntary motion, not to the involuntary movements of heartbeat and pulse caused by *virtus vitalis*, these faculties do not seem to include *virtus vitalis*, despite Aricenna's contrary opinion. Yet if this *virtus vitalis* is not a virtue of the soul, but consists instead of a virtue with which the *spiritus* is endowed before the reception of the soul, how can it be the source of life, since life comes from the soul? Turisanus himself came to the conclusion that the essential nature of the *virtus vitalis* is *spiritualis*, and that its function is to enrich the blood with *spiritus*. (Supposedly, *spiritus* is a highly refined substance that flows through the arteries; some medical writers, of whom Taddeo was one, held that there are three separate varieties of *spiritus*, each distributing one of the three virtues—*vitalis*, *animalis*, and *naturalis* —through the body.)[56]

[55] "videtur quod virtus vitalis non possit comprehendi sub aliqua istarum 3 potentiarum anime. nam non videtur quod possit contineri sub vegetabili, quia dicit Avicenna quod ista virtus non inest plantis: ergo non est sub anima vegetabili. Preterea, neque sub anima sensibili, nam sensibilis anima aut apprehendit aut movet voluntarie, sed ista virtus non apprehendit neque movet voluntarie. ergo non est sensibilis. Preterea neque videtur rationalis: quia rationalis est separabilis. hec autem non est talis. Ad hoc dico quod ista virtus non est proprie sub aliqua istarum trium: sed est radix ad omnes has virtutes prout sunt in homine. et fundantur in ea omnes," Taddeo, *Isagoge*, fol. 359r.

[56] On the evolution of the concept of *spiritus*, or *pneuma*, see Siegel, *Galen's System of Physiology and Medicine*, chaps. 1 and 2; G. Verbeke, *L'Évolution de la doctrine du Pneuma, du stoicisme à S. Augustin*; and E. Ruth Harvey, *The Inward Wits*. According to George P. Klubertanz, *The Discursive Power*, the division of the virtues into *vitalis*,

In the course of tackling the question whether or not this spiritual virtue (*virtus spiritualis*) gives life to the whole, Turisanus paused to consider the nature of life itself. His exposition ran in part as follows.

According to Aristotle, "life" means both the power to perform vital functions and the actual performance of those functions; the soul is not life itself, but life's cause. If, therefore, Turisanus went on, one could identify an operation of the soul that continues uninterrupted so long as the soul is in the body, that operation would no doubt be the one through which life is given; but the only operation to fit this description is the process of giving off heat by the heart through the *spiritus*, the heart being like the sun of the body and the *spiritus* like its sunlight. In animals, life lasts only as long as heat, *spiritus*, and the consequent pulsation are produced; and, according to Avicenna, it is *spiritus* that prepares the limbs for sense and motion, which however are not essential to life in the way that the vegetative functions and, in animals, *spiritus* are. Vague though the concept of *spiritus* may appear to be, it was intended to provide a *physical* explanation of the phenomenon of life, as may be seen from Turisanus's critique of the definition of life supplied by Albertus Magnus in his commentary on *De anima*.[57] Turisanus understood Albertus to have maintained that life is an act of the soul that is somehow different and separate from any corporeal manifestation of life. He found this definition unsatisfactory because it provides no physical criteria for ascertaining the presence or absence of life: if life can be identified only as a certain light flowing from the soul, and is not tied to any particular physical manifestation, then the cessation of all the body's operations is not conclusive proof that the light of the soul has been shut off. The objection is a natural one, coming from a physician whose primary concern was no doubt to establish acceptable medical definitions of human life and death, a problem that is still debated among physicians (and theologians and lawyers) in the last quarter of the twentieth century.

The foregoing examples are representative not only of some of the general philosophical issues discussed by Taddeo and Turisanus, but also of their normal practice of engaging in such discussion only when it served

---

animalis, and *naturalis* may have been taken over by later medical writers from the *Pantegni* of Constantinus Africanus.

[57] Turisanus, *Plusquam,* fols. 30v-31r; see Albertus Magnus, *De anima* 2.1.1 (ed. Borgnet, 5:191-192), and also idem, *Liber de morte et vita* 1.2 (ed. Borgnet, 9:346-348), "Digressio declarans essentialem diffinitionem vitae et explanatio ejusdem."

a specific purpose in the teaching of medical theory. Moreover, I must emphasize once again that material in this, the first of the three categories of medical philosophy posed at the beginning of this chapter, constitutes but a small proportion of the generalized discussion of medical theory by Taddeo and Turisanus, two of the most philosophically inclined members of the group; and it represents only a minuscule part of the medical output of the group as a whole. Nor does it appear from the examples presented above that either Taddeo or Turisanus were deeply involved in current philosophical debates, although a few of Turisanus's positions may have been somewhat controversial. On a good many issues they shared a tendency to follow lines laid down by Avicenna, who was no doubt recommended to them as a philosopher by his status as the "prince" of physicians. Both cited Averroes freely as a philosophical authority, but it is doubtful if, in their eyes, he ever rivaled the status of Avicenna as an authority of equal weight in both philosophy and medicine. (Averroes's chief medical work, the *Colliget*, was not translated into Latin until 1285[58] and therefore could not have been known to Taddeo for most of his career; even in the generation of Turisanus, the *Colliget* was probably not as universally consulted and revered in the schools of the West as was the far more comprehensive *Canon*.)

Yet there is, of course, one famous passage that suggests a very different picture of the place of philosophy in the medical writings of Taddeo Alderotti, and perhaps therefore also in the works of those influenced by him. In his commentary on the *Isagoge*, Taddeo went far beyond any conceivable requirements of the medical context in incorporating a detailed and well-informed account of the Averroist theory of the unicity of the human intellect. Showing an uneasy awareness of the recent episcopal condemnation of that theory at Paris in 1277, Taddeo refused to pronounce on the merits of the Averroist case or to give his own opinion on monopsychism; he frankly owned to a certain "timidity" in the face of ecclesiastical censure.[59] Nonetheless, as already noted, the very

[58] See the *explicit* of the work in Cesena, Biblioteca Malatestiana, MS Pluteo D[estra] xxv item no. 3, fol. 27v. The dates 1255 or 1289 found in various printed sources stem from misreadings of this explicit. I am grateful to Professor Michael McVaugh for supplying a photocopy of the leaf in question.

[59] Taddeo, *Isagoge*, fols. 360v-361r; the passage is also printed in B. Nardi, "L'Averroismo bolognese." The view that the rational soul is one in all men was regarded as heterodox because of its consequences for the Christian doctrines of personal immortality and individual reward and punishment after death.

presentation of the Averroist theory in this passage was enough to convince so eminent a student of medieval Italian Aristotelianism as the late Bruno Nardi that Taddeo shared the position he was describing.[60]

But it cannot be taken for granted that the boldness of Taddeo's approach in this passage to a genuinely—and dangerously—controversial philosophical topic is the first sign of a general penetration of radical Aristotelian views into the Bolognese faculty of medicine, or even that it reflects a lifelong commitment to philosophical concerns on the part of Taddeo himself. Taddeo's interest in fundamental philosophical questions, which he displayed in the early commentary on the *Isagoge* and the presumably even earlier commentary on Avicenna's chapter on ingested substances (since portions of it were, as noted, included in abbreviated form in the commentary on the *Isagoge*), is not particularly characteristic of the rest of his medical output. The Hippocratic commentaries written later in his career contain little material of the same kind.

The sources of Taddeo's own knowledge of heterodox Aristotelian, or Averroist, teaching regarding the intellect must presumably be traced to the controversies that engulfed the *studium* of Paris in the 1260s and 1270s.[61] Taddeo's account of the Averroist position appears to have been written before the sojourn of his pupil Gentile da Cingoli in Paris; it may, indeed, have been Taddeo who fostered Gentile's interest in Parisian philosophy in the first place, and who sent him to its fountainhead (see chapter two). But since contacts between French and Italian centers of intellectual life were numerous in the thirteenth century (one has only to think of the travels of various celebrated thinkers and writers of Italian origin, especially in the friar orders), and since the Parisian condemnations of 1277 soon became widely known outside France,[62]

---

[60] See notes 4 and 5, above.

[61] For an account of these disputes and of the events leading up to the celebrated condemnation of theses including that of the unicity of the intellect in 1277, see Steenberghen, *Aristotle in the West*.

[62] See Kuksewicz, *De Siger de Brabant à Jacques de Plaisance*, p. 97. A set of condemnations, probably those of 1277, were described as "well known" at Bologna in the mid-fourteenth century; see William J. Courtenay, "John of Mirecourt and Gregory of Rimini on Whether God Can Undo the Past," *Recherches de Théologie Ancienne et Médiévale* 40 (1973):170. I am grateful to Professor Edward Mahoney for this reference. The relative rapidity with which, in the thirteenth century, disputes at Paris could find an echo at Bologna is suggested by a papal letter of September 24, 1257, addressed to the bishop of Bologna and forbidding the scholars there to hear William of St. Amour if the latter should attempt either to preach or to lecture in the city (Denifle and Chatelain, *Chartula-*

there is probably no need to seek any special channel of information peculiar to Taddeo.

During the academic ascendancy of the generation of Taddeo's pupils, although the influence of Parisian philosophy no doubt continued to be felt, the faculty of arts at Bologna was beginning to develop as a center of radical Aristotelianism in its own right, under the guidance of Gentile da Cingoli and such other masters of arts as Taddeo da Parma and Gentile's student Angelo d'Arezzo.[63] Direct evidence of the influence of contemporary philosophical debate, however, whether at Paris or at Bologna, is hard to find in the work of Taddeo's pupils, largely because, despite the notable exception of Turisanus's references to Albertus Magnus, they did not ordinarily cite recent nonmedical Latin writers by name. Unquestionably, though, the Bolognese medical faculty studied works by members of their contemporaries in the faculty of arts. This is sufficiently demonstrated not only by the joining of arts and medicine in a common student university and doctoral college and by the requirement that medical students know arts and philosophy, but also by the fact, already alluded to, that Gentile da Cingoli's *reportatio* of the *quaestiones* on *De generatione animalium,* by the Parisian arts professor Johannes Vath, is contained in the same manuscript with, and written in the same hand as, medical works of Bartolomeo da Varignana and other members of the Bolognese school; and by the fact that, as already noted, works of Taddeo da Parma and Cecco d'Ascoli were written for the benefit of medical students.[64]

---

rium, vol. I, pp. 367-368, no. 318). In the course of a series of quarrels, culminating in the early 1250s, between Franciscan masters and certain secular masters of the University of Paris, William had written a treatise condemning mendicancy as a religious ideal; this work was condemned by ecclesiastical authority in 1256.

[63] See note 6, above; regarding the early growth of Bolognese Aristotelianism see also Grabmann, "Gentile da Cingoli," and "L'Aristotelismo italiano"; Anneliese Maier, *Die Vorläufer Galileis im 14. Jahrhundert,* pp. 251-278; Charles Ermatinger, "Averroism in Early Fourteenth-Century Bologna," *Mediaeval Studies* 16 (1954):35-56; and idem, "Some Unstudied Sources for the History of Philosophy in the Fourteenth Century," *Manuscripta* 14 (1970):3-23, 67-87; Zdzisław Kuksewicz, *Averroisme bolonais au XIVᵉ siècle.*

[64] In addition BAV, MS Vat. lat. 2366, contains Taddeo's commentary on the *Isagoge* and other medical works along with Cecco d'Ascoli's commentary on the *Sphere* of Sacrobosco; see P. Micheloni, *La medicina nei primi tremila codice del Fondo Vaticano Latino;* MSS Vat. lat. 3066 and 3144, which formerly constituted one codex, contain a medical and philosophical miscellany including, in addition to works by the mid-fourteenth century English logicians Burley, Kilvington, and Heytesbury, medical works by Mondino, Dino, and Turisanus, and philosophical questions by Matteo da Gubbio, Antonio da Parma, and Johannes de Casali, another member of the Bologna faculty of arts in the second

If the philosophical influence of the school of arts is hard to trace in the medical works of the members of Taddeo's school, it is even harder to evaluate how much concern, if any, these physicians felt for the possible theological implications of their philosophical positions. Their normal practice, as already noted, was to exclude discussion of such matters; Taddeo's own reference to the Paris condemnations is unusual in that respect. Their reticence is more likely to have been due to their concept of the proper concerns of natural and medical science than to indifference to religion or hostility to orthodox doctrine, although scientific detachment conceivably could have served to mask either or both of the latter.

One possible test of the extent to which radical or heterodox philosophical ideas actually penetrated the medical works of the members of Taddeo's circle is an examination of the extent and nature of their treatment of the human soul, a theologically sensitive subject on which much thirteenth-century philosophical debate centered. All masters learned in theoretical medicine had to be familiar with current philosophical doctrines concerning the soul, since the soul was held to affect the body: according to Aristotle, the vegetative and sensitive faculties of soul supplied the human body with, respectively, powers of nutrition and growth, and powers of motion, sense, and emotion.[65] Moreover, in certain passages Aristotle appeared to indicate his belief that the soul was in some special way linked with the heart.[66] As a result, from time to time one finds some discussion of the soul or its faculties and virtues in three specific contexts in medieval medical works: first, in the course of general accounts of physiological "virtues and operations" (pulsation, respiration, sensation, local motion, digestion, and so forth); second, in discussions of the heart, where physicians occasionally inquired whether the heart is the seat of the soul, or made an attempt, as we have seen, to fit the idea of

quarter of the fourteenth century. Although this collection was compiled some years after the period in which Taddeo and his pupils flourished, there is no reason to suppose that it reflects any fundamental change in the relationship of arts and medicine in the curriculum since their day; see Charles Ermatinger, "The Missing Leaves of Codex Vaticanus Latinus 3066," *Manuscripta* 2 (1958):152-162.

[65] *De anima* 2.2-4, 413a30-416b30. For concepts of psychology and sense perception in Taddeo's circle, see chapter seven, below.

[66] See, for example, *De partibus animalium* 3.5, 667b15-30; *De juventute et senectute* 2, 468a20-21. In *De anima*, however, the soul is treated as the principle of organization of the body, with no mention of any physical location. For discussion of Aristotle's changing views on the soul, see the editor's introduction to Aristotle, *Parva Naturalia*, trans. David Ross (Oxford, 1955), pp. 3-10.

virtus vitalis emanating from the heart into the Aristotelian division of the vegetative, sensitive, and rational faculties of the soul; and third, in passages on generation where a physician's attention was drawn to the problem of the origin of the soul in connection with discussions of the animation of the fetus. Thus, the philosophically inclined physician had legitimate opportunities to discuss the soul if he chose to do so, and these opportunities could be enlarged. Taddeo, as already noted, expounded the doctrine of the unicity of the intellect (which has to do with the rational, not the vegetative or sensitive aspect of the soul) in a discussion of "virtues" in the human body. How, then, was the subject of soul treated by his colleagues and pupils?

Among Taddeo's associates, only Dino del Garbo and Turisanus seem to have given any extended consideration to the subject of the soul. The topic arises neither in the medical works of Guglielmo da Brescia, which are mostly practical in import, nor, apparently, in the specialized treatises on Galenic medicine by Bartolomeo da Varignana. Although Mondino de' Liuzzi wrote a lengthy general introduction to medicine in his commentary on Galen's *Tegni*, he chose to focus his attention therein mainly on symptomology and to avoid philosophical excursions about the soul or anything else. Some account has already been given of Dino's ideas about the faculties of the soul expressed in his philosophical commentary on a poem of Guido Cavalcanti. It may be recalled that the emergence of controversy over whether "Averroist" leanings are to be attributed to Guido, or to Dino, or to neither, or to both, has led to diligent scholarly examination of Dino's teaching on the soul in this work, without bringing to light any clearly heterodox views expounded, let alone maintained, by Dino.

In their medical works, both Dino and Turisanus tackled the problem of the animation of the fetus, thus confronting a question on which there was a wide range of opinion among thirteenth-century Latin philosophers and theologians; Bruno Nardi has identified no fewer than eight distinct theories held by generally orthodox Christian thinkers about the precise relationship of divine creation and parental generation in forming new human souls.[67] In Nardi's view, the explanation advanced by Dino in his commentary on Hippocrates' *De natura fetus*[68] resembles that espoused

---

[67] Bruno Nardi, *Studi di filosofia medievale* (Rome, 1960), pp. 12-24, the opinion of Averroes making a ninth view.

[68] Dino, *De natura fetus*, fols. 45-89r. The discussion of the soul is at fols. 51r-52r, and 59v.

by Alfredus Anglicus a century earlier.[69] Dino held that, at the time of conception, the semen of the father becomes imbued with *spiritus*, which conveys vegetative, sensitive, and motive powers to the embryo. This *spiritus* is simultaneously a natural endowment of the father and the instrument of divine power, namely, of the intelligences acting through the heavenly bodies. The soul of the father, he believed, acts upon the embryo through the *spiritus* in the semen in the same way that the intelligences act upon things here below through the heavenly bodies. Just as the intelligences do not themselves provide the forms of the heavenly bodies, but are instead their movers and their givers of their operations, so the soul of the father acts through the sperm without being contained within it as a form (an opinion Dino attributed to Averroes). The action of the celestial bodies aids in all generation here on earth, but the father, not the stars, determines that a man will be produced rather than something else. Dino concluded his account by emphasizing once again that, although the *spiritus* borne by the sperm is of a higher order than the natural, and though it conveys sensitive and motive as well as vegetative powers, yet it is nonetheless "in the first place and primarily the organ of a natural virtue."[70] Thus, Dino claimed that the father generates the vegetative and sensitive soul of his offspring in cooperation with the conscious and purposive creative force of divine power transmitted through the stars.[71] Evidently he subscribed to the view that intelligences

[69] Nardi, "Noterella polemica," pp. 52-54.

[70] "Hic spiritus est instrumentum primo et principaliter est organum naturalis virtutis; et tamen altioris quam naturalis," Dino, *De natura fetus*, fol. 52r.

[71] "ideo opportuit concurrere in generatione illa calidum naturale quod est organum alicuius forme determinate: tale autem calidum terminatum est ipse spiritus: et ideo necesse fuit intercipi spiritum: et includi in ipso spermate, et quia hic spiritus generat virtute duplicis agentis, scilicet universalis et particularis, universalis quidem ut corporis celestis digerentis et mensurantis ipsum spiritum in suis actionibus. . . . Tunc dico quod hic spiritus in generatione corporum vivorum est organum alicuius virtutis cognoscitive. Cuius ratio est quia ut sic est organum intellective virtutis, utputa intelligentie, et quia intelligentia agit virtute divina: ideo ultimo est organum virtutis divine. Quod autem sit organum virtutis cognoscitive declaratur, quia omne organum agens propter finem terminatum aut cognoscit finem illum aut dirigitur a cognoscente finem illum; necessario oportet hoc, aliter enim non ageret determinate hoc magis quam illud sed a casu, nam sagitta ipsa determinate feriens in signum, licet non cognoscat de se, tamen dirigitur a sagitante qui signum cognoscit, sed spiritus in spermate exiens agit determinate et propter finem; ergo de necessitate oportet quod aut cognoscat aut dirigatur a cognoscente; sed hic spiritus non cognoscit, ut patet quia non est animatus, cum anima sit actus corporis organici et spiritus non sit organizatus; ergo dirigitur ab eo qui cognoscit omnes formas mixtorum et species omnium formarum naturalium que sunt in mente divina," ibid., fol. 51v.

moving the celestial bodies served somehow as intermediaries in the continuing work of creation.[72] Beyond making it clear that only vegetative and sensitive powers were received directly from the father, Dino avoided the question of the origin of the rational soul. He seems to have believed that the rational soul organized and unified the developing fetus and presumably, therefore, held that this aspect of soul was infused by divine power at the moment of conception.[73]

The somewhat similar account provided by Turisanus seems to have derived, unsurprisingly, chiefly from Avicenna.[74] According to this theory, semen is imbued with *virtus informativa*, and by this means vegetative and sensitive life is imparted to the embryo; however, the rational soul is subsequently infused from without and is the work of God. Turisanus also held that the embryo experiences repeated generation and corruption of forms, each new form being more perfect than the predecessor that it replaces; in addition, he maintained that the semen, aided by heat from the heavenly bodies, is somehow active in preparing and organizing the body to receive the infused rational soul. The concept that successive acts of generation and corruptions of form occur in the embryo, which was also adopted by Thomas Aquinas,[75] served to preserve the unity of the soul and its unique position as the single form of the body at all times, while allowing both for the physical transmission of the principle of life from the parents and for the subsequent divine creation of the rational soul. The notion that the semen and the influence of the stars combine to "organize" the body for the reception of the rational soul may be thought to push naturalistic explanation as far as is possible if any role at all is to be reserved for direct divine intervention. But, as appears from the summary of Dino's views, the action of the stars could itself be regarded as the work of heavenly intelligences and therefore as somehow divine. Despite the similarities in Dino's and Turisanus's accounts of the process of animation, the differences are sufficient to indicate both that,

[72] A view widely held, in one form or another, in the thirteenth century; see for example Nardi, *Studi*, pp. 27-28, for the version maintained by Albertus Magnus. Aristotle could be called upon in support of these views, since he had held that intelligences moved the heavenly bodies (*Metaphysics* 12.8, 1073a13-1074b14) and that the sun, at any rate, played a part in all sublunary coming to be and passing away (*De generatione et corruptione* 2.10, 336a32-336b20).

[73] Dino *De natura fetus*, fols. 59v-60r; see also B. Nardi, "Noterella polemica." pp. 52-54.

[74] Turisanus, *Plusquam*, fol. 59v.

[75] ST 1, q. 118, a.1, ad 3; see Nardi, *Studi*, pp. 18-20, for discussion.

whatever Dino may have plagiarized from Turisanus, he did not plagiarize his description of the origin of the soul; and that, in this instance as in others, one cannot speak of philosophical doctrines common to Taddeo's school.

Turisanus also considered whether the soul has any special connection with the heart.[76] He noted that, since the substance of the soul is one, it is necessary to suppose that one organ rules the body as the soul's deputy; and that "all the Peripatetics," as well as anatomy and experience, sustain the idea that the organ in question is the heart. The relationship of soul and heart Turisanus described in terms of the physiology of elemental qualities, saying that the soul moves the body, but movement is impeded by cold, and the heart is the fount of bodily heat. He also noted that operations of the soul, such as the generative action of *virtus informativa*, in parts of the body other than the heart are, according to Aristotle, not the work of the soul's essence but of its powers, which flow out from the heart and are borne to the rest of the body by the *spiritus*, which also emanates from the heart. This concept, Turisanus remarked, involves an apparent impossibility, namely the separation of the essence of the soul from its powers, and has consequently given rise to much debate. According to Turisanus, those who were chiefly concerned to justify Aristotle (*salvantes philosophum*) usually maintained that the virtues, or powers, of the soul always depend upon the essence of the soul, just as sunlight depends upon the sun; thus, the powers of the soul can no more be described as separate from the soul than sunlight can be called separate from the sun. In their opinion, therefore, it was satisfactory to state that the soul is present in organs of the body other than the heart only in its virtues, not in its essence. As a negative proof of this concept, they were accustomed to point out that if the essence of the soul were present in, say, the eye, then the soul would be extinguished when an eye is put out. This opinion was, to Turisanus's mind, untenable. He preferred the explanation of others who were "investigating more subtly" (*subtilius indagantes*); these thinkers claimed that the soul is not joined to the body through any intermediary, whether an organ or powers, but is united directly with the whole body. They put forward a number of considerations to support their view: first, the soul is the form of the body, and every form is joined directly to its matter; second, the body of man is not like a house, which is a composite of the separate form and matter of

[76] Turisanus, *Plusquam*, fols. 27v-29v.

every one of its materials, but is a single, natural entity with one form for the whole; it follows therefore that every part of a man (and of an animal) receives its being and species from the soul, its own form; and third, Aristotle speaks of the soul as the act of an organic body, but if the soul were located only in the heart, it would be the act of the heart, not of the whole body, and the other parts would presumably be perfected by other forms. In short, according to the view endorsed by Turisanus, the soul is in the whole body and in every part of it—or rather, the whole perfection of the soul is in every part, but not necessarily all its virtues (presumably what he meant is that, say, the power of seeing, which is a virtue of the sensitive soul, resides only in the eye, not in every part of the body). Thus, Turisanus stated, the powers and the essence of the soul are not separated; yet he went on to conclude that in both aspects the soul resides principally in the heart, whence its instruments (heat and *spiritus*), rather than its powers, flow.

The account of the soul provided by Turisanus appears entirely orthodox in its insistence upon the union of the soul with the whole body, rather than with a particular organ, and in the distinction but not separation of the essence and the powers of the soul. Moreover, it may be possible to detect a specifically Thomist influence in the assertion that the soul is the one substantial form of the body.[77] In this passage Turisanus, far from being a stubborn and radical Aristotelian, showed himself ready to criticize what he took to be an opinion of Aristotle and his defenders (elsewhere, as we shall see, he displayed very considerable reservations, on physiological grounds, about the Aristotelian doctrine of the primacy of the heart). Ultimately, however, he proved unable totally to renounce the view that the soul is in some way "principally" in the heart, perhaps because he was aware that Albertus Magnus had asserted that rejection of the primacy of the heart is tantamount to accepting the belief that a separate soul exists in each of three principal organs: heart, brain, and liver.[78]

The few passages in the works by members of Taddeo's school that

[77] Cf. ST 1, q. 76.1, 76.4.3, 77.1; but see also Callus, "Origins," passim, for the earlier antecedents of the idea. See also note 43, above.

[78] See Albertus Magnus, *De animalibus*, ed. Herman Stadler, 3.1.6, *Beiträge zur Geschichte der Philosophie des Mittelalters* 15 (1916):302-303; *De spiritu et respiratione* 1.2.1 (ed. Borgnet 9:231-232).

touch upon controversial philosophical issues do not suggest that heterodox views made any significant penetration beyond Taddeo himself. All of Taddeo's pupils, it is true, were less overtly concerned about the theological implications of their ideas than was, say, Albertus Magnus when writing on some of the same topics; but Albertus was a theologian and natural philosopher, not a physician. For the most part, the members of Taddeo's circle simply went about the intellectual business of the learned physician, which was primarily to be zealous in gathering and sifting through naturalistic explanations, from the best available authorities, of psychological and physiological phenomena. One feels inclined to suggest that, when Taddeo and his pupils paid tribute to the usefulness of philosophy for medicine (insofar as such tribute was anything more than a rhetorical genuflection to tradition), they had in mind Aristotle's biology rather than "Averroist" ideas about the possible intellect, the eternity of the world, or other dangerous subjects. Taddeo's own undoubted interest in heterodox speculation was expressed only in an early work and probably gave way to more strictly professional concerns later in his career. Much that is known about these men—Taddeo's proverbial wealth, Guglielmo's career at the papal court, the opposition of Dino and Mondino to astrological excesses, Turisanus's late monastic vocation—suggests that, as a group, they were characterized chiefly by a concern for professional advancement that was allied with conservative religious views, an orientation that makes them unlikely exponents of heterodox philosophical trends. One may note too that, despite the involvement in professional rivalries and the attendant muckraking recorded of Taddeo, Bartolomeo, Dino, and Turisanus (see chapter two), no contemporary or immediately posthumous reputation for unorthodoxy appears to have hung over any of them (as it did, for example, over Peter of Abano).[79] On the contrary, as we have already noted, a close associate of Dino del Garbo was himself involved in 1311 in launching accusations of heresy against a colleague, the radical Aristotelian philosopher Angelo d'Arezzo. Whatever Taddeo's own intellectual and personal relationship with Gentile da Cingoli, the development in the first forty years of the fourteenth century of Bologna as a major center of philosophical speculation remarkable for its radical or "Averroist" tendencies cannot be satisfactorily traced in the medical writings of those trained in the school of Taddeo.

[79] See Thorndike, *History of Magic*, 2:938-947.

GENERAL SCIENCE AND NATURAL HISTORY

Although miscellaneous information drawn from natural science and natural history was incorporated into some of their medical works, Taddeo and his pupils kept it, like philosophical speculation, within bounds and, on the whole, fairly well subordinated to their overall medical purpose. No member of this group carried his interest in general science and natural history so far as to merit Petrarch's famous gibe at Guido da Bagnolo, a Bologna-trained physician of the mid-fourteenth century who was obsessed with Aristotle's *Historia animalium*, Pliny, and the encyclopedists: "he has much to tell about wild animals, about birds and fishes: how many hairs there are in the lion's mane; how many feathers in the hawk's tail; . . . that elephants couple from behind and are pregnant for two years. . . . All of this is for the greater part wrong."[80] Guido was, of course, following a well-established tradition; physicians had for centuries made a practice of discussing "natural questions" on a wide variety of topics having to do with meteorology, zoology, and assorted marvels of nature, as the accumulation of the famous collection known as the Salernitan Questions demonstrates.[81] If anything, the general scientific interests of physicians tended to broaden and deepen during the later Middle Ages; in the fourteenth century some of them made contributions to sciences and branches of technology as diverse as clock making, astronomy, and military engineering.[82] On the whole, however, the work of Taddeo and his associates does not show many signs of interest independent of medical purposes in the details of other sciences. It is clear, for example, that they incorporated questions on climate and the seasons in their medical works perhaps partially because such material occurred in earlier collections of "natural questions," but chiefly because they believed, following Hippocrates, that regional and climatic conditions affected human health and development.[83]

[80] *De sui ipsius et multorum ignorantia*; the translation is that of Hans Nachod in Ernst Cassirer, P. O. Kristeller, J. H. Randall, Jr., eds., *The Renaissance Philosophy of Man* (Chicago, 1948), pp. 57-58. On the identification of Guido, and his career, see Paul Oskar Kristeller, "Petrarch's 'Averroists': A Note on the History of Aristotelianism in Venice, Padua, and Bologna," *Bibliothèque d'Humanisme et de Renaissance* 14 (1952):63-64. See also idem, "Il Petrarch, l'umanesimo e la scolastica a Venezia," in *La civiltà veneziana del Trecento*, pp. 149-170.

[81] Lawn, *The Salernitan Questions*, pp. 16-49.

[82] See Lynn White, "Medical Astrologers and Late Medieval Technology," *Viator: Medieval and Renaissance Studies* 6 (1975):295-308.

[83] *Airs Waters Places* 2, *Prognostica* 4. See also note 64 to chapter five, above.

Where Taddeo, Turisanus, and the rest touched upon natural phenomena that do not directly affect human health, they did so almost invariably because they believed them to provide a medically useful analogy: thus, for example, if certain medicines act by specific form, an understanding of other phenomena caused by specific form will be an aid to the comprehension of the action of medicines.[84]

Apart from the fundamental concepts of Aristotelian physics, discussed in the preceding section, the general scientific idea most pervasive in the works of Taddeo and his school was probably that of the terrestrial influences of the heavenly bodies. This, while supported by (and, as a recent scholar has pointed out, "inextricably involved with" Aristotelian cosmology),[85] was nonetheless based upon a science of astronomy that was considered to be distinct from natural philosophy and that was derived from a separate learned tradition; *astrologia* has therefore been treated as a separate, ancillary science earlier in this work. Here it need only be recalled that, while numerous passing references point to the general acceptance by Taddeo and his pupils of the universal influence of the heavens on things here below, these authors devoted relatively little space in their medical works to astrological exposition and, unlike other physicians of the period, are not known (with one possible exception) to have written any astronomical or astrological works. Moreover, Dino, Mondino, and Gentile da Cingoli are on record as opponents of excessive reliance on astrology. Upon other, very disparate, scientific subjects they touched from time to time, and an account of the treatment of optical theory, under the rubric of the sense of sight, will be found in the following chapter. Here we may note discussions of magnetism called forth by the subject of medicaments, which were supposed to have special powers of attraction; a lengthy disquisition upon the reproduction of plants as compared with human reproduction; treatments of climate and geography in connection with their effect upon human health; and information about the phases of the moon and the length of the solar year provided in connection with the concept of "critical days" in illness.

Magnetism was discussed in some detail by both Taddeo and by Tu-

---

[84] On the history of the use of analogy in medicine, see Lester S. King, "Evidence and Its Evaluation in Eighteenth-Century Medicine," *Bulletin of the History of Medicine* 50 (1976):174-190.

[85] Lemay, "Teaching of Astronomy," p. 197.

risanus and was alluded to by Guglielmo da Brescia.[86] As has been noted, the power of the magnet was a standard example of the action of specific form, a type of action also attributed to certain medications. All three authors treated magnetism as parallel to the power of particular medicines to attract one or another of the humors. Taddeo inquired whether the property in the magnet that attracts iron is the same as or different from the property in the iron that causes it to be drawn to the magnet. In his view, the possible alternatives are either that the two substances possess the same property, with the magnet having it to a stronger degree, or that they have different but complementary properties. Taddeo's preferred solution is that the magnet and the iron are alike in matter and in the influence that they receive from the stars, but differ in their degree of perfection. If so, he asked, which is the more perfect, the magnet or the iron? If the magnet, then what benefit does it receive from drawing a less perfect object to itself? (Some benefit there must be, since nature does nothing in vain.) Yet how can the iron be the more perfect when it is the patient, and the magnet the agent? Taddeo declared that it is the drawing force, not the ultimate benefit, that is stronger in the magnet than the iron. He accepted without question that a magnet does not attract a magnet, but queried the assertion that iron does not attract iron, because he himself had owned a knife that did attract other metal objects; however, he concluded that this was because it had been tempered in water in which *calamite* was dissolved.[87]

Turisanus's discussion of the magnet occurred in a general discussion of attraction as a category of motion, which he prefaced to an account of the "attractive and opening power" of laxative medicines.[88] As is often the case, his theoretical framework seems more elaborate, philosophically sophisticated, and "scientific" than that of Taddeo. Turisanus explained that "attraction" is a type of motion that can take two forms: either violent, or partly violent and partly natural. (Since attraction presupposes that the thing attracting is outside the thing attracted, a wholly natural motion of attraction is not possible.) The first of these forms requires the physical contact of the attracting and attracted bodies and is an action

---

[86] Guglielmo, *Questiones de tyriaca*, in McVaugh, "Theriac at Montpellier," p. 134. McVaugh comments (pp. 126-127) that Guglielmo appears to have been the first at Montpellier to equate medicinal and magnetic action; it appears likely, however, that he derived the idea from his master at Bologna, Taddeo.

[87] Taddeo, *Quod comeditur*, BAV, MS Palat. lat. 1246, fols. 92r-93r.

[88] Turisanus, *Plusquam*, fols. 122v-124r.

wholly violent; an example is the pulling of one thing by another. But, Turisanus continued, the second kind of attraction occurs without physical contact and requires that the thing attracted have itself some virtue that cooperates in making it responsive to the attracting body (this kind of attraction fills the description of being partly natural and partly violent because the force exerted by the attracting body is violent, while the virtue inherent in the attracted body is natural); an example of this second kind of attraction is the movement of iron toward a magnet.[89] Thus Turisanus managed to smuggle action at a distance into a generally Aristotelian explanation of motion, being induced to do so primarily by his desire to explain the real or supposed effects of certain medicines or medical procedures.

Turisanus subdivided attraction of the "partly natural and partly violent" kind into three categories: that caused by vacuum, that caused by heat, and that caused by the action of specific form (magnetism and the effect of laxatives are examples of the last). Regarding the first category of attraction, Turisanus raised and disposed of the problem that a vacuum, because it is nothing, cannot have an effect. He explained that the suction that leads to the immediate replenishment of a vacuum (Turisanus, naturally, accepted the Aristotelian doctrine that a vacuum is impossible in nature) is more properly attributed to the matter that was evacuated to make the vacuum than to the vacuum itself. He then proceeded to demolish, to his own satisfaction, the contention of Galen and Avicenna that the drawing power of heat is essentially the same as that of a vacuum. Those authors, he said, had maintained that when the wick of a lamp burns the substance of the wick disappears, a vacuum is created, and oil or wax are drawn up to replace it. Turisanus held instead that the heat of the wick turns the oil or wax into vapor, which naturally moves upward, and that this effect should therefore be attributed to gen-

[89] "Sed dicamus nunc quot modis fiat attractio: et que sit virtus medicine attrahentis et aperientis: et quis modus purgandi attrahentium [BAV, MS Urb. lat. 244, fol. 148v: attractum]: dico ergo quod attractio alicuius ab aliquo aut est tota violenta aut partim violenta et partim naturalis. tota autem naturalis esse non potest cum principalis eius causa sit principium extra id quod attrahitur, in totam autem violenta est illa que sequitur motum attrahentis contactum habentis ad attractum nihil conferente attracto. . . . Propterea Averroes in 7° physicorum exemplificans de motu violento dixit quod motus violenti sunt attractio impulsio vectio et vertigo; est autem et alia attractio in qua licet principium attrahens sit extra attractum non tamen proficit: nisi aut attractum habeat etiam virtutem qua sine contactu currat in attrahens ut contingit in attractione qua ferrum attrahitur a magnete aut ubi attrahens faciat dispositionem in circuitu attracti," ibid., fol. 122v.

eration rather than to the drawing power of a vacuum. Heat does indeed exercise its own distinct form of attraction, according to Turisanus, as one can readily see from the action of *tapsiam*, which draws up a swelling on any part of the body; the attraction of heat works either by changing liquids into vapor or by thinning them out so that, in either case, they can move more easily.

Turning to attraction by specific form, Turisanus declared that this is always direct and without the mediation of any quality or substance. Actions of this kind are more properly termed supernatural than natural. A magnet does not attract iron by heat or cold, but simply because it is a magnet; moreover, once the magnet and the iron are in contact, there is no joint action that they perform as agent and patient, nor is the iron absorbed by the magnet. The action of the latter is comparable to that of the fish called *stupefactor* or *torpigo*, which paralyzes the hand of the fisherman who takes it in the net without his touching it directly. One could argue that the air between the iron and the magnet, in the case of magnetism, and the net, in the case of the *stupefactor* fish, act as intermediaries by which the force is transmitted; but this does not seem to be the case, since the air and the net, respectively, are not affected by the action of the magnet and the fish. After remarking that the power of a magnet can be removed by rubbing garlic on it (a traditional belief), Turisanus concluded his discussion of magnetism by pointing out that the magnet requires only the presence of the iron for the exercise of its power, whereas laxative medicines need the heat of the body to enable them to work on the humors; and that is why laxatives do not work when they are outside the body.

One might expect physicians whose medical practice consisted very largely in the prescription of herbal remedies to show a special interest in the natural history of plants. In fact, although the medicinal properties of various plants are frequently referred to in almost all the works of members of the group, and although at least three of them produced works specifically on (mostly herbal) remedies,[90] the only extended treat-

---

[90] Namely, Guglielmo da Brescia's *Practica*, Taddeo's *Tabula de remediis*, and Dino's *Compilatio emplastrorum et unguentorum*; Dino's commentary on Book 2 of the *Canon* is, of course, also mainly concerned with herbal remedies, and sometimes circulated under the title *De virtutibus medicamentorum*. I have not explored the connection, if any, between the last named work and the *Compilatio emplastrorum et unguentorum*, which also claims to be based, in part, on Book 2 of the *Canon*. For manuscripts and editions, see Bibliography.

ment of botany to be found occurs in quite another setting. Following
the example of the Hippocratic author on whom he was commenting,
Dino del Garbo introduced the subject of plant reproduction and growth
into his work on the fetus.[91] The main purpose of Dino's lengthy discussion of this subject, which almost constitutes a separate treatise within the
larger work, is to examine the parallels and differences between mammalian and vegetable reproduction and development. His approach is
"philosophical" in the sense that he laid down general principles and
avoided particulars wherever possible.[92] In sharp contrast to the usual
medical treatment of plants in herbals and in works on remedies, Dino
here made no mention of any particular plant species, or of their medicinal properties and balance of elemental qualities. Instead he examined
such factors affecting plant growth as planetary influences and variation
in the temperature of the soil at different times of year, and he compared
the planting of the seed in the ground and the ramification of roots and
branches to human conception and the development of the embryo. He
also inquired whether a seed puts out roots or branches first, and whether
plants that grow from seeds can in some circumstances be generated
without seeds. Among the differences noted between the reproductive
systems of plants and of mammals were the capacity of plants to be multiplied by division and transplantation, and the ability of perennials to
renew themselves. Dino further remarked, by way of apology for the
Hippocratic author's deviation from content appropriate to a medical
treatise, that Hippocrates' knowledge of natural philosophy is demonstrated by his discussion of the reproduction of trees, a subject he had
treated "better than any other author we have, no matter who he may
be."[93]

---

[91] Dino, *De natura fetus*, fols. 72r-82r.

[92] One is reminded of the attitude expressed by Albertus Magnus in the introduction to
the catalogue of individual plant species that fills Book 6 of his *De vegetabilibus et plantis*:
"In hoc sexto libro *Vegetabilium* nostrorum, magis satisfacimus curiositati studentium quam
philosophiae: de particularibus enim etiam philosophia esse non poterit" (ed. Borgnet,
10:159).

[93] "et melius tractat de istis plantis quam alius auctor quem habeamus quicunque sit
ille," Dino, *De natura fetus*, fol. 82r. The only work specifically on plants cited by Dino
is the pseudo-Aristotelian *De plantis* (ibid., fol. 73v, where, however, the citation of
Averroes as the author of this work is a printer's error; BAV, MS Vat. lat. 4464, 14c,
fol. 111, reads "auctoris libri de plantis," in place of "Averr. libri de plantis" in the printed
version).

Climate, the seasons, and the lunar and solar calendar were subjects to which Taddeo returned in several of his major works. In the commentary on the *Isagoge*, he discussed changes in the air (one of the six "non-natural things" affecting human health, according to medieval Galenic theory) brought about by changes of season, by the rising and setting of particular stars and planets, by the prevailing winds, and by altitude. He incorporated and amplified some of the same material in his commentary on the *Aphorisms*, where he also discussed the calendar, as he did in his commentary on the *Prognostica*.[94]

Taddeo noted that astrologers describe the seasons in precise terms, according to the days of the months and the movement of the sun through the zodiac; whereas physicians simply refer to climatic change. He explained that seasonal variations in temperature occur because of variations in the angle of the sun's rays, a point also made by Turisanus, who introduced a somewhat similar discussion of climate into a section of the *Plusquam commentum* dealing with factors affecting the complexion of the brain.[95] Turisanus understood that latitude as well as season had to be taken into account in any discussion of the obliquity or directness of the solar rays, and he seized this opportunity to refute those who claimed that the equatorial region is temperate in climate, thus no doubt showing his awareness, and disapproval, of the doubts that were coming more and more frequently to be cast on the ancient theory of the uninhabitability of the equatorial regions because of their excessive heat.[96]

Turning to variations in temperature caused by altitude, Taddeo came to the conclusion, after lengthy discussion, that lowland is warmer than highland and not the other way about. He also noted the cooling and humidifying effect of the proximity of the sea, although pointing out

---

[94] Taddeo, *Isagoge*, fol. 373r; Taddeo, *Aphor.*, fol. 78v.

[95] Taddeo, *Aphor.*, fol. 78v; cf. Turisanus, *Plusquam*, fols. 40r-v, 43r.

[96] Turisanus, *Plusquam*, fol. 40v. The belief that the equatorial regions were uninhabitable, transmitted from antiquity by Macrobius (*In somnium Scipionis* 2.5.16-17) and other authors, was challenged in the thirteenth century by Robert Grosseteste and others on the basis of various Arabic authorities; see G.H.T. Kimble, *Geography in the Middle Ages* (New York, 1968, repr. of 1938 ed.), pp. 162-164; by the latter part of the thirteenth century the accounts of recent travelers were also available to refute the notion of the uninhabitability of the equatorial zone. As a result, Peter of Abano, for example, claimed that the equatorial regions were not only habitable, but so favored by nature as to have been the probable site of the Garden of Eden (*Conciliator*, differentia 67), basing his assertion both on travelers' tales and learned authority. It is conceivable that Turisanus was specifically concerned to refute Peter's opinion.

that southern coasts, such as that of Sicily, are warmer than more northerly ones.[97] Both Taddeo and Turisanus also gave a good deal of attention to winds, which Taddeo defined as vapors originating from the earth. Taddeo's account of winds includes the Aristotelian four causes of winds, the names of various winds, the complexion of winds (with the explanation that winds are dry and cold by nature, but absorb moisture when they cross marshy places and are heated by the sun), and the strength of winds from various directions at various seasons.[98] The source of most of his material on climate was no doubt Aristotle's *Meteorologica*, although Taddeo also drew fairly extensively from passages on climate in earlier medical texts.

In considering Taddeo's comments on the effect of the stars upon seasonal temperature, one is at a loss whether to categorize this material as natural philosophy or astrology, for it draws upon the resources of both sciences. Taddeo held that the temperature at different times of year is governed by the rising of particular fixed stars, for instance the Pleiades in spring and the Dog Star in summer, as well as by the planets. He believed, moreover, that all the stars, rather than just the sun, are the source of heat and light from the heavens, although their lesser lights cannot be seen when they are near the sun.[99] It is clear from another passage that Taddeo believed the effect of the stars on seasonal temperatures to embody two of the three kinds of celestial action, namely, the general effect of the heat and light of the heavenly bodies upon everything on earth, attested to by Aristotle and agreed to by "all philosophy" as well as by experience; and the particular heating effect of certain among the heavenly bodies, most notably the sun. Taddeo was careful to explain that the air serves as intermediary for these kinds of action, thus removing the objection, raised on the basis of Aristotelian physics, that the action of the stars on terrestrial things is impossible because there is no direct contact between mover and moved, or agent and patient. The third kind of celestial action postulated by Taddeo is by specific form and affected nativities, critical days of illness, and so on.[100] Thus Aristotelian cosmology, meteorology, and teaching on generation and corruption were brought into harmony with astrology and made to support one another in a unified system.

[97] Taddeo, *Isagoge*, fol. 375r; Taddeo, *Aphor.*, fol. 78v.

[98] Taddeo, *Isagoge*, fols. 374r-v; Turisanus, *Plusquam*, fol. 43r.

[99] Taddeo, *Isagoge*, fol. 374r.   [100] Taddeo, *Aphor.*, fol. 49r.

Taddeo's interest in the calendar appears to have been, for the most part, a byproduct of his concern to expound the concept of critical days in illnesses: a usable system of calculating critical days would require both exactness and agreement among physicians on the calendrical system to be used. Taddeo accordingly explained to his readers that the medicinal month (*mensis medicinalis*) is 26 days and 22 hours long. This figure he obtained by averaging the 26½ days in which the moon is visibly waxing and waning (*mensis manifeste apparitionis*) with the 27⅓ days taken for its passage through the zodiac "on account of the days it stays in conjunction" (*propter dies in quibus stet apud conjunctionem*). He noted that the entire month (*mensis lunaris integer*) is 29½ days long, but pointed out that the moon can exercise no influence when it is not visible.[101] Regarding the length of the year, he noted the difference of one fiftieth of a day between the estimate of Galen and that of Ptolemy and Albumasar; rejecting the former as erroneous, he observed that one should always prefer the word of a specialist in any particular discipline.[102]

ARISTOTELIAN BIOLOGY AND THE HIPPOCRATIC-GALENIC TRADITION

For Taddeo and his circle, as for other physicians of their day, Aristotle's biological works provided much information on a variety of anatomical and physiological topics, and especially on the heart, reproduction, and sense perception. Yet their examination of Aristotle's teaching and of the available interpretative material revealed that, on important issues, the Philosopher differed from the chief ancient medical authorities, and most notably from Galen. Among the subjects on which Aristotle and the Hippocratic-Galenic tradition differed were the anatomy of veins and arteries, the anatomy and function of the heart, whether or not the heart is the first organ to be developed in the fetus, the function of the brain, whether the semen is the product of the whole body or only of a part, and the function of the testicles.[103] Two differences stand out as more

---

101 Ibid., and *Pronost.*, fol. 237v, with cross-references to his commentaries on Galen, *De creticis*, and on the *Aphorisms*.

102 Taddeo, *Pronost.*, fol. 237v; a similar remark about Galen's inadequacy as an astronomical authority was made by Peter of Abano, *Conciliator*, fols. 149v-150r, differentia 104.

103 Aristotle's teachings on mammalian biology in general and the biology of man in particular are scattered throughout the works on animals, and especially in *Historia animalium*, Books 1, 3, 6, and 7; *De partibus animalium*, Books 2, 3, and 4; and *De generatione*

fundamental and more inclusive in their implications than the rest. The first is the Aristotelian doctrine of the primacy of the heart, as contrasted to Galen's teaching on the three principal members. Aristotle held the heart, the source of heat and life, to be the primary organ of the whole body, and he therefore repeatedly claimed that the heart controls not only the arterial and venous systems (between which he did not distinguish), but also sense and motion.[104] The Galenists, however, taught that there are three principal organs in the body—heart, brain, and liver (the testicles being sometimes added as a fourth)—all of which are equally necessary to life. Moreover, since Galen, on the basis of empirical investigations carried out by himself and his medical predecessors, was aware both of the distinction between veins and arteries and of the role of the brain and spinal cord in controlling sense and motion, he postulated three bodily systems, each controlled by one of the principal organs: the nerves, originating in the brain; the arteries, originating in the heart; and the veins, originating in the liver.[105] The second major discrepancy between Aristotle and Galen has to do with sexual reproduction. Aristotle held that the active principle in conception is supplied entirely by the male, the female providing merely the passive matter acted upon by the male formative agent.[106] In order to account for the fact that hereditary characteristics can be acquired from both parents, however, Galen found it necessary to postulate that both contribute actively to the formation of the fetus. He therefore maintained the existence of female as well as male sperm, the former being sometimes identified with vaginal secretions emitted during sexual intercourse.[107]

---

animalium, Books 1 and 2. Galen's system of anatomy and physiology is described in numerous treatises among his very copious works (19 volumes in the nineteenth-century Kühn edition); a comprehensive account is to be found in *Galen on the Usefulness of the Parts of the Body,* trans. May. On the extent of the knowledge of these aspects of the work of Aristotle and Galen in the Middle Ages, see below.

[104] *De partibus animalium* 3.4, 666a6-666b1; 3.5, 667b15-30; and elsewhere.

[105] A brief statement, no doubt known to all thirteenth-century learned physicians, is found in the medieval Latin version of the *Tegni*: "Principalis igitur sunt cor, cerebrum, epar, et testiculi. Ab illis vero exorta sunt et illis famulantur nervi et spinalis medulla cerebro, Cordi vero arterie, Vene epati, Seminalia vasa testiculis," *Tegni Galieni* 2.28-29, in *Articella nuperrime impressa* (Lyon, 1515), fol. cxi^r. Elaborations of the concept, are of course, worked out in *De usu partium* and other longer treatises by Galen. For a recent general account (not always very satisfactory) of Galen's physiology, see Siegel, *Galen's System of Physiology and Medicine.*

[106] *De generatione animalium* 1.19-20, 727b6-729a35, and 2.4, 738b20-739a23.

[107] *On the Usefulness of the Parts* 14.6-11, trans. May, 2:628-646; *De semine* and *De*

The first author to point out some of these discrepancies was Galen himself, who took Aristotle severely to task for certain of his views.[108] But in the medieval Latin West, an understanding of the differences between Aristotle and Galen was achieved only slowly over the course of the thirteenth century. The nature of this understanding was, inevitably, conditioned by the way in which the teachings of Aristotle and Galen reached Latin physicians. Together with the Hippocratic medical tradition, a simplified version of Galen's teaching on anatomy and physiology was available in the West, as we have seen, long before the reception of Aristotle's work on those subjects. Yet the serious and minute study of any of Galen's authentic longer treatises in Latin translation was probably still something of a novelty when Taddeo undertook a detailed comparison of two translations of *De interioribus* sometime during the last four decades of the thirteenth century. Furthermore, as noted above, Galen's anatomy was known only through abbreviations or at second hand. Thirteenth-century Latin physicians thus fell heir to a medical tradition in which Galen's teachings were compressed, mediated, and sometimes distorted; nonetheless, there is no doubt that most of the information received about anatomy and physiology, both from Constantinople and Alexandria in late antiquity and via the Islamic world in the eleventh and twelfth centuries, was Hippocratic and Galenic in its essentials. By contrast, Aristotle's biological ideas, known only after the translation into Latin of the *Parva naturalia* (ca. 1200) and, later, of the works on animals, were a relative novelty.[109] They formed part of an enormously impressive philosophical system that could be studied from much fuller texts than could Galen's work.

Guidance in evaluating the relative merits of the physiological and anatomical systems of Aristotle and Galen was provided by Avicenna,

foetuum formatione, ed. Kühn, 4:512-702. For discussion and comparison of the views of Aristotle and ancient medical authors on conception, see Howard B. Adelmann, *Marcello Malpighi and the Evolution of Embryology* (Ithaca, N.Y., 1966), 2:734-747, and Joseph Needham, *A History of Embryology*, pp. 31-74.

[108] For example in *On the Usefulness of the Parts* 7.14, trans. May, 1:362-363, and *De placitis Hippocratis et Platonis* 1.8-10 (ed. Kühn, 2:200-210). According to Ynez Violé O'Neill, "The Fünfbilderserie Reconsidered," *Bulletin of the History of Medicine* 43 (1969): 241-245, *De placitis* may have been translated into Latin by Constantinus Africanus, although no such translation appears to survive.

[109] As noted above, some twelfth-century physicians seem to have had a (probably indirect) acquaintance with Aristotelian natural philosophy, but this apparently did not include any of the contents of the biological works.

both in his *Canon* and in his compendium *De animalibus* (translated into Latin before 1232),[110] and by Averroes in a brief chapter *De corde*, which appeared in Latin about 1230.[111] Avicenna often tended toward reconciliation, although he was sometimes very critical of Galen.[112] Averroes at crucial points rejected Galen entirely, although he did not always accept Aristotle's view either.[113] On philosophical grounds (since he believed Galen to have entertained unacceptable beliefs concerning the human soul), Albertus Magnus, whose influential *De animalibus* was probably written around 1260, also supported Aristotle's physiology over Galen's.[114]

Thus, the earliest Latin writers who examined the differences between Aristotle and Galen, a staple subject of Latin medical (and some philosophical) literature from about 1225,[115] found both that the details of Aristotle's teaching were often easier to come by than those of Galen's and that a growing body of authoritative opinion tended to favor Aristotle on points where the two authors conflicted. As a result, although in medicine as in other medieval learned disciplines the goal was the reconciliation of authorities rather than the definitive victory of any one of them, reconciliation was frequently achieved by saving the Aristotelian system as a whole (particularly the primacy of the heart), while fitting into it as many of the details of the teaching of "Galen and all the *medici*" as possible.

Nonetheless, the Hippocratic-Galenic tradition was still extremely vigorous, and it was central to the historical identity and self-image of the medical profession. Later in the thirteenth century, as already noted, the modest beginnings of a revival of the study of Galen were evident in the circle of Taddeo and elsewhere. Although Taddeo and his associates appear to have concentrated much of their interest on treatises dealing with disease, and although the major anatomical works remained unknown to

---

[110] *Aristoteles Latinus*, 1:81.

[111] Ibid., 1:108; Vaux, "La première entrée d'Averroès," p. 225. Albertus Magnus incorporated the whole of this work of Averroes into his *De animalibus* 3.1.5, ed. Stadler, *Beiträge*, 12:295-301. A brief work attributed to Averroes and entitled *De concordia inter Galenum et Aristotelem de generatione* is to be found in BAV, MS Vat. lat. 4454, a fourteenth-century medical and philosophical miscellany including works by Dino del Garbo, Bartolomeo da Varignana, and Taddeo da Parma, at fols. 109r-110v.

[112] See for example note 134 to this chapter.

[113] See Albertus Magnus, *De animalibus* 3.1.5., ed. Stadler, *Beiträge*, 15:295-301.

[114] Ibid., 3.1.6, 9.2.2-4, ed. Stadler, *Beiträge*, 15:301-306, 710-722.

[115] The first work in which the theme is developed at all extensively appears to be the *Anatomia vivorum*.

them, it seems reasonable to assume that as a result of these studies they obtained an understanding of Galen's system of anatomy and physiology superior to that of many of their predecessors. The text of Mondino's *Anatomia* also suggests that the author carefully studied such admittedly inadequate sources of Galen's anatomical teaching as were then available. Therefore, Taddeo and his pupils were probably better equipped to judge between Aristotle and Galen than most of the Latin scholars who came before them. Such, at any rate, was the view of their mid-fourteenth-century successor, the physician Gentile da Foligno, who noted that the "true opinion" of Galen, distinguished from an opinion ascribed to him, was to be found in the writings of Bartolomeo da Varignana, Dino, and Mondino.[116]

Their judgment, of course, rested on the application of philosophical and scientific principles to the analysis of texts. One cannot find any evidence in their work of their awareness that some of the discrepancies between Aristotle's and Galen's mammalian anatomy and physiology might be due to the accumulation and classification of empirical knowledge, or to the superiority of Galen's own research. That Aristotle had lived before Galen was presumably known in Taddeo's circle. According to Mondino, Galen of Pergamum (which, he felt obliged to warn his readers, should not be confused with Bergamo) lived at the time of Christ and visited Him in order to investigate miraculous healing.[117] Yet one cannot therefore attribute to Taddeo's circle any sense of anatomy and physiology as cumulative sciences. Nor was their intellectual or their technical equipment capable of effective empirical testing of the concepts set forth by Aristotle and Galen.

But it would be a mistake to dismiss their efforts as insignificant because their goal was reconciliation and their tool was the analysis of texts

[116] "7ᵃ opinio que vere fuit in mente Galeni intellecta a Dyno . . . est opinio quam Dynus postquam magis profecit in medicina perfecte declaravit. . . . Istam autem opinionem ut credo ponit Dynus alios sequens, nam invenio ipsam in quibusdam collectionibus Bartholomeo da Varignana attributis. Et invenio ab [*sic*] Antonio et tandem a Dyno. Et Mundinus etiam predicat ipsam post istos," Gentile da Foligno, *Questiones et tractatus extravagantes*, fol. 65v. It is not certain that the Mundinus here referred to is Mondino de' Liuzzi.

[117] "Causa autem efficiens fuit Galenus . . . fuit etiam de civitate quadam que dicitur pergamum, non de pergamo quod est in lumbardia sed de pergamo quod est in asia, et dicitur quod ipse fuit coetaneus Christo; et dicitur in cronicis quod ipse audiens miracula que faciebat Christus de sanatione infirmorum venit ad ipsum," Mondino, comm. *Tegni*, BAV, MS Vat. lat. 4466, fol. 57r.

without reference to empirical observations. For one thing, their fundamental assumption that the teachings of natural philosophy and of medicine about the human body should be regarded as comparable descriptions of physical phenomena is in itself worthy of note, since other modes of reconciling apparently conflicting scientific authorities were from time to time employed by some of their contemporaries. Thus, for example, it was fairly common to suggest that different sciences had different methods, different subject matter, and different authorities, and hence yielded variously expressed, and even apparently contradictory, truths. Hence, one way of explaining the differences between the account of the heavens provided by Aristotle and by Ptolemy was to maintain that the goal of the astronomer was to provide the mathematics that would "save the appearances," while that of the natural philosopher was to describe the physical universe. Some authors seemed to imply that a similar type of reconciliation was possible between natural philosophy and medicine. Albertus Magnus not only distinguished theology (which, naturally, he regarded as superior to any secular science) from philosophy, but also philosophy from medicine: "Augustine is to be preferred rather than the philosophers in case of disagreement in matters of faith. But if the discussion concerns medicine, I would rather believe Galen or Hippocrates, and if it concerns things of nature, Aristotle or anyone else experienced in natural things."[118] For physicians, the enormous authority of Avicenna was, on certain issues at least, thrown behind reconciliation of this type; Avicenna, as we shall see, in effect instructed his readers to accept Aristotle's views about the brain as the "ultimate" or "higher" truth, but to follow Galen's when practicing medicine (see note 124 below). Another way of dealing with the differences between Aristotelian and Galenic physiology was to treat them as part of the larger conflict between Platonism and Aristotelianism. Albertus Magnus, for example, repeatedly associated Galen's ideas about the principal members of the body and their virtues with the Platonic conception of the soul.[119] This removed the judgment between the rival physiological systems from a physical to a philosophical, even a theological, plane. By contrast, Taddeo and his colleagues, like other contemporary medical writers, usually strove to provide a fully integrated account of the human body. They

[118] *In 2 Sent., distinctio* 13, C, art. 2 (ed. Borgnet, 27:247).
[119] *De animalibus* 3.1.6., ed. Stadler, *Beiträge*, 15:304; *De spiritu et respiratione* 1.1.1 (ed. Borgnet, 9:231-232).

would confront the differences between philosophical and medical authorities and, using physical descriptions of specific physiological functions, reconcile or choose from among them.

Taddeo himself strongly asserted both the general primacy of the heart and its specific dominance over sense and motion.[120] Citing Aristotle and the compendium *De animalibus* of Avicenna, he stated that the heart is the first of the members and the one in which the soul is founded. He added that the expression "principal member" can be understood in two ways: if it is interpreted as "principal instrument of operation" (*instrumentum principale operationis*), there are four such members in the human body; if it is understood as the "first root" (*prima radix*) of the virtues, then there is only one, namely, the heart. In answering the related question "whether the origin of the nerves is in the heart or in the brain,"[121] Taddeo noted that "all the *medici*" place the origin of the nerves in the brain and thus contradict Aristotle. However, he pointed out that, since the nerves are hard (which suggests that he was among those who failed to distinguish nerves from tendons),[122] it is more likely that they originate in a hard organ like the heart than in a soft one like the brain; moreover, nerves are found within the heart itself but not within the brain. His conclusion is that "the nerves simply and according to truth have their origin in the heart, as Aristotle said,"[123] but, when they come from the heart, they are instruments only of imperfect sense and motion; only from the brain do they become instruments of perfect sense and motion.

The younger physicians did not necessarily share Taddeo's dogmatically Aristotelian approach. Avicenna, after all, had asserted in the

---

[120] Taddeo, *Isagoge*, fols. 350v-353r.

[121] "an sit origo nervorum ab eo [i.e., cerebro] vel a corde," ibid., fols. 352v-353r.

[122] One may compare the somewhat superior treatment by Peter of Abano, who declared: "Nomen siquidem nervi iuxta 2ᵐ interiorum et Haly tripliciter accipitur. Une quidem pro substantia subalbida ad flectendum habilis et ad separandum dura qua organum sensus secundum medicos existit et motus. Cuius ortus apud eos ad cerebrum est vel nucca [*sic*] . . . Alterque pro substantia priori magis indurata subalbida etiam visibilis ex ossibus nata ipsa in adinvicem coniungens ac continens similiter que musculum cum reliquo corpore, et ideo dicitur ligamentum. Tertio vero est corda nascens ex musculo sed eius alterum maxime extremum ex nervo et ligamento composita," *Conciliator*, differentia 41, fol. 59r.

[123] "nervi simpliciter: et secundum veritatem ortum habent ex corde sicut dicit Aristoteles," Taddeo, *Isagoge*, fol. 353r.

Canon that, for all practical purposes, the brain is the source of the nerves of motion and sense and that, although true, it is of no concern to the physician that the heart is in some ultimate sense the primary source of activity for the whole body.[124] His example no doubt fortified the Galenism of some other physicians. For instance, Mondino de' Liuzzi, after explaining, in his commentary on the *Tegni*, Galen's concept of the virtues emanating from each of the four principal members, added that Aristotle taught that all virtues are possessed by one principal member. Far from attempting an elaborate reconciliation of the two theories, Mondino simply remarked curtly that "it is established that the opinion of Aristotle is the cause of much error in medicine, and because of this the opinion of Galen should instead be believed," whence he passed on to the next topic.[125] Describing dissection of the brain in his *Anatomia*, Mondino referred to that organ as the source of the nerves of motion and sense, without any mention of the Aristotelian view.[126] Bartolomeo da Varignana seems to have made little use of Aristotelian ideas on the body in his medical commentaries, which, as several times noted, are all, with one exception, on works of Galen. Among the works expounded by Bartolomeo, *De interioribus* contains a clear and detailed statement of Galen's views on the brain and nervous system; Bartolomeo made almost no comment on this portion of the work, however, and provided no corresponding exposition of Aristotle's views, although it is possible that this may have been because he was working with a defective text.[127]

124 "Debet autem scire et credere in diversitate prima, quod non est ei curandum: utrum cor sit principium sentiendi et motionis cerebro et virtutis nutrientis hepati, aut non sit. Cerebrum namque sive per se sive post cor habeat, principium animalium actionum existit comparatione aliorum membrorum," Avicenna, *Canon* 1.1.5 (Venice, 1507, repr. Hildesheim, 1964), fol. 7v.

125 "sedit quod sententia Aristotelis est causa multi erroris in medicina propter quod magis est credendum Galieno quam Aristoteli" Mondino, comm. *Tegni*, BAV, MS Vat. lat. 4466, fol. 68v.

126 Mondino, *Anatomia*, in Singer, ed., *Fasciculo di Medicina*, 1:91-94. In describing the anatomy of the heart, however, Mondino following Avicenna, made an effort to combine the accounts of Aristotle and Galen; ibid., pp. 82-84 and notes.

127 Galen, *De interioribus* (*De locis affectis*) 3.8 (ed. Kühn, 8:168-170). Since both known manuscripts of Bartolomeo's commentary on *De interioribus* (BAV, MSS Vat. lat. 4452 and 4454) are written with lemmata, not a complete text, of the work commented upon, it is difficult to judge whether or not his copy of the treatise was complete; in the copy of his commentary contained in MS Vat. lat. 4454, book and chapter divisions are clearly indicated, but the chapter divisions do not correspond with those in the Kühn edition. Apparently Bartolomeo (or the version from which he worked) compressed the material contained in 3.1-8 in Kühn into three chapters; the five remaining chapters of

Turisanus also expressed grave reservations about Aristotelian teaching on the nerves and their relation to the heart, although his general philosophical orientation led him into long-winded attempts to reconcile the Aristotelian and Galenic systems considered as a whole. Turisanus, as we have seen, certainly maintained that the heart is the primary organ of the body and in some special way associated with the soul, and that heat and lifegiving *spiritus* flow to the rest of the organs from the heart. Yet in the same passage he was careful to remind his readers that the brain (with the spinal cord) is the source (*principium*) of sense and motion for the rest of the members, offering as proof the assertion that all the nerves are physically connected with the brain and spinal cord, not with the heart, and that blocking the nerves that lead to any particular part of the body leads to a loss of sense and motion in that part.[128]

In a later chapter, Turisanus treated at some length the by then standard question of the origin of the nerves.[129] He began by expounding with approval Aristotle's theory that the function of the brain is to cool and thus to regulate the flow of heat from the heart, but continued, "this much being conceded to him [Aristotle], his statement that it [the brain] is in no way the principle of sense is not conceded."[130] He then devoted two folios to a systematic demonstration of the dependence of the nervous system on the brain and a refutation of its dependence on the heart. Among his arguments were that the "common sense" (a separate faculty that organizes the messages received from the five external senses), on account of the versatility of its operations, requires a soft and flexible organ, namely the brain; that cool, subtle, and pure blood, by Aristotle's own account, fosters greater sensibility, intelligence, and prudence; and it is obvious that the blood around the brain is more subtle, purer, and colder than elsewhere in the body; that the heart, being fleshy, contains nerves responsive to touch, and it cannot simultaneously be an organ of a particular sense and of the common sense (if so, one would be able to perceive sweetness and whiteness by touch, which is impossible); and

---

Book 3 in the manuscript cover the same topics as 3.9-15 in Kühn, although the breaks between chapters seem to occur at different places. On fol. 62v, in part of his 3.3 corresponding to 3.8 in Kühn, Bartolomeo briefly set forth the "opinio Platonis" regarding the location of the various divisions of the soul in brain, heart, and liver as an explanation for Galen's position regarding the function of these organs. There appears to be no reference to Aristotle's views in this passage.

[128] Turisanus, *Plusquam*, fol. 28v.   [129] Ibid., fols. 34v-35r.

[130] "Sed hoc ei concesso non conceditur ei quod dicit ipsum non esse aliquo modo principium sensus," ibid., fol. 34v.

that the nerves, with their specialized sensory and motor functions, do not all ramify from a single nerve center, but, he reiterated, are all physically linked to the brain and spinal cord. In defense of Galen and of the control of brain and spinal cord over the nervous system, Turisanus was prepared to oppose not only Aristotle, but also Avicenna, the "prince" of physicians. Of a remark "in contradiction to Galen" supposedly made by Avicenna in his *De animalibus*, to the effect that the first principle and the instrument of a virtue necessarily emanate from the same place, Turisanus observed that this is true of the arteries, which serve merely as channels for *spiritus*, but not of the nerves, which are not just vehicles for sense and motion, but actually the source. He concluded his discussion with the announcement, "We are not in any doubt whatsoever that the brain has some kind of domination over sense and motion."[131]

In setting forth Galen's principles on the brain's function, Turisanus made repeated reference to Galen's authority, but cited none of his works by title. Since he did provide the titles of philosophical works by Aristotle and Avicenna, this perhaps suggests that he, unlike Taddeo and Bartolomeo, still derived his own knowledge of Galen's views from brief introductory works and from Avicenna, rather than from studying any of Galen's longer works.

The subject of conception seems to have been less controversial among Taddeo and his students than that of the nervous system. On the whole, Aristotle's views were accepted without demur; Taddeo, Turisanus, and Dino differed only in the extent to which they were prepared to explain away Galen's views as the result of semantic confusion rather than to reject them out of hand. In part, again, this attitude was no doubt a reflection of the state of the sources. Aristotle treated mammalian (and specifically human) reproduction exhaustively and at length, not only in *De generatione animalium* but also in Books 6 and 7 of the *Historia animalium*. The chief available medical discussions of the subject, if we judge by the citations provided by Taddeo, Turisanus, and Dino, seem to have been the brief *De natura fetus* (*De natura pueri*) ascribed to Hippocrates; a work of Constantinus Africanus (*De coitu*); sections of the *Canon* of Avicenna; and, in the case of Dino alone, the *Colliget* of Averroes (after its translation in the 1280s).[132]

---

[131] "nullo modo dubitamus cerebrum habere aliquem principatum super sensum et motum," ibid., fol. 35v.

[132] *Canon* 1.1.5.1 (Venice, 1507, repr. Hildesheim, 1964), fol. 8r; *Colliget* 2.10 (Venice,

Both Avicenna and Averroes reported the conflict between Aristotle and Galen over generation, although Averroes proffered the advice—certainly ignored in Taddeo's circle and by other western physicians—that it is not necessary to discuss these differences in works on medicine (as distinct from natural philosophy). In addition to his authentic *De semine*, or *De spermate*, translated into Latin by Niccolò da Reggio (active from about 1308), Galen was the supposed author of another *De spermate*, a translation of which, existing in a number of manuscripts, is sometimes attributed to Constantinus Africanus.[133] Neither of these works, however, seems to have been relied upon by the members of Taddeo's school. No such title is included in the list of thirty-nine works of Galen compiled by Bartolomeo da Varignana (see Appendix Two) or in the collection of Galenic treatises in which Taddeo's version of *De interioribus* is to be found. Furthermore, Dino del Garbo expressed his dissatisfaction with the existing state of knowledge of Galen's authentic teaching on reproduction as follows: "Avicenna in Book 9 of *De animalibus* said that he [Galen] thought he knew a lot about the branches of natural science, but in reality knew nothing; but by God he knew more than Avicenna. For we do not have Galen's treatise *De spermate*, and so the one attributed to him is taken for his, [which is] like [a work] of Brunellus [the ass], and Avicenna attributed many things to him that I do not think he said."[134] Taddeo also cited Galen's opinion via Avicenna, while noting that Avicenna strongly reprehended it.[135]

There may be reasons other than a lack of authentic Galenic texts that

---

1531), fols. 24v-26 (misprint for 25)r. On the sources and development of medieval views on conception, see M. Anthony Hewson, *Giles of Rome and the Medieval Theory of Conception*. Neither Taddeo in the *Isagoge*, nor Turisanus, nor Dino in his commentary on the Hippocratic *De natura fetus* referred by name, however, to the *De formatione humani corporis* of Giles of Rome. Some discussion of medieval conception theory is also contained in Vern L. Bullough, "Medieval Medical and Scientific Views of Women," *Viator: Medieval and Renaissance Studies* 4 (1973):485-501.

[133] Durling, "Corrigenda and Addenda to Diels' Galenica," p. 472; V. Tavone Passalacqua, ed., *Microtegni seu de spermate, Traduzione e commento . . . Istituto di Storia della Medicina dell'Università di Roma* (Corpus Scriptorum Medicorum infimae latinitatis et prioris Medii Aevi, Rome, 1958).

[134] "Et hec est ratio in qua se fundavit Galenus, ut dicit Avicenna 9° de animalibus, 'qui putavit se multum scire de ramis scientie naturalis et nihil scivit,' sed per deum ipse plus scivit quam Avicennam, quia libellum Galeni de spermate non habemus, et ita ille qui ei imponitur est suus, sicut Brunelli, et multa imponit sibi Avicenna que non credo quod dixerit," Dino, *De natura fetus*, fol. 49r.

[135] Taddeo, *Isagoge*, fol. 357v.

explain why Aristotle's teaching on conception was received more uncritically than his theory of the nervous system. Since Galen's understanding of the relationship of brain, spinal cord, and nerves was in fact
superior to Aristotle's, it seems likely that the practical experience of physicians (for example, with patients suffering from injuries resulting in
partial paralysis) would, from time to time, confirm some of Galen's
views. But as far as conception was concerned, neither Aristotle, nor
Galen, nor their medieval successors knew of the existence of spermato-
zoa, ova, or chromosomes. The only way to choose between Aristotle,
who restricted the active formative role in generation to the male, and
Galen, who believed that both parents emit generative semen, was to
reason and to consult philosophy. And reason and philosophy, not to
mention the manifold experiences of daily life, naturally tended, in the
Middle Ages as in antiquity, to support a scientific view that gave the
female a secondary and passive role. Galen's case for an active role in
conception essentially rested on the capacity of offspring to acquire hereditary characteristics from the mother as well as from the father, and on
his belief that vaginal secretions during intercourse constitute the emission of generative female sperm. The latter contention was easily disposed
of by the correct observation that such secretions are not indispensable to
impregnation; the former failed to stand alone against the accumulated
weight of philosophical counterargument.

Thus, when Taddeo, Turisanus, and Dino each in turn considered the
questions "whether females emit sperm" and "whether the sperm of a
woman has active, generative power," they reached somewhat similar
conclusions.[186] Taddeo, rather confusedly and hesitantly, followed Avicenna in identifying female sperm with vaginal secretions and in stating
that although they possess heat and spirit, these do not have active generative power. Among the standard arguments Taddeo used against the possibility of generative female sperm was the one that if woman were both
to have active generative power and also, as Aristotle said, to provide the
matter of conception, there would be no reason why parthenogenesis
should not take place. But the reading he gave to statements by Constantinus and Avicenna led Taddeo simultaneously to accept the idea that the

---

[186] Ibid., fols. 357r-358r; Turisanus, *Plusquam*, fols. 58v-59r; Dino, *De natura fetus*,
fols. 46v-47v. The titles of the questions as given in Dino's treatise are "Utrum mulier
habeat sperma" and "Utrum in spermate mulieris sit aliqua virtus activa in generatione
fetus."

so-called female sperm plays some kind of secondary role in conception, although he admitted it is difficult to determine what this might be, since Aristotle assigned to retained menstrual blood the function of providing the matter for conception and nutriment for the fetus. Taddeo suggested that female sperm might constitute a kind of prime matter (*prima materia*) of the fetus "before the menstrual blood is drawn to the womb," the menstrual blood subsequently providing for fetal nourishment and growth.[137] He concluded with a flourish of argumentation in which his contradictory sources are not so much reconciled as thoroughly muddled:

> But it is better to say that woman has sperm, but not really; because her sperm adds little to the menstrual nature, as Avicenna says in 3, and Aristotle in 18 [*De animalibus*][138] says that the first matter is of the menstrual nature, hence when Aristotle denies that this female sperm plays a part in conception, he says this about the nature of the sperm, as if he were to say that female sperm is of no account where there is real sperm, but only insofar as it is menstrual in nature; and yet it should be noted that this female sperm, although it is menstrual in nature, yet adds to the menstrual blood something . . . proceeding from further decoction than that possessed by the menstrual blood, and on account of this decoction it constitutes the prime matter of the spermatic members;[139] while the menstrual blood is the matter of nourishment; and thus this solution, along with what was said before, solves the question completely.[140]

[137] "antequam sanguis menstruus adducatur ad matricem," Taddeo, *Isagoge*, fol. 358r.

[138] Apparently *De generatione animalium* 2.4, 738b5-27; if so, this numbering indicates that Taddeo was using the translation of the works on animals by William of Moerbeke, from the Greek, rather than the older Arabo-Latin version of Michael Scot. But at least one manuscript, NLM, MS 492, 1, fol. 67v, gives "xv°" in place of "xviii" found in the 1527 edition.

[139] Decoction was the supposed process whereby nourishment was progressively refined, first to blood and then to sperm; the spermatic members were the bones, sinews, and other parts whitish in color and hard in texture.

[140] Aut dic [*sic*] melius quod mulier habet sperma sed non verum: quia eius sperma parum addit super naturam menstruam . . . unde quando negat Aristotelis ipsum sperma mulieris ingredi generationem dicit hoc in natura spermatis quasi dicat sperma mulieris non competit ubi sit verum sperma sed in quantum in eo est natura menstrui, et tamen nota quod istud mulieris sperma licet sit de natura menstrui tamen addit super menstrua, scilicet albedinem quam fecit et delectationem [*sic*: delactationem?] que procedit ex aliqua decoctione maiori quam sanguis menstruus habeat et ob hanc . . . fit materia prima membrorum . . . et sic hec solutio cum priori solvet complete," Taddeo, *Isagoge*, fol. 358r.

The rather better-organized discussion by Turisanus touched on many of the same points. As usual, Turisanus showed a greater readiness than Taddeo to make a clear choice from among his authorities and, unlike his master, had no hesitation in repudiating the views of Aristotle, as well as those of Galen, when occasion demanded. Turisanus asserted, contrary to Aristotle, that the "principle of generation in the male seems to reside in" the testicles (which Aristotle had believed merely to retard excessively rapid discharge of semen, comparing them to weights hung on a loom to balance it).[141] Nonetheless, the picture Turisanus presented of conception itself was wholly Aristotelian. "Generative virtue" (*virtus generativa*) he held to inhere in both sexes, but more strongly in the male; if male and female sperm were equal in dignity, this would imply that the female role in conception is more important than that of the male, since conception takes place in the womb, a female organ—an obviously impossible proposition, since female nature is by definition colder and more imperfect than male nature. Turisanus went on to give his readers a succinct exposition of the Aristotelian theory of the roles of semen and menstrual fluid: menstrual fluid in the female is the equivalent of sperm in the male, but, since the female is weaker and colder, the female secretion is less digested (or concocted) than that of the male, and consequently more abundant and red rather than white in color. The equivalence of sperm and menstrual fluid Turisanus proved by the "facts" that the emission of both starts and stops at about the same age in men and women, that women have increased sexual appetite during menstruation, and that at this time their eyes are disturbed, the eyes obviously being affected by venereal excess. The last proof is presumably a reference to the belief, widely held in the Middle Ages, that the gaze of a menstruating woman will cloud a mirror. But, Turisanus continued, if menstrual fluid is the female equivalent of the male emission, then evidently women can produce no other spermatic fluid. Moreover, if vaginal secretions at the time of intercourse contribute to the matter of the fetus, they must be drawn inward to the womb, rather than discharged outward; yet to suppose that the same secretion is first discharged and then drawn back is to abandon the principle that nature does nothing in vain. Thus the vaginal secretions are not sperm, contribute nothing to the matter of the fetus, and are not even to be found in all women. Therefore, although Galen

---

[141] *De generatione animalium* 1.4, 717a13-717b14.

claimed that the male and the female sperm are each both efficient and
material causes of the fetus, and that from their mixture are made bones,
cartilage, and other so-called *membra radicalia* (or *spermatica*), whereas
only flesh and fat are made from menstrual blood, it is preferable to
follow Aristotle in believing that the female contributes only passive
matter to conception and that menstrual blood is the sole source both
of the matter and of the nourishment of the fetus.

Dino del Garbo may be regarded as having a more specialized interest
in the subject of generation than either Taddeo or Turisanus, since he
was the author of an entire work on the subject, namely, his commentary on the *De natura fetus* ascribed to Hippocrates.[142] This interest does
not appear to have been the fruit of any kind of specialization in his practice. If anything, his discussion of the differences between Aristotle and
Galen on the female role in conception is more philosophical, scholastic,
and abstract than that of either Taddeo or Turisanus. Dino treated the
discrepancy between Aristotle and Galen as essentially semantic, pointing
out that "sperm" can be understood in two ways: either as any white,
viscous fluid emitted with pulsation and pleasure, or as the fluid that
causes generation. Thus, according to Dino, women secrete sperm in the
broader of the two senses, but their so-called sperm is not necessary to
generation. Dino joined Turisanus, though in more philosophical language, in denying that female sperm, understood in the sense of vaginal
secretions, is either an active or a passive (material) ingredient in conception. An important purpose of vaginal secretions, in Dino's opinion, is to

[142] This work was printed in Venice in 1502 as part of a collection of treatises on
embryology (see note 68, above), which also includes, at fols. 17v-32v, a commentary on
Avicenna, "De generatione embrionis" (that is, *Canon* 3.21.1), ascribed to Dino and accepted as his by Hewson (*Giles of Rome*, pp. 201-233). I have based my own discussion of
Dino's ideas about conception solely on his commentary on *De natura fetus*, because the
attribution to Dino of the commentary on "De generatione embrionis" seems to me, as it
did to the sixteenth-century editor of the text, uncertain. Dino is referred to by name
as an authority a number of times in the work and is also disagreed with therein (fol.
19v): "Hanc rationem conatur solvere dinus dicens quod agentia universalia sunt duorum
modorum. . . . Ista solutio non valet"; furthermore, the author identified himself as a
pupil of Gentile da Foligno ("Gentilis de fulgineo doctor meus," fol. 19v); it is highly
improbable that Dino, who died in 1327, studied under Gentile, whose earliest recorded
teaching was in 1322 and who died in 1348 (see note 4 to the Introduction). The only
other member of the group of authors now under discussion to produce an entire work on
conception was Mondino de' Liuzzi, who wrote an exposition of Avicenna, "De generatione embrionis," contained in BAV, MS Reg. lat. 2000, fols. 1-23v. According to the
explicit, the *reportator* was Mondino's pupil Bertruccio, and the work is dated 1318. It is
not the same as the commentary on the same text ascribed to Dino.

aid in lubrication and to enhance pleasure (one of his very few remarks that does not echo themes developed by Taddeo, Turisanus, and doubtless other authors). The only sense in which women can be said to have sperm that is necessary to generation is if the decocted menstrual blood, which participates in the material formation of the fetus in the womb, is described as sperm with passive, not active, virtue. It is impossible for active virtue to be present in either the menstrual blood, decocted or undecocted, or the vaginal secretions. Dino bolstered his conclusion with the usual arguments about parthenogenesis and the need for generative sperm to be drawn inward to the womb. From the *Colliget* of Averroes Dino claimed to have derived an elaborate disproof of the possibility that the female might have active generative virtue and still need to mix her sperm with that of the male for generation to occur. Dino, like Taddeo and others, explained away resemblances of offspring to their mother with the cliché that this is due to weakness on the part of the paternal sperm, which is in certain cases unable to overcome the mother's disposition.

The reconciliation of philosophers and physicians was a task that seemed urgent to Taddeo and his associates, as it did to their contemporary, Peter of Abano. Their imperative appears reasonable when rephrased as an insistence that medical teaching cannot ignore or flout either the basic principles of physical science as currently understood, or the work of the best biologist known. The physicians of Taddeo's day could have ignored Aristotelian natural philosophy only at the risk of taking medicine out of the mainstream of learned scientific activity. The foregoing account has demonstrated that Taddeo and his colleagues responded in several intelligent ways to the challenge that the influx of Aristotelianism into western scientific thought presented to medicine: the most consistently and determinedly Aristotelian member of the group was Taddeo himself, possibly followed in the next generation by Dino; among Taddeo's pupils and younger successors Turisanus, Mondino, and perhaps Bartolomeo were ready to range themselves against the Philosopher on issues of some importance. Obviously, insofar as these and other medical masters attempted reconciliation of authorities without reference to external criteria, their efforts were doomed to fruitlessness; yet by such efforts Turisanus, Mondino, and perhaps some of their colleagues learned that contradictions between respected authorities had to be confronted and could not be explained away. Even though, unlike certain Italian physicians who flourished later in the fourteenth century,[143] Taddeo and his associates produced relatively few independent contributions of any significance to current logical and philosophical debate or to general scientific activity, their achievements in making use of natural philosophy should not be minimized. They based their medical learning firmly upon contemporary philosophy and science and were remarkably adept in applying specific parts of those disciplines to medical theory; they fostered the study of Galen, perhaps as a conscious response to the prevailing Aristotelianism; and they retained and developed independence of judgment in choosing among conflicting authorities.

[143] For example, the clockmakers Jacopo and Giovanni Dondi, or Jacopo da Forlì, who wrote at length about the intension and remission of forms, to choose only two instances of practical and theoretical accomplishment.

CHAPTER SEVEN

MIND AND SENSE

Rather than attempting a survey of every aspect of the medical and physiological science of Taddeo and his fellow physicians—an undertaking that would strain the patience of the reader to its limits and expand the size of this volume far beyond the practicable—it seems preferable to take a closer look at their teaching in a single area. Several aspects of their thought on the structure, functioning, and disorders of the mind, and on its interaction with the body, suggest the mind and senses as suitable topics.

The relationship of mind and body, of perennial concern to all physicians, was a subject to which Taddeo and some of his associates gave a good deal of attention. In particular, problems of psychology (in the sense of the structure and functioning of mind) and of sense perception absorbed Taddeo himself and, to a somewhat lesser extent, Turisanus. Although their interest may have been unusually strong, it was not in itself idiosyncratic. Discussion of such subjects as cognition, the way in which the soul and its powers or "virtues" cooperate in bodily processes, the physical effects produced by the emotions, the organization of the senses, and the process of vision was part of an already time-honored tradition among natural philosophers, theologians, and physicians.[1] But the interest of Taddeo and the others in these and related subjects was by no means wholly philosophical and analytical: these heirs of Hippocrates were well aware of the role of the mind in causing physical disease, in treating it, and in establishing a satisfactory regimen for health; and, as will become evident, their practice included both the diagnosis and the treatment of the afflictions of the mind, as well as the identification of external stimuli for those afflictions. From passages in their writings pertaining to mind, sense perception, and emotion we can learn both how they analyzed consciousness and the role they assigned to psychology and

---

[1] For a general account of the treatment of psychology by medieval theologians, see O. Lottin, *Psychologie et morale au XII* *et XIII* *siècles*, vol. 1, *Problèmes de psychologie*. Regarding the internal and external senses, vision, and the passions among natural philosophers and physicians, see notes 16 and 21, below.

to the treatment of mental conditions in medical practice.[2] The same passages may perhaps yield a glimpse of how human nature itself was understood among a group of learned, professional men at the dawn of Italy's humanist age.

Before turning to the medical works of Taddeo and his colleagues, we may note an extended discussion of some of these topics by the only one among Taddeo's pupils who appears not to have become a physician, namely, the philosopher Gentile da Cingoli. Gentile's question "whether a sensible or intelligible species has the virtue of altering a body toward heat or cold" is, indeed, a striking example of the way in which the concerns of philosophers and physicians overlapped. It is a discussion of Galen's statement, made in his (Galen's) commentary on the *Prognostica* of Hippocrates, to the effect that a physician is more likely to effect successful cures when his patients have confidence in him; in his comments, Gentile assumed that he was dealing with a physiological phenomenon, for which he attempted to find an explanation consonant with natural philosophy. Both subject matter and procedure recall many similar endeavors of Taddeo, Turisanus, and Dino.

As far as Gentile (following Galen) was concerned, disease is equivalent to a disturbance in the body's *complexio*, that is, in its balance of the elemental qualities of hot, cold, wet, and dry; cure is effected by a restoration of the *complexio* to normal, that is, by another shift in the balance of qualities. If confidence in the physician produces or aids a cure, this must mean that confidence, a nonmaterial trace (*species*) left in the senses or intellect as a result of the impression made by the physician on the senses, or the intellect's interpretation of that impression, is capable of affecting the matter of the body by changing its complexion. Not only was this supposition apparently incompatible with Aristotelian ideas about motion and change in matter; it also gave rise to the objection that plainly not all "species of sensibles" have any such property, since the perception of sound and tastes, for example, does not alter the body.[3]

---

[2] A fairly large body of medical literature was available that dealt with the analysis of personality in complexional and regional terms, with the physiology of the brain, and with mental disease. In addition to sections in the medical encyclopedias of Haly Abbas and Avicenna that summarize the antique tradition, mention may specially be made of Hippocrates, *Airs Waters Places*, and Constantinus Africanus, *Liber de oblivione*. The thirteenth-century encyclopedias of Bartholomeus Anglicus and Vincent of Beauvais also included sections touching on some or all of these topics.

[3] "Questio magistri Gentilis de Cingulo. Questio est utrum species sensibilis vel intelli-

The elucidation of this problem led Gentile into a long discourse on the physical mechanism by which the mind and sense can affect the body. He further extended the discussion to provide similar explanations of various examples of the effect of mind on a remote body and vice versa, and of the effect of one body on another without apparent physical contact. Gentile considered the evil eye to be an example of the first category, the influence of the heavenly bodies on the human mind an example of the second, and the power of the glance of a menstruating woman to cloud a mirror an example of the third. He was mainly concerned to fit these supposed phenomena into the framework of Aristotelian physics, which denied action at a distance and required that every motion involve a mover. Gentile pointed out that the Philosopher had himself asserted in *De motibus animalium* that fantasy and intelligence have "the virtue of things: and hence of producing alteration in bodies"; moreover, Gentile continued, the power of sensible or intelligible species to heat or chill the human body is a matter of common, nay universal, experience, since the mechanism that produces emotional change in man is, in fact, an alteration of the balance of heat and cold in the body. Thus, he pointed out, anger is nothing but a certain rising of blood around the heart, and this rising is caused by heat; similarly, what we call joy is a diffusion of heat throughout the body. Gentile went on to explain, in a passage closely paralleling the explanation of emotions provided by Turisanus in his commentary on the *Tegni*, that other emotions, such as fear, are con-

gibilis habet virtutem alterandi corpus ad caliditatem vel frigiditatem, quia Galenus vult circa principium libri pronosticorum, quod ille medicus plures sanat . . . ," edited in Grabmann, "Gentile da Cingoli," pp. 68-88. ". . . multe sunt species aliorum sensibilium, que non habent virtutem alterandi ut sunt species sonorum, saporum et sic de aliis. . . . Preterea si species habet virtutem alterandi aut hoc habet facere, quia sit talis formaliter aut quia sit talis effective. Non formaliter, cum actu non sit calida neque effective, quia omnis actio fit per contactum. . . . Preterea movens et motum oportet esse distinctum loco et subiecto. Sed species sensibilis est unum subiecto faciens cum sensitivo. Ergo non habet ipsum movere. . . . Preterea omne quod movet aliud movetur. Si igitur species [movet] corpus, ipsa movetur. Sed ipsa non potest moveri cum non sit corpus," idem, "Gentile da Cingoli," pp. 68-70. Gentile's answer to the last point was, startlingly, "Ad aliud, cum dicitur: Omne quod movet aliquid movetur, dico, quod falsum est," idem, "Gentile da Cingoli," p. 87. Gentile accepted that it is the *species* of objects that impresses itself upon the senses and that the *species* is separate from the form of a perceived object (p. 74), although the opposite view was later strongly defended by some learned physicians, including Dino's son Tommaso del Garbo; see Edward G. Smith, "A Disagreement on the Need of a Sensible Species in the Writings of Some Medical Doctors in the Late Middle Ages" (Ph.D. diss., St. Louis Univ., 1974).

nected with cold. And since the mere apprehension of something causing delight or sorrow is enough to produce emotional change, it is clear that this apprehension itself changes the balance of heat and cold in the body.

Having established that the body is altered by impressions (*species*) existing in the sense or intellect, it remained for Gentile to expound just how this alteration takes place. This feat he accomplished to his own satisfaction by pointing out that anything generated retains some of the virtues by which it was generated (as shown by the astrologers' assertion that men conceived under a malevolent sign are malevolent and by the teaching of magicians that images made under a certain constellation retain the virtues of that constellation—examples adduced by Gentile without hesitation or apology), and that this principle applies in the generation of matter, in the compounding of mixtures from simple or composite ingredients, and in nourishment.[4] Thus, for example, something of the virtue of milk remains in anything nourished by it. It is, furthermore, axiomatic that all qualities perceptible by sense—color, taste, odor—are generated from a mixture of the primary sensible qualities, namely, heat, cold, humidity, and dryness. Hence, any impression made on the senses must retain and convey something of the primary qualities to the *sensus communis* and, at second remove, to the intellect, whence, in turn, something of those qualities is transmitted to the body. In discussing the powers of sense, Gentile showed himself a convinced Aristotelian, stressing the primacy of the heart with the remark that one should say not that the eye sees and the ear hears, but rather that the heart sees by means of the eye and hears by means of the ear; he made no mention of Galen's views on the role of the brain.

The explanation of the beneficial physical effects of confidence in one's doctor is now clear: the confident patient imagines he is getting better; the primary sensible qualities play a part in creating the mental image (*deserviant imaginem*), and the image acquires the power to improve the balance of the qualities in the body. For the effect of the glance of a

---

[4] "omne quod generatur ab aliquo per se et non secundum accidens, retinet aliquo modo virtutem illius. . . . Iterum hoc potest declarari in hiis, que fiunt in arte astrologie. Volunt enim Astrologi, quod illi, qui generantur sub signo benivolo [*sic*], sunt benivoli et qui generantur sub malivolo sunt malivoli. Iterum secundum intentionem magycorum hoc habet veritatem. Volunt enim, quod in ymaginibus quibusdam, que fiunt sub aliqua determinata constellatione. In illis enim remanet secundum ipsos virtus constellationis, sub qua fiunt et ex hoc contingit, quod ille ymagines habent eandem operationem sicut constellationes sub quibus fiunt," Grabmann, "Gentile da Cingoli," pp. 72-73.

menstruating woman, Gentile rejected as un-Aristotelian Avicenna's suggestion that the virtue of the soul can, by imagination, act at a distance without any medium. Gentile instead maintained that the menses are distributed throughout a woman's body, including her eyes; the eyes, however, are provided with subtle veins (*pleni venarum subtilium*) through which some of the finer parts of the menses seep out and infect the air around the eyes, thus causing the appearance of a bloody mass in the mirror. Gentile's explanation, although more elaborate, is identical with that given by Taddeo in his commentary on the *Isagoge*,[5] and it is derived from Aristotle's own.[6] But Gentile held, in addition, not only that the menses can in certain cases exude imperceptibly from the pores of the entire body, but also that other harmful substances can similarly exude. The notion that the glance of a sick person can transmit disease by exuding harmful matter from the eyes was a variant of the Galenic idea that communicable diseases spread through corruption of the air. In the case of the damaging glance, what was postulated was, in effect, a localized corruption of the air. The idea explained an apparent action at a distance in the (really bacterial or viral) transmission of disease from one person to another.[7] In Gentile's words: "And through this means, certain diseases that exist in one person [*uno*—thus indicating that he conceived of other agents of infection besides menses] infect another."[8] Gentile similarly believed that one's bad intentions toward an enemy can physically infect the surrounding air and hence inflict bodily damage. This he held to be particularly likely when old women, being very cold and dry in complexion and much given to imagination, cast their evil eye (*fascinatio*) upon impressionable and weak-complexioned children.

[5] Taddeo, *Isagoge*, fol. 363r.

[6] See *De somniis* 459b27-460a26. On this belief, mentioned by both Aristotle and Pliny, see further Marshall Clagett, ed., *Nicole Oresme and the Medieval Geometry of Qualities and Motions* (Madison, Milwaukee, and London, 1968), pp. 457-458. I owe this reference to Professor Bert Hansen.

[7] Corruption of the air is heavily emphasized in the contemporary medical accounts of the immediate causes of bubonic and pneumonic plague in the middle and later fourteenth century, which are summarized in Anna M. Campbell, *The Black Death and Men of Learning* (New York, 1931), pp. 48-56. Campbell also provides several examples of fourteenth-century medical writers who more or less tacitly accepted the notion of infection or contagion from person to person along with that of corruption of the air, and quotes an anonymous plague tractate from Montpellier to the effect that *spiritus* streaming from the eyes of the sick infects those about them (pp. 60-61).

[8] "Et per huncmodum quedam egritudines existentes in uno inficiunt alium," Gentile da Cingoli, *Questio*, in Grabmann, "Gentile da Cingoli," p. 80.

In discussing the ways in which the stars can affect man, Gentile found himself obliged to counter the objection that the human soul is nobler than the stars and therefore cannot be influenced by them. While admitting the truth of the proposition that the soul is nobler than the stars, he asserted that the stars undoubtedly affect bodies here below; in human beings, therefore, since the mind is involved with the body, the heavenly bodies greatly affect the mind *per accidens*.

The complex ramifications of Gentile's speculations about the effects of a patient's confidence in his physician may be contrasted to Mondino de' Liuzzi's pragmatic treatment of the same subject.[9] Mondino, like Gentile, believed that confidence aids cure; but, unlike Gentile, he denied that this takes place through any physical alteration of the body brought about directly or indirectly by the emotion of trust. Instead, he offered the relatively simple suggestion that patients like the remedies prescribed by a doctor in whom they have faith and follow his orders more closely, and that this positive attitude makes it easier for nature to play its part in working a cure.[10] Mondino's opinion may seem to have the ring of medical experience—whether one relates his remarks, in modern terms, to the effectiveness of a placebo or to psychotherapy—whereas Gentile's contribution remains embedded in the vocabulary of medieval speculative philosophy. But, as we have already indicated, it would be unwise to generalize about the different approaches of a philosopher like Gentile and a learned physician like Mondino from this instance. In fact, little distinguishes Gentile's treatment of problems about the interaction of mind and body from the handling of similar subjects by Taddeo himself or by several of the physicians who were Gentile's fellow students under Taddeo. Indeed, although the edition of Gentile's question about the effect of

---

[9] Mondino, comm. *Pronost.*, BAV, MS Vat. lat. 4466, fol. 2r: "utrum confidentia infirmi de medico sit causa sanitatis."

[10] "Dico ad hoc quod confidentia infirmi de medico est causam [*sic*] sanitatis dupliciter; potest intelligi uno modo principaliter et immediate, alio modo mediate et ex consequenti. primo modo non est causa sanitatis, et causa huius est quod dicta est iam, quod non alterat corpus nec est contrarium egritudinis non est causa sanitatis . . . Si autem intelligatur 2° modo, dico quod confidentia est causa et huius ratio est duplex. prima est scilicet id est quodam modo causa sanitatis quod facit ad hoc quod medicine exhibite infirmo et universaliter instrumenta medici melius regularentur a calore naturali et a natura, sed hoc facit confidentia . . . confidentia est causa quod infirmus se probat medico secundum quod oportet et ideo facit omnia quod dicit medicus, et accipit farmaciam cum delectitudine magis. medicine autem accepte cum delectitudine magis, magis regulantur a natura et virtute sicut etiam cibi cum delectatione accepti melius operantur," ibid.

mental impressions upon the body was based upon a manuscript copy found among a collection of theological and philosophical treatises, another, anonymous, version of the same text appears in a collection of medical treatises. In the latter version of Gentile's work, presumably in order to stress its medical significance, the opening sentence about intelligible species has been omitted so that the question begins: "Because at the beginning of his commentary on the *Prognostica* Galen expressed the opinion that the physician cures more patients. . . ."[11] In this manuscript, Gentile's question follows Taddeo's commentary on Avicenna's chapter on things eaten and drunk, a juxtaposition that is perfectly appropriate, since, as we have seen, Taddeo treated, in philosophical terms, the effect of other bodies (namely, ingested food and medicine) on the animal body. The single most striking difference between Gentile's production and those of contemporary learned physicians trained in the same school is his omission of any reference or allusion to Galen's ideas about the role of the brain in sensation, an omission no physician would have been likely to make. But, as will become apparent, the relationship of mind, sense, and body was an area of investigation that brought philosophy and medicine very close. The philosopher Gentile's exposition of a problem that, after all, relates primarily to medical practice—since it has to do with the interaction of doctor and patient—is an excellent example of that closeness.

Of the physicians under consideration, Taddeo and, later, Turisanus wrote most extensively on the nature of the mind. Taddeo incorporated a lengthy discussion of the subject into a chapter concerning the virtues of the soul in his commentary on the *Isagoge*.[12] The virtues of the soul are, according to his definition, "the power[s] of the soul whereby the soul carries out its actions"; he explicitly equated *virtus* and *potentia* and stated that "the soul is the substance in which the virtues are rooted."[13] As we have seen, Taddeo divided the virtues of the soul into *virtus vitalis*, or *spiritualis*, proceeding from the heart; *virtus naturalis*, associated with

---

[11] BAV, MS Palat. lat. 1246, fols. 97v-112v, inc. "Quia Galenus vult circa principium libri pronosticorum quod ille medicus plures sanat. . . ." The remaining contents of this codex include, besides Taddeo's commentary on Avicenna, a lengthy anonymous commentary and *dubia* on Avicenna's chapter on the formation of the embryo.

[12] Taddeo, *Isagoge*, fols. 354v-366v.

[13] "dicitur virtus pro potentia anime qua anima agit suas actiones: et hoc modo accipitur virtus in hoc capitulo," ibid., fol. 354v; also "bene vocatur virtus potentia" and "anima est substantia in qua radicuntur virtutes," ibid.

the organs and processes of growth, nutrition, excretion, and reproduction; and *virtus animalis*. Despite his Aristotelian insistence on the ultimate primacy of the heart over the nervous system, Taddeo denied any association of *virtus vitalis* with the sensitive faculties of soul.[14] He therefore placed both sensation and cognition under *virtus animalis* and, in this passage, discussed cognition and the reception of sense impressions as located in the brain.

Taddeo went to some pains to assemble a satisfactory definition of *virtus animalis*. He insisted that it was so called because it distinguished animals from plants; he explicitly excluded from his argument the concept of virtue of the soul "in the sense that the word soul is accepted among philosophers but not by physicians." He dismissed as inadequate the statements of various authors who defined *virtus animalis* as consisting of "all virtues over and above the natural" (including *virtus vitalis*); or as the source of motion and sense (but not cognition); or as the source of cognition (but not motion and sense). He was also critical of Avicenna's definition on the grounds that it did not include intellectual activity among the functions of *virtus animalis*. His own formulation, which, he stressed, "is not given by any author that I know of"—but which he had put together from several—was that *virtus animalis* is the power producing voluntary motion, sense perception, and intellect.[15]

Cognition and sense perception Taddeo described as the products of an aspect of *virtus animalis* termed *virtus apprehensiva*, and this in turn he

[14] "videtur quod virtus vitalis non possit comprehendi sub aliqua istarum 3 potentiarum anime . . . neque sub anima sensibili, nam sensibilis anima aut apprehendit aut movet voluntarie, sed ista virtus non apprehendit neque movet voluntarie. ergo non est sensibilis." Ibid., fol. 359r.

[15] "dico quod hoc vocabulum, scilicet, virtus animalis accipitur in 4 modis. nam uno modo comprehendit in se omnes virtutes que sunt in anima. est enim dicere virtus animalis idest virtus anime secundum quod anima accipitur apud philosophos et non prout accipitur apud medicos. . . . dico quod ista virtus diffinitur ab Avicenna tamen illa diffinitio non comprehendit virtutem intellectivam et est talis diffinitio in 6° de naturalibus. virtus animalis est perfectio prima corporis naturalis instrumentalis secundum hoc quod comprehendit particularia [NLM, MS 492, 1, fol. 68v: per ipsam] et movetur voluntarie. et quia hec diffinitio non comprehendit totam istam virtutem, ideo pono aliam collectam ex diversis auctoribus que talis est. virtus animalis perfectio est animalis activa vel passiva, et dicitur hec virtus perfectio animalis, nam ipsa complet animal, et separat ipsum a plantis. Item dicitur potentia activa: quia motiva semper agit et non patitur, et passiva dicitur pro anima apprehensiva sensibili. nam dicit Galenus et Aristotele quod sentire est pati. Item intellectus dicitur agere et pati. agit quidem intellectus agens et patitur materialis. ergo dicitur bene virtus passiva et activa. hec quidem diffinitio non est posita ab aliquo auctore quem ego sciam, sed collegi eam ex dictis eorum," ibid., fols. 359r-v.

divided into interior and exterior, the latter, obviously, being the five
senses. Taddeo adopted a triple division (ultimately based on Aristotle as
interpreted by Galen)[16] of *virtus apprehensiva interior* into *phantasia,
virtus rationalis,* and memory. *Phantasia* he located in the anterior ventricle of the brain, and he stated it to comprise both the *sensus communis*
(which organizes the impressions received from the five senses and conveys them to the other mental faculties) and a power that retains those
impressions (which he termed *virtus formans* or *formativa*). He denied
that the latter power should be termed *imaginativa*,[17] apparently because
he identified *imaginatio* with the faculty termed *intellectus passivus* by
Averroes and thus included it under *virtus rationalis*.[18] The subdivision of
imagination into retentive imagination (Taddeo's *virtus formans*) and
into human, or animal compositive, imagination (which can create new
images based on sense perception or distortions thereof, as opposed to
merely retaining sense impressions); the placing of retentive imagination
with common sense in the anterior ventricle of the brain; and the location
of compositive imagination in the middle ventricle—are all to be found
in the *Canon* of Avicenna, whom Taddeo cited as his source.[19] But Taddeo departed from Avicenna's account in his treatment of the power
termed (by Taddeo, not Avicenna's translator) *virtus rationalis*. While he
distinguished between *ratio* and *intellectus*, Taddeo apparently intended
to include under *virtus rationalis* (which, as we have seen, he regarded
as a subdivision of *virtus animalis*) the entire Aristotelian-Averroist structure of the passive, material, and agent intellects, and the power of speculation as well as that of abstraction.[20]

[16] See Harry A. Wolfson, "The Internal Senses in Latin, Arabic, and Hebrew Philosophical Texts," *Harvard Theological Review* 28 (1935):72-73; also Harvey, *The Inward
Wits*, passim.

[17] "virtus phantastica est virtus que omnia sensu percepta percipit et conservat post
recessum sensus. hec ergo diffinitio complectitur totam phantasiam prout hec ponitur. quod
autem sub phantasia hic posita non concludatur virtus imaginativa sic probatur. dicit Avicenna quod sedes virtutis imaginative est medius cerebri ventriculus, et iste auctor dicit
quod sedes phantasie est forma [NLM, MS 492, 1, fol. 69r: frons]. quare non clauditur
imaginatio sub ea, sed potius sub ratione," Taddeo, *Isagoge*, fol. 359v.

[18] "potest etiam poni quartus intellectus qui vocatur intellectus passivus, et hic est idem
quam imaginatio sicut dicit Averroes," ibid., fol. 360v.

[19] Wolfson, "The Internal Senses," pp. 95-100.

[20] "ratio ab intellectu in hoc differt, quia ratio confert causam cum effectu, et universale
cum particularibus, sed intellectus comprehendit solum causas. . . . dicitur intellectus alius
materialis alius agens et alius adeptus sive speculativus," Taddeo, *Isagoge*, fol. 360r (and
see note 18, above). For Taddeo's insistence that *intellectus* is among the powers of *virtus
animalis*, see note 15, above.

Taddeo's threefold division of the internal faculties was, in a sense, an old fashioned one. Although an essentially similar division into imaginative, cognitive, and memorative powers had been adopted from Galen by John Damascene and Nemesius of Emesa and was still used (along with other schemes of division) by Albertus Magnus,[21] on this subject, as on so many others, the reception of the *libri naturales* of Aristotle and the works of Aristotle's Moslem commentators, especially Avicenna and Averroes, encouraged Latin writers to develop new formulations. Following Avicenna and Averroes, such influential scholastic authors as Albertus Magnus and Thomas Aquinas subdivided and recombined the internal faculties into various fourfold and fivefold schemes of classification.[22] Taddeo was evidently reluctant to abandon the triple classification sanctioned by its Galenic antecedents and by current conceptions of the physiology of the brain, but he nevertheless sought to combine the threefold scheme with some of the more refined definitions of the internal faculties contrived by medieval Latin and Islamic philosophers.

But the most unusual feature of Taddeo's account of the internal faculties is his apparent intention to include human rational activity among the powers of *virtus apprehensiva interior*. Medieval philosophers (Moslem, Jewish, and Christian) debated which, if any, specifically human mental abilities might be included among the internal faculties of the brain, or "internal senses"; but they generally agreed that since these faculties are powers of the sensitive aspect of soul, reason, as such, is not to be numbered among them.[23] Taddeo not only spoke of *virtus rationalis* as a subdivision of *virtus animalis*, but also provided an account of its powers, which included abstraction and speculation, offering only the (heterodox) alternative that the agent intellect might be one in all men and come from outside. Taddeo's description of one of the internal senses as *rationalis*, like his retention of the older, threefold classification, may simply represent the routine preservation of a medical tradition distinct from philosophical tradition, since both Galen and Constantinus Africanus had used similar terminology.[24] But Taddeo's insistence that *virtus*

[21] See Nicholas H. Steneck, "Albert the Great on the Classification and Localization of the Internal Senses," *Isis* 65 (1974):197-198.

[22] Ibid., passim; Wolfson, "The Internal Senses," pp. 114-124.

[23] See (in addition to the cited works of Wolfson, Steneck, and Harvey), Klubertanz, *The Discursive Power*, passim. Klubertanz emphasizes that Thomas Aquinas considered sensitive and estimative faculties in man to be *influenced* by reason.

[24] For example, in *De symptomatis differentiis* (included in the medieval *De accidenti et*

animalis includes intellect, his selection of aspects (but only some aspects) of the account of the internal faculties provided by Avicenna, and his consciousness of the originality of his own definition—all suggest considerable deliberation. It may well be that, despite his adoption of the threefold classification rather than the fourfold division favored by Averroes, Taddeo's general picture of mental processes owes more to Averroes than to any other single source. In passages in both his epitome of the *Parva naturalia* and his long commentary on *De anima*, Averroes had indicated that he took the internal sense often termed "cogitative" to include human thought.[25] Furthermore, as Harry Wolfson pointed out, in the medical *Colliget* (which, however, is not cited by Taddeo in the passage under discussion, and was probably not known to him) Averroes employed a triple, rather than his usual fourfold, division of the internal faculties, and named *ratio* among them.[26] Whether or not Taddeo's views on mind can be described as unambiguously Averroist, they can legitimately be termed radical, not only because of his inclusion of the famous discussion of the unicity of the agent intellect, but also because of his willingness to include man's rational intellectual activity in an exposition of the powers of *virtus animalis*, defined as the characteristic that separates animals from plants.

Although he too adopted a triple division of the internal apprehensive faculties, the account of them given by Turisanus is at once philosophically more conservative and more physiologically and medically oriented than that in Taddeo's commentary on the *Isagoge*.[27] Turisanus held that the correct and authentically Aristotelian (as opposed to the views of Moslem commentators on Aristotle) classification of "the three principal

---

morbo) 3, Galen stated: "Reliqua vero animae functio, quae a principe facultate procedit, in imaginatricem, rationatricem et recordatricem dividitur" (ed. Kühn, 7:56). Regarding the views of Constantinus Africanus and their source, see Judith S. Neaman, *Suggestion of the Devil*, p. 9.

25 Wolfson, "The Internal Senses," pp. 108-109. Klubertanz, however maintains that although Averroes sometimes included human reason when he spoke of cogitative power, this is an infrequent usage and not representative of the general tendency of his thought (*The Discursive Power*, pp. 115-122). Whatever the intentions of Averroes, Taddeo could clearly have found texts in Averroes's works that would support the placing of reason among the powers of *virtus animalis*.

26 Wolfson, "The Internal Senses," pp. 109-110. As noted, the *Colliget* was not translated into Latin until 1285 (see note 58 to chapter six, above); so the Latin version postdates Taddeo's commentary on the *Isagoge*, written between 1277 and 1283.

27 Turisanus, *Plusquam*, fols. 36v-38r.

apprehensive virtues of the brain" is into *virtus imaginativa* (also known as *fantasia* or *virtus informativa*), *virtus cogitativa*, and *virtus memorativa*; he specifically rejected Avicenna's concept of a distinct estimative power.[28] Impressions originally received directly from the senses pass from the common sense to the internal apprehensive faculties, which are able to grasp these impressions without direct contact with the sensed objects. The analogies that sprang to Turisanus's mind as he strove to illuminate this process for his readers were those of a projectile that continues to move after leaving the hand of the thrower and of a fire that heats objects near it.[29] Turisanus was careful to preserve the distinction, which Taddeo had obliterated, between cogitative power and reason: he explained that when Galen said that ready understanding is a sign of rarefied brain tissue (*substantia subtilis cerebri*) he was not talking about the operation of *virtus rationalis*, which has no physical organ, but about the virtue whose task it is to compose and divide the images brought to it by the fantasy from the common sense—this virtue being the *virtus cogitativa* located in the middle ventricle of the brain.[30] He also noted that the internal apprehensive faculties are rightly said to be the ruling ones in an animal, since all animal motion is caused by *appetitus*, which is the

[28] "Sed hec imaginativa seu fantastica secundum arabes movet distinctivam quam princeps [that is, Avicenna, the "prince" of physicians] vocat existimativam. . . . Abiectis ergo in hoc sententiis arabum dicemus secundum Aristotelem quod he sunt tres virtutes alterius modi ab eo quem dicunt . . . ," ibid., fol. 37r.

[29] "virtutes cerebri principales apprehensive sunt in genere tres, scilicet, sensus communis, imaginativa, cogitativa, et rememorativa. . . . Est autem hec passio que est alteratio sensitivorum facta a sensibili similis passioni eorum que projiciuntur. non enim ulterius contangente eo quod primo movuit moventur proiecta: illud enim quod primo movet impulit aerem quemdam: et hic aliud: donec stet violentia: similiter est in omnibus alterationibus, calidum enim ut ignis proximum calefacit: et hoc aliud donec durat violentia calefactionis: ita ergo procedit alteratio facta a sensibus cum enim sensus moventur a sensibilibus movetur alius intus virtute cum suis organis," ibid., fol. 36v.

[30] "in facilis intellectus esse est signum substantie subtilis cerebri: maxime tamen medii ventriculi cui attribuitur hec operatio. et volebat [Galenus] per intellectum non operationem virtutis rationalis que est sine organo ex qua nihil est discernere de cerebri complexione secundum se: sed operationem virtutis quam diximus componere et dividere et conferre. hanc enim quidam intellectum vocaverunt. Potest autem fortassis per intellectum intelligere operationem virtutis rationalis que dicitur apta vel inepta, facilis vel difficilis, per aptitudinem vel ineptitudinem fantastice distinctive et clare ostendentis sibi formas a quibus abstrahet suum objectum, scilicet, universale, quia erit isto modo per illius virtutis operationem devenire in cognitionem complexionis cerebri per accidens: est autem facilitas operationis apud cogitativam aptitudo componendi et dividendi fantasmata et conferendi ea ad intentiones sine multo scrutinio. Apud autem anime rationalis particulam facilitas intellectus sollertia dicitur . . . ," ibid., fol. 38r.

same in substance as fantasy and imagination, although different from reason.[31]

Somewhat more than Taddeo, Turisanus stressed the physiological aspects of brain function. Turisanus, who took a generally more Galenic position on the relationship of brain and nervous system than Taddeo had done, emphatically stated that, *pace* Aristotle, the brain, not the heart, is the site of the apprehensive faculties. He offered two proofs of this proposition: the consideration that if it were not so, every disease affecting the heat of the heart (presumably, that is, every case of fever) would produce insanity; and the fact that when insanity does occur physicians apply remedies to the head, not the heart.[32] Furthermore, he stressed that sense perception is a process requiring the participation of the brain: "it is obvious therefore from what has been said that sight is not primarily in the pupil, nor hearing primarily in the ears, and so on, but they are primarily in the sensitive *spiritus*."[33] Turisanus also devoted attention to the location of the various internal faculties, taking the conventional position that common sense and *fantasia* belong to the anterior ventricle of the brain, with memory in the rear. His discussion once again makes clear the literal and physical way in which he and his contemporaries understood mental activity: common sense and fantasy are in the anterior part of the brain because this part is soft and humid and therefore receives impressions easily "as wax does a seal," whereas memory is in the rear where the firmer tissue holds impressions better. Turisanus evinced an interest, which he apparently did not get from Taddeo, in explaining variations

[31] "hic [appetitus] autem cum fantasia et imaginatione idem est subiecto: ratione autem differens," ibid., fol. 36v.

[32] "Sed quid sit organum harum virtutum dubium est: sicut enim ex supradictis patet Galenus ponit cerebrum esse propter id quod diximus. Aristoteles autem vult organum istarum virtutum esse cor: dicens enim cerebrum factum esse ut adequet cordis calorem: subiunxit quod si amplius debito calefiat: vel infrigidetur ipsum cerebrum non faciet proprium opus, que est adequare cordis calorem, sed sicut dicit aut non infrigidabit aut coagulabit: unde aut dementias faciet et mortes: quod enim in corde calidum sicut dicit velociter simul passivum est patiente eo quod circa cerebrum sanguine: ergo videtur velle quod dementia sit propter pati cor sicut organum mentis: pati autem propter non equari a cerebro. Sed si ita esset tunc oporteret omnem cordis distemperentiam esse causam dementie: cuius contrarium videmus in multis febribus, in quibus calidum cordis adventum [*sic*] valde usque in mortem dementiam non efficit, quod dicendum ob aliud non sit, nisi quia cerebrum non est passum. ergo non est dicendum cor esse illarum organum sed cerebrum, quod manifestat dementiarum sanatio per medicinas illi appositas et non cordi," ibid., fol. 37v.

[33] "Manifestum est ergo ex his quod visus primus non est in pupilla: neque primus auditus in auribus: et sic de aliis: sed sunt in spiritu primo sensitivo," ibid., fol. 37r.

in the level of intelligence from one person to another; this, too, he believed to be at least partially determined by the consistency of the brain
—subtle and clear tissue making for ready penetration of the *virtus* and
spiritus, which bring forms to the brain to be abstracted by the *virtus
rationalis*. However, Taddeo had explained variations in the power of
memory in an essentially similar manner: according to him, a good
memory follows when the complexion of the rear ventricle of the brain
is dry enough to hold a good impression.[34]

Both Taddeo and Turisanus, following Aristotle, agreed that the internal faculties of the brain function primarily in response to stimuli from
the external senses. (Both authors, however, took the position that *imaginatio* can on occasion conjure up phantasmata that are "imaginary" in the
modern sense of the word, and Taddeo further held that "the intellect
that understands itself" does so without benefit of phantasmata, that is,
without calling forth images derived from sense experience).[35] Accordingly, it seems appropriate to turn next to their understanding of sensation and the functioning of the individual senses.

The general picture of sense perception drawn by Taddeo, Turisanus,
and doubtless also their fellow physicians was mainly derived from Aristotle's *De anima* and Avicenna's commentary thereon.[36] Taddeo, and
later Gentile da Cingoli and Turisanus, explained that the senses receive
the *species* of the thing sensed, not its matter; that sensation is essentially
passive; and, according to Turisanus, that it involves both potency and
act, potency being the continuous presence of the power of sense in an
organ and act the operation of that power. Taddeo's emphatic endorsement of Aristotle's assertion that only potential and not actual sensation
exists during sleep is noteworthy for its basis in personal experience:
Taddeo believed that sensation does not occur during sleep because he

---

[34] "illi qui habent complexionem cerebri in posteriori ventriculo siccam melius memorantur [*sic*]: sed illi qui habent humidam, male memorantur [*sic*]: quia impressio in re
sicca firmius adheret quam in re molli," Taddeo, *Isagoge*, fol. 361v. The idea that subtle
substances are more readily penetrated and the metaphor of wax and seal were both
well-worn conventional formulations deriving from ancient sources.

[35] Turisanus, *Plusquam*, fol. 37r; Taddeo, *Isagoge*, fol. 360r: "dico quod phantasia
postest esse de vero et falso; potest enim quis imaginari chimeram que nihil est secundum
veritatem"; fol. 360v: "an contingat intelligere sine phantasmate, vel non. . . . omnia cum
phantasmate dico intelligi preter intellectum, cum ipse seipsum intelligat. nam iste cum
non oporteat ipsum esse in virtute imaginativa non indiget phantasmate ut intelligatur.
ipse enim per seipsum sufficit movere se ad intelligendum seipsum."

[36] *De anima* 2.5, 416b32-3.2, 427a15.

himself, while sleepwalking, had fallen to the ground from a height of four feet without any awareness of having done so until after he woke up.[37]

Rather than attempt a complete, and necessarily repetitive, survey of the teaching of Taddeo and Turisanus on each of the five senses, we shall follow their own lead in concentrating upon the sense of sight, to which both of them devoted much more space than to any of the other four.[38] For Taddeo, indeed, sight seems to have served as a model of all sense perception, since in discussing both hearing and touch he made constant comparisons with the process and organs of seeing.[39] The reasons for this special interest in vision are not hard to find: not only was sight traditionally considered to be the noblest of the senses, but in addition, in the course of the thirteenth century, the science of optics had risen to a position of importance among the disciplines studied by scholars in the Latin West.

Yet in examining what Taddeo and Turisanus had to say on vision, one is struck by their relatively restricted range of reference and interest. By the thirteenth century, Latin scholars had gained access to three major bodies of writing about the eye and vision: the views of the philosophers of Greek antiquity and especially Plato and Aristotle (Plato's thoughts on vision being contained in the *Timaeus* and thus early available in the West) and of the Islamic natural philosophers Avicenna and Averroes; those of medical writers, beginning with Galen but importantly enriched by Islamic physicians, notably Johannitius; and those of students of geometrical optics, beginning with Euclid and Ptolemy, but much advanced by the Moslem mathematician Alhazen. The reception of this material had inspired the well-known interest in optics of such thirteenth-century Latin writers as Albertus Magnus, Roger Bacon, Witelo, Pecham, and Theodoric of Freiberg—all of whom wrote at length on the subject.[40]

---

[37] Taddeo, *Isagoge*, fol. 362r.

[38] Ibid., fols. 362r-363v; Turisanus, *Plusquam*, fols. 45r-46v.

[39] For example, "Et per hoc tangit illud quod facit idem in auditu quod facit humor cristallinus in visus, quia sicut in humore cristallino est quedam armonia et temperantia gratia cuius meretur esse instrumentum visus, ita est in illo aere quedam temperantia gratia cuius fit auditus: collectum [*sic*] in concavitate nervi obtici [*sic*], per hoc tangit instrumentum auditus," Taddeo, *Isagoge*, fol. 363v; and "dico quod triplex est instrumentum tactus sicut supra dictum est, nam quoddam est instrumentum solum recipiens sicut cristallina in visu et caro in tactu . . . ," idem, *Isagoge*, fol. 365r.

[40] On the sources, reception, and development of optical theory in the medieval West, see David C. Lindberg, *Theories of Vision from Al-Kindi to Kepler*, pp. 1-146.

But the writings of Taddeo and Turisanus gloss over mathematical optics in the most cursory and casual way, and they are innocent of citations of Alhazen or any of the recent Latin writers, with the exception, in the case of Turisanus, of Albertus.[41] Only the natural philosophical and the medical traditions concerning vision aroused interest in Taddeo's circle; he and his students tended to treat this, as they treated so many subjects, chiefly by exploring the differences between the teaching of Aristotle and that of (Plato and) Galen.

Taddeo's principal authority in his lengthy discussion of vision was Avicenna's commentary on *De anima* (known as Avicenna, 6 *De naturalibus*). From this source as well as from *De anima* itself (2.7, 418a26-419a24), he drew his definitions of *lux* (the light of a luminous body, such as the sun or fire), *lumen* (reflected light, as the light of the moon), radiation, and color. Although Taddeo treated a whole series of miscellaneous problems on vision, ranging from whether or not sight occurs instantaneously, through the reasons why some animals can see at night and why man, the noblest of animals, does not have this gift, to the old favorite about the menstruating woman and the mirror, his interest was evidently focused on the question of whether sight occurs by intromission or extramission. This problem had of course long been debated in both the Islamic world and the West. Its main attraction for scholastic physicians such as Taddeo was that Aristotle had opted for the intromission theory, stating that in the presence of external light and color the air serves as a medium to carry forms from objects to the eye, whereas Galen had claimed that vision takes place through the extramission of visual *spiritus* from the eye. The proponents of vision by extramission could also claim the support of Plato, who wrote in the *Timaeus* of fire streaming from the eye. (Plato considered that it was essential for the extramitted fire or light to fuse with daylight for vision to occur; so his was a modified theory of extramission.)[42] Although Galen's views were propagated among physicians by Johannitius (Hunain ibn Ishaq), whose writings on optics and ophthalmology are said to have been widely influential in the West,[43] both Avicenna and Averroes vigorously reasserted the Aristotelian theory.

[41] Turisanus, *Plusquam*, fol. 46v.

[42] For further discussion and detailed citations of the authors named, see Lindberg, *Theories of Vision*, pp. 1-11, 33-57.

[43] According to Lindberg, "it was chiefly through Hunain that medieval ophthalmologists in the west obtained their Galen" (ibid., p. 34); this is no doubt generally true, but

Leaning on the authority of Aristotle and Avicenna, Taddeo announced himself a believer in the intromission theory and adduced arguments drawn largely from Avicenna, *De naturalibus*, in its support. The chief of these ran as follows: if vision is by extramission, then what is extramitted must be either a body or not a body; yet for a variety of reasons it is impossible to postulate that a body emerging from the eye can reach the stars. But if what is emitted is not a body, it cannot be an instrument that goes forth and returns, because no instrument can cross from the sublunar to the celestial world and back again. Nor can one suppose that something is emitted from the eye that assists the air to become the instrument of sense, because then the air would be able to see by itself. Nor can light or heat emitted from the eye (a reference to Plato's ocular fire) be itself the medium of vision, since the light of the sun is obviously much greater than any possible light from the eye, while if heat is the crucial factor one would not be able to see when it is cold. Thus, Taddeo concluded, there is no way in which sight by extramission can satisfactorily be explained. Taddeo treated Plato's statements in the *Timaeus* as the chief source of the extramission theory. He referred to Plato's followers in this belief, including Galen, as heretics, and he soundly denounced them: "Whosoever therefore he (or they) may be who holds the opinion of Plato, let him be expelled from the academy and excluded from our parish, but with candles extinguished and bells tolling let him be banned from the company of those wise in philosophy."[44]

Turisanus, too, endorsed vision by intromission, characterizing the Platonic opinion as empty (*"supervacue et importune dicitur a Platonicis"*);[45] his position on sight may be regarded as generally Aristotelian, in that he also took pains to justify Aristotle's view that color is an essential

---

both Taddeo and Turisanus cited Galen's views on extramission from his commentary on the *Prognostica* of Hippocrates; see Taddeo, *Isagoge*, 1527, fol. 362v; Turisanus, *Plusquam*, fols. 45v-46r. Turisanus also referred to *De iuvamentis membrorum* in this connection. In discussing vision Taddeo does not appear to cite the ophthalmological works of Johannitius at all; they are mentioned once by Turisanus (*Plusquam*, fol. 46v).

44 "plato in Timeo: et sui sequentes voluerunt quod nos videremus extramittentes . . . et multi philosophi secuti sunt eum: et puto quod Isaac et Galenus sint tales heretici. . . . quicunque ergo illi vel ille sit qui habeat scilicet platonis opinionem abiiciatur ab achademia [NLM, MS 492, 1, fol. 71v: inmitatur sit anothomia (*sic*)] et non sit de nostra parochia, sed extinctis candelis et pulsatis campanis a consortio sapientium philosophie excludatur," Taddeo, *Isagoge*, fol. 363r.

45 Turisanus, *Plusquam*, fol. 45r.

component of vision. However, he provided a much more detailed and sympathetic account of Galen's views than Taddeo had done. He pointed out that just as it is impossible to see without external light, so too it is impossible to see without the eye; and he further maintained that Averroes had been mistaken in supposing that the luminous quality in the eye is a reflection of external light. He concluded that Galen had been right to suppose that the *spiritus visibilis* within the eye is itself a source of light, and that this light is somehow necessary for sight.[46] Thus on this issue Turisanus, unlike Taddeo, achieved a compromise by managing to declare the truth of the intromission theory without outright repudiation of Galen.

Yet, as already noted, neither Taddeo nor Turisanus chose to expound at any length or any detail the most convincing and thorough demonstration of the case for intromission—namely, that of Alhazen, who is said to have been the first to combine the intromission theory with geometrical optics.[47] This omission is unlikely to have been due to ignorance; it seems clear that both authors had some knowledge of Alhazen's views, perhaps via the work of one of his Latin followers (most likely Bacon or Witelo), since both of them conjoined the concepts of the visual pyramid and of intromission.[48] Taddeo provided a vague and highly compressed description of the image of the heavens as coming to the eye "under angles" and along lines.[49] Turisanus, in a somewhat more specific reference to the theory of punctiform radiation developed by Alhazen and his followers, wrote that "the way in which a colored thing comes to the eye is under straight lines from every part of the colored thing proceeding to the sight,

---

[46] "Sciendum est quod sicut non est videre sine lumine exteriori: ita et sine lumine intrinsecus oculi. . . . Manifestum ergo est quod non sine causa vocat Galenus predictum humorem [within the eye] lumen visibile," ibid., fol. 46r.

[47] Lindberg, *Theories of Vision*, p. 78.

[48] Witelo was active in Italy, first at Padua and later at the papal curia at Viterbo; Bacon's works were dispatched to the papal court; Witelo's familiarity with Bacon's writings on optics has also been demonstrated from internal evidence. See ibid., pp. 117; and, for Witelo's career, Agostino Paravicini Bagliani, "Witelo et la science optique à la cour pontificale de Viterbe (1277)," *Mélanges de l'école française de Rome* 87 (1975):425-453, and bibliography there cited.

[49] "dico quod totum idolum celi non venit ad oculum secundum quod est in celo, sed res veniunt sub angulis ad oculum, unde illa magna imago celi acuitur sub angulis et veniunt hoc modo visibilia ad oculos: hoc autem probatum est per artem de speculis, quomodo enim posset aliter in parvo speculo formari mons aut turris nisi sub angulis res viderentur . . . iudicat per expansionem id quod intrat oculum ut in expansione linearum et termini ad quem perducuntur," Taddeo, *Isagoge*, fol. 363r.

and for this reason their progress is under the figure of a pyramid whose base is in the angle of the thing seen. . . .[50] The brevity and imprecision of these passages is no doubt explained by a general lack of concern with mathematical optics on the part of writers absorbed in the natural philosophical and medical aspects of the subject.

The interest in the analysis of vision shown by Taddeo and Turisanus should not lead one to suppose that these learned physicians were indifferent to practical medical and anatomical considerations pertaining to the eye and to sight. Both Taddeo and Turisanus provided their readers with a short account of the internal structure of the eye, with its humors and tunics.[51] Both also gave some attention to the function of the various parts of the eye: Taddeo inquired whether the optic nerve or the lens is the principal organ of sight and decided that both are;[52] Turisanus attempted to explain how a single image is seen by the action of two eyes.[53] Turisanus also showed some interest in defective vision, referring to the difficulty in reading experienced by the aged (which he explained on the basis of complexion theory as due to the general loss of moisture with advancing years, a process especially damaging to a naturally humid organ like the eye), and also referring to blindness caused by the presence of too thick a tunic over the pupil—perhaps meaning a cataract.[54]

Another of Taddeo's students, Guglielmo da Brescia, displayed a sensitive awareness of the way in which optical, mental, and general physiological factors can interact in a problem involving the eyes. In his *consilium* for a patient who saw nonexistent things in front of his eyes (*ad*

[50] "oportet scire quod color non movet visum sine presentia materie. materia autem non est presens oculis nisi per directas lineas, quare processus colorati in oculum fit sub lineis rectis ab omni parte colorati procedentibus in visum, quare processus eius sub figura pyramidis cuius basis est res visa, conclusio autem anguli sit versus oculum. quum ergo immutatio oculi sit in puncto in quo concluduntur linee predicte fiet iudicium quantitatis rei vise secundum quantitatem anguli conclusi in oculo secundum punctum. hic autem angulus est magnus vel parvus, primo secundum distantiam linee que est in summo ad eam que in infimo apud basem: si enim est magna, tunc angulus fiet obtusior, quare et maior. si autem parva tunc erit acutior, quare minor," Turisanus, *Plusquam*, fol. 45v.

[51] Taddeo, *Isagoge*, fols. 370r-v; Turisanus, *Plusquam*, fol. 46r.

[52] "que sit ibi principalis particula in oculo," Taddeo, *Isagoge*, fol. 370v.

[53] "Sed dicet aliquis quod omne unum visibile debeat videri duplex: quia formatio eius fit in duplici oculo, et dextra rei vise debet videri sinistra . . . et econverso," Turisanus, *Plusquam*, fol. 45v.

[54] "Quod autem alii sunt qui eminentius nihil vident, quo minus clare intuentur, non est causa positio chrystallini in profundo, sicut putat Albertus, que sicut patebit est causa contrarii, scilicet, videndi a remotis, sed est causa huius, sicut dicit philosophus, spissitudo tunice que est super pupillam," ibid., fol. 46v.

appariciones fantasticas oculorum), Guglielmo stated that the symptoms were produced by the heat of certain vapors in the crystalline lens and in front of the grapelike tunic of the eye; when these vapors were perceived by the *virtus visiva*, the soul shaped them into images.[55] Sometimes illusions of this kind were insignificant and would soon disappear, as when the patient perceived motes dancing in the air or when he "saw stars" following vomiting or rage. However, if the images were larger and persisted, then they were caused either by the brain or the stomach. Much the more dangerous, Guglielmo asserted, are those caused by the brain, for they presage the descent of watery humor from that organ onto the pupil of the eye. He then proceeded to list signs whereby the physician can determine whether a particular patient's symptoms come from the brain or the stomach: images caused by the stomach appear before both eyes, those caused by the brain in front of one only; if the symptom persists for six months or more, this is a good sign, for, if the cause is in the brain, watery humor will block the pupil long before that time; moreover, if the pupil itself appears clear, without any turbidity or darkness, this also indicates that the cause of the problem lies in the stomach, as does intermittent presence and absence of the symptoms; continuity and stability of the symptoms suggest that the cause lies with the brain. Finally, if the symptoms respond to treatment of the stomach by emetics or other means, then obviously that was where the trouble lay. Guglielmo decided that the symptoms in the case in which he had been consulted emanated from the stomach, and he prescribed accordingly; fortunately so, for the commonest condition to produce the symptoms he attributed to a malady of the brain is a torn or detached retina, an irreparable eye injury in his day and for many centuries thereafter.

Thus, in Taddeo's circle, understanding of sense perception in general and of vision in particular was not grounded solely is speculative philosophy, but was also shaped by practical experience. For a final, and telling, example of the way in which theoretical analysis and professional experience combined to explain sensation, we may turn to the treatment of a type of sensation fundamentally and intimately involved with all medical practice, namely, pain.

Taddeo, Turisanus, and Bartolomeo all produced analytical or "theo-

---

[55] Guglielmo da Brescia, *Ad appariciones fantasticas oculorum*, edited in Erich Walter Georg Schmidt, *Die Bedeutung Wilhelms von Brescia als Verfasser von Konsilien*, pp. 26-37.

retical" discussions of pain; but whereas Taddeo and Turisanus speculated about its essential nature, Bartolomeo's purpose was to classify different varieties of pain as an aid to diagnosis.[56] In his commentary on
Book 2 of *De interioribus*, Bartolomeo followed Galen's lead in categoriz-
ing pain as dull (literally, freezing—*congelativus*), throbbing (*pulsati-
vus*), or acute (*aggravativus*). Besides this primary classification he also
discussed piercing (*perforativus*), corrosive (*corrosivus*), stabbing (*pun-
gitivus*), and gnawing (*mordicativus*) pain and explained how knowledge of varieties of pain can guide the physician in his estimation of
specific internal diseases and injuries. Bartolomeo's list of different kinds
of pain, somewhat reminiscent of the elaborate descriptions of variations
in pulse also developed by Galen and his followers,[57] may be arbitrary
and academic; but its origins lie in the experience of the working physician (whether Galen or Bartolomeo or both), and its purpose is to help
practice. Its ramifications do not grow from a system based on the principles of natural philosophy, but rather from the formalization of the
sensitivity that the best ancient and medieval physicians must have developed toward the smallest variation in the diagnostic signs available to
them.

However, although standard medical sources contained fairly detailed
discussions of pain from a diagnostic standpoint (discussions which constituted a standing invitation to elaboration in commentary), philosophical inquiry among physicians into the nature of pain and the way in
which it is perceived by the senses was apparently something of a new
departure. Such, at any rate, was Taddeo's view: on two separate occasions he explained that his own solution to a question on pain was tentative or provisional, once "on account of the novelty of the question,"[58]
and the second time because the problem was "difficult and left un-
touched by everyone in my time."[59] As one might expect, the accomplish-

[56] BAV, MS Vat. lat. 4454, fols. 59v-61r (Vat. lat. 4452, fols. 88r-89v); at fol. 59v:
"in hac particula docet ipsa loca paciencia cognoscere ex accidentibus que sumpta sunt a
membris ut agunt actionem animatam. et hoc non est aliud quam docere cognoscere loca
paciencia interiora ex speciebus dolorum."

[57] See N. G. Siraisi, "The Music of Pulse in the Writings of Italian Academic Physicians
(Fourteenth and Fifteenth Centuries)," *Speculum* 50 (1975):695-697, and bibliography
there cited.

[58] "Hic tamen attende: quod etiam in ista solutione propter novitatem questionis ego
multum dubito, et propter hoc si et quando mihi sententia verior occurrerit eam sine
pudore mutarem" Taddeo, *Aphor.*, fol. 31r.

[59] "Ad hanc autem difficilem et intactatam ab omnibus meo tempore questionem deter-

ment of Taddeo and Turisanus in this area consisted of reconsidering
traditional medical accounts of pain in the light of Aristotelian sensation
theory. Thus Taddeo adopted, from *De interioribus*, Galen's definition of
pain as "injurious sensation" (*sensus nocivus*).[60] Turisanus, like Bartolomeo, explicitly accepted the Galenic dictum that all pain is produced
by one of two underlying causes—namely, either by disorder in the balance of elemental qualities (*mala complexio*) on the body, or by sudden,
usually traumatically induced, physical change (*solutio continuitatis* or
continui).[61] But how is pain, thus caused and thus defined, actually experienced by the five senses, and in particular how is it distributed amongst
them? On this question Turisanus focused his attention, pointing out that
since delight can be experienced by every sense—by the eye in seeing
beautiful colors, by the ear in hearing sweet melody, and so on—it is
conceivable that pain can be too. His conclusion was, however, that pain
is exclusively a function of the sense of touch, which is more retentive of
both pleasant and unpleasant sensation than any of the other senses.[62]

The two fairly lengthy disquisitions on pain that Taddeo incorporated
into his commentary on the *Aphorisms* address problems of more immediate medical relevance. In both cases, however, Taddeo's purpose was to
provide a philosophically (that is, scientifically) acceptable explanation of
phenomena described by medical authorities. The first question—whether

---

minandam cum quadam dubitatione accedam . . . ex hac distinctione plenarie intellecta
patet veritas questionis et solutio obiectorum. universis autem inspicientibus locum hunc
supplico ut carior sit eis veritas quam vana victoria, et propter hoc antequam ad iudicium
procedant diligenter examinent et huiusmodi scrupulosam questionem subiiciant scrutinio
rationis et si vera dixi confirment si autem veritatem non dixi saltem viam aperui ad in-
daginem veritatis," ibid., fol. 172v.

[60] Ibid., fol. 31r, citing *De interioribus* 2.2.

[61] Turisanus, *Plusquam*, fol. 73r; and "diceret aliquis frater tu dixisti in pluribus locis
omnem dolorem fieri aut a solutione continuitatis, aut a malicia complexionis diverse.
modo dicis dolorem fieri ex pluribus aliis . . . respondet et dicit quod omnes ille cause
faciunt dolorem aut solvendo continuitatis aut introducendo malam complexionem . . . et
sic habemus quod Galenus posuit esse duas causas doloris et etiam ponit in tegni. Unde
Avicenna inconvenienter ipsum reprehendit," Bartolomeo da Varignana, comm. *De interioribus*, BAV, MS Vat. lat. 4454, fol. 60r (Vat. lat. 4452, fol. 88v).

Citing Galen in *De accidenti et morbo*, Turisanus (*Plusquam*, fol. 73r) provided some
examples of *solutio continuitatis* as follows: "in quolibet sensu videtur esse dolor ex solutione continuitatis, sicut in visu ex lumine splendidissimo cuius est dispergere spiritum
visibilem, in auditu ex voce magna aspera et acuta, in gustu ex sapore amaro acetoso pon-
tico et acuto, in odoratu ex fumis salientibus ad cerebrum a talibus saporibus; quoniam
sicut dicit de natura omnium talium sensibilium est solvere continuam in suis sensibus."

[62] Ibid.

it is possible to suffer pain without being aware of it—was raised in
Taddeo's mind by the Hippocratic author's statement, amplified in
Galen's commentary, to the effect that the insane sometimes appear unaware of pain-causing conditions. Here, Taddeo defended Hippocrates
against an apparently persuasive medico-philosophical argument running
as follows: pain is especially harmful to the tactile virtue, but because it
inflames the *spiritus*, it also damages all the other virtues, including the
virtus sensitiva; once the *virtus sensitiva* becomes aware of pain, there is
no way that the sensation cannot be carried to the soul, since the *virtus
sensitiva*, by definition, knows itself to feel. Because Taddeo conceived of
pain as invariably inflammatory, he was obliged to add the rider that pain
as an existing entity, not the cause of pain, directly affects the *virtus sensitiva*; this explains how pain can be produced by cold, which in and of
of itself gives rise to congelation rather than inflammation. As a possible
justification for Hippocrates' words, Taddeo rather hesitantly suggested
that pain should be defined as consisting of two things, namely, sensation
and injury; in a given case the former might be absent on account of a
defect in the patient's *virtus apprehensiva*, while the latter would still be
present. He ended his discussion with the observation that, while apparent insensitivity to pain might sometimes be a symptom of mental derangement, one cannot go on to assume that all mental illness causes
anesthesia; on the contrary, maniacs usually feel both pain and touch.[63]

Taddeo also attempted to provide adequate theoretical grounds for the
medical doctrine of *condolentia*, that is, "sympathetic" pain felt in one
part of the body when another part is injured or diseased (as when a
digestive upset is thought to be the cause of a headache).[64] That such
pain is felt had been taught, with examples, by both Galen and Avicenna,
but a satisfactory explanation of how pain is transferred from one part
of the body to another was lacking. Taddeo rejected the ideas that the
pain extends itself like a rod; that *solutio continuitatis* or its cause is
multiplied by generation; that injury to one part can suddenly produce
mala complexio in another; and that not the pain itself but its *species*
passes to the organ secondarily affected. The last he found unacceptable
on the grounds that touch, like the other external senses, is only activated
by the presence of matter; the internal mental faculties of the common
sense and *imaginatio* can respond to the *species* of a sensible object without directly encountering its matter, but, when they respond to the *species*

<hr>

[63] Taddeo, *Aphor.*, fols. 30v-31r.   [64] Ibid., fols. 172r-v.

of something causing pain, the result is sadness or anxiety, not pain in another part of the body.

In attempting to resolve this issue, Taddeo pointed out that not all simultaneous pain in different parts of the body can be described as *condolentia*, since unrelated injuries might occur at the same time by coincidence. Furthermore, some cases of *condolentia* he held to be caused by material vapors emanating from the injured part and reaching another organ. Then, too, the same circumstances might simultaneously produce *solutio continuitatis* in one part and disturbed complexion in another. But true *condolentia* (he gave as an example pain and itching felt at the head of the penis by men suffering from stones in the bladder) Taddeo believed to be most probably the result of contraction or distention of the nerves or ligaments connecting the seat of primary injury with the other organ where pain was felt.[65]

Not only cognition and sense perception but also the emotions had a place in the picture of normal human psychology traced by Taddeo and his fellows. Physicians had long placed the *accidentia anime*, or passions of the soul, among six "nonnaturals" (the others being, as noted previously, diet, air, exertion or its absence, sleeping and waking, and evacuation and repletion) that inevitably affect human life.[66] Turisanus quoted the assertion of Haly that the physician should not speculate about or evaluate the *accidentia anime*, although he should make use of them in effecting cures. In Turisanus's own view, since the passions most certainly affect health, it is the physician's duty to watch carefully for their influence "although what they are, and whence, he should take on trust from the natural philosopher."[67] Experience would teach the physician the ap-

[65] "si membrum principaliter dolens ex fortitudine doloris recipiat contractionem vel repletionem ex materia ita quod membrum sibi colligatum extendatur et trahatur propter contractionem vel repletionem fientes in membro principaliter dolente, v.g. propter contractionem, ut si fiat dolor in ore stomachi ex solutione continui, tunc utique propter fortitudinem doloris contrahetur os stomachi: et trahet nervos colligatos cum cerebro, quibus contractis miringe cerebri extendentur: et fiet in eis solutio continui, faciens dolorem . . . et sicut cum solvitur continuum in collo vesice per lapidem fit contractio nervorum virge: et fit dolor et pruritus in capite eius . . . sicut contingit in apostemate epatis, nam cum apostemate epar fit dolor in pectore quia ligamenta epatis trahuntur inferius . . . ," ibid., fol. 172v.

[66] On the nonnaturals see note 46 to chapter five, above.

[67] "Dicit autem Hali quod super hoc loco medicus non contemplatur in arte sua in accidentibus anime neque mensurat illa ad conservationem sanitatis, licet utatur eis: ut dicit ad curationem egritudinis: sed dicit quod speculatio et mensuratio eorum ad illud est

propriate emotional balance for each of his patients. Turisanus found that
the passions could reflect the state of physical health as well as influence
it; in particular, he found the elemental qualities in the bodies of some
people to be so well balanced that they experienced only temperate and
beneficial emotions. Naturally, the physician need do nothing about the
emotional health of such fortunate individuals. For others Turisanus suggested that the doctor prescribe a regimen of the passions and, rather opti-
mistically, recommended that the patients discipline their wills to follow
it. He did admit, however, that the physician's advice is unlikely to make
much impact upon established bad habits, which must be left to philosophy, laws, and punishments for correction. Similarly, in patients with
temperaments naturally disposed to passionate excess, the physician can
only strive to inculcate better habits and to improve the patient's complexion.

In the passage just described, Turisanus apparently had foremost in his
mind the regulation of sexual activity on medical grounds, since this was
the topic to which he next turned his attention. Although he believed that
excess could be damaging and bring on premature old age (his definition
of excess being that point at which the individual felt himself to be
weakened in *virtus*), he reserved his direct warnings for the dangers of
abstinence: this could cause epilepsy and syncope in men, "suffocation of
the womb" in women, and loss of appetite and pains in the head and
kidneys in both sexes.[68] Nonetheless, when Turisanus insisted on the need
for medical supervision of the *accidentia anime*, he was not referring exclusively to amorous passion and concomitant sexual activity. The *accidentia anime*, as he elsewhere made clear, include the whole range of
human emotion—joy, delight, sadness, anguish, anger, jealousy, and
shame. All of these were the physician's concern because the presence of
any of them indicated change in the *complexio* of the body. Thus, Turisanus asserted, the perception of something pleasing causes an abnormal
amount of heat and *spiritus* to radiate from the heart to the extremities
and surface of the body, thus producing joy and delight. This centrifugal
motion of heat and spirit, although more intense than usual, is essentially

---

philosophiam [*sic*] et legem [*sic*]. Hoc autem repugnans est hiis que Galenus supradixit
. . . Adhuc autem palam est quod medicus scrutatur de effectibus horum accidentium in
corpore humano, quid autem sint et unde sint philosopho naturali credit," Turisanus,
Plusquam, fol. 87v.

[68] Ibid., fol. 87v-88r.

natural, and hence joy is usually harmless or beneficial to the body; but people with weak hearts who are already deficient in heat and *spiritus* could die as a result of the sudden flight of all their *spiritus* from the heart, which follows the unexpected announcement of good news. Opposite emotions have opposite physical causes: the perception of sad things causes the *spiritus* to move toward the center of the body, and also results in the loss of *spiritus* in the form of tears. And, as we have already seen from Gentile da Cingoli's account, anger was accounted for as the result of a sudden boiling up of the blood around the heart.[69]

In a somewhat similar vein, Dino del Garbo devoted a short *tractatus*, or *questio*, to an investigation of the physical causes of laughter.[70] Dino expressed his dissatisfaction with Aristotle's treatment of the topic, which he claimed, is not only undesirably brief but also describes laughter merely as a function of the *virtus tactus*, that is, as a result of being tickled. It is obvious, Dino asserted, that laughter is also aroused by means of the mind's apprehension of messages brought by the sight and hearing, and when this occurs it indicates *spiritus* especially apt to receive cheerful impressions.[71] This cheerfulness can be induced, as Avicenna had noted, by the moderate consumption of good wine. Indeed, the disposition to laugh is so strong in those who have imbibed, and in children, that they are apt to break into laughter on very slight pretext, a disposition that, if found in sober adults, is a sign of stupidity. Dino explained laughter following physical titillation as the result of a diffusion and dilation of *spiritus* toward the surface touched; laughter at ludicrous sights or sayings is the result of an excessive humidity of the *spiritus*, which weakens the operation of cognition and intellective virtue. He carefully explained that the laughterlike spasm that results from wounds to the diaphragm is not true laughter and cannot be classified with the other two kinds.

Crude though this physiological psychology of the emotions may seem, it served to rationalize and justify the concern of physicians for the mental well-being of their patients. One suspects that, if only for pragmatic reasons, the psychological component of the medicine practiced in Taddeo's circle must in any case have been considerable, corresponding inversely to its limited physical effectiveness. In theory, however, all were

[69] Ibid., fol. 83.

[70] Munich, Bayerische Staatsbibliothek, CLM 7609, 14c, fol. 140 (139)r, part of a set of miscellaneous medical *questiones*, inc. "Ad solvendum dubitacionem scilicet cuius virtutis risus sit passio . . ."; expl. "dynus de florencia. . . ."

[71] Regarding the concept of *spiritus*, see note 56 to chapter six, above.

agreed that it was the task of the physician to heal the body, leaving the soul to philosophy and religion. Hence the medical claim to a practical understanding of the physical causes of mental and emotional conditions provided the essential sanction for a broad interpretation of the physician's authority and professional scope.

Perhaps, too, a larger significance may also be attributed to the physicians' propagation of an essentially Galenic description of the natural, physical origins of the passions. This explanation was not in itself new; but, with the expansion of systematic medical education in the north Italian university centers and elsewhere, the revival of Galenic studies, and the reception of the medicine of Avicenna, the medical theory of emotions was, from the later thirteenth century, undoubtedly more widely disseminated than ever before in the West. We have, indeed, already seen that Dino del Garbo's naturalistic analysis of the passion of love reached out beyond the schoolroom to a wider, nonmedical audience. Medical discussions of the passions can perhaps be allowed a place, alongside literary and religious explorations of the inner life, and alongside the study of ethical systems deriving from classical antiquity, among the sources of the focus on man's nature usually thought of as characteristic of Renaissance humanism. The unique feature of the medical discussions just considered is their lack of overt moralization, whether pre-Christian or Christian. But of course, it is also true that to the extent that physicians propagated not only the idea that violent emotions and bodily appetites have physical causes, but also the notion that their free indulgence is likely to produce adverse physical consequences, they lent their science to the tacit support of traditional morality. Galen himself had drawn upon the Stoic tradition, with its demands for self-restraint, in his discussion of the passions; similarly there is no reason to suppose that the morality consciously espoused by thirteenth- and fourteenth-century physicians was other than conventional.[72]

As already indicated, the physicians of Taddeo's circle and their contemporaries did not limit themselves to the understanding and attempted regulation of normal cognition, sensation, and emotion. They had, in addition, clearly defined concepts of several varieties of mental abnormality. The current emphasis among medical, social, and literary historians upon the social and ideological roots of any society's concept of madness has

---

[72] I owe this point to the insight of Dr. Judith Neaman.

tended to concentrate scholarly attention upon the religious sources of medieval ideas about deviancy.[73] Yet, while it is true that medieval theologians, devotional writers, and poets tended to treat madness as a moral rather than a medical category, and while it is equally true that the resources of society did not permit the enforced segregation of all those defined as insane, medieval physicians nonetheless thought of mental disturbance as a disease. Like other diseases, it was thought to have natural, physical (that is, complexional) causes; like other diseases, it was most appropriately treated by a learned physician; and furthermore, it could be expected to respond to medical treatment. For a systematic and fairly detailed account of the understanding and classification of mental disabilities current among the group of physicians here under discussion we may turn once again to Turisanus.[74]

The single feature that emerges with greatest clarity from Turisanus's handling of mental illness is his belief, apparently shared by the other pupils of Taddeo who wrote on the subject, that all forms of insanity and mental defect are the immediate result of physical disease or of a constitutional inadequacy of the brain. These writers ascribed insanity to a complexional imbalance, usually the brain's excessive frigidity or, in the

---

[73] See for example, Penelope B. R. Doob, *Nebuchadnezzar's Children: Conventions of Madness in Middle English Literature* (New Haven, 1974); and Thomas S. Szasz, M.D., *The Manufacture of Madness: A Comparative Study of the Inquisition and the Mental Health Movement* (New York, 1970). The latter author makes the startling claim that the persecution of supposed witches in late medieval and Renaissance society occupied the position filled by the diagnosis, confinement, and treatment of the supposedly mentally ill in modern society; in so doing, he completely ignores the existence of medieval medical concepts of mental illness. He is, however, justly skeptical of the claim that "witches" were themselves mentally ill, pointing out that they were victims of persecution whose confessions were wrung from them under torture.

A balanced, brief account of medical, religious, and legal concepts of madness in the Middle Ages and of the treatment of the insane is provided in Neamen, *Suggestion of the Devil*. Neaman stresses that despite current recognition of the near impossibility of producing a definition of madness that is not primarily a product of the definer's socially determined concepts of normality, "certain hard-core diagnoses and definitions of diseases considered forms of the forbidden disease physicians are loath to call 'insanity' survive and bear marked resemblance to medieval forms of madness" (p. 149). See also George Rosen, *Madness and Society* (New York, 1969), pp. 71-150, regarding medical concepts and social treatment of insanity in classical antiquity and the Middle Ages. A useful summary of some of the medieval descriptive and prescriptive literature on mental illness is contained in Basil Clarke, *Mental Disorder in Earlier Britain*, pp. 82-111. Fundamental is the account of the historical development of the concept of melancholy in Raymond Klibansky, Erwin Panofsky, and Fritz Saxl, *Saturn and Melancholy*, pp. 3-123.

[74] Turisanus, *Plusquam*, fols. 69v-70r.

case of mania, excessive heat.[75] Complexional and emotional factors were, of course, closely linked (for example, anger was associated with heat, and fear with frigidity). The idea that insanity is a divine punishment for sin, so prevalent in the religious and secular literature of the period,[76] is, as far as I know, nowhere discussed by them, although there is no evidence that they would have rejected it. Insofar as emotional or physical excess could be equated with sin, the scientific concepts of these physicians were consistent with popular religious notions. Nonetheless, Turisanus, Bartolomeo da Varignana, and Guglielmo, the members of the group of physicians under consideration who discussed mental illness most extensively, all indicated that the emotions themselves have physical (complexional) causes, and all concentrated their attention upon insanity considered as a disease of the brain.

The principal theoretical problem that they faced was to fit observed facts and medical traditions about various forms of insanity into a philosophically acceptable description of the various internal faculties of the mind and their location in different parts of the brain. Thus, Turisanus asserted that, in theory, any one of the parts of the brain housing the interior faculties of common sense and *fantasia*, cognition, and memory can become disordered: if the patient suffers from forgetfulness, then the power of memory is at fault, and the trouble is in the rear of the brain; if his judgment is deranged so that he thinks an enemy a friend or vice versa and is irrationally hopeful or fearful, then disease of the central portion of the brain has affected his cogitative power; if he has hallucinations but is able to describe them rationally, then only the front of the brain, the seat of fantasy and common sense, is afflicted. But, Turisanus went on to point out, the lucid scheme just outlined is deceptively oversimplified, in that more than one part of the brain might be, and usually is, affected at once; indeed, Averroes taught that affection of one part might itself induce derangement of another, so that someone who has delusions that he is in the presence of an enemy might think and speak

[75] "egritudines cerebri declarantur lesionibus operationum suarum . . . operationes autem que in eo sunt principales sunt quatuor sicut superius ostendit, scilicet, operatio fantasie, cogitationis, et memorie, et quarta operatio imperantis motum, scilicet, appetitus ergo declaratur cerebrum esse egrum ex lesionibus istarum," ibid., fol. 69v.

"ablatio [actionis cerebri] vero que universaliter litargia vel taciturnitas dicitur frigiditatem cerebri preter naturam comitatur, et similiter nocumentum et diminutio actionis que dormitatio mentis vocatur," ibid., fol. 70r.

[76] See Doob, *Nebuchadnezzar's Children*, passim.

accordingly. In the last instance, the defect in imagination would be so fixed and strong that the cogitative power would be unable to overcome it.[77]

The same problem of distinguishing disorders of the individual internal faculties also attracted the attention of Bartolomeo da Varignana, who considered it in a passage expounding Galen's views on mental alienation (*alienatio*). Casting his opinion into the form of a discussion of the questions "whether the cogitative power can continue to function if the imaginative power or the memory has been destroyed,"[78] Bartolomeo declared that, in the absence or malfunctioning of the other internal faculties, the cogitative power cannot possibly function. Turisanus would probably have had Bartolomeo's support for his suggestion that, in the context of mental illness, it might be preferable to retain Galen's single term mind (*mens*) for the various faculties of *sensus communis, imaginatio*, cogitation, memory, and *appetitus* (the last governing voluntary motion), and to speak either of loss of mind, producing the condition known as *litargia* or *taciturnitas*, or of diminution of the mind resulting in the state called "sleep of the mind" (*dormitio mentis*).[79]

Mental illness was also discussed in works on medical practice. Thus, the *Practica* attributed to Guglielmo da Brescia, which lists treatment for 129 forms of disease or injury, includes chapters on *stupor*, sleeplessness, frenzy (*frenesis*), drunkenness, falling in love, and melancholy. The author reserved his most detailed exposition for the subject of melancholy. According to him, there are numerous subspecies of melancholia: some melancholics laugh, others weep; some are suicidal, others fear death; some are silent, others talkative; some strike themselves and others; some

---

[77] Turisanus, *Plusquam*, fol. 70r.

[78] [Bartolomeo da Varignana], comm. *De interioribus*, BAV, MS Vat. lat. 4452, fol. 90v: "utrum ablatio memorie possit esse cum cogitatione. . . . ad hoc dico propter rationem factam quod totaliter ablatio memorie cum cogitatione esse non potest. . . . . utrum ablatio ymaginationis possit esse cum cogitatione et dico quod non totaliter. . . ." The passage quoted is part of about forty lines that are present in Vat. lat. 4452, but have been omitted from the corresponding folio of Vat. lat. 4454, namely 62v, where a half-line gap occurs shortly before the point of omission.

[79] "Post hoc autem dicemus quod tres virtutes [sc. imaginativa, cogitativa, memorativa] que presunt predictis tribus operationibus dicuntur a Galeno uno nomine mens sive virtus anime regitiva: eo quod ex eis procedit omne regimen animalis . . . Sed in actione virtutis anime regitive, ut in summa est dicere tria contingunt accidentia: sicut dicit Galenus in libro *De morbo et accidenti* quorum unum est ablatio actionis, secundum vero est nocumentum sive diminutio, tertium vero a cursu sue nature mutatio," Turisanus, *Plusquam*, fol. 70r.

fear that the heavens will fall on them, others that the earth will swallow them up; some have visual hallucinations, others imagine themselves to be kings, or wolves, or demons, or birds, or fragile vases; some keep a hand closed because they think they are holding the world within it; others think they are roosters and stretch their wings when they hear one crow.[80] It seems likely that this list of symptoms of derangement has literary antecedents; similar lists were provided by Arnald of Villanova (d. 1311) and other writers.[81] This, of course, does not exclude the possibility that Guglielmo encountered some of these manifestations in the course of his own practice.

Under melancholy, Guglielmo seems to have assimilated both the severe psychoses suggested by his list of symptoms and also relatively mild forms of depression. Thus, as examples of cures, he cited the case of a woman who became melancholic when her lover left and recovered when he returned, and of a man who was melancholic because of money worries—it is unclear whether these were real or imaginary—and recovered when the doctor brought several people to give him money (amounts not stated). He admitted, however, that he himself had been unable to cure a case of persistent delusions.[82]

From the foregoing, it will have become evident that the specific symptoms of mental illness recognized by Turisanus, Bartolomeo, and Guglielmo, and doubtless by their associates include catatonia, paranoid delusions, hallucinations, amnesia, and depression. Bartolomeo also referred to congenital mental defects (*stolliditas* or *stultitia*), which he regarded as the result of a deficiency in the *virtus rationalis*. Symptoms of mental disturbance were fitted into the broad categories of melancholy and frenzy. Melancholia, which embraced a much wider range of behavior than "depression," was thought to be the result of the clouding of the mind by melancholic humor, although, as Bartolomeo da Varignana was careful to point out, this occurred only in certain individuals who were predisposed thereto.[83] "Frenzy" was apparently used to describe any

---

[80] Guglielmo, *Practica*, fol. 20v.

[81] See Neaman, *Suggestion of the Devil*, pp. 18-19.

[82] Guglielmo, *Practica*, fol. 21v (and see also chapter nine, below).

[83] Bartolomeo da Varignana, comm. *De interioribus*, BAV, MS Vat. lat. 4454, fols. 63r, 64r-v (Vat. lat. 4452, fols. 91r, 92r-v); at fol. 64r: "in parte ista in quadam passione ipsius [cerebri] que in communi dicitur allienatio secundum autem proprium nomen dicitur melancolia, docet in ista cognoscere . . ."; (fol. 64v) "non vult Galenus quod in cerebro sit una anima que videat illam obtenebrationem que fit ab humore melancolico quia nullus

manic state; Mondino de' Liuzzi, for example, was at pains to distinguish delirium during fever and wandering of the mind during the last stages of illness, both described by Hippocrates, from "true frenzy."[84]

The physical treatments recommended for mental disturbances seem on the whole to have been fairly mild. Taddeo recommended various herbal medicines for frenzy, melancholia, and *litargia*.[85] Guglielmo assembled a catena of authorities recommending very different approaches to the melancholic and the frenzied, in which melancholics definitely had the better part of the bargain. They were to be kept in clear temperate air, take moderate amounts of exercise in pleasant, natural surroundings, hear melodious music, wear clean, sweet-smelling clothes, take warm baths, and in general do anything pleasing to the senses (except engage in coitus) and likely to produce joy and lightheartedness. The frenzied, on the other hand, were to be kept confined, in the dark and the cold, in somber clothing (bright colors being thought exciting), without pictures to look at, without noise, and without visitors.[86] Perhaps the exalted social standing of many of the patients of our group of learned physicians saved them, if not from bloodletting and cautery, then at least from flogging and confinement in bonds. (The latter treatments were inflicted upon the insane from time to time in the Middle Ages, although not with the universality and organized support that, in a later and more "enlightened" age, made it impossible even for kings to escape them.)[87]

---

hoc diceret, sed vult sic intelligere. Nam sicut apparet in exterioribus homines exeuntes in tenebris timent propter duo, scilicet, quia non vident quod debent, unde causatur in ipsis quidam modus contristationis in anima [?] aut etiam quia natura ipsorum apta est ad timorem ita etiam [quando humor melancolicus vadit ad cerebrum quia fit ex ipso tenebratio, Vat. lat. 4452, fol. 92r] in spiritu fit timor et hoc ex proprietate quadam illius vel etiam quia natura et complexio patientis est disposita et apta ad timorem." For further details regarding the scholastic medical analysis of melancholy, see Klibansky et al., *Saturn and Melancholy*, pp. 82-108.

[84] Mondino, comm. *Pronost.*, BAV, MS Vat. lat. 4466, fol. 6r: "sciendum est quod frenesis non vera dicitur tripliciter. . . . apparet etiam solutio ad quemdam aliam dubitationem quare, scilicet, distinxit dolorem a frenesi."

[85] The "tabula magistri thadei de bononiense [*sic*] de remediis omnium egritudinum in generali" contained in BAV, MS Palat. lat. 1363, 14c, at fols. 168r-171r (inc. "[C]um nostra corpora diversis et occultis proprietatibus"), includes four herbal remedies for *frenesis*, six for *melancolia*, and eight for *litargia*.

[86] Guglielmo, *Practica*, fols. 15v-16r, 21r.

[87] Confinement in bonds was recommended, for the prevention of injury and not as a punishment, by the thirteenth-century encyclopedist Bartholomeus Anglicus in a succinct popularized account of current medical views on the diagnosis, symptoms, and treatment of insanity; this passage of Bartholomeus's *De proprietatibus rerum* is most readily available

Despite the summary nature of the foregoing review of the concepts about mind, sense, and emotion, and of mental normality and abnormality found in the circle of Taddeo, enough has been said to indicate the important position of these topics in their thought. Moreover, in this area, more than in many others, their desire for theoretical understanding seems to have grown directly out of their experience as medical practitioners. As a learned man, a physician of course turned to *theoria* for explanations in all branches of his discipline; but every physician must inevitably have encountered many instances in which knowledge of the most advanced scientific teaching available—that of Aristotle and his commentators and of the Hippocratic-Galenic tradition—appeared to have little immediate application to the medical problem at hand. But, faced with such universal and nonspecific problems in his patients as pain, fear, and desire, the physician might find his philosophical and medical learning of genuine practical use, since his psychology, however incorrect the physiology on which it was based, taught the naturalness of the emotions and stressed the inextricable, mutual involvement of physical with emotional reactions. Obviously, physicians who advocated moderate self-restraint for reasons of health, and the binding of the mad because they could *not* restrain themselves, shared to a greater or lesser extent the prevailing ideological emphasis upon the power and duty of mind and soul, in all except the insane, to dominate the body. Nonetheless, the medical emphasis upon man's physical and animal nature and upon the physical origins of his emotions did not lend much support to an ideal of ascetic spirituality.

The influence of medical thought upon views of human nature should not be overestimated. As we have seen, learned physicians themselves shared, and no doubt by oral exhortation reinforced in their patients, the religious and moral preconceptions of the age. Moreover, learned physicians cannot have been very numerous, and they treated chiefly the relatively small proportion of the population that happened to be wealthy or to dwell in cities. The intellectual, social, and institutional influence of these doctors never even remotely resembled that achieved by medical professionals in the western world in the nineteenth and twentieth cen-

(in English translation) in Jan Ehrenwald, M.D., ed., *The History of Psychotherapy: From Healing Magic to Encounter* (New York, 1976). Regarding flogging, see Rosen, *Madness and Society*, p. 140. The supposedly therapeutic beatings to which George III was subjected by his attendants are well known.

turies. Nonetheless, the significance of medical attempts to regulate the passions and prescribe for mental disturbances in the Middle Ages should not be minimized. Those who had access to treatment by learned physicians also had some degree of access to a body of thought that, contrary to many prevailing currents, did not lay primary stress upon the sinfulness of the victim as the cause of either physical disease or irrationality. This is surely a matter of some moment.

However, it would be as grossly misleading to imply that the practice of Taddeo and his colleagues consisted chiefly in the provision of psychological reassurance as it would be to imply that philosophical speculation was their chief intellectual concern. For a more rounded view of their activities as teachers and practitioners we may turn to the next two chapters.

CHAPTER EIGHT

FAVORITE TOPICS OF DISCUSSION: THE SCHOLASTIC *QUESTIO* AS A TOOL OF MEDICAL TEACHING

As the preceding chapters show, the life work of Taddeo and his pupils fits into a variety of contexts. In one way or another, their activities and writings help to illuminate the rise of the university system in Italy, civic life in the north Italian cities, the growth of secular professions, the origins of Italian humanism, vernacular culture in the age of Dante, the development of concepts of scientific method, and the study of Aristotelian philosophy in the schools of Bologna. Yet to examine their work in the light of themes that have proved of lively interest to twentieth-century historians is not necessarily to reveal the priorities of Taddeo and those he influenced; an examination along the lines of our own interests, however useful in itself, may sometimes mask those priorities. For a full understanding of the world of thought inhabited by Taddeo and his pupils, we need also to determine what topics and ideas they themselves considered to be of primary importance. Unfortunately, however, the very qualities of their work—its copiousness, repetitiveness, and, in large measure, derivativeness—constitute a barrier to such understanding.

Happily, a tool is at hand that allows us to identify with reasonable accuracy and objectivity some of the subjects that Taddeo and those he trained discussed most frequently. Presumably these are the subjects that they found most important or engaging. This tool is provided by the lists of *questiones* contained in their commentaries (such lists were appended to some of the commentaries in both manuscripts and early editions) and by the subjects of various *questiones* and sets of *questiones* by members of the group that survive in manuscript. A unified register of question titles from all these sources appears in Appendix One. Guided by the frequency with which various topics crop up in this register, we shall see in this chapter some of the main themes favored by Taddeo and his students and colleagues. In this way, we may hope to obtain a firmer grasp of their own conception of the chief intellectual, scientific, and medical problems confronting the learned physician. Furthermore, insight may be gained into some of the ways in which pedagogical method helped to shape thought, since by Taddeo's day the posing and discussing of *questiones* in scholastic form had emerged as a central feature of higher medical education. For him and his pupils, as for their successors down to at least the end of the fifteenth century, medical education without disputed *questiones* and the resolution of *dubia* within commentaries would have been inconceivable. The uses that Taddeo's circle made of the question method therefore merit serious consideration in their own right.

It is hard to distinguish the practice of formulating and discussing *questiones*, in medicine or in any other discipline, from the development of the so-called scholastic method as a whole, since the clear identification of a problem, the citation of various opinions thereon, and the provision of a solution based on a combination of authority and syllogistic reasoning are essential characteristics of that method. Thus, the prototypical product of medieval scholasticism, the *Summa theologiae* of Saint Thomas Aquinas, is broken up into parts, which are in turn divided into units entitled "*questiones*," each of which is resolved in the manner just indicated. This method of approaching a subject, which is rooted in pedagogical practice, grew up in the late eleventh- or early twelfth-century cathedral schools and reached the height of its development in the thirteenth century, in the milieux of the universities and of the *studia* of the orders of friars. Its immediate origins have been thought to lie in the amalgamation of the practice of assembling opposing opinions on the same topic (the *Sic et non* of Abelard being an early and celebrated example) with the syllogistic mode of argument derived from first the Old and subsequently the New Logic of Aristotle, and with the custom of oral academic debate. Its earlier antecedents are complex: they have been variously sought in Carolingian biblical exegesis and the work of Alcuin; in developments in canon law in the late eleventh century; in the writings of Photius, patriarch of Constantinople (d. 886); among Islamic theologians; and elsewhere—these suggestions not necessarily being mutually exclusive.[1]

---

[1] The standard work on the subject is Martin Grabmann, *Die Geschichte der scholastischen Methode*. The literature is conveniently summarized and a perhaps not wholly convincing case made for the importance of Islamic influences in George Makdisi, "The Scholastic Method in Medieval Education: An Inquiry into Its Origins in Law and Theology," *Speculum* 49 (1974):640-661.

Hitherto, most investigations into the origins and growth in the medieval Latin West of the scholastic method of inquiry have concerned the disciplines of theology and philosophy. Developments in medicine, which were often parallel with those in other disciplines, have been much less fully and systematically treated. Although much scattered information about the structure of medical teaching and the influences between medicine and other disciplines is available, a satisfactory synthesis is still lacking.[2] It is clear, however, that the use made of *questiones* by our group of learned physicians in the schools of Bologna and elsewhere in the years around 1300 not only reflected the general developments in pedagogy alluded to above, but also continued a distinct and ancient scientific tradition—the custom among both physicians and natural philosophers of posing and attempting to answer "natural questions" on a variety of subjects, both medical and pertaining to other branches of science. The antecedents of this practice are to be found in such compilations of late classical antiquity as the *Natural Questions* of Seneca and the pseudo-Aristotelian *Problemata*, and its medieval continuation was ensured by Adelard of Bath and by those physicians of Salerno responsible for the compilation of the famous collection known as the *Salernitan Questions*.[3] These and other collections of natural and medical questions originally represented the reduction to writing of oral teaching in which an individual master either posed problems to his pupils and then provided his own solution, or else responded informally to questions from students. As time went on, a good many of the subjects became traditional and were reiterated; moreover, it appears probable that the practice of posing and solving questions in writing, without prior oral debate necessarily having taken place in each separate instance, also developed. While oral teaching by the question method undoubtedly continued, there is no need to suppose that every question in the twelfth-century collections is a record of oral discussion, in or out of the classroom.

University-trained physicians of the High Middle Ages thus inherited not only the scholastic methodology common also to theology and philosophy, with its heavy emphasis on breaking down material into question form; they fell heir, too, to a living tradition of medical question-litera-

---

[2] Most of the available discussions are cited in the notes to chapter four, above, q.v. But see also Luke Demaitre, "Scholasticism in Compendia of Practical Medicine, 1250-1450," in *Science, Medicine, and the University, 1200-1550: Essays in Honor of Pearl Kibre*, ed. N. Siraisi and L. Demaitre, *Manuscripta* 20 (1976):81-95.

[3] Lawn, *The Salernitan Questions*, chaps. 1-5, passim.

ture. The continued interest of university physicians in discussing collections of questions on miscellaneous scientific and medical topics is probably best illustrated by the commentary on the pseudo-Aristotelian *Problemata* by Peter of Abano (completed ca. 1310);[4] but the practice of casting inquiry in the form of such questions and the reiteration of some of the same subject matter continued until the sixteenth century.[5] By the thirteenth century it was also standard practice both to introduce medical questions into commentaries and to write sets of questions on particular texts, as can be seen from the works of both Albertus Magnus and the physician Petrus Hispanus (d. 1277 as Pope John XXI). Albertus, for example, produced a set of questions *De animalibus* (that is, on Aristotle's books on animals) that includes a number of medical questions deriving from the Salernitan collections or other sources.[6] Questions associated with a particular work tended to have somewhat more unity of theme (the theme being dictated by the content of the work commented on) than did the twelfth-century question miscellanies, but, as we shall see, it would be easy to overstate the extent of this systematization. Albertus and Petrus were, however, leaders in extending the range of subject matter and in treating medical and natural questions in the light of the newly received Greek and Arabic scientific learning, according to the scholastic method that had developed in the schools of the West.

The discussion of *questiones* at Bologna and the other *studia* in which Taddeo Alderotti and his pupils taught medicine was also affected by yet another development, namely the role given to formal disputation in university education. In the schools of the medieval West, the practice of oral debate long antedated the rise of universities; but the general formal structuring of education that accompanied that rise, together with the need for appropriate exercises that would serve as steps toward the completion of a "degree," led in the course of the thirteenth century to the institution and regulation of disputation as an essential part of the course

---

[4] *Aristotelis stagirite philosophorum summi problemata atque divi Petri Apponi Patavini eorundem expositiones* (Mantua, 1475; Klebs 776.1). There are other early editions. For discussion, see N. G. Siraisi, "The *Expositio Problematum Aristotelis* of Peter of Abano," *Isis* 61 (1970):321-339.

[5] Lawn, *The Salernitan Questions*, chaps. 8-10.

[6] See, on Petrus's commentary on the Aristotelian books on animals, Wingate, *The Mediaeval Latin Versions of the Aristotelian Scientific Corpus*, p. 79, and Lawn, *The Salernitan Questions*, p. 77; and for Albertus, his *Quaestiones super de animalibus*, ed. Ephrem Filthaut, O.P. (in his *Opera Omnia*, ed. B. Geyer, 12:77-351), and Lawn, *The Salernitan Questions*, p. 85.

of study in the various faculties at Paris, Oxford, Bologna, and elsewhere.[7]
Public disputations conducted by masters constituted both a useful forum
for the investigation of questions of current intellectual concern and an
effective means of training students in techniques of rational argument;
hence successful participation in such disputations came to mark the
achievement of a certain stage in the student's academic career. Both
regularly scheduled disputations on previously fixed topics and more infrequent quodlibetal disputations at which questions could be raised at
will early emerged as standard parts of the university curriculum in almost all disciplines. Attendance and participation were required of masters and would-be masters in arts and philosophy, in canon and civil law,
in theology—and in medicine. We find, for example, that the statutes
drawn up in 1405 by the student University of Arts and Medicine at
Bologna contain a whole series of provisions regulating the conduct of
medical disputations.[8] One official disputation was to be held each week
by a doctor or master, with each of the doctors or masters performing this
duty in rotation. The disputing master was to reserve his determination
(that is, his own solution of the problem) until the following week, when
he was to deposit a copy of his disputation and its determination with the
university stationer for student use. Medical disputations were to be held
both on theory and on practice. In addition, doctors teaching medicine
were to conduct quodlibetal debates twice a year. At least four scholars
were to take part in each hebdomadal disputation on medicine, students
being eligible to participate only after a year's study of medicine. Rather
elaborate regulations ensured fair distribution of a chance to argue among
those qualified to do so. No scholar was permitted to be the principal
respondent in a regularly scheduled disputation unless he had studied for
at least two years. Four of the ten questions composing each quodlibetal
debate were to be contributed by scholars; but in order to be the respondent at a quodlibetal disputation a scholar must have studied medicine at
Bologna for three years or more, unless he was already a doctor in arts,
in which case two years of medical study were sufficient. The statutes go
on to provide for regular and quodlibetal disputations in arts—namely,
grammar, logic, philosophy, and astronomy-astrology (which, as noted, is

---

[7] See Rashdall, *Universities*, 1:450-462, 476-486, and Palémon Glorieux, *La littérature
quodlibétique de 1260 à 1320*, 1:1-59 and 2:1-50.

[8] Malagola, *Statuti*, pp. 260-266, nos. 54, 55, 56, 57, 61; for disputations in the law
schools at Bologna, see pp. 107-109. Regarding the requirements for disputations in all
faculties at Paris, see Glorieux, *La littérature quodlibétique*, 2:19-22.

shown by the texts required to have included arithmetic and geometry)—and to ensure that scholars participated in each of these only after studying the particular art or science in question; scholars and masters of philosophy were also bidden to attend disputations given by the lectors of the orders of friars.

The practices recorded in these regulations of the Bologna University of Arts and Medicine closely parallel those demonstrated to have existed in the Parisian faculties of arts and theology and in the *studia* of the friars from about 1260 or before;[9] they may therefore be presumed to have been for the most part already of long standing when the Bologna statutes were compiled in 1405. We have no way of knowing whether the whole of the elaborate regulatory structure just outlined governed the conduct of disputations at Bologna while Taddeo or his pupils were there; it is, however, clear from their writings that the custom of disputation was already well established in the faculty of medicine, as it was in the faculty of arts and no doubt also the faculty of law in the same period.[10] Although the existence of sets of questions on particular works (such as Mondino's questions on the chapter on generation in the *Canon* of Avicenna)[11] and the universal prevalence of questions embedded in commentaries may suggest that *disputatio* and *lectio* were not always clearly distinguished in the teaching of these masters, independent questions also survive that are described as "determined" or "disputed" "in the schools."[12] In these independent questions the academic standing of

[9] Glorieux, *La littérature quodlibétique*, 1:1-20 and 2:22-27.

[10] Philosophical *questiones* from Bologna in the same period (including those embedded in commentaries on philosophical works) are indexed in an inventory of unstudied and incompletely studied philosophical works by masters of arts in the European universities during the period 1270-1350, which has been compiled by Professor Charles Ermatinger of St. Louis University from the extensive holdings of microfilms of Vatican manuscripts in the Pius XII Memorial Library of St. Louis University, and which may be consulted there; see C. J. Ermatinger, "Projects and Acquisitions in the Vatican Film Library," *Manuscripta* 12 (1968):170-175, for a description of this inventory. Comparison of the question titles in Appendix One, below, with the St. Louis inventory, which I have not so far attempted, might suggest lines for further research on the relationship of philosophy and medicine in the period in question. It may be noted that on occasion medical and philosophical questions were assembled in the same codex; see, for example, note 64 to chapter six, above. Regarding the use of disputed questions in the teaching of law at Bologna in the fourteenth century, see Manlio Bellomo, *Aspetti dell'insegnamento giuridico nelle Università medievali. Le "quaestiones disputatae."*

[11] BAV, MS Reg. lat. 2000, fols. 1-23r.

[12] For example, Dino del Garbo, comm. *De malicia complexionis diverse*, BAV, MS Vat. lat. 2484, fol. 196v: "fuit questio disputata in scolis primo anno nostre lecture in civitate

the author is not always indicated, but, where it is, he is described as "master." This, taken with the absence of interjections of the kind found by Glorieux in some of the Parisian quodlibeta of the same period[13] (which represent the presence of several participants), suggests that the surviving independent questions by Taddeo and his associates record the second stage of debate, namely, the master's *determinatio* some days after the conduct of the disputation itself.

Compared to the very large number of *questiones* embedded in their commentaries, surviving independent *questiones* by Taddeo and members of his circle are very few (see Appendix One). Only a minute portion of the output of these writers can therefore be said with any degree of certainty to be a direct record of oral debate in the setting of a formally organized academic disputation. Nevertheless, the use of questions was for Taddeo and his pupils very far from being merely a literary device, taken over from earlier scholastic commentaries in natural philosophy or medicine and from the various existing collections of medical and natural *questiones*. Not only in formal disputations, but also in their lectures, it was a living and pervasive pedagogical method. Thus the term *questio* was employed without inconsistency by the copyists of their works to describe both the separate records of arguments "disputed in the schools" and brief statements of opinion incorporated into commentaries, sometimes with little or no "scholastic" apparatus of opposing arguments, syllogistic reasoning, and so on. The *questiones* in commentaries may indeed often have been the ultimate distillation of longer questions that were actually orally disputed or, at any rate, were the subject of an independent treatment in full scholastic form, although this is impossible to determine except in rare instances, such as Taddeo's treatment of specific form in his commentary on the *Isagoge*.[14] Duly indexed under question headings in that work, this treatment is, as already noted, a drastically compressed version of thirteen rather lengthy and complex questions on specific form included in his commentary on Avicenna's chapter on things eaten and drunk and referred to admiringly by the copyist of the

---

senarum"; anonymous question, with questions of Dino and probably by him, MS Vat. lat. 4454, fol. 101r: "Questio disputata in scolis fuit utrum complexio naturalis possit permutari"; question of Mondino, MS Vat. lat. 3144, fol. 12r: "determinatio secundum M. Mundinum de Bononia."

13 Glorieux, *La littérature quodlibétique*, 1:18-20.
14 Taddeo, *Isagoge*, fols. 378r-v.

latter as "*pulchra dicta Tadei.*"[15] Not all *questiones* in commentaries were
so abbreviated, however; treatments as detailed as some of those surviving
in independent form are also to be found therein, such as, for example,
Taddeo's handling of the problem "Utrum videamus extramittentes vel
intus suscipientes," that is, whether sight is by the emanation of rays from
the eye to the perceived object or vice versa (for his views, see chapter
seven, above).[16]

Moreover, "treatise" (*tractatus*), "commentary," and "question" were
not always as clearly distinct from one another as the terms would indicate; so while in some instances traces of treatment in independent question format may have been lost, in others it may have been imposed.
Thus, for example, the *Practica de febribus* of Taddeo and the commentary on Book 1, *fen* 4 (also on *practica*) of the *Canon* of Avicenna by
Guglielmo da Brescia are included in one manuscript as groups of items
in a numbered list of miscellaneous questions.[17] In another manuscript,
a work of Mondino's is referred to as a "*tractatus seu questio de cerussa.*"[18]

In commentaries, *questiones* proliferate—227 are listed in one manuscript of Dino del Garbo's *Dilucidatorium totius practice medicine* (a
commentary on Avicenna, *Canon* 1.4), and 335 in a manuscript of Turisanus's *Plusquam commentum.*[19] In some instances passages of literal commentary on the text are followed by sets of questions or *dubia*; in others
questiones are scattered apparently at random through the commentary.
Naturally the subject matter of questions in commentaries was suppos-

---

[15] BAV, MS Palat. lat. 1246, fols. 83-97v, attribution on fol. 97v.

[16] Taddeo, *Isagoge*, fols. 362v-363r.

[17] Padua, Biblioteca Universitaria, MS al numero provvisorio 202, medical miscellany,
14c, contains a set of 118 numbered *questiones* on fols. 31-97r and 107r-125r (a list of
the question titles occurs on fols. 28v-29r); however, *questiones* nos. 82-86, fols. 107r-115r,
actually constitute the *Practica de febribus* of Taddeo. *Questio* no. 82 begins "Quoniam
nihil melius ad veritatis indagationem," the incipit given for that work, from other manuscripts, in TK 1288; at fol. 113r are the words "Explicit practica honorabilis doctoris medicine thadei disputata." Similarly, *questiones* nos. 88-117, fols. 117v-124v, are actually a
commentary by Guglielmo da Brescia on Avicenna, *Canon* 1.4; *questio* no. 88 begins
"Dicemus quod res medicationis etc. Sciendum hoc quod instrumentum medici est duplex,"
this incipit being the same as that of the work in Milan, Biblioteca Ambrosiana MS C115
Inf. (ex Q), fol. 60v (described in Astrik Gabriel, *A Catalogue of Microfilms of One
Thousand Manuscripts in the Ambrosiana*, p. 59, no. 74). At fol. 124v the Padua MS has
"Expliciunt questiones 4e fen libri primi avicenne recollecte sub provido viro . . . magistro
Guilielmio de Brixia."

[18] BAV, MS Vat. lat. 4455, fol. 41r.

[19] Dino, *Dilucidatorium*, BAV, MS Vat. lat. 2484, fols. 182v-184v; Turisanus, *Plusquam*,
BAV, MS Vat. lat. 4472, fols. 19v-20v.

edly determined by the subject matter of the text commented upon; but the text was not always a limiting factor in practice, both because the subject of such frequently commented texts as the *Tegni* and the *Isagoge* is the whole of medicine, and because Taddeo and the other authors were accustomed to use both very general statements and very minor points in their texts as pegs on which to hang lengthy treatments of questions in which they felt a special interest. The scope thus opened for varying personal tastes is well illustrated by the fact that the same brief passage of the *Tegni* (2.35) provided the pretext for Taddeo to expatiate upon the mutability of innate complexion, with yet further references to his favorite subject of specific form, and for Turisanus to introduce scathing criticism of Galenic theories about pulse. (For the content of their views on these topics, see chapter six, and below.) Similarly, there is little in the section on food in the text of the *Isagoge* that seems to demand the series of questions on specific form inserted at that point by Taddeo as a result of his reflections on Avicenna.

As the examples above and the later witness of the Bologna university statutes of 1405 indicate, scholastic *questiones* were employed not only in the study of *theoria* but also in that of *practica*. The general assumption of the almost universal validity of the question method is exemplified by a somewhat ambiguous statement in the preface of Taddeo's *Practica de febribus*. Taddeo there announced that, since nothing is more helpful for the investigation of truth than the exercise of skilled disputation, he would dispute on the cure of fevers in order to bring opposing views on the subject into harmony, but he would do this "armed with the scythe of authority and not vacillating in sophistical appearances."[20] This looks like a contradiction in terms, since the main effect of the use of the disputation format is usually held to be the fostering of, precisely, reliance upon logical argumentation and *sophystice apparentie*. It is quite probable that Taddeo actually thought the considered opinions of medical authorities, which were presumably based on their clinical experience as well as on their academic learning, more valuable in a practical work on fevers than conclusions reached via the logical subtleties encouraged by scho-

[20] "Quoniam nihil melius ad veritatis indagationem compertam existit quam providere [?] disputatione exercitatos ideo de cura febrium disputare propositum ut diversarum dicta que sibi repugnare videntur plerunque ad plenam reducantur concordiam ut tempora faciendarum medicinarum earum motus distinguantur et hoc totum auctoritate falcite et non sophystice apparentie vacillans," Taddeo, *Practica de febribus*, Padua, Biblioteca Universitaria, MS al numero provvisorio 202, fol. 107r.

lastic modes of debate; even so, he felt obliged to endorse the value of the question method and of disputation as such.

A special value naturally attached to questions disputed by celebrated medical masters, which were carefully collected and studied; thus, for example, a certain Paulus, who was a medical student or master at Padua in the 1340s, copied for his own use a series of questions by leading learned physicians of his own and the previous generation, including Mondino de' Liuzzi, Dino del Garbo, Dino's son Tommaso, and Gentile da Foligno.[21]

The importance attached to *questiones* as a tool of medical instruction is further attested by the very practice of compiling lists of the questions that were embedded in commentaries. Such lists occur in both manuscripts of the fourteenth and fifteenth centuries and in printed editions of the fifteenth and sixteenth centuries with sufficient frequency to lead one to suppose that they were regarded as valuable references by medieval and Renaissance students of medicine. Obviously the lists serve as detailed tables of contents to the works to which they are appended, but the presentation of the contents in this form suggests that those who studied these particular commentaries regarded them primarily as aggregates of *questiones*. Of interest in this connection is an edition of Turisanus's *Plusquam commentum* printed at Venice in 1557, which contains both a question register and an alphabetically arranged "Index of those things in the *Plusquam commentum* that seem to be specially worthy of note."[22] Evidently, in the mid-sixteenth century a question register was still thought worth printing, but it by then required the supplement of a modern subject index; the transition is one among many signs that medical scholasticism was at last nearing the end of its long life.

No consistent principle seems to have determined which commentaries would be provided with question registers. Probably the extent of the

[21] BAV, MS Vat. lat. 3144, where the medical questions occur mostly between fols. 11r and 38v. On the history of this codex, see note 64 to chapter six, above. The copyist, who appended his name and the date to several questions (see, for example, fols. 10v, 11v) also included marginal notes indicating the source of some of them; for example, at the foot of fol. 20r: "istam questionem habeo in libro questionum medicinalium in cuius principio est anatomia mundini."

[22] *Plusquam commentum in parvam Galeni artem Turisani Florentini Medici Praestantissimi* . . . (Venice, 1557). Both the "Index digressionum et dubitationum [all beginning "Utrum"] contentarum in Plusquam commento" and the alphabetically arranged "Index eorum quae in Plusquam commento adnotatu digna visa sunt" are placed at the beginning of the volume.

author's reputation counted for a great deal; thus the major commentaries of Dino, Taddeo, and Turisanus, which were still sufficiently in demand to merit printing some two centuries after their authors' lifetimes, are almost all equipped with question registers either in manuscript, in print, or both (see Appendix One). The commentaries of Mondino on Hippocratic and of Bartolomeo on Galenic works, which were never printed, are not accompanied by question registers either (although question titles are sometimes noted in the margins of the manuscripts). The existence of a question register in manuscript, however, is no guarantee of its subsequent appearance in print. For example, Dino del Garbo's *Chirurgia*, a commentary on the surgical portions of Book 4 of the *Canon*, is replete with lengthy *questiones* accorded full scholastic treatment (such as a discussion of whether *medicina generativa carnis* ought to be drying "beyond natural dryness," in which the author proceeded through a whole series of propositions, "*objecta in oppositum*," "*argumenta*," and "*responsiones*").[23] In a manuscript dated 1400 in the Biblioteca Estense, this work is accompanied by a register of 124 *questiones*,[24] but no register is to be found either in a manuscript in the British Library[25] or in the edition printed in Ferrara in 1489.

Question lists appear to be the work of copyists or editors rather than of the authors of the commentaries, since the lists sometimes vary in different manuscripts or editions of the same work, even though the text of the work remains substantially the same. For example, the list of 230 "*dubitationes*" (all beginning "*Utrum*") and "*digressiones*" appended to the edition of Turisanus's *Plusquam commentum* printed in Venice in 1512 differs from the longer list of 335 "*questiones*" found with the copy of the same work in MS Vat. lat. 4472.[26] Thus, the voluminous discussion of resolution and composition summarized in chapter five above is listed in the edition of 1512 under the following headings (the numbering is my own):

1. Digressio de processibus doctrinarum et sufficientia istarum
2. Utrum diffinitio habeatur per viam divisionis vel demonstrationis
3. Utrum doctrina resolutiva contineat omnia capitula huius libri.

[23] Dino, *Chirurgia*, sig. l[4r]-m3v.
[24] Modena, Biblioteca Estense, MS lat. 710 (alpha V.7.21), fols. 1r-102r, register of questions at fols. 101r-102r.
[25] London, British Library, MS Harley 4087.
[26] Cf. Turisanus, *Plusquam*, in the edition of Venice, 1512, fols. 137r-138r, with MS Vat. lat. 4472, fols. 19v-20v.

The copyist of MS Vat. lat. 4472 indexed the same discussion as follows:

1. Quare resolutiva fiat ex notione finis
2. Utrum via qua provehimur ad diffinitionem sit demonstratio divisio compositio vel aliquid aliud
3. Utrum per divisionem possit invenire diffinitio
4. Utrum ex doctrina resolutiva facile habeatur memoria. . . .

The titles found in the manuscript index occur in the text of the work in both manuscript and edition (for example, heading 2 in the manuscript list is found, word for word, in the text on fol. 4v of the 1512 edition); the sixteenth-century editor, either on his own initiative or following a separate manuscript tradition, simply preferred slightly broader titles (and fewer of them). Both lists accurately reflect the content of the work; and from the point of view of the reader, whether of the fourteenth, sixteenth, or twentieth century, there seems little to choose between the two versions.

As we turn to survey the subject matter of the *questiones* discussed by Taddeo and the other authors, as revealed in the approximately two thousand titles in the cumulated question register in Appendix One, it must be emphasized that question titles, even in this formidable quantity, are not infallible signposts to the scope and emphasis of thought in Taddeo's circle. As already noted, not all commentaries are provided with question registers; furthermore, question titles obviously tell us nothing about works in which the question method was not employed—for example, the *consilia* and collections of remedies that are the subject of the next chapter. In addition, the reader is once again reminded that the term *questio* is used in the registers to embrace both major pieces of analysis, to which their authors evidently devoted much thought and effort, and brief passing statements of opinion. Again, similar question titles may refer to very different kinds of discussion, while essentially parallel discussions may be concealed under different titles. Nonetheless, as will become apparent, the fourteenth- and fifteenth-century copyists and Renaissance editors were substantially justified in their assumption that question registers constitute an excellent introductory guide to and overview of the teaching of learned physicians.

On looking over the *questiones* of Taddeo and his colleagues, one is simultaneously struck by the prevalence of common themes and the absence of standard titles. The same broad topics are treated over and over again by different authors, but the duplication of question titles in exactly or almost exactly the same words is relatively rare. Rarely, too, did an author repeat the same questions in his different works, although Taddeo himself had a thrifty fondness for reusing the same questions in different commentaries and did so on a number of occasions.[27] The same question titles sometimes appear independently and in commentaries; titles that are repeated are frequently stock queries (such as the various questions about the existence and powers of "female sperm") that can also be found in the works of other authors outside the circle of Taddeo and cannot be in any special way linked with particular interests or trends of thought within it.[28] Obviously, repetition of question titles in any case says nothing about the independence or lack of independence of the argument itself.

Most of the questions by Taddeo and the others, and particularly those in their commentaries, are evidently a routine teaching device: standard, central aspects of medical learning such as complexion theory or the doctrine of the four principal members are argued in such a way as to acquaint the reader with the main lines of thought and authorities on the matter, but without any real polemics. A few questions, such as Turisanus's treatment of pulsation and Bartolomeo's rejection of Taddeo's views on the way in which the powers of medication are released in the body, are genuinely controversial in intent.[29] A still smaller number apparently reflect idiosyncratic interests of their authors—an example is Dino's discussion of laughter,[30] a subject that was also treated by Albertus Magnus[31] but was apparently not picked up by Taddeo or his other pupils.

The topics discussed by Taddeo and the other physicians under consideration provide abundant evidence that the use of *questiones* in medical

[27] For example, "Utrum omne aromaticum sit calidum et siccum," Taddeo, *Isagoge*, fol. 364v, and "Utrum maxima pars aromatum sit calida et sicca," Taddeo, *Aphor.*, fol. 136; "Utrum aqua possit digeri," Taddeo, *Isagoge*, fol. 379v, and "Utrum aqua digeratur," Taddeo, *Aphor.*, fol. 135; "Utrum morituri sint dietandi," Taddeo, *Aphor.*, fol. 8, and Taddeo, *Reg. acut.*, fol. 306v.

[28] For example, the question "Utrum solus sanguis nutriat," found in Taddeo, *Isagoge*, fol. 348v, recurs among the independent questions of Dino del Garbo (BAV, MS Vat. lat. 3144, fols. 13v-14v); the same question is to be found in Albertus Magnus, *Quaestiones super de animalibus*, ed. Filthaut, 3.20.

[29] Turisanus, *Plusquam*, fols. 47v-48v; Bartolomeo da Varignana, comm. *De complexionibus* (excerpt in Puccinotti, *Storia della medicina*, vol. 2, pt. 1, cxiii-cxv).

[30] "Ad solvendum dubitacionem, scilicet cuius virtutis risus sit passio," Munich, Bayerische Staatsbibliothek, CLM 7609, fol. 139 (140r).

[31] Albertus, *Quaestiones super de animalibus*, ed. Filthaut, 13.18.

teaching, even in a university faculty of arts and medicine, was by no means inseparably associated with an interest in abstract problems, with philosophically oriented subject matter, with a methodology derived from Aristotle's logic, or even, as already noted, with medical *theoria* rather than with *practica*. The *questio* was frequently a tool of practical medical instruction. Thus about two-thirds of the questions included in Appendix One concern the causes, nature, symptoms, course, and treatment of various kinds of disease and injury; this proportion excludes questions on astrological causation and the Aristotelian four causes and general questions on "signs" that do not refer explicitly to disease in the title. The 283 questions listed in one edition of Dino's *Dilucidatorium totius practice medicine* (that is, his commentary on *Canon* 1.4) are almost entirely given over to treatment, a subject examined in down-to-earth detail by means of such inquiries as "Whether vomiting should be provoked on two successive days."[32] Moreover, even Taddeo's commentary on the *Isagoge* and Turisanus's *Plusquam commentum*, both general introductory works by authors notably devoted to speculation and philosophical method, also contain large bodies of material on *practica*. Taddeo's Hippocratic commentaries, too, are almost wholly given over to the discussion of disease—its nature, diagnosis, and cure. These commentaries demonstrate the extent to which the continued study of the Hippocratic works, lacking as these were in a theoretical superstructure such as that of Aristotelian biology and psychology or Galenic physiology and complexion theory, perpetuated a tradition that was essentially practical.

Of the remaining questions, over five hundred concern the specifics of physiology and anatomy, and more than another hundred deal with signs and with healthful regimen. Another relatively large group examines basic definitions, some of which are discussed in chapter five above—definitions of medicine, health, sickness, the physician's task, and so on. By comparison, the number of questions devoted to subjects such as those treated in the foregoing chapters—the fundamentals of natural philosophy (form, matter, the elements, and so on), human psychology, meteorology, and astrology—is small indeed.

Sickness and injury, then, were the first concerns of these academically trained and philosophically inclined physicians; anatomy and physiology

---

[32] Dino, *Dilucidatorium*, chap. 13, q. 3. The question register in this edition, at fols. [62r-64r] following the separately foliated edition of Dino's *De virtutibus medicamentorum* bound with this printing of the *Dilucidatorium*, is fuller than that accompanying the *Dilucidatorium* in BAV, MS Vat. lat. 2484 (see note 19, above).

were the second. We must turn to a closer examination of these categories to gain a better idea of their main interests.

The questions on disease and trauma identify by name a fairly wide
range of specific conditions, including (among others) anthrax, apoplexy,
cancer, deafness, dropsy, dysentery, epilepsy, fractures, frenzy, hydropho-
bia, ophthalmia, pleurisy, stones in the kidney and bladder, retention of
urine, and wounds. As one might expect, however, a good deal of attention was also devoted to such broad categories as *apostemata* (any ulceration or tumor) and, above all, to fever. Following the tradition of the
ancient medical writers, fevers were elaborately classified into such categories as hectic, ephemeral, and periodic; and they were more frequently
discussed than any other named disease or condition.

In their rather infrequent investigations of the causes of diseases (some
eighty questions), the writers of course gave due weight to the humors,
complexions, and qualities; but they also considered such other factors as
the season and weather, overeating and overexertion, putrefaction, and
obstruction of the pores. Writing in an age relatively free of massive epidemics, they gave little attention to their causes; only a very few titles
refer to epidemics, pestilence, or corruption of the air. Dino del Garbo,
moreover, responded in the negative to the question whether pestilence
constitutes a distinct category of fever.[33] He held that pestilence can result
from corruption of the air brought about by hot, humid weather, but that
only those individuals will be affected whose bodies are already predisposed to this kind of sickness.

The question titles further indicate that a physician was expected to
monitor a variety of bodily processes and excreta for symptoms of disease,
including the density, color, odor, and turbidity of urine; the odor and
consistency of feces; the color of and presence or absence of blood in
sputum; and perspiration, breathing, appetite, and regularity of menstruation. Rather surprisingly, in view of Galen's prolix treatment of the
subject, there are few signs of any special attention to variations in pulse
as a symptom of ill health.

Much attention was given to treatment; it is clear from looking over
the numerous questions on this topic that physicians never questioned

---

[33] Dino, *Scriptum de differentiis febrium*, BAV, MS Vat. lat. 4450 (TK 1072), fols.
1-21v; the discussion of pestilential fever occupies fols. 4v-5v: "et sic apparet quod febris
pestilentialis debet reduci ad genus putridi et humoralis, verum est tamen quod pestilentialis febris potest esse aliquando effimera," fol. 5v.

that they commanded a variety of effective remedies. However, serious thought had to be given to the choice of treatment for particular categories of disease. As the tag went, practical medicine consisted of diet, medication, and surgery (*dieta, potio, chirurgia*); and each of these divisions is well represented in the question lists. Diet and other items in the regimen of the sick, such as bathing, seem to have attracted the least attention of the three types of treatment (that is, as far as *questiones* are concerned—diet and regimen were heavily emphasized in *consilia*, as will become apparent from the next chapter). Taddeo himself inquired about the role of diet in chronic and acute diseases and in cases of fever; and he also asked whether the food of those suffering from acute diseases should be salted, and how diet should be adjusted at different stages of illness. Turisanus, too, wrote briefly on the diet of the sick, and Dino on the timing of meals.[34] Much of the emphasis in discussions of treatment was placed on the concept of *evacuatio*—that is, ridding the body of harmful qualities, humors, or substances. *Evacuatio* was conceived as essentially a natural process in recovery from disease and was often carried out by means of the normal processes of elimination. If a physician succeeded in bringing about *evacuatio* he could, as several questions of Taddeo's pointed out, be thought of as in some sense imitating nature.[35] Artificially induced *evacuatio* could be achieved either by *potio* or by *chirurgia*: in addition to the administration of laxatives or, according to Dino, emetics, it could also be brought about by bloodletting, the subject of over sixty questions in Dino's *Dilucidatorium* and of briefer discussions by Taddeo and Guglielmo. That physicians were aware that *evacuatio*, whether natural or provoked, could be excessive is demonstrated by Dino's discussion of the appropriate treatment for simultaneous diarrhea and vomiting, and by Guglielmo's and Taddeo's questions on the signs to watch for during and after phlebotomy. Discussions of medicinal substances are also frequent: in addition to general questions about the complexions of medicines, the effectiveness of medication in particular diseases, and the circumstances in which medication should be prescribed, other questions categorize medicines as strong or weak, laxative, stupefacient, or emollient—and inquire precisely when and how they should be administered.

[34] Dino, "Quaestio famossimi Dini de Florentia de Coena et Prandio," in *Opera Andreae Thurini Piscaensis* . . . , fols. 149r-153v. The question is "an in prandio conveniat plus de cibo, quam in coena, an econverso."

[35] On the role attributed to nature by medieval physicians, see Luke Demaitre, "Nature and the Art of Medicine in the Middle Ages," *Medievalia* 2 (1976):23-47.

Individual medicinal substances are also sometimes discussed, although actual recipes are not very often found in works in which the question form plays a significant part.

Besides the particulars just reviewed, fundamental questions about disease and treatment were also raised; and definitions of what constitutes disease were carefully explored. Turisanus, for example, inquired whether starvation and overeating can be considered diseases, and Taddeo solemnly discussed whether the loss of a finger should be regarded as an affliction (*morbus*) in number or in quantity. More comprehensible to a modern reader, perhaps, is Taddeo's interest in questioning whether nature can cause sickness, whether one can be born sick, whether putrefaction can occur in the living body, and whether every disease in fact has its contrary (much medical treatment was based on the theory that diseases are cured by contraries). Dino devoted a lengthy question "proposed in the schools" to the subject of whether disease can be hereditary.[36] Some of the questions posed about treatment show a remarkable readiness to examine basic assumptions. Both Taddeo and Turisanus inquired about the relative importance of the activities of the physician compared with the body's own recuperative powers; Taddeo further discussed whether medical treatment can cure mortal sickness; Guglielmo asked "whether medication is useful";[37] Turisanus wanted to know if it is necessary to remove the cause of a disease for a cure to take place; and Guglielmo wondered whether a physician can cure a disease he does not understand (and whether, if he does effect such a cure, he can be said to know medicine). In most instances, however, the raising of these issues served to provide an opportunity for a qualified and cautious but nonetheless definite endorsement of the kind of medical activities described above. Thus, for example, Guglielmo's questioning of the usefulness of treatment by medication is based not on doubts about the effectiveness of known medical compounds, but on fears about the excessive strength of purgatives. He pointed out that the physician should never prescribe anything either dangerous or prematurely aging, and that medicinally in-

---

[36] "Questio proposita in scolis nostris fuit, utrum aliquis morbus qui esset in patri posset hereditari in filio," BAV, MS Vat. lat. 4454, fols. 99v-101r, with questions of Dino and probably his (a question with the same title is identified as Dino's in Paris, Bibliothèque de la Sorbonne, MS 128, fol. 113v, and in Munich, Bayerische Staatsbibliothek, CLM 13020, fols. 187v-188v).

[37] "Utrum farmacia competat," Guglielmo da Brescia, questions/commentary on *Canon* 1.4, Padua, Biblioteca Universitaria, MS al numero provvisorio 202, fol. 121v.

duced purging could be both. (The aging qualities attributed to purgatives presumably derived from the supposition that they provoke loss of radical moisture.) Other, safer ways of evacuating harmful humors were at hand in the shape of good regimen, massage, gentle medicines, and phlebotomy, the last of which Guglielmo, citing the authority of Galen, claimed to be safer than medication. He contended that there is indeed a place for strong purgatives in medical treatment, but that it is the physician's responsibility always to consider other modes of treatment, to use purgatives only when there was no alternative, and to mitigate their ill effects as far as possible.[38]

What is revealed in Guglielmo's discussion of this question is not skepticism about the effectiveness or usefulness of the medications known to him, but a generally modest (and realistic) level of expectation about results. The effects of good regimen, massage, and gentle medicines—amounting essentially to skillful nursing accompanied by soothing herbal drinks—he evidently regarded as the best that could normally be hoped for (for treatments prescribed in individual cases, the reader is referred to the following chapter). In many cases, these effects would of course have been far from negligible, but by contrast even the use of a strong purgative seemed an heroic remedy. The claim that purgatives are more dangerous than bloodletting perhaps implies that even the latter was in Guglielmo's practice usually a fairly restrained procedure.[39] In most instances, medical intervention could have had only a minor impact upon the course of a disease; and the expectations of physicians, and no doubt of their patients, were shaped accordingly.

Overlapping the two main categories of disease and injury on the one

[38] "id non competit nec debet a medico exhiberi quod inveterascit. . . . Item id quod est periculosum non debet exhiberi. . . . Item si possumus uti via securiori non debemus uti farmacia sed possumus uti via securiori ad evacuationem humorum ut bono regimine et fricationibus et resolventibus et medicinis non dando medicinas fortes. . . . Item si possumus uti via securiori non debemus uti periculosiori, sed via securior est flobotomia . . . apparet per G[alenum] secundo regiminis, dicit enim quod flobotomia est via secura evacuanda farmacia autem periculosa. . . . debemus ea farmacia uti restringendo eam ab eius malicia," ibid.

On the duty of the physician to preserve and extend life, see further McVaugh, "The 'Humidum Radicale,'" passim; and for the similar caution about phlebotomy of Bernard of Gordon, see Demaitre, "Nature and the Art of Medicine," p. 32.

[39] But Dino del Garbo's question "Utrum liceat cum farmaco evacuare usque ad sincopim, sicut cura flobothomia (*Dilucidatorium* 3.23) indicates that the approach was not always so cautious.

hand, and physiology and anatomy on the other, is a large group of questions on complexion theory and the qualities.[40] The concept of *complexio* (that is, the balance of the qualities of hot, cold, wet, and dry) was, as we have already seen, fundamental to physiological explanation and also to much medical treatment. The theory of *complexio* was an all-embracing one that on the whole provided a flexible and satisfying general explanation of many kinds of physical, physiological, and even psychological changes; but its practical applications were elusive and gave rise to endless discussion. Questions about it range from the highly philosophical and abstract (Taddeo's "Is complexion to be identified with specific form?") to the apparently pragmatic (Bartolomeo's "Can bad complexion [*mala complexio*] be identified by touch?").[41] The ramifications of the theory were almost limitless. For example, not only did each individual human being have his or her own *complexio innata*, but the parts of the body all had *complexiones* of their own. Not only had the latter *complexiones* to be determined (for example, by Taddeo's "Is the liver of cold complexion?"), but the effects of the *complexio* of one organ upon that of another had to be considered (as by Turisanus's question "whether the brain [traditionally of cold complexion] can work against the hot heart"). Again, the functioning of an individual organ was presumably affected by its complexion, a consideration that led Bartolomeo to inquire whether a temperate or a hot stomach performs digestion better. The theory of complexion and of the qualities was of course also intimately involved with humoral physiology. The general pattern of associations between the qualities and humors was established by long tradition (for example, phlegm is cold and wet, choler hot and dry); but the precise complexional makeup of each humor could still be the subject of discussion, as when Taddeo inquired whether black bile is drier than choler.

The effects of complexion on bodily states and activities, and vice versa, also had to be taken into account. Accordingly, physicians wrote various questions about the effect of the emotions, of sexual intercourse, and of exercise on complexion; about the relationship of parental complexion to

[40] For a recent account of some major aspects of complexion theory in this period, see McVaugh's introduction to Arnald of Villanova, *Aphorismi de gradibus* (vol. 2 in his *Opera Medica Omnia*).

[41] For the Latin, and location, of this and other question titles quoted in this chapter see Appendix One. Separate annotation is provided only when the content of a question is discussed or when the English translation is not obvious.

the sex of offspring; and about the way individual complexion affects the functioning of the nervous system and leads to stoutness or emaciation. Complexion was also held to be age- and sex-linked; discussion in this area tended to debate the possible limits of individual variations. For example, a standard question discussed both by Taddeo and Dino and by various other authors outside the group with which we are here concerned was: Given that women are generally colder in complexion than men, can any woman ever be hotter in complexion than any man?[42] Questions touching on changes in complexion produced by age ranged from Dino and Turisanus's inquiries about which complexion is most productive of longevity to Taddeo's practical concern with the appropriate variation in diet for different age groups.

External factors affecting human complexion were believed to include climate, disease, and ingested substances. Different ailments not only disturbed the complexion of the afflicted patient, they also had complexions of their own. Numerous questions classify illnesses as *frigidi* or *calidi*; and a fair number refer to the complexion of named conditions, most notably and obviously fever, but also apoplexy, *ptisis*, and wounds. The celebrated difference of opinion between physicians about whether wounds should be kept dry or moist was no doubt perceived by those involved as concerning a practical application of complexion theory. (Both Taddeo and Turisanus followed the Bolognese tradition and opted for dry.)[43] Yet other questions explore the association of named symptoms—vomiting, bad blood (*sanies*), *suffocatio*, cold sweats, among others—with particular kinds of complexion.

The imbalance in complexion produced by disease might be treated by the prescription of medicines that not merely affected but also possessed complexion. The physicians of Taddeo's circle discussed the complexion of various medicinal substances (Taddeo followed his Hippocratic sources

---

[42] For example, by Albertus Magnus, *Quaestiones super de animalibus*, ed. Filthaut, 15.6.

[43] "Utrum omne vulnus debeat desiccari vel non" and "Utrum dato quod omne vulnus debeat dessicari et dessicantia debeant esse sicca in tertio gradu," Taddeo, *Isagoge*, fol. 398r; "Utrum universaliter in vulnere complexio servetur per exiccantia," Turisanus, *Plusquam*, fol. 113r. From antiquity until centuries after Taddeo's day many physicians held that the use of moist salves and unguents on wounds was beneficial because this treatment was observed to encourage the formation of "laudable pus"; the belief that some pus was a necessary concomitant of healing no doubt arose because almost all wounds became infected to a greater or lesser extent, so that a mild infection was perceived as part of the healing process; see Guido Majno, *The Healing Hand*, pp. 183-184.

in giving much attention to wine in this connection) and the relative usefulness of medicines with different qualities. However, they seem to have given only limited attention to the question of determining degree or intensity of qualities in medicines, a subject that some of the physicians of Montpellier treated at length.[44]

In addition to exploring specific questions raised by complexion theory, Taddeo and his associates also reconsidered the fundamentals of the theory itself, in an apparent attempt to eliminate some of its vagueness, inconsistency, and awkwardness. In defining *complexio* both Taddeo and Mondino reminded their readers that the term should be used in practice only as a comparative, not as an absolute: they pointed out that the only way to define a particular complexion is to describe its relative intensity ("hot and wet in the second degree," and so on), to compare it with the ideal for the species or individual, or to compare complexion in life with complexion after death in the same species or individual.[45] Efforts were also made to determine exactly how the complexion of medicines and the complexion of those who ingested them interacted; thus Bartolomeo asked whether the powers of medicine are released by the heat of the human body, and whether, if so, the effect of cold medicine is changed by its encounter with bodily heat; Turisanus inquired whether a medicine hotter than the body can be actuated by it. Bartolomeo's discussion of the problem led him vigorously to repudiate Taddeo's views on the same subject.[46] At least two subsequent authors who treated the general topic of "the reduction of medicine to act" (that is, the release of the powers of medicine in the human body)—namely, Tommaso del Garbo and Gentile da Foligno—drew heavily upon these discussions in the circle of Taddeo. Tommaso, who lost no opportunity of proclaiming himself the son of *"olim famossimi medici Dini,"* expounded his father's views; Gentile, as we have already noted, summarized the opinions of every author treated in the present work—Taddeo, Gentile da Cingoli, Gu-

[44] See Michael R. McVaugh, "Quantified Medical Theory and Practice at Fourteenth-Century Montpellier," *Bulletin of the History of Medicine* 43 (1969), 397-413. One of the few questions by Taddeo that does touch on "degree" is cited in the preceding note.

[45] Taddeo, *Isagoge*, fols. 347r-v; Mondino, comm. *Tegni*, BAV, MS Vat. lat. 4466, fol. 64v. Of the two, Taddeo is the more explicit about the need always to specify with what standard any actual complexion is being compared.

[46] Bartolomeo da Varignana, comm. *De complexionibus*, excerpt in Puccinotti, *Storia della medicina*, vol. 2, pt. 1, pp. cxiii-cxv.

glielmo da Brescia, Bartolomeo da Varignana, Turisanus, Dino, and Mondino—referring to each of them by name before proceeding to his own exposition.[47]

But the principal difficulty connected with *complexio* was that it appeared to be simultaneously an immutable and a mutable characteristic. Its close association with concepts of specific and even of substantial form meant that *complexio* was often thought of as almost identical or identical with the essential determining, identifying, or active quality that made each complexioned thing (species, compound, organ, and individual human being) what it was.[48] Yet, as the foregoing account of questions asked about particular aspects of complexion shows, the complexion of individual human beings was at the same time thought of as something that changed with age, with the attack of disease, with the administration of medicines, and even with changes in the weather. How were these two ideas about complexion reconcilable? Taddeo, and in the next generation Turisanus and Dino, all addressed themselves to this central concern; some of their arguments are outlined below.

In a question that both survives in independent form and is also incorporated into his commentary on the *Tegni*, Taddeo inquired "whether innate complexion can be changed."[49] In his exposition, Taddeo first assembled an impressive list of authorities who had claimed that innate complexion cannot be changed—including, besides the assertions of various medical authors, a statement of Aristotle's to the effect that anything that inheres in something by nature cannot be changed into its contrary.

[47] Tommaso del Garbo, . . . *Summa medicinalis . . . Tractatus eiusdem de reductione medicinarum ad actum* (Venice, 1506), fol. 117v: "Gentilis enim de Fulgineo in questione quam disputavit de hoc longitudinem fecit quam plurimam tediosam . . . Galienus autem pro certo est opinatus si quis attente inspicit eius dicta, et primo 3° *De simplici medicina* et 3° *De complexionibus*, quem Dynus sequitur sicut evangelium et eius mentem perfecte dilucidat in 2° *Canonis* et nimis prolixe." The last thing that would occur to a modern reader is to praise Dino for his brevity, but all things are relative. For Gentile's use of our authors, see the Introduction, above.

[48] Despite the association of complexion with specific form, medieval physicians normally assumed that in human beings complexion and the balance of humors were individual characteristics, inasmuch as one person might be described as more or less choleric, phlegmatic, etc., than another.

[49] BAV, MS Reg. lat. 2000, fols. 115v-116v, explicit "Explicit questio determinata per magistrum tadeum in septimo terapeutice"; cf. *Thaddei Florentini . . . in C. Gal. Microtechnen Commentarii . . .* (Naples, 1522), fols. 107v-110v. The printed version includes additional material at the end of the question and the parallel passages have numerous variants, but there is no doubt that the text is substantially the same.

He noted that, according to Avicenna, each individual has his own unique complexion, which prepares him for the reception of specific form, which is immutable. Moreover, if complexion could change at all, it would certainly be changed by a fever; but this would not be possible without a change in the natural complexion of all the blood, since fever is in the blood. But if such a change took place, life could not continue. Furthermore, the *virtus vitalis*, which produces life, is received in the organs only by the mediation of *spiritus*; and *spiritus*, again according to Avicenna, has complexion. If this complexion were changed by fever, life would end. On the other side of the case were: the universal assumption of medical authors that human complexion can be affected by external conditions, especially disease, attack, and treatment; the logical argument that whatever can be intensified or diminished is variable; the known fact that complexion alters with age (if it did not, man could live forever, which is patently false); and an anecdote of Galen's about a poisonous tree that lost its venom on being moved from Persia to Egypt, thus showing that its specific form and hence its complexion had changed. Taddeo's solution was to postulate two kinds of complexion: one is a balance of qualities that can be disturbed by sickness and other factors, the other something that comes into being in the body as a result of the mixture of spermatic moisture and menstrual blood at the time of conception. Nobody, Taddeo asserted, doubts that complexion in the first sense can change; hence the argument concerns only complexion in the second sense. Some people absurdly say that complexion in this sense cannot change but can only be corrupted, thus applying to *complexio* something true only of substantial form. Taddeo's own opinion was that complexion in both senses is subject to change when change occurs in the substance in which the complexion exists; any other solution is frivolous.[50]

[50] "an complexio innata permutetur. . . . Ad evidentiam huius questionis est notandum quod complexio innata dicitur dupliciter, uno quidem modo dicitur complexio bona secundum quam animal perficit suas operationes . . . et resultat talis complexio ex debita proportione qualitatum. . . . Dicitur alio modo complexio innata complexio que sequitur prima componentia corpus [*sic*] scilicet humidum spermaticum et sanguinem menstruum: *et hanc complexionem non solum habent membra spermatica sed etiam sanguinea.* . . . Et de hac dubitaverunt quidam quod non posset permutari, sed ponebant eam corrumpi quod est valde absurdum. Nam sola forma substantialis est illa que corrumpitur et non alteratur. Ego autem dico complexionem in natum [*sic*] secundum utrunque significatum alterari secundum alterationem subiecti in quo est . . . et concedo omnes rationes ad hanc partem adductas, et si locus concederet destruerem omnes solutiones frivolas que fuerunt adducte per quosdam," Taddeo, comm. *Tegni* (Naples, 1522), fols. 107v-108v.

Turisanus, who included in his *Plusquam commentum* the question "whether permutation from the natural complexion is possible," used some of the same authorities and arguments put forward by Taddeo. Dino's discussion of the subject is to be found both in his commentary on *De malicia complexionis diverse*—which in fact rehearses a question "disputed in the schools in the first year of our lectureship in Siena" whether the complexion of all parts of the body is affected by the *mala complexio* associated with fever[51]—and in his independent question, also "disputed in the schools" (year unstated), "whether natural complexion can be changed."[52] In the latter, after citing some of the same authorities noted by both Taddeo and Turisanus, Dino listed several reasons why it might be supposed impossible that complexion could change, among them the fact that complexion is a *prima passio* of the thing in which it exists and hence derives from *principia naturalia* and is immutable; moreover, if it were possible to change the natural complexion, then life could be prolonged indefinitely (he noted that the proponents of the immutability of complexion did not allow that the loss of radical moisture throughout life, which was generally agreed to cause the process of aging, constituted a change in natural complexion). The arguments presented by Dino in favor of the possibility of change in complexion have to do, once again, with disease and treatment. His own conclusion was that in one

[51] "Quia intencio est nostra est [*sic*] edere tractatum quendam de malicia complexionis diverse in quo dilucidatur intencio Galieni in libro de ma [*sic*] malicia complexionis . . . ut melius cognoscatur eius natura, ideo fuit questio disputata in scolis primo anno nostre lecture in civitate senarum: Utrum in febre in qua est mala complexio diversa, complexio in omnibus partibus tocius corporis . . . leditur. . . . Explicit tractatus de malicia complexionis diverse disputata per dinum de florencia medicine scientie doctorem mcccxxvii in civitate senarum," BAV, MS Vat. lat. 2484, fols. 196v-210r. Presumably this means that Dino went back to a question he had disputed early in his professorship at Siena and reworked it into his commentary on *De malicia complexionis diverse*—an interesting glimpse of method.

[52] [101] "Questio disputata in scolis fuit utrum complexio naturalis possit permutari. . . . [101v] respondeo ad questionem cum queritur utrum complexio naturalis possit permutari quia aut loqueris de complexione naturalis que insequitur preparacionem principiorum corporis . . . [102r] aut loqueris de complexione naturali que insequitur proporcionem principiorem. . . . Si quidem loqueris de prima dico quod illa complexio permutatur ymo non solum permutatur ymo necessario permutatur . . . nam videmus quod complexio pueritie non manet. . . . Si autem loqueris de secunda complexione naturali . . . aut est sermo de complexione que in individuo inest principaliter propter formam specificam quantum in ea cadit diversitas in qua unus dicitur flegmaticus, alter collericus, alter sanguineus, alter melancolicus, alter vero temperatus, aut loqueris de complexione naturali que inest individuo ex parte conditionum materialium . . . de prima dico quod illa permutari non potest," Dino, question, BAV, MS Vat. lat. 4454, fols. 101(131)r-102(132)r.

sense complexion not only does change but changes of necessity, as the child grows into the youth and the youth into the man. He further distinguished two additional meanings of complexion: on the one hand there is a kind of complexion linked with specific form, referred to when one man is described as phlegmatic, another as choleric, and so forth, and this does not change; on the other hand complexion is something present in the individual in connection with matter and the condition of matter, and complexion in this sense can and does change as that condition changes.

After complexion, the governing forces in the body were considered to be the humors (the balance of which was, of course, in some sense at once the manifestation, product, and cause of complexion), *spiritus*, and the various virtues. Questions about the humors as such are, however, very much fewer in number than those about complexion, even if all questions about the nature and function of blood are included under the category of humor. General inquiries about the humors include whether any humor is found in the human body in pure form (twice asked by Taddeo), whether the humors are generated solely in the liver, and whether a humor receives its species from matter. Of the individual humors, choler and blood were more frequently discussed than phlegm or melancholy. Questions about choler dealt with the way in which it was produced, its location in the body, and its role in the digestive process. The principal enigmas concerning blood appear to have been the nature and source of frothy blood (*sanguis spumosus*), which Taddeo connected with the lungs and Turisanus with the heart; the possibility of the putrefaction of blood, explored by the same two authors; and whether nutrition is carried out by means of blood alone, a question asked by both Taddeo and Dino.

Of *spiritus*, the substance that supposedly flowed through the arteries distributing the force of life through the body, Taddeo asked whether it is the vehicle of *virtus animalis* (the power of the sensitive soul associated with the brain) as well as of *virtus vitalis* (the lifegiving power associated with the heart). He concluded that, according to the physicians (*secundum medici*), there are three separate forms of *spiritus*, each carrying one of the three virtues: *vitalis*, *animalis*, and *naturalis*. (The thrust of a discussion by Turisanus about the relation of *spiritus* to *virtus vitalis* has already been indicated in chapter six.) Other problems connected with *spiritus* included whether or not it could putrefy, whether it existed in insensible things, whether *spiritus vitalis* was more rarefied (*subtilior*) than *spiritus animalis*, whether blood flowed in the arteries along with *spiritus*, and how *spiritus* was nourished. The most salient feature of these question titles is their assumption of the essentially corporeal nature of *spiritus*, an assumption which, as already noted, had since antiquity distinguished medical from philosophical or theological treatments of the *pneuma*. Most discussions of the virtues explained how particular bodily functions were carried out by an appropriate virtue (such as digestion by a *virtus digestiva*), but there are also to be found a few general questions about the virtues as such. Into this category, for example, fall the inquiries by Taddeo and Turisanus already discussed (in chapters six and seven, above) concerning the respective functions of *virtus vitalis, animalis,* and *naturalis,* and considering whether any one permanent virtue lasts throughout life.

Complexion, the humors, and virtues provided the basic theoretical structure of Hippocratic-Galenic physiology. The application of these concepts was often arbitrary or confusing, in Galen's own case as well as in that of his medieval followers. But Galen's own exposition of his theories had been accompanied by close observations of both anatomy and function in men and animals. In the case of Taddeo and his colleagues, however, even if the questions on complexion, humors, and virtues are set aside, a survey of the remaining question titles on physiological and anatomical topics supports the conclusion that they found it more important to attempt to provide an intellectually coherent account of the chief bodily processes and functions than to engage in anatomical description. Within the general category of physiology and anatomy the two most frequently discussed topics were reproduction and the whole process of nourishment, digestion, excretion, and growth.

Many of the questions on reproduction reflect the debate over the respective merits of the Aristotelian and Galenic accounts of generation described above in chapter six. Thus the female role in conception (whether women generate sperm and to what end, and whether their sperm is endowed with *virtus activa*) was the subject of questions by Taddeo, and subsequently Turisanus, Dino, and Mondino—every one of the writers in the group who is known to have discussed the physiology of reproduction at any length. The inheritance of parental characteristics, another standard component of the Aristotelian-Galenic debate over male and female roles in generation, was treated by Taddeo, Dino, and Mondino. Taddeo, Dino, and Turisanus each inquired into the function of the testicles; Dino and Turisanus both asked the related question whether the semen is the product of the whole body or only of a part of it. Taddeo and Dino discussed the Aristotelian supposition that the heart is the first organ to be formed in the fetus and further inquired whether the male sperm actually becomes part of the matter of the fetus (or whether, as in Aristotle's view, it acts as a solidifying agent upon the matter provided by the mother, as rennet curdles milk).

Other standard questions on reproduction that were treated by the group include the ancient query whether an eighth-month child could survive (Dino and Mondino), and another old favorite used, one imagines, to brighten the monotony of many a lecture—"Whether man or woman takes more pleasure in sexual intercourse" (Mondino and Taddeo).[53] The remainder of the questions on reproduction vary widely in topic, although most of them repeat the subject matter discussed by earlier authors, most notably by the author of the Hippocratic *De natura fetus*, but also by Aristotle, Avicenna, and Albertus Magnus. Dino and Turisanus inquired into the role of the various virtues, *spiritus*, and the soul; Dino, Taddeo, and Mondino all investigated the reasons for and process of sexual differentiation of the fetus *in utero*; Dino and Taddeo discussed lactation; and, as noted above, Dino (following the Hippocratic text on which he was commenting) asked several questions about plant reproduction. Also discussed were the causes of multiple births, the possibility of successive conception, the reasons for the color of the menses, puberty, sterility, and pain in childbirth. One does not, however, receive the impression of any special interest in practical obstetrics, a skill no doubt largely left to midwives, except perhaps from Taddeo's questions about abortifacients and the proper means of calculating the months of pregnancy, and from his inquiry whether sneezing brings on labor.

A synthesis of philosophical and medical teaching regarding the process of nutrition and its relationship to the preservation of life and to growth was achieved in the Latin West in the course of the thirteenth century,

[53] Cr. Albertus Magnus, *Quaestiones super de animalibus*, ed. Filthaut, 5.4. Other authors also discussed this question, including Peter of Abano.

largely owing to the work of Albertus Magnus.[54] The philosophical aspects of nutrition continued to fascinate Taddeo and some of his pupils, as may be seen from the outline in chapter six above of their discussions of form and matter. Various questions about the "ages" into which human life is divided should also be fitted, for the most part, into the context of discussion of growth and the maintenance of life. Speculation about the fundamental nature of nutrition and growth further took the form of inquiries about the location and powers of the *virtus nutritiva* (which, following Galen, was usually held to reside in the liver) and of the *virtus augmentativa*. Taddeo asked whether the two virtues are in fact one and the same; Turisanus speculated whether nutrition is a form of generation. Other questions on the subject included Taddeo's "whether nutrition is through the contrary or the similar" and "whether any food is pure nourishment [without mixture]" and his more prosaic "whether the hair receives nourishment." Still other questions reflect the general belief in a threefold process of digestion, each stage progressively refining away more impurities and providing a yet purer nourishment than the last; thus Mondino inquired whether sediment in urine is a product of the second digestion or the third, and Taddeo wanted to know if it is the byproduct of the conversion of food into blood.

Apparently excretion fitted into the overall picture of nutrition and growth only with difficulty, if we judge by Taddeo's "whether we ought to excrete fully digested material" and "whether good *habitudines* should finally be evacuated." The problem no doubt arose from the desire to find a common rationale for the excretion of body wastes and of semen, the latter being regarded as the ultimate and most refined product of the third digestion. A related problem, raised by Dino and Mondino, was whether vomiting could be regarded as a natural and therefore beneficial means of evacuation. Much attention was paid to urine, perhaps largely because variations in its appearance were regarded as an important diagnostic tool; the questions asked include whether urine represents the evacuation proper to any particular member (presumably in the sense that vomiting could be regarded as an evacuation of the stomach), whether it is the residue solely of ingested fluids, and not of solids, whether the color of urine is produced by *alteratio* or *permixtio*, and

---

[54] See Joan Cadden, "The Medieval Philosophy and Biology of Growth: Albertus Magnus, Thomas Aquinas, Albert of Saxony, and Marsilius of Inghen on Book I, Chapter v of Aristotle's *De generatione et corruptione*," Ph.D. diss., Indiana Univ., 1971.

which came first, color or density. Urinary sediment was much discussed, being the subject of a lengthy independent *questio* (in effect a short treatise) by Turisanus.[55]

After generation, nutrition, and growth, the aspect of physiology that attracted most attention seems to have been sense perception. The views of Taddeo and his associates on the physiology and psychology of the senses have been discussed at some length in chapter seven above and will not be further examined here. A very small number of questions also touch upon respiration, the voice, and the effects of exercise.

Turning to discussions of particular parts of the body, and again excluding questions about complexion, one finds that the emphasis is still on explanation of function rather than description of form. Questions were asked about a fairly large number of different organs and body parts, including the heart, brain, spinal cord, liver, testicles (see the remarks on reproduction above), flesh, bones, muscles, nerves, arteries, veins, stomach, spleen, nails, and hair. Much of the treatment of the heart, brain, liver, arteries, veins, and nerves concerned the Aristotelian-Galenist dispute over whether there are one or four principal members in the body (and the related questions whether the nervous system is dominated by the heart or the brain and the venous system by the heart or the liver), a controversy that has already been discussed in an earlier chapter. Other questions about these organs concern their origin, as in Taddeo's "whether the brain is generated from menstrual blood" and "whether the liver is a spermatic member"—that is, an organ formed in the fetus from the substance of the paternal sperm rather than from the matter contributed by the mother. The pulsation of the heart and arteries, the subject of two brief *questiones* by Taddeo, was a topic of special interest for Turisanus, who devoted to it a lengthy *"digressio"* and three questions.[56]

As we have seen, Turisanus discussed at length the belief of "Galen and almost all the school of physicians" (*medicorum schola*) that the heartbeat and pulsation are caused by a virtue of the soul and constitute the first, lifegiving operation of the soul in the body (see chapter six, above). His account of pulsation must be placed in the context of his opinion of the Galenic idea that pulsation is a manifestation of *virtus vitalis*. According to Galenic physiology, pulsation and respiration are

---

[55] "Quesito de ypostasi," printed with Turisanus, *Plusquam*, fols. 138r-141r.
[56] Turisanus, *Plusquam*, fols. 47v-48v.

essentially similar in nature and purpose, since both serve to draw puri-
fying and cooling air into the system (in respiration, via the lungs, and
in pulsation, via imperceptible pores [*insensibiles poros*]); in pulsation,
the dilation and constriction of the vessels not only brings in air to purify
the *spiritus* pouring out from the heart into the arteries, but also regulates
its flow. In one of the pithiest statements to be found of the criteria behind much physiological speculation, Turisanus admitted that the Galenist
explanation of pulsation saves the appearances and contains no falsity of
a kind liable to hinder the physician in his work;[57] nonetheless he himself rejected the explanation as untrue, largely on philosophical grounds.
Turisanus pointed out that if pulsation is caused by a virtue of the soul,
this obviously is not by rational or sensitive virtue and cannot even be
by vegetative virtue (the last must be excluded because pulsation is
neither generation, nor growth, nor alteration). That leaves only *virtus
appetitus*, the only virtue of the soul capable of causing local motion. Yet
it is not clear that the movement of pulse can properly be described as
local, since it does not cause any body or part of a body to move from
its place. Some, Turisanus continued, attribute pulsation to the same form
of *virtus appetitus* that causes somewhat similar motions in other body
parts, namely Galen's *virtus attractiva* and *expulsiva*, which he made
responsible for digestive and puerperal contractions. Turisanus rejected
this hypothesis, pointing out that contractions of the kind supposedly
caused by the *virtus attractiva* and *expulsiva* are incidental to particular
bodily functions and occur only when needed, whereas pulsation and
heartbeat go on all the time. He also refused to accept the idea that
pulsation serves to regulate the flow of *spiritus* through the arteries, main-
taining that *spiritus* does not flow through the inner cavities of the arteries, but is transmitted along their outer walls, a theory he derived from
the analogy of the nerves, which have no apparent inner cavity to transmit *virtus sensitiva* through the body. Turisanus himself opted for the
Aristotelian explanation that pulsation is the result of a mechanical ebul-
lition occurring when the blood is heated, a process comparable to the
boiling up of any other fluid when heat is applied—and he firmly denied

[57] "Sed nos istis opinionibus [BAV, MS Urb. lat. 244, fol. 88r: positionibus] non in
totum consentimus: quamvis enim ab eis sufficienter apparentium cause demonstrentur;
neque per eas ullo modo impediatur medicus in suis operationibus, nihilominus tamen
falsitatem habent," ibid., fol. 47v.

that the process is in any way connected with soul.[58] Turisanus's rejection of part of the Galenic system of virtues and his preference for a mechanistic explanation of physiological function seems almost to foreshadow seventeenth-century developments,[59] but more to the point is the example that his discussion provides of the fruitful results that could on rare occasions be achieved in physiological investigation by the use of the scholastic *questio* and the application of principles of Aristotelian natural philosophy.

The foregoing brief review of the way Taddeo and his colleagues used the *questio* format reveals them as physicians whose primary interest was in understanding and treating disease, that is, in *practica*. But their *practica*, although more eclectic and pragmatic than their *theoria*, was nonetheless grounded in large part on the authority of ancient and Arabic writers and organized in scholastic fashion for purposes of teaching and discussion.[60] The chief function of *theoria* emerges as the provision of intellectually respectable accounts of basic bodily functions: reproduction, digestion, excretion, sense perception, and so forth. Many of the *questiones* on *theoria* illuminate the way in which this branch of medical science was at once more systematic and cohesive and yet more open to speculation and intellectual exploration than was *practica*; the boundaries of hypothesis were usually only that explanations be rationally coherent, justified by reference to ancient authority, and, as Turisanus put it, that they save the appearances without misleading the physician into harmful treatment. It simply was not possible, in most instances, to demonstrate whether or not an explanation that saved the appearances

---

[58] "non erit talis motus [of pulse] rationabiliter attributus alicui virtutum anime. Adhuc autem cum talis motus sit passio quedam similis ebulitioni: sicut dicit Aristoteles si autem invenire [*sic*] talem motum in quocumque humido exteriori calefacto ubi non est anima, non poterimus iuste nec proprie tribuere anime: sicut attribuimus motum attractionis et expulsionis per villos factum: quorum simile non est reperire in non animatis," ibid., fol. 48r.

[59] I am grateful to Professor Jerome Bylebyl of the Institute of the History of Medicine of The Johns Hopkins University for helpful observations regarding the significance of Turisanus's views on pulse.

[60] Further discussion of the role of scholasticism in medical works given over to *practica* is to be found in Demaitre, "Scholasticism in Compendia of Practical Medicine," and idem, "Theory and Practice in Medical Education at the University of Montpellier in the Thirteenth and Fourteenth Centuries," *Journal of the History of Medicine and Allied Sciences* 30 (1975):103-123.

was also physically true. Physicians had practical operations to carry out that would be hindered by a theory that was too grossly erroneous; but the allowable margin, from the point of view of practice, was wide indeed. Despite the formulations produced by Taddeo and the other authors about the interdependence of theory and practice (see chapter five, above), and despite their serious attempts to base prescriptions in individual cases on sound theoretical grounds (see chapter nine, below), it is clear that there were broad areas of physiological science that did not provide and were not expected to provide much guidance when it came to deciding on treatment. The strongest link between physiological and pharmacological theory and medical practice was probably complexion theory, a consideration that may do much to explain the importance attached to the latter. In medical teaching, it was largely the question method itself that joined *theoria* and *practica*, giving to both a common structure and system.[61] But how did medical teaching, of both *theoria* and *practica*, affect practice itself? For the answer to that question we must turn to the next chapter.

[61] For recent views of the relation between theory and practice at Montpellier in the same period, see McVaugh, "Quantified Medical Theory and Practice," and Demaitre, "Theory and Practice." McVaugh points to certain disjunctions between theory and practice, especially in pharmacology, while Demaitre notes the links between them. The two authors are, however, dealing with different aspects of a complex situation.

CHAPTER NINE

THE PRACTICE OF MEDICINE

According to *Bartolomeo de Varignana, who was repeating a commonplace, all medical learning is ultimately practical in purpose.*[1] *There can be no question that the treatment of the sick and the* regulation of the regimen of the healthy was the goal of the medicine studied and taught by Taddeo and his colleagues and pupils. As far as they are concerned, at any rate, nothing is further from the truth than the idea that scholastic medicine was a closed intellectual system in which the treatment of patients played little part; on the contrary, beyond the institutional, intellectual, and pedagogical system so far surveyed always lay the final reality of the confrontation of doctor and patient. The economic importance of practice for university teaching physicians has already been noted. But practice meant much more than economic return, even though the extent to which the medical learning of the schools was actually employed in the treatment of patients is not always clear: recent scholarship has demonstrated that, in the period with which this study is concerned, certain of the current refinements of academic medical teaching had little impact upon the actual practice even of learned physicians.[2] But, as will become apparent, the teaching of the schools plainly did help to shape clinical practice in important ways, just as the physician's personal familiarity with sick bodies did, if not always overtly, affect his medical and indeed his philosophical learning. Obviously, too, the social and intellectual influence of the medical profession sprang in part from the relations between doctors and patients; analysis of the nature of practice may reveal more clearly the basis of that beneficial confidence in the physician that Gentile da Cingoli and Mondino de' Liuzzi labored to explain.

Yet it must be admitted that the precise nature of the practice of Tad-

---

[1] See chapter five, above.

[2] See McVaugh, "Quantified Medical Theory and Practice," pp. 397-413. For a somewhat negative evaluation of the impact of medical scholasticism on practice, see also John M. Riddle, "Theory and Practice in Medieval Medicine," *Viator: Medieval and Renaissance Studies* 5 (1974):157-183.

deo and those associated with him, and of other medieval learned physicians, is in many respects elusive. The problem does not lie in an absence of sources; on the contrary, written works attesting to their practice by Taddeo and other members of the group are fairly numerous (as are passing allusions to their own practice in their other writings).[3] All of them other than Gentile, who was not a physician, and Turisanus, whose limited or unsuccessful practice was sufficiently unusual to become a matter of comment, left surviving material in one or more of the categories—collections of remedies, *experimenta* (that is, tried and tested medicaments), regimens of health and *consilia* for individual patients, and works with the word "*practica*" in the title—that give specific and detailed recommendations for the treatment of various complaints.[4]

What is difficult to determine is the extent to which these works describe what was actually observed and done. Let us first consider the type of work that is presumably the most accurate historical record of the individual patients and complaints actually treated by Taddeo and the other physicians here discussed—that is, the *consilium*. A *consilium*, as the name suggests, purports to be professional advice written down in response to an individual request for counsel. While Taddeo has occasionally been credited with inventing the genre in medieval medical writing, this is unlikely; Michael Scot produced at least one similar description of an individual case in which he had been consulted while residing at Bologna in 1220.[5] The evolution of medical *consilia* at Bologna parallels, and was probably influenced by, that of legal *consilia*; the latter be-

---

[3] Thus, for example, Mondino, in discussing "apostematum in stomacho" in his commentary on Hippocrates' *Prognostica*, remarked, "vidistis alio anno quod quidam habuit apostematum in stomacho quod fuit ruptum ad interiora, administrari feci lavativa et abstersiva et liberatus fuit. sed nunquam vidi quod rumperetur [*sic*] ad exteriora quod quis liberaretur," Mondino, *Pronost.*, BAV, MS Vat. lat. 4466, fol. 10r. Similarly, Guglielmo da Brescia described what he claimed was his own experience with two patients who suffered delusions of having swallowed frogs, in his *Practica*, fol. 21r. Despite its title, this work contains much learned theoretical discussion and was most likely written as an academic textbook for the school study of *practica*. Although there are literary antecedents (see Neaman, *Suggestion of the Devil*, pp. 1-2), Guglielmo's claim to personal experience may probably be accepted as genuine, both because he recorded his failure rather than his success and because the delusion of having swallowed a small living creature is apparently a fairly common symptom of mental disturbance.

[4] For titles, manuscripts, and editions, see Bibliography.

[5] Michael's description of the case appears, in English translation, in Thorndike, *Michael Scot*, p. 73. The case is discussed in Ynez Violé O'Neill, "Michael Scot and Mary of Bologna: A Medieval Gynecological Puzzle," *Clio Medica* 8 (1973):87-111 and 9 (1974): 125-129.

gan to appear in the twelfth century and to proliferate at the end of the thirteenth.[6] It is true, however, that the earliest medical *consilia* to survive in any quantity appear to be those emanating from the circle of Taddeo: at least 185 are ascribed to Taddeo himself,[7] 21 to Guglielmo da Brescia,[8] 18 to Mondino, and there are a a few by Bartolomeo and Dino.[9] Some of the longer *consilia* provide sufficient information about the patient and his or her symptoms to be loosely categorized as case histories, with the result that Taddeo has sometimes been accorded praise, not altogether merited, for encouraging the growth of clinical medicine based upon direct personal observation.

But in truth even the most detailed *consilia* are not case histories in the sense that the term may be applied, say, to the justly famous day-by-day records of the progress of diseases contained in the Hippocratic *Epidemics*. The following considerations may demonstrate this point. In a number of cases where the fact is explicitly stated, and perhaps in more where it is not, the author of a *consilium* was responding as a consultant to a request for advice written by the patient's physician (who doubtless wished to draw upon the learning of such celebrated professors as Taddeo and the others), and had not necessarily seen the patient himself.[10] More-

[6] See Peter Riesenberg, "The Consilia Literature: A Prospectus," *Manuscripta* 6 (1962): 3-22, and Guido Kisch, *Consilia: Eine Bibliographie der juristischen Konsiliensammlungen* (Basel-Stuttgart, 1970). It seems more likely that legal *consilia* influenced the development of medical *consilia* than the other way round, given the fact that the earliest known examples from Bologna are legal, not medical, and given the superior age and standing of the universities of law over the university of arts and medicine. In both law and medicine, professors at Bologna pioneered the *consilium* form in the Middle Ages.

[7] Taddeo, *I "Consilia,"* ed. Giuseppe M. Nardi (Turin, 1937). This is the only complete edition. For earlier partial printings, see Bibliography under Petella, and below, note 14.

[8] A complete list of Guglielmo's *consilia* and the texts of a selection of them appear in E. Schmidt, *Die Bedeutung Wilhelms von Brescia*.

[9] "Consilia Mundini," CLM 77, fols. 46r-59v; and "Consilia Mundini Bononiensis," CLM 23912, fols. 208r-247r. Mundinus, "Consilium ad retentionem menstruorum," Vienna, Nationalbibliothek, MS 2300, fols. 84v-85r (TK 1218); Bartholomaeus de Vagana [*sic*], "Lavate post cibum in estate extremitates corporis . . . ," Munich, Bayerische Staatsbibliothek, CLM 23912, fols. 253r-254v (TK 814); "Consilium Dini de Florentia," CLM 205, fols. 246r-v (TK 1345). For Mondino's *consilia* see also B. Vonderlage, *Consilien des Mondino dei Luzzi aus Bologna* (Leipzig, 1922), to which, however, I have so far been unable to gain access.

[10] For example, "Quoniam ut michi scripsistis, in tumore mamillae illius dominae, percipiuntur calor . . . ," Guglielmo, *Consilia,* in E. Schmidt, *Die Bedeutung Wilhelms von Brescia,* p. 12; and "Provido et discreto viro, magistro Inglisco, Guillermi [*sic*] bononiensis archidiaconus salutem. . . . Vestrarum litterarum intellecto tenore de diligencia cognicionis egritudinum et curationis sororis et nepotis . . . ," p. 13. That master Ingliscus was a

over, the primary purpose of a *consilium* was not to record observations but to recommend treatment; many of them therefore contain no detailed description of the patient's condition and no account of the process whereby diagnosis was arrived at. Thus, of Taddeo's 185 *consilia*, over 100 are simply brief medicinal recipes. Of the remainder, only about half give any description of the patient's symptoms and then often only in extremely laconic terms, such as, for example, "this patient suffers from pain in the joints caused by excessive complexional heat."[11]

Furthermore, a good many *consilia* have reached us in a form that suggests they have undergone considerable editing. While some of them survive as individual items in manuscript miscellanies, the *consilia* of famous physicians, including Taddeo's, Mondino's, and Guglielmo's, are found gathered into collections. The fact that such collections were made and recopied (there are at least fourteen complete and partial manuscripts of Taddeo's *consilia*)[12] suggests that an important secondary purpose of the genre was to serve as aids to teaching and study. A few *consilia* may indeed have originated as written records of oral teaching sessions at the patient's bedside; Taddeo's, in which he is frequently referred to in the third person, were perhaps collected by one of the students or junior physicians who were accustomed to accompanying him when he attended patients. The subsequent use of *consilia* as written aids to study and as guides to similar cases is exemplified by Guglielmo da Brescia's instruction to a fellow doctor, who had written for advice about a case of cancer (*cancer*) of the breast, to be diligent in studying two of his (Guglielmo's) "*consilia* or treatises" on the subject.[13] The publication of the names of noble patients gives rise to the perhaps unduly cynical supposition that another purpose in forming a collection of written *consilia* was to advertise the expertise and the distinguished clientele of the physician who treated the case. This in turn strengthens the probability that the

---

physician as well as a concerned relative is indicated by Guglielmo's instructions that he study certain medical works.

[11] "Hic infirmus patitur dolorem articulorum de causa calida," Taddeo, *1* "Consilia," no. 6, p. 11.

[12] Based on TK.

[13] "Licet autem ad hoc multa et diversa, quae in consilio "Ad sclirosim" iam dudum transmisso collegerem [*sic*].

Similiter etiam in consilio "Ad cancrum" multa ad hoc conferencia conscripserem [*sic*]. Unum in illis duobus consiliis vel tractatis [*sic*] studere non pigeat," Guglielmo, *Consilia*, in E. Schmidt, *Die Bedeutung Wilhelms von Brescia*, p. 13.

shortage of references to any unfavorable outcome of treatment is not accidental. In short, it must be assumed that the *consilia* that survive are, for the most part, highly self-conscious and probably carefully selected and revised productions.

Moreover, *consilia* compiled in Latin for an audience of other learned physicians or medical students certainly do not give us much direct information about the interaction of physician and patient. Just about the only surviving production of Taddeo's circle to reflect the way doctors communicated with the laymen who consulted them is the contemporary Italian version (perhaps by Taddeo himself) of Taddeo's health manual (*regimen sanitatis*) for Corso Donati.[14]

Thus, about all that can be claimed with any confidence for the *consilia* is that the treatments recommended therein are indeed those that the authors thought most appropriate for the conditions in question, and that the cases alluded to were in most instances real, not fictitious. When this degree of uncertainty surrounds the extent to which even the *consilia* reflect the social and technological realities of medical practice, it is no surprise to find that the similar problems surrounding collections of remedies and works labeled "*practica*" or "*practica de*" . . . are of even greater magnitude.

We have already seen that works with the word *practica* in their titles can take the form of commentaries upon the standard medical authors studied in the schools, and that their content can include scholastically argued *questiones*; an example several times alluded to is the *Dilucidatorium totius practice medicine* of Dino del Garbo, which is a commentary on a portion of the *Canon* of Avicenna and includes 283 questions. However much of himself and his own experience as a practitioner Dino may have put into this work, it remains, obviously, a carefully composed academic textbook and a record of activity in the classroom, not at the bedside. The same is true of Dino's *Chirurgia* and his *De virtutibus medi-*

[14] For manuscripts and editions of Taddeo's Latin *regimen sanitatis* and its relation to the thirteenth-century Italian version entitled *Libello per chonservare la sanità del corpo*, see Bibliography. The Italian text has been several times printed, most recently in G. Spina and A. Sampalmieri, "La lettera di Taddeo Alderotti a Corso Donati e l'inizio della letteratura igienica medioevale," XXI *Congresso Internazionale di Storia della Medicina, Siena, 1968*, Atti, 1:94-99. No scholarly apparatus is provided, however. The tract for Corso may have been written in 1293, when Corso was in Bologna, but of course the aging learned physician and the tumultuous young nobleman could also have met in their native Florence. The probability that the Italian version is Taddeo's own work is suggested by his translation of the *Ethics*.

camentorum, both also commentaries on Avicenna, which constitute, respectively, a guide to the treatment of ulcers, wounds, and fractures of the skull; and a directory to the usage of different types of medication. Works with such subject matter were evidently put to practical professional as well as academic use; but with what degree of regularity or accuracy their prescriptions were followed, either by their authors or by subsequent medical readers, it is impossible to say.

Other works labeled *"practica,"* such as the *Practica de accidentibus* attributed to Mondino,[15] the *Practica in cyrurgia* of Guglielmo,[16] or the *Introductorium ad practicam* of Taddeo,[17] can be called "less academic" in the sense that they are shorter, do not take the form of commentaries, and proliferate in recipes or specific directions for treatment rather than in *questiones;* but their relationship to the clinical situation is no clearer than that of the longer works.

Even more ambiguous are the origins and uses of collections of remedies. In this category the most widely used work produced by a member of Taddeo's circle seems to be the *Compilatio emplastrorum et unguentorum,* usually ascribed to Dino del Garbo. There are at least sixteen complete or partial manuscripts of this work, and it was several times printed in the fifteenth and sixteenth centuries. It is a collection of recipes for ointments, plasters, and powders for external application in connection with surgical treatment (understood as treatment of ulcers and wounds) and purports to be based on Book 5 of Galen's *De simplicibus medicinae* and Book 2 of the *Canon* of Avicenna.[18] However, it is neither an edition of nor a commentary upon those works, and it includes recipes that are claimed to be of recent origin, such as a prescription said to have been

---

[15] Mondino dei Liuzi [*sic*], *Practica de accidentibus,* ed. G. Caturegli (Pisa, 1966). This work is ascribed to "Mundinus" in four manuscripts, to Mundinus de Lentiis in one, to Mundinus de Forolivio in one, and to John of Paris in one (see TK 278); Caturegli maintains that it is definitely the work of Mondino de' Liuzzi (*Practica,* pp. 7-8).

[16] Preface and table of contents printed in Sudhoff, *Beiträge zur Geschichte der Chirurgie,* 2:419-21.

[17] BAV, MS Palat. lat. 1284, fols. 143r-154v: "Tu scis quod sanitas non est nisi equatio humorum. . . . Et sic est finis illorum tractatuum et capitulorum excerptorum ex introductorio ad practicam magistri thadei. . . ."

[18] *Compilatio emplastrorum et unguentorum Magistri Dini florentini artium et medicine doctoris excellentissimi. Et primo de repercussivis* (Ferrara, 1489; Klebs 336.1; the copy at the New York Academy of Medicine is bound separately from Dino's *Chirurgia* (Ferrara, 1489), with which it was apparently printed. For manuscripts and other, early editions, see TK. The work is attributed to Mondino in one manuscript (see TK 1348). The incipit in the edition of Ferrara, 1489, is "Commemoratio. . . ."

given to Pope Boniface (presumably VIII) by Master Anselmus of Genoa.[19] Variations in the manuscripts and early editions[20] suggest the possibilities of substantial later interpolation and excision in Dino's compilation, but the extent and nature of such changes, together with the precise relationship of Dino's compendium to the treatises of Galen and Avicenna, or rather to their medieval Latin manuscript tradition, must await the appearance of critical editions of all three works. In general, the very fact that works listing remedies continued to be put to practical use by generation after generation of physicians increases the probability of deliberate interpolation. But even if these problems are set aside for a time, what is one to make of Dino's claim that his recipes are "according to Galen"? It would be farfetched to assume that all of Galen's ingredients were correctly recognized, available, and used in fourteenth-century Italy. Omissions and substitutions surely took place, but it is usually impossible to find out what was left out and on what basis substitutions were made (whether consciously or unconsciously, systematically or at random, and whether by similarity of name or supposed similarity of action). Furthermore, the foregoing problems often vitiate any attempts to assess the probable effectiveness of medieval herbal remedies.[21]

For all these reasons, no systematic exposition of the pharmacology of Taddeo and his school will be attempted here. The whole subject of medieval herbals and remedy collections, including ancient remedy collections used in the Middle Ages, is so vast and still so scantily explored that it seems best left to specialists.[22] Regardless of whether it is practical to

[19] Dino del Garbo, *Unguenta* (i.e., the same work as that cited in the preceding note), Rome, Biblioteca Angelica, MS 1489, 14c, fol. 211 (219)r. In the edition of Ferrara, 1489, sig. [B7v], the passage occurs with the name of the pope omitted, presumably in the interests of modernization.

[20] For example, the incipit appears variously as "Commemoratio," "Memoratio," and "Rememoratio"; see TK 866, 1348, and note 18, above.

[21] Some of the problems are indicated in Jerry Stannard, "Medieval Herbals and Their Development," *Clio Medica* 9 (1974):23-33. A valuable assessment of ancient pharmacology is contained in Majno, *The Healing Hand.* See especially pp. 61-64, 184-188, 215-227, 349-353, 369-370.

[22] The standard guide to medieval botany is still Hermann Fischer, *Mittelalterlichen Pflanzenkunde* (Munich, 1929, repr. Hildesheim, 1967). On medicinal botany, see further Jerry Stannard, "Botanical Data in Medieval Medical Recipes," *Studies in History of Medicine* 1 (1977):80-87. On the transmission of herbal medicine from antiquity, see John M. Riddle, "The Latin Alphabetical Dioscorides," *Actes du XIIIᵉ Congrès International d'Histoire des Sciences, 1971,* 3-4:204-209; Linda E. Voigts, "A New Look at a Manuscript Containing the Old English Translation of the *Herbarium Apulei,*" *Manuscripta* 20 (1976): 40-60.

hope for the emergence of a generation of scholars who will combine the necessary paleographical and editorial skills with a sophisticated understanding of herbal pharmacology, I do not feel qualified to undertake even a small segment of this formidable task.

Despite the caveats just given, *consilia* (and to a lesser extent works entitled *practica* and remedy collections) are a rich source of information about certain aspects of the practice of medicine in the circle of Taddeo. They can be made to yield insights into the social context of practice, the range of conditions treated, methods of diagnosis and their foundations in medical theory, and the nature and basis of recommendations for treatment. What follows regarding these categories is based chiefly on the sets of *consilia* by Taddeo, Guglielmo, and Mondino; on Taddeo's regimen for Corso Donati; on Mondino's *Practica de accidentibus*; on portions of Dino's *Chirurgia*; and on Taddeo's *Tabula de remediis omnium egritudinum in generali.*[23]

THE PATIENTS

Consilia convey a good deal about the social context of the professional practice of learned physicians, since the name, rank or occupation, place of residence, age, and sex of the patient are quite frequently included. Thus, out of the approximately seventy-five *consilia* by Taddeo that consist of more than just recipes, one or more the above facts is found in thirty-four cases. The amount of information in any individual instance varies from the simple grammatical indication of sex ("*infirmus*") to "a certain man from Ferrara . . . forty years of age, and his trade was buying and selling wine."[24] Not surprisingly, this small sample reveals those on whose behalf Taddeo was consulted as predominantly male and predominantly upper class. The thirty men and youths (the age of the patient is given in a total of nine cases of either sex, and ranges from fourteen to the sixties) treated included the doge of Venice;[25] two bishops, one of

[23] BAV, MS Palat. lat. 1363, fols. 167v-171r.

[24] "Conquestus fuit quidam ferrariensis, macri corporis et coloris citrini quantum ad totam habitudinem colerice complexionis, in etate 40 annorum—eius ars erat emere et vendere vinum—de fluxu sanguinis narium," Taddeo, I "Consilia," no. 147, p. 196.

[25] Ibid., no. 62, p. 129. The holders of the office of doge during Taddeo's professional career were Ranieri Zen, 1253-1268; Lorenzo Tiepolo, 1268-1275; Jacopo Contarini, 1275-1280; Giovanni Dandolo, 1280-1289; Pietro Gradenigo, 1289-1311 (A. Cappelli, *Cronologia, cronografia e calendario perpetuo* [3d ed., Milan, 1969], pp. 346-347).

whom was the famous surgical writer Theodoric of Lucca;[26] two counts;[27] a member of the house of Malatesta,[28] and nine other individuals whose social status was sufficiently elevated to rate the sometimes ambiguous honorific *dominus*;[29] a priest;[30] the wine merchant; and one artisan, a twenty-five-year-old smith (*faber*).[31] From other sources we learn, as already noted, that Taddeo's patients included the Black Guelf leader Corso Donati, and perhaps Pope Honorius IV. Of the seven women treated (counting only cases in which the patient is named, described, or grammatically indicated as female, and not including unannotated recipes obviously meant for women, such as a potion to bring on menstruation), three merited the title of "lady" (*domina*).[32] Hence it looks as though Taddeo found a good deal of occasion to use his special "laxative for the noble and delicate."[33] The cases in which rank and occupation are noted do not necessarily reflect the actual pattern of Taddeo's practice, since his amenuensis may have found only relatively high social position worth recording. A similar bias in reporting probably lies behind the identification of only two patients in the edited *consilia* of Guglielmo da Brescia: the brother of the bishop of Brescia,[34] and the lord of that city.[35] It prob-

[26] "Circa curam egritudinis domini nostri episcopi," Taddeo, *I* "*Consilia*," no. 49, p. 117; "Emplastrum ad scrofulas episcopi Cerviensis," ibid., no. 29, p. 66.

[27] Bartholocus T. (ibid., no. 11, p. 24), and Bertholdus (ibid., no. 24, p. 57).

[28] "Ad arteticam. Pro domino Malatesta," ibid., no. 18, p. 42.

[29] Ibid., no. 10, p. 19; no. 22, p. 52; no. 41, p. 86; no. 44, p. 98; no. 46, p. 103; no. 127, p. 165; no. 128, p. 171; no. 150, p. 201; no. 167, p. 221.

[30] Ibid., no. 23, p. 56.   [31] Ibid., no. 153, p. 204.

[32] Ibid., no. 139, p. 189; no. 146, p. 195 ("domina theotonica"); no. 156, p. 209.

[33] "Ad laxandum nobiles et delicatos," ibid., no. 68, p. 136.

[34] Guglielmo, *Consilia*, in E. Schmidt, *Die Bedeutung Wilhelms von Brescia*, p. 13. The bishops of Brescia during William's career were Berardo de' Maggi, 1275-1309, and Federico de' Maggi, 1309-1317, two members of the city's seignorial family; Percevallo Fieschi, 1317-1325; and Tiberio Torriani, 1325-1335 (Conrad Eubel, *Hierarchia catholica medii aevi* [Regensburg, 1913], 1:147).

[35] "Ad facilitandum vomitum. Pro domino brixiensi," Guglielmo, *Consilia*, in E. Schmidt, *Die Bedeutung Wilhelms von Brescia*, p. 17. In Guglielmo's lifetime, Brescia was under the lordship of Charles of Anjou from 1269 until 1281, of Bernardo de' Maggi from 1298 until 1308, and Matteo de' Maggi from 1309 until 1311. Henry VII occupied the city between 1311 and 1313, and Robert the Wise of Naples and Sicily was its overlord between 1319 and 1330 (Cappelli, *Cronologia*, p. 341). All things considered, it is perhaps most likely that Guglielmo had been the client of the de' Maggi, a local noble family, and retained connections with them. If "dominus brixiensis" is interpreted as "a nobleman (or gentleman) of Brescia," rather than as "lord of Brescia," then of course Guglielmo's *consilium* could have been written for a member of the city's upper class during its republican periods, 1281-1298 and 1313-1319.

ably also explains why the one known surviving *consilium* definitely attributable to Bartolomeo da Varignana is for the Emperor Henry VII.[36] Nonetheless, it is probably true that attendance upon noble patrons provided the single most important source of income for learned physicians, and was of greater economic significance to them than any or all of the other types of remunerative position available: service to urban governments, professorial appointments in the *studia*, and practice among a citizen clientele.

There may also be a bias in favor of reporting the treatment of males in the *consilia*, since the large number of gynecological remedies and cosmetics included in Taddeo's *Tabula de remediis* perhaps implies an extensive practice among women and a situation in which upper-class males were prepared to spend frequently and generously for the medical treatment of their wives and daughters. It must be admitted, however, that the balance of remedies in different categories in this and similar collections may equally well have been determined by the content of existing collections of remedies used as sources.

Taddeo's patients and those on whose behalf he was consulted came from all over northern and north-central Italy: cities and regions mentioned included Lucca, Mantua, Venice, Ferrara, and the March of Ancona.[37] In most instances, there is no way of telling whether the patient came to Taddeo at Bologna, whether Taddeo traveled to the patient, or whether the consultation was by letter; however, Taddeo certainly spent some time in Ferrara and Venice (see chapter two) and probably attended the patients in those cities in person. Guglielmo's *consilia* for patients in Brescia suggest that he maintained ties with his native city long after he had left it permanently to study, teach, and practice in Padua, Bologna, Avignon, and Paris, and that news of his growing medical fame continued to reach his former home.

THE CONDITIONS TREATED

Diseases have their own history, but little is at present known of the actual nature and incidence of disease in the Italy of Taddeo and his pupils (that is, at the beginning of an apparent European population

[36] See note 9, above, and Bartolomeo's biography in chapter two.
[37] Taddeo, *I "Consilia,"* no. 5, p. 8; no. 22, p. 52; no. 23, p. 56; no. 48, p. 112; no. 62, p. 129; no. 147, p. 196; no. 150, p. 201.

contraction after the great twelfth-century expansion and before the Black Plague).[38] Although the *consilia* ascribed to the circle of Taddeo cast some light upon this problem, their usefulness is limited. These documents are too few in number (though over two hundred of them exist), they often describe diseases too ambiguously, and they reflect the ailments of too small a segment of society to be the basis of any general conclusions about disease patterns. It is not to the *consilia* written for and about Taddeo's privileged patients that one can turn for information about general health conditions in a society that has been described as having a "huge population, massive poverty, [and] endemic malnutrition,"[39] and in which subsequent population losses have been perceived by some scholars as essentially Malthusian.

Nevertheless, *consilia* and certain remedy collections do provide a useful overview of the conditions that academically trained physicians were most commonly called upon to treat. The range of diseases for which Taddeo, Guglielmo, and no doubt their colleagues prescribed was as catholic as their range of patients, who, as already noted, included both sexes and all ages from puberty on. The *consilia* include scant reference to surgery for wounds and fractures (although here they are almost certainly misleading, as we shall see) and apparently refer to no pediatric cases. Little else was excluded.

Thus Guglielmo, a cleric who spent most of his career as a papal physician, treated both gynecological problems (if we can judge from the fact that he wrote on breast cancer and tumors of the breast on five separate occasions)[40] and problems of sexual dysfunction.[41] His *consilium pro*

[38] An excellent summary of the literature on this topic that pertains to Italy and an analysis of population trends in one Italian commune is found in David Herlihy, *Medieval and Renaissance Pistoia* (New Haven and London, 1966), pp. 55-77, 102-120.

[39] Ibid., p. 114. Cipolla, *Public Health and the Medical Profession*, pp. 81-83, points to the wide distribution of university-trained physicians, even in rural areas, in early seventeenth-century northern Italy. But ca. 1300, although even quite small Italian towns commonly provided medical services for their citizens (citizens being, at least, to some extent, a privileged class), it is doubtful if learned physicians spent much time treating the rural population—other than members of the nobility or clergy—or the urban poor in large cities. For the development of medical services in a small Mediterranean city that made use of Italian university physicians in the fourteenth century, see Susan M. Stuard, "A Communal Program of Medical Care, Medieval Ragusa/Dubrovnik," *Journal of the History of Medicine and Allied Sciences* 28 (1973):126-142.

[40] Guglielmo, *Consilia*, in E. Schmidt, *Die Bedeutung Wilhelms von Brescia*, pp. 12, 13; and in Guglielmo, *De tyriaca*, ed. McVaugh; in one of the *consilia* edited by Schmidt, Guglielmo referred to *consilia* that he had written "Ad sclirosim" and "Ad cancrum"

quodam qui carebat spermate includes a lengthy series of questions to be put by a doctor to infertile couples among his patients, as well as two tests for virginity, both (wisely) hard to fail. Taddeo, who in the secular society of Bologna presumably had a wider gynecological practice, prescribed in his *consilia* for a good many ailments peculiar to women (for example, pain in the breasts, retention of an aborted fetus, uterine cramps, amenorrhea);[42] and he displayed sensitivity to the problems of pregnancy in his insistence that pregnant women be dosed sparingly and then only with gentle medication.[43] Taddeo, too, concerned himself with problems of fertility, and incidentally with sexual dysfunction; he gave detailed recommendations for the achievement of simultaneous orgasm, apparently because he thought it an aid to conception and especially to the conception of males.[44]

Other specific conditions or symptoms that Taddeo was frequently called upon to treat (if we judge by his *consilia*) included fevers (at least fifteen *consilia*); various pulmonary and respiratory complaints including coughs, asthma (*asma*—this and other terms do not, of course, necessarily indicate the condition today called by the same name), phthisis (*ptisis*),

---

(p. 13). These do not appear to survive in the form of *consilia*, but there are chapters on these subjects in his *Practica in cyrurgia*; see the table of contents edited in Sudhoff, *Beiträge zur Geschichte der Chirurgie*, 2:420. One is reminded again that the boundaries between different genres of medical writing were far from firmly fixed.

[41] Guglielmo, *Consilia*, in E. Schmidt, *Die Bedeutung Wilhelms von Brescia*, pp. 22-25.

[42] Taddeo, I "*Consilia*, no. 3, p. 5; no. 60, p. 128; no. 88, p. 140; no. 130, pp. 177-179. A total of ten of Taddeo's 185 *consilia* concern gynecological problems, although, as noted, his practice among women was probably larger than this proportion suggests.

[43] "Egritudo istius mulieris talis est, ut videtur: habet enim febrem putridam, ex materia coniuncta ex flegmate et colera, et febrem ethicam vel dispositionem, et habet screatum pauci sanguinis, cum rasacatione et interdum cum tussi; et habet etiam fistulam in extremitate longaonis, et super omnia dicit se esse pregnantem. Quia ergo egritudines sunt contrarie inter se, medicamina que uni prosunt, alteri nocent, et impregnatio prohibet multa medicamina que secundum egritudinis naturam fieri deberent; etiam quia delicata, non possumus in ea fortia medicamina facere," ibid., no. 37, p. 75. Taddeo made a similar point in his *Introductorius ad practicam*, in which he explained the humoral basis of medicine and discussed various considerations (the age, sex, and habits of the patient; the weather; the position of the heavenly bodies; and so on) that the physician should take into account in prescribing medicine: "in pregnantibus in primis tribus mensibus neque in tribus ultimis ipsas farmacare non debemus forti medicina, in mediis vero . . . oportet plus quam si non essent pregnantes," BAV, MS Palat. lat. 1284, fol. 144r. We may assume that the woman whose treatment was recorded in *consilium* 37 was in the first or the last trimester of her pregnancy.

[44] Taddeo, I "*Consilia*," no. 13, pp. 33-34.

catarrh (*catarrum*), pleurisy (*ad pleureticos*), and spitting blood;[45] gen-
ito-urinary problems of various kinds, especially blood in the urine, burning urine, the stone, and pains in the kidneys;[46] pains in the stomach,
digestive problems, and diarrhea;[47] and arthritis (*artetica*), pains in the
joints, and gout (*podagra*).[48] Taddeo also treated skin conditions (termed
scrofula, *lepra*, and *scabies*);[49] dental problems, gum disease, and oral
infections and abscesses;[50] defective vision and hearing;[51] hernia,[52] dropsy
(*ydropisis*),[53] and epilepsy;[54] and hemorrhoids.[55] On occasion his professional dignity did not bar him from providing his patients with recipes
for mouthwash, hair restorer, hair dye, and cosmetic facewashes; nor
were such recipes found unsuitable for inclusion in his collected *consilia*.[56]
The psychological problems he treated included melancholy (on several
occasions), sleeplessness, and loss of memory.[57]

In addition to the various ills named above (some of which were, of
course, symptoms of disease entities unrecognized in the thirteenth century), many of Taddeo's patients were described as suffering from complaints of the internal organs that cannot now be even vaguely identified.
Thus, Taddeo's confident (and doubtless correct) assertions that one patient had blood in his urine or that another had a cough were paralleled
in other cases by equally confident assertions that the problem was "bad
disposition of the liver," "obstruction of the spleen and liver," or "exces-

---

[45] Ibid., no. 28, pp. 63-66; no. 38, pp. 78-81; no. 97, p. 142; no. 98, p. 143; no. 99,
p. 143; no. 109, p. 145; no. 127, pp. 165-170.

[46] Ibid., no. 11, pp. 24-27; no. 43, pp. 94-97; no. 47, pp. 110-112; no. 62, pp. 129-135;
no. 71, p. 137; no. 83, pp. 139-140; no. 85, p. 140; no. 86, p. 140; no. 123, pp. 154-158;
no. 145, p. 195; no. 152, pp. 203; no. 153, pp. 204-206; no. 160, p. 211; no. 161, p. 212;
no. 178, p. 235.

[47] Ibid., no. 7, pp. 15-17; no. 48, pp. 112-116; no. 70, p. 136; no. 82, p. 139; no. 155,
pp. 208-209; no. 176, p. 234; and several others.

[48] Ibid., no. 6, pp. 11-15; no. 18, pp. 42-44; no. 19, pp. 44-49; no. 20, pp. 49-50; no.
164, pp. 216-218; no. 165, pp. 218-219; no. 177, pp. 234-235.

[49] Ibid., no. 29, pp. 66-68; no. 33, p. 71; nos. 105-107, pp. 144-145; nos. 142-144,
pp. 191-195.

[50] Ibid., no. 21, pp. 50-52; no. 25, p. 62; no. 39, p. 82; no. 119, pp. 147-148.

[51] Ibid., no. 1, pp. 1-3; no. 2, pp. 3-4; no. 5, pp. 8-11; no. 91, p. 141; no. 92, p. 141;
no. 158, p. 210; no. 159, pp. 210-211; no. 172, p. 233.

[52] Ibid., no. 40, pp. 82-86; no. 163, pp. 212-216.

[53] Ibid., no. 15, pp. 37-39; no. 41, pp. 86-91.

[54] Ibid., no. 12, pp. 27-33.   [55] Ibid., no. 65, p. 135.

[56] Ibid., no. 30, p. 68; no. 51, pp. 125-126; no. 52, p. 126; no. 133, p. 186; no. 146,
pp. 195-196.

[57] Ibid, no. 1, pp. 1-3; no. 22, pp. 52-56; no. 102, pp. 143-144, no. 103, p. 144.

sive heating of the liver with heat and coldness of the kidneys"; other sufferers were said to be in need of "purging of the brain" or "cooling and opening of the liver."[58] In most instances we have no clues to the actual conditions such descriptions record, nor is it possible to know whether doctors used disease identifications of this type with any degree of precision or consistency. Nor is it clear whether the physicians themselves perceived their ability to recognize, say, an unsatisfactory complexional state of the liver as any different in quality from their ability to recognize diarrhea or a nosebleed. A certain skepticism about diagnoses of the former kind is engendered by the advice that Taddeo's younger contemporary Arnald of Villanova, who was associated with the medical school of Montpellier, offered to his fellow physicians: "you may not find out anything about the case, then say that he has an obstruction in the liver . . . and particularly use the word obstruction [*oppilatio*], because they do not understand what it means, and it helps greatly that a term is not understood by the people."[59]

Another glimpse of the relative frequency with which various types of complaint cropped up in Taddeo's practice may be provided by his "table of remedies for every kind of disease in general," which is preserved in a Vatican manuscript.[60] This table lists 170 different ailments and indicates simples held to be effective against each. The number of remedies listed for any one disease varies from 42 for "obstruction of the spleen and liver" to one for apoplexy. A total of 100 remedies is listed for gynecological conditions, 26 of them being for repletion of the womb (*de repletione matricis*), 17 for vaginal discharge (*de fluxu matricis*), and 15 for expelling a dead fetus. Presumably the simples in the first and third categories were conceived of as having abortifacient properties, although whether in most cases they were deliberately prescribed as such one cannot say. A wholly unambiguous attitude to contraception, however, is expressed in the opening passage of a "*consilium* for preventing pregnancy" attributed to Mondino in one manuscript. There the author asserts that the prevention of pregnancy is, in certain circumstances, as much a part of the

---

[58] "De mala epatis dispositione in qua humores aduruntur," ibid., no. 35, pp. 73-75; "De calefactione epatis cum caliditate et frigiditate renum," no. 150, pp. 201-202; "De oppilatione epatis et splenis cum habundantia humorum grossorum," no. 167, pp. 221-225; "Ad purgandum cerebrum," no. 93, pp. 141-142; "Ad infrigidandum et aperiendum epar," no. 173, p. 233.

[59] Translated in Grant, ed., *A Source Book in Medieval Science*, p. 751.

[60] BAV, MS Palat. lat. 1363, fol. 168r-171r.

physician's art as the facilitation of conception is in others. He pointed out not only that pregnancy can for some women be dangerous to health, but also that it is a lesser evil to assist a woman who has been sexually active outside marriage to avoid pregnancy than it is to terminate her pregnancy when it occurs. This avowal drew upon Mondino the disapproval of a later annotator of his *consilium*, who wrote austerely and unsympathetically in the margin of the manuscript: "a stupid *consilium*; women who should not get pregnant should not engage in sexual intercourse."[61] Perhaps unfortunately for his patients, Mondino's contraceptive technology was not as advanced as his principles; neither herbal potions nor suffumigants were likely to be very effective measures. But he did suggest a kind of pessary or suppository made of vegetable ingredients that might have offered some protection.

Taddeo's remedies against various kinds of fever number forty-five, while cosmetic preparations (facewashes, depilatories, hair dyes, hair restorers, deodorants, dentifrices, mouthwashes) mount to fifty. Nongynecological conditions with more than twenty remedies each are syncope and heart disease (*de syncope et cardiaca passione*), coughs, stomachaches, asthma, indigestion, worms, hardness of the spleen and liver (*de duricia splenis et epatis*), pain in the bowels (*de dolore intestinorum*), diarrhea (*de fluxu ventris*), dysentery (*de dissenteria*), hemorrhoids, ar-

---

[61] "Quia non sufficit in arte inferre virtutes sed oportet vicia exstirpare, ideo manifestum quod ad artem medicine non solum requiritur notificare que impregnacionem inducunt et corroborant, sed oportet constrare [?] que impregnacionem impugnant ut evitentur. Et non solum propter istam causam, sed et . . . ut impregnacio prohibeatur in hiis que sunt inapte ad conceptionem ex dispositione naturali, ut in puellis et parvis mulieribus in quibus impregnacio est timorosa propter partum periculosum, vel in hiis que sint inapte ad conceptionem propter dispositionem accidentalem ut in habentibus apud vesice vel ulcera vel alteras passiones et aliorum membrorum ut matricis etc. Et etiam ut impregnacio prohibeatur propter eas que illicite coeunt vel a natura coguntur et infestantur coyre, et eas non est licitum impregnari, propterea in eis licet peccatum sit prohibere conceptionem, minus tunc malum est quam fetum conceptum abortire," Mondino, *Consilia*, Munich, Bayerische Staatsbibliothek, CLM 77, fol. 58r; explicit, fol. 58v: "finis consilium ad prohibicionem impregnacionis." The marginal addition on fol. 58r reads: "stultum consilium; que non debent impregnari non debent inniri." In regard to medicaments "to bring on the menses," C. Mohr (*Abortion in America: The Origins and Evolution of National Policy, 1800-1900* [New York, 1978], p. 4) points out that prior to the development of reliable tests for early pregnancy, these could be prescribed and taken more or less in good faith. Regarding legal and theological positions on the prevention and termination of pregnancy in the Middle Ages, see John T. Noonan, *Contraception, A History of Its Treatment by the Catholic Theologians and Canonists* (Cambridge, Mass., 1965), pp. 86-91, 157-158, 232-233.

thritis (*arthetica*), ulcers, and tenesmus (*de tenasmone*). Various mental conditions—*frenesis*, melancholia, *litargia*, and loss of memory—collectively rate twenty-two remedies. Some of the nongynecological conditions against which more than ten remedies each are listed are headaches, gas in the stomach, dropsy, bladder stones (? *de vicio lapidis*; *vicio* may be a corruption of *vesica*), *scabies*, and paralysis.

If the distribution of remedies in Taddeo's tables bears any relation at all to the actual incidence in his practice of the different complaints mentioned and does not simply reflect pharmacological tradition, the conclusion seems clear that among the criteria for the selection of cases for his collected *consilia* were the avoidance of excessive repetition, the inclusion of cases considered to be of particular medical interest (sometimes for their rarity), and perhaps the social distinction of the patient.

THE PROCESS OF DIAGNOSIS

As the foregoing section demonstrates, a modern interpretation of medieval medical diagnoses presents problems of considerable complexity. Relatively few medieval descriptions of disease can be translated into twentieth-century medical terminology or identified with specific conditions with any degree of certainty. This point is well illustrated by the debates over the nature of the disease or diseases known in the Middle Ages as *lepra*. The question whether this term referred to leprosy (Hansen's disease), to syphilis or a related infection such as yaws, or to any or all of various disfiguring skin conditions that were uncritically lumped together is unlikely ever to be definitively resolved by further analysis of the literary evidence, even though medical writers on *lepra* provided their readers with long lists of striking symptoms.[62] The hazards of attempts to identify vaguer descriptions are even greater. Thus, to choose an example relating to the circle of Taddeo, G. Caturegli's insistence that the reference in Mondino's *Practica de accidentibus* to "scabiem grossam, flematicam, melicam [*sic*], cum epatis malitia, movet ad sellam" is a description of syphilis is a case of reading a precise meaning into very gen-

---

[62] For a recent summary of the state of the argument as to the nature of medieval "leprosy" and the related question of the European or American origins of syphilis, see William H. McNeill, *Plagues and Peoples*, pp. 174-180, 218-220, and bibliography there cited. The prevalence of different disease organisms at different times and places in human history can be and has been traced, to some extent, by the study of skeletal remains; but this of course does not identify or differentiate the conditions described in literary sources.

eral terminology.[63] The interpretation is not necessarily incorrect, but it lays more weight on the evidence that it can reasonably bear. Of course there are cases where the identification of a medieval description with a particular disease is much less open to doubt; yet even in such cases the use of twentieth-century technical terminology (with its implied assumptions of bacterial or viral classification of diseases and its linkage of symptoms which were not understood to be related in the Middle Ages) may construct a misleading frame of reference. It seems preferable, therefore, simply to examine the process of diagnosis in the terms revealed in the *consilia*.

As already noted, most *consilia* provide no diagnosis beyond a brief identification of the patient's complaint. In a substantial minority of cases, however, both Taddeo and Guglielmo described the patient's symptoms at some length and gave some indication of the way in which their diagnosis was reached.

The first basis of diagnosis was a physician's observation of the patient, although, as we have seen, the authors of *consilia* were ready to pronounce on written reports about patients whom they had not personally examined. In some instances at least, the doctor's own observations were supplemented by interviewing the patient. Thus, of one case Taddeo remarked: "this patient is suffering from pain in the joints caused by excessive complexional heat, judging by the symptoms [*accidentia*] that he suffered earlier, and that were revealed by interrogation of the patient; but we cannot find signs of this condition in the present state of his disease, because he does not have the paroxysms from which we can assume its presence."[64] In another instance Taddeo distinguished, perhaps intentionally, between a swelling of the tongue, "which the patient feels," and a "descent of matter from the rear part [of the tongue or mouth], which the patient *says* he feels" (italics added).[65]

[63] Mondino, *Practica de accidentibus*, ed. Caturegli, pp. 34, 71-72, 77-80. In support of his argument Caturegli points out that the term *scabbia* was used for syphilis in a fifteenth-century Italian account (p. 77).

[64] "Hic infirmus patitur dolorem articulorum de causa calida, iudicando per accidentia que precesserunt, assumpta ab interrogatione infirmi; per ea vero que apparent in egrotante, non possumus assumere signa per ea, quia non habet paroxismus [*sic*, ed. Nardi] a quo possum assumere signa presentia" Taddeo, I "*Consilia*," no. 6, p. 11.

[65] "Signum autem quod ex tali humiditate lingua impediatur, est multitudo salive et etiam aliqualis grossities lingue, quam sentit infirmus, et etiam descensus reumatis a parte posteriori quam infirmus dicit sentire," ibid., no. 24, p. 58.

Descriptions of symptoms varied greatly in the amount of detail included. In some instances an obvious effort was made to report every aspect of the patient's condition. Thus, for example, *dominus* F. was said to be suffering from "multiple diseases"—that is, "excessive heat of the liver without obstruction of the spleen and of the whole body, with a slow fever that is increasing the production of choleric humor and producing granular tissue [*tericiam*], severe bleeding hemorrhoids with pain in the anus, and a fistulous wound at the lower extremity of the intestine, leading for the most part to weakness of the whole body, to syncope, and to loss of appetite; these results are also due to the bad complexion of the humors lying together in the substance of the stomach and to diseases of the bile system [*zinarie*], which further lead to dropsy and hectic fever."[66] In other cases, a much simpler account sufficed: "I say therefore that his ailment is diminution of the voice with some alteration to a certain hoarseness and sharpness."[67]

The causes of disease are mentioned in only a few of the *consilia* of Taddeo and Guglielmo and then frequently in cautious and undogmatic terms; expressions such as "I think the cause of this to be," "I presume the cause of this is," and "this seems to have happened to him because of" recur.[68] Usually explanations of causation are brief to the point of being cryptic, like Taddeo's curt statement that *dominus* Decanus suffered from a cardiac complaint "because of bad humors in the stomach."[69] Much less characteristic is the careful discrimination, found in one of Guglielmo's *consilia*, between different possible causes of floating objects seen in front of the eye (see chapter seven). However, Taddeo, too, was

[66] "Egritudo domini F. multiplex est, scilicet calefactio epatis sine oppilatione splenis et totius corporis, cum lenta febre multiplicante coleram et faciens tericiam, et immoderatus fluxus emoroidarum cum dolore ficteris et vulnere fistuloso extremitatis intestini, perducente plurimum ad debilitatem totius corporis et ad sincopim et ad defectum appetitus, consequens ad predicta et etiam ex malitia humorum concubitorum in substantia stomachi et ex egritudinibus zinarie, in ydropisim et ethicam," ibid., no. 46, p. 103. I owe the suggested translations of *tericiam* (*pterigium* or *pterygion*) and *zinarie* to the courtesy of Dr. Adrian Zorgniotti, M.D.

[67] "Dico ergo quod egritudo eius est vocis diminutio cum aliqua alteratione ad aliquam raucedinem et acuitatem, et hec est species morbi," ibid., no. 10, p. 20.

[68] "cuius causam arbitror esse . . . ," ibid., no. 11, p. 24; "Hoc autem sibi evenisse videtur . . . ," no. 24, p. 57; "Causam huius presumpsi fore . . . ," no. 147, p. 196. Other examples of similar language could be cited.

[69] "Egritudo domini Decani est cardiaca, propter malos humores existentes in stomacho," ibid., no. 44, p. 98.

aware that the same or very similar symptoms might arise from widely different causes. Thus, he attributed the bloody urine passed by Count Bartholocus T. to rupture (? *refrecationem*) of the veins near the kidneys and bad condition of the kidneys. Similar but more severe symptoms in the doge of Venice he believed to be the result of a lack of physical and an excess of mental exertion "because he multiplied thoughts and cares beyond his normal custom; and, as a result of these, bad digestion of the blood in the liver and veins took place."[70]

As the foregoing examples indicate, the causes of disease were frequently, although not invariably, explained as changes in the balance of the humors and complexional qualities. Although the language of humors and complexions undoubtedly lent itself on occasion to rhetorical and unduly abstract speculation about purely hypothetical phenomena— "I think the cause to be a certain bad disposition in the liver and veins, burning the humors and converting them to green choler and burnt melancholy"[71]—the terms were also used very concretely. Not only were the humors physical substances, but the hot, the cold, the wet, and the dry were thought of, at least ideally and some of the time, as physically perceptible states. For example, a woman who was unable to eat because of constriction of the throat (although her appetite remained normal) was said by Taddeo to be thus afflicted either because of dryness (*siccitas*) of the throat or because of the presence of thick and viscous phlegmatic humors.[72]

Taddeo and Guglielmo based their diagnoses firmly upon medical theory. In their *consilia*, not only are diseases explained in terms of complexions, humors, and virtues, but citations of learned medical (but seldom philosophical) authorities abound; furthermore, some *consilia* either specifically cite or are clearly related to passages in academic works by the same author. Thus, when recommending theriaca as a remedy for

[70] Ibid., no. 11, p. 24, and: "patitur enim micturam puri sanguinis in magna quantitate. . . . Dico ergo quod arbitror hunc sanguinem venire a membris que sunt supra membra mingendi, scilicet ab epate et a toto corpore; et arbitror causam huius esse, quia homo iste consuevit habere emunctionem per emoroidas et restricta sunt, et quia dimisit exercitium corporale et augmentavit animale, scilicet quia multiplicavit cogitationes, sollicitudines supra consuetudinem, et ex his mala digestio sanguinis in epate et venis," no. 62, p. 129.
[71] "causam arbitor esse quamdam malam dispositionem in epate et venis, adurentem humores et convertentem eos ad coleram viridem et in humorem melancolicum adustum," ibid., no. 35, p. 73.
[72] Ibid., no. 66, pp. 135-136.

breast cancer, Guglielmo da Brescia referred to his own question on theriaca.[73] Similarly, Taddeo's interest in the problem of *condolentia* (see chapter seven) was either stimulated by or reflected in his careful attention to the case of Count Bertholdus, for whom he produced one of his longest and most detailed *consilia*. This unfortunate nobleman suffered from a speech impediment owing to "softness of the tongue," which Taddeo believed to be itself a secondary result of a disease of the genitals. In Taddeo's view the immediate cause of the indisposition of the tongue lay in the brain: either excess humidity of the brain had affected the nerves connecting brain, tongue, and genitals (as evidence for a specially close connection between brain and genitals Taddeo referred to the Hippocratic idea that sperm descends from the brain to the testicles); or else the disease was originally in the genitals, whence vapors produced by the excess of melancholy humors had risen to the brain. In setting forth these alternatives, Taddeo cited the *Aphorisms* and *Epidemics* of Hippocrates, the section of the *Canon* "on the anatomy of the nerves of the brain," and Serapion.[74] No doubt this learned analysis and discussion was primarily intended to be read by Count Bertholdus's physician or Taddeo's trainees; one wonders how much of it was transmitted to the patient. In contrast, the vernacular version of Taddeo's regimen for Corso Donati, which presumably was intended for the patient's own eyes, stresses in the opening section that it is the product of a "master of science and art" and is based on "the sayings and books of the ancient philosophers"; but it contains no citations of authorities and no theoretical discussion.

Further evidence of the close connection between the *consilia* and the theoretical writings of their authors is provided by Taddeo's three *consilia* on *lepra*,[75] which was also the subject of his commentary (*lectura*) on a portion of the *Canon* of Avicenna.[76] Two of the three *consilia*, both of which give a regimen and recipes for medication for those afflicted with the disease, contain material without parallel in the *lectura*; however, the third, which lists the signs of *lepra* (in general and without reference to a particular case), covers exactly the same subject matter as a portion of the commentary. The two works are entirely distinct, the list of symptoms in

---

[73] Guglielmo, *Consilia*, in E. Schmidt, *Die Bedeutung Wilhelms von Brescia*, p. 12.

[74] Taddeo, *I "Consilia,"* no. 24, pp. 57-62.

[75] Ibid., nos. 142-144, pp. 191-195.

[76] Florence, Biblioteca Medicea Laurenziana, MS Ashburnham 217, fols. 91v-93r, inc.: "Lepra est infirmitas mala. A principio huius fen 3e"; explicit: "Explicit lectura super tractatum de lepra secundum tadeum." The passage commented upon is *Canon* 4.4.3.1-3.

the *consilium* being considerably longer; nonetheless, both agree that
lepra produces in the sufferer a reddening of the eyes, hoarseness, obstruction of the nostrils, gooseflesh, falling hair, altered facial appearance, and
a thickening of the blood. To this common core the commentary, following Avicenna closely, adds the loss of parts from ulceration (beginning
with the cartilage of the nose), loss of the nails, the appearance of prominent veins in the face, difficulty in breathing, and mental alienation. The
consilium lengthens the list to include insensibility of the extremities,
formication or itching in the face and elsewhere, muscular wasting, shin-
ing skin (*cutis etiam luciditas*), irritability, abnormal sensitivity to changes
of temperature, and foul-smelling breath, sweat, skin, and blood. The
reference to foul smell comes from the *Canon*, but the other symptoms
listed in the *consilium* but not in the commentary were either drawn
from a different source or noted by Taddeo in his own patients.

The relative fullness and detail of the *lepra* symptomology in Taddeo's
consilium may well be the result of observations carried out not just on
one individual but over a number of cases. Conceivably, his purpose may
have been to provide a description of *lepra* that could be used as a basis
for deciding whether particular individuals should be legally segregated
as lepers; according to Marsiglio of Padua, who studied medicine around
1315, probably in Padua, the certification of lepers was part of the duties
of a "physician or college of physicians."[77] But equally careful is Taddeo's
account of the symptoms of *ruptura sifac*, that is, in all probability, in-
guinal hernia; this *consilium*, too, is general and not attached to advice
for any particular patient. Taddeo stated that the causes of this kind of
rupture can be either internal or external: the external causes are such
things as a blow, lifting too heavy a weight, or engaging too strenuously
in coitus; the internal causes include vehement coughing, shouting, and
violent sneezing. The presence of such a rupture is shown by a lump in
the groin; when the patient lies on his back the lump becomes smaller,

[77] "medicus aut medicorum collegium iudicio primae significationis indicare habent de
morbo corporali, propter quem debet quis ne alios inficiat, ut leprosus, ab aliorum consortio
separari," *The Defensor Pacis of Marsilius of Padua*, ed. C. W. Previté-Orton (Cambridge,
1928), 2.6, pp. 169-170. The medical references in the *Defensor Pacis* are discussed in
George Rosen, "The Historical Significance of Some Medical References in the *Defensor
Pucis* of Marsilius of Padua," *Sudhoffs Archiv für Geschichte der Medizin* 37 (1953):
35-56. "Leprosy" was a widespread social and medical problem in the Middle Ages; lepers
were banned from the community, being, in some cases, housed in *leprosaria*; see Saul N.
Brody, *The Disease of the Soul*, for an account of medical theory and treatment, religious
responses, and social practices, as well as of literary uses of the theme of leprosy.

but it reappears if he coughs. In this way, Taddeo added, rupture can be distinguished from various other conditions producing swelling in the groin, including the application of medicaments and ligatures, bruising resulting from breaking of blood vessels, and fleshy tumors.[78]

For Taddeo, Guglielmo, and doubtless their colleagues, diagnosis was therefore a serious and demanding process. The best examples of this art that survive among their *consilia* are the work of physicians thoroughly familiar with every external manifestation of disease or injury in their individual patients. To gain this information they drew on a variety of skills and resources developed only in the course of medical practice: their accumulated personal experience, their own and others' powers of observation, and their ability to gain the confidence of patients in an interview. Naturally, they were often unsuccessful in relating such external manifestations as paroxysms, fever, abnormal excretions, lesions, swelling, and local pain to diseases of the internal organs, the condition of which they could mostly only guess at. But they showed great skill in drawing upon theoretical, academic learning in concrete situations and in classifying and analyzing the untidy phenomena of life in terms of the vast and complex body of medical science as they knew it.

TREATMENT

In the *consilia* advice for treatment, like diagnosis, is for the most part carefully organized to fit into theoretical categories. Treatment is discussed under the headings of regimen (or diet) and medication, or it is divided under diet, potion, and surgery. Both "regimen" and "diet" usually include advice about all six of the Galenic nonnaturals (that is, about air, sleep, exercise, repletion and inanition, and the passions of the soul, as well as food and drink). Medicines, characterized as internal or external, and preventative or curative, are further classified according to their supposed action: altering the complexion (*alterativa*), evacuating superfluities (*evacuativa*), and strengthening various parts of the body (*confortativa*). The learned, academic aspect of treatment is further emphasized by Taddeo's habit of prescribing remedies found in the works of authoritative writers—often simply by citing the passage where the physician who had sought him as a consultant could look up the actual rec-

[78] Taddeo, *I "Consilia,"* no. 163, pp. 212-216.

ipe.[79] Despite this orientation toward theory and system, Taddeo paid little or no attention in his *Tabula de remediis* to the concepts of complexional quality and "degree" (*gradus*, that is intensity) of medicines. Regarding degree, Taddeo perhaps shared the view, subsequently expressed by Turisanus, that "the degrees of medicine are only distinguished in respect of the effects they have on a body that is in perfect complexional balance, as may be seen from the fact that physicians say (and indeed it seems to be true) that a certain medicine is hot for Plato, but not for Socrates; hence it is that the authorities often differ among themselves about degree in medicines, because it was difficult for them to find a perfectly balanced body in which they could try them out."[80]

A short essay variously attributed to Dino and Mondino attempts to solve what must have been a major practical difficulty in prescribing remedies made up from recipes found in the works of medical authorities. In this little "treatise on weights and measures" the author attempted to explain to his readers the various systems of measurement used by pharmacological and medical writers and to relate these to the current usage of physicians at Bologna and elsewhere. His complaints about the imprecision inherent in the use of such measures as "a grain," given the difference in weight of the grains of different cereals and the regional variations in the weight of a grain of any one cereal, indicate a degree of appreciation of the scientific usefulness of quantitative exactness and consistency still quite rare in the early fourteenth century.[81] It must be re-

---

[79] For example, "Et si aliquando patitur ardorem urine, utatur tragea posita in Almansore, de ardore urine," ibid., no. 11, p. 27. Other instances could be cited. The reference is to the *Liber Almansoris* of Rasis, a much-used medical encyclopedia.

[80] "gradus medicine non distinguuntur nisi respectu operationis ab ea facte in corpore optime temperato cuius signum est quia sepe dicunt medici et verum videtur quod aliqua medicina est calida respectu socratis que non est calida respectu platonis: inde etiam est quod sepe discordare inveniuntur auctores in gradibus medicinarum: quia difficile fuit eis reperire corpus optime temperatum in quo experirentur eas," Turisanus, *Plusquam*, fol. 100v.

[81] "diversitas forte pervenit ex diversitate ponderis ordei vel frumenti; nam forte plus ponderant lx grana frumenti quam ordei, et plus ponderat frumentum et ordeum in una regione et una parte quam in alia, et ideo forte per grana non potest haberi ita precise quantitas pondorum sicut crederetur," *Tractatus Dini de ponderibus et mensuris* (Venice, 1499; Klebs 336.3; printed with Dino's *Chirurgia* and other works), fol. 152r. The work is discussed in Mary C. Wellborn, "Studies in Medieval Metrology: The *De Ponderibus et Mensuribus* of Dino del Garbo," *Isis* 24 (1935-1936):15-36. Regarding the attribution of this work, see note 163 to chapter two, above. For an account of the elaborate theoretical discussions, and restricted use in practice, of concepts of degree in pharmacology by ap-

marked, however, that actual recipes attributed to physicians trained at Bologna seldom or never show evidence of this kind of concern. Those found in Taddeo's *consilia*, for example, frequently and confidently indicate amounts of ingredients and dosages in pounds (*libra*), ounces (*unzie*), drams (*drachme*), and grains (*grana*) without any allusion to the regional diversity or local lack of standardization of these measures. Probably almost as often recipes are given in terms of proportion ("take equal parts of," or "boil in ten parts of wine and one of vinegar"), or with no quantitative indications at all. In Dino's own *Compilatio unguentorum et emplastrorum*, indications of quantity seem to be somewhat less frequent than in Taddeo's *consilia*; conceivably, their very omission may be credited to Dino's awareness of the problem.

A "regimen for sickness" (*regimen egritudinis*)[82] forms part of many of Taddeo's longer *consilia*, although it is not characteristic of those of Guglielmo's that have been edited. Taddeo's regimens for the sick differ relatively little in substance from his "regimen for health" (*regimen sanitatis*) for Corso Donati, although the latter is organized according to the seasons of the year rather than according to the six nonnaturals and contains, as the *consilia* usually do not, simple rules for personal hygiene (comb the hair, brush the teeth, and wash the hands and face upon arising). Corso's regimen contains not only a rule for daily living, but also advice on possible health hazards, the chief of which in Corso's case Taddeo seems to have thought to be overeating and sexual excess in summer.[83]

Furthermore, while some effort was obviously made to tailor each regimen for sickness to the needs of the patient, similar rules for living were handed down to sufferers from widely different diseases. This was especially true, of course, in advice regarding the passions of the soul, since few patients, whatever their disease, could fail to benefit from the almost uniform admonition to avoid sadness, care, and wrath, and to induce joy and happiness by engaging in their favorite pastimes as far as possible.

---

proximately contemporary physicians at Montpellier, see McVaugh, "Quantified Theory and Practice," *passim*.

[82] "Regimen huius egritudinis duplex est, scilicet previsum et curativum," Taddeo, *I* "Consilia," no. 6, p. 11.

[83] Taddeo, *Libello per chonservare la sanità del corpo*, in Spina and Sampalmieri, "La lettera de Taddeo Alderotti a Corso Donati," pp. 94, 96, 98.

In similar vein, Corso Donati was urged to adorn himself with fine clothes "because the soul rejoices in them."[84]

Much repetition and homogeneity is also to be found in the recommendations for air, sleep, exercise, and diet. Thus hot, dry air, fumigations with myrrh and other substances, and a fire in the room all day, especially in rainy or cloudy weather, were prescribed by Taddeo for patients suffering respectively from cataract, hoarseness, and "softness of the tongue."[85] One may conclude that Taddeo thought this the best environment for people afflicted with complaints of the head.

For diet, Taddeo recommended in case after case that patients avoid bread hot from the oven, cheese, some or all fruit, fish from standing water, beef, and pork; his preferred diet included poultry, veal, a moderate use of vegetables and herbs, with "subtle and fragrant" white wine to drink. His concern for his patients' diet extended to prescribing cooking methods (he was usually rather suspicious of stews and broths, recommending dry cooking instead) and seasoning. In the carefully measured mixtures of spices he devised to improve the savor and digestibility of his patients' food, the line between culinary and medicinal recipes becomes hard to distinguish.[86]

On the whole, medical treatments were more closely tailored to the patient and the specific nature of his or her illness than were regimens for sickness. Taddeo tempered his treatments according to the age and general condition of his patient; he believed, for example that a fistula in a pregnant woman who was also suffering from fever and a cough could only be cured by cutting and cautery, but that her condition made it impossible to perform either this operation or the phlebotomy and purgation of the head that she also needed.[87] In another instance, he hesitated to perform phlebotomy on a male patient who was over sixty.[88] The purpose for

[84] "Anche adornerai la tua persona di begli vestimenti, però che l'animo se ne ralegra," ibid., p. 94.

[85] Taddeo, I "Consilia," no. 5, p. 8; no. 10, p. 20; no. 24, pp. 57-58.

[86] For examples of diets incorporating most or all of these recommendations see ibid., no. 5, p. 8; no. 6, p. 12; no. 7, p. 15; no. 10, pp. 20-21; no. 11, pp. 24-25; no. 12, p. 28; and many more; also Libello per chonservare la sanità del corpo, in Spina and Sampalmieri, "La lettera de Taddeo Alderotti a Corso Donati," p. 95 (although Corso was advised to drink soup). These dietary rules were, of course, in no sense peculiar to Taddeo and, indeed. have ancient antecedents; see Majno, The Healing Hand, p. 189.

[87] Taddeo, I "Consilia," no. 37, pp. 76-77.

[88] Ibid., no. 62, p. 129. As a "gentler" substitute for phlebotomy the patient (the doge

which a particular medicine was intended, and its relation to the causes and manifestations of disease, were usually carefully noted. For example, a case of asthma was treated with an evacuative medicine to relieve the "repletion of the lungs and their passages that are near the heart and brain," which was the cause of the disease; with a medicine to correct the bad complexion caused by that repletion; and with a medicine to strengthen the heart and brain. In addition, Taddeo prescribed a special medicine to be administered during an actual attack, when the patient should be taken into fresh cool air and massaged on the extremities and chest.[89]

Moreover, the choice of medicines was clearly thought of as determined for the most part by medical theory. For example, Taddeo enumerated as "rational" various medications for epilepsy: a lotion for bathing the hand (since this was thought to be "the root of the disease"), an inhalant for altering the condition of the brain, theriaca and other medicines for internal consumption, and ointments and plasters.[90] Most of the ingredients in the recipes were herbal, although at least one animal component—dove's dung—and at least one mineral—antimony sulphide (*antimonium*)—were also included.[91] Remedies prescribed on grounds other than "reason" were, at least on occasion, clearly distinguished by Taddeo. Thus, at the end of the list of rational remedies for epilepsy, he remarked: "having seen the cure prescribed by reason, it is now necessary to see the cure by empirically derived remedies that have been demonstrated by experience and work by specific form."[92] What follows casts a new light on Taddeo's learned discussions elsewhere of the relationship between specific and substantial form. It will be remembered that specific form was called upon to account for any real or supposed actions of particular substances that were inexplicable by currently accepted scientific principles. The remedies for epilepsy placed in this category by Taddeo include a concoction of burned human bones, wine, and peony juice, and pills hav-

---

of Venice) was subjected to deliberate aggravation of his hemorrhoids, an alternative that does not seem greatly preferable.

[89] Ibid., no. 38, pp. 79-81.

[90] Ibid., no. 12, pp. 27-31.

[91] According to Robert P. Multhauf (*The Origins of Chemistry* [New York, 1966], p. 402), early references to "antimony" should usually be interpreted as meaning "antimony sulphide."

[92] "Viso de cura per rationem, videndum est de cura per empirica experimenta, per formam specificam operantia," Taddeo, I "*Consilia*," no. 12, pp. 31-32.

ing among their ingredients the gallbladder of a beaver and bear's testicles. Yet another recipe made use of the liver of a wolf, the hoofs of an ass (burnt and ground up), and the blood of a tortoise. Still another form of treatment called for the sufferer to wear an emerald ring in which was inserted some peony root and hairs from a white dog.[93]

While the remedies put into the specific form category in this particular *consilium* consistently call for slightly more bizarre ingredients than those in the "rational" category, it is by no means obvious on what basis assignment to one or the other of the two categories was made. It is tempting, but almost certainly erroneous, to suppose that the remedies said to act by specific form were grouped together (and distinguished from "rational" remedies) as a first step toward discarding certain medicaments and forms of treatment as useless. Taddeo was emphatic in his assertion that remedies owing their action to specific form worked and were indeed tested by experience. Moreover, there is absolutely no evidence to suggest that all the ingredients from which fairly uniform and readily perceptible results might in fact have been expected by the physicians of Taddeo's day (since the medieval pharmacopeia was far from consisting wholly of inert substances) were systematically or consistently assigned to either the "rational" or the "specific form" category. Predictability as we define it did not seem to be a criterion for assignment to one category or the other. Thus, in the *consilium* under discussion, Taddeo twice listed sulphide of antimony among the ingredients of a "rationally" determined remedy; but Turisanus discussed the action of laxatives as an example of specific form. In another of Taddeo's *consilia*, moreover, the remedies said to work by specific form are not random—apparently—collections of exotica, but herbal simples with recipes cited from the *Canon* of Avicenna.[94]

In a few cases, the assignment to the "specific form" category is readily understandable. Thus, in the case of the emerald ring prescribed against epilepsy, the vegetable and animal substances inserted into the ring came into no direct contact with the diseased body, either by ingestion or external local application to the afflicted parts; and "specific form" was sometimes used, as we have seen earlier, as an explanation for action at a distance, as in the case of the magnet. No doubt, too, herbal ingredients were assigned to the "rational" category when their use was determined

93 Ibid., p. 32.
94 Ibid., no. 24, p. 62.

by complexional reasoning, although, as noted, Taddeo seldom mentioned either the complexion or the degree of simples and remedies. Taddeo himself claimed that medicines that did not work by specific form
were open or manifest in their operations, as opposed to the occult virtues
of specific form; as he said, "there are two kinds of medicine for effecting
a cure of this condition, for some of them work through manifest virtue
—but I call manifest virtue every common alteration—whereas some of
them work through hidden virtue, that is, specific form. Of those working manifestly, some are evacuative medicines, some alterative, and some
strengthening."[95]

Of the various parts that might make up a *consilium*—description of
the patient and his or her symptoms, a regimen of sickness, prescriptions
for medication, and recommendations for *chirurgia*—medicinal recipes
are the one essential element that is never omitted. The prescription of
medicines—that is, of recipes for medicines to be taken internally, and for
enemas, inhalants, lotions, plasters, and ointments—lies at the heart of
the *consilia* of Taddeo and Guglielmo and of the *Practica de accidentibus*
attributed to Mondino. Surgical treatment was much less consistently
emphasized. In the *Practica de accidentibus*, among a host of herbal remedies for ailments of every part of the body there are two references to
bleeding from a severed vein or artery.[96] Taddeo included recommendations for *chirurgia* in a substantial number of his *consilia*, but this almost
always refers to either phlebotomy or cautery. The *consilia* do not include
advice on bonesetting or the bandaging or suturing of wounds, although
it is clear that at least the supervision (and perhaps the direct handling)
of cases of this kind—presumably the bread-and-butter of medieval surgical practice—was undertaken by Taddeo and no doubt also by his colleagues. This much is evident from Taddeo's prescriptions for medication
for a dog bite, for a lotion to minimize scarring, and for "an excellent
powder against every kind of fracture," as well as from his reference to
the value of alcohol for cleansing wounds.[97] Taddeo also referred to
couching for a cataract, stating that the case on which he had been called

[95] "Medicinarum autem ad hoc facientium duplex est genus; quedam enim operantur per
manifestam virtutem—appello autem manifestam virtutem omnem communem alterationem
—quedam vero operantur per virtutem occultam, scilicet formam specificam," ibid., p. 60.

[96] Mondino, *Practica de accidentibus*, p. 22.

[97] Taddeo, I "*Consilia*," no. 79, p. 139; no. 50, p. 125; no. 56, p. 127; no. 180, p. 238.

to pronounce had not yet reached a sufficiently advanced stage to permit this procedure.[98]

In his *consilia* Taddeo showed almost as little interest in phlebotomy as he did in the surgery of wounds and fractures; his relative neglect of the subject is in striking contrast to the heavy emphasis thereon not only in his own *Introductorius ad practicam*,[99] which appears to survive in a single manuscript, but also in one of the most widely used academic works on *practica* by a learned physician of his circle, namely Dino del Garbo's *Dilucidatorium*.[100] On the other hand, cautery has a prominent place among the surgical treatments advised by Taddeo. He urged its use for specific existing lesions (a fistula, for example)[101] and as a general treatment for the evacuation of superfluities. He used the term *cauterium* to refer both to cautery properly so called and to blistering. Thus he included cautery of the hand among the treatments he prescribed for epilepsy; it was to be carried out either by caustic medications or by instrument, and in the latter case the wound was to be kept open until much matter had evacuated.[102]

The surgical practice of Taddeo and his associates was undoubtedly more extensive than their *consilia* and Mondino's *Practica de accidentibus* suggest. These men were actively involved in carrying on the Bolognese surgical tradition: this much is clear from the place of surgery in the medical curriculum; from Taddeo's discussion in one of his commentaries on dry healing versus the encouragement of "laudable pus"; and from his account of a way of closing wounds "which I have not found described by any author but which I saw my uncle use";[103] from Mondino's dissections[104] and his celebrated anatomical textbook; from Dino's textbook on

---

[98] Ibid., no. 5, p. 11.

[99] Discussion of phlebotomy takes up more than half this work; see BAV, MS Palat. lat. 1284, fols. 147v-153r.

[100] In this work, Dino devoted the whole of chapter 21, in which 68 *questiones* are discussed, to the subject of phlebotomy.

[101] Taddeo, *I "Consilia*," no. 21, pp. 50-52.

[102] Ibid., no. 12, p. 32.

[103] "Item debes scire quod si vulnus non sit nimis magnum potest fieri sutura non in substantia carnis: sed in peciis positis in labiis vulneris si optime cum aliquo glutine inviscentur pecie in labiis: et postea fiat sutura in substantia panni: et cum pulvillis triangularis fiat constrictio undique: hunc autem modum ab auctore scriptum non inveni: sed vidi eum a quodam meo patruo," Taddeo, *Isagoge*, fol. 398v.

[104] For a strong defense of the proposition that Mondino did his own dissecting and

surgery and his collection of remedies for wounds and ulcers, both many times copied and, subsequently, printed; from Guglielmo's brief *Practica in cyrurgia*, which devotes a chapter each to wounds and fractures;[105] and from detailed recommendations for treating wounds that are even to be found in Turisanus's otherwise highly theoretical and abstract *Plusquam commentum* (for example, for large deep wounds whose margins could not easily be drawn together Turisanus recommended the temporary use of small triangular pads with a bandage—*ligatura*—on top).[106] Some of these works certainly seem to imply the personal performance of surgery, not just its supervision: thus, Dino wrote angrily about the practice of "stupid surgeons" who expose a patient with head injury to pain and danger by unnecessarily laying bare the bone; such an incision should be made, he believed, only after the presence of an actual fracture has been demonstrated by careful palpation.[107]

Moreover, the duties of the *medici condotti* on the Bologna city payroll, of whom Bartolomeo da Varignana was certainly one, included examining those who claimed to be victims of assaults and examining the corpses of those whose death was unexplained or suspicious, in order to determine whether their injuries were the result of crimes. These medico-legal experts had to be able to decide whether apparent injuries were mortal, and in some instances they resorted to autopsy to determine the cause of death. Thus Bartolomeo reported in 1307 that he had diligently examined by anatomical investigation the body of a certain Ghiseta and found her to have died of a wound in the upper body, which, after it was closed, continued to cause internal bleeding in the chest. In another instance Bartolomeo pronounced that Tomasino di Castel San Pietro had not died of a wound in the right side of his chest, even though this had penetrated the thoracic cavity, because "he could always breathe without difficulty, without coughing, without loss of blood by mouth or from below, without secretion of bad blood, and even without pain"; rather, Tomasino had been the victim of dysentery "in the same way that many others have

---

did not delegate the task to an assistant (as in the famous frontispiece to the *Anatomia* in Ketham's *Fasciculo di medicina* of 1493), see Ongaro, "Il metodo settorico di Mondino de' Liucci," passim.

[105] Sudhoff, *Beiträge zur Geschichte der Chirurgie*, 2:420-421.

[106] Turisanus, *Plusquam*, fol. 112r. His recommendations appear similar to, and may be derived from, those of Taddeo quoted in note 102, above.

[107] Dino, *Chirurgia*, sig. x[6r]-y1v.

recently perished of a similar disease, as they are still doing at present." In yet another case, Bartolomeo joined a Master Tommaso in reporting that a recipient of wounds in the head and nose would recover if he had good care.[108] It is possible, although surely excessively cautious, to argue that Bartolomeo most likely restricted his involvement in these cases to supervision, leaving any surgical treatment of survivors, along with any actual dissection, to assistant surgeons. Such an arrangement may be reflected in the composition of the panel of medical men who reported on the wounds of Azzolino di Domenico in 1302: Bartolomeo and another master are each termed *doctor physice,* and two of the other members *medici in cyrurgia.*[109] On the basis of the reports just summarized, however, there can be no doubt that Bartolomeo was fully cognizant of contemporary surgical practice and directed the treatment of surgical patients.

It is indeed hard to see how the boundaries between medicine and surgery could have been very sharply drawn in practice, whatever may have been the case in theory.[110] The age was one in which much surgery was doubtless wound surgery, and many wounds doubtless became infected and were medicated as ulcers.[111] Furthermore, the surgical procedure of phlebotomy and cautery were prescribed for ailments of every possible description. And quite apart from any other considerations, it appears highly unlikely that Taddeo and his associates would have excluded a lucrative staple from their practice.

The virtual omission of surgery, other than recommendations for cautery and some phlebotomy, from the *consilia* is unlikely, therefore, to be the result of a systematic shunning by these particular learned physi-

[108] Münster, "Alcuni episodi," pp. 207-213, where the documents are printed on pp. 210, 213: "Dico et affero non fuisse mortuum propter illud vulnus, eo quia non apparuunt [*sic*] accidencia indicancia mortem sequi ex illo vulnere et quia semper fuit sine difficultate anelitus, sine tussi, sine emissione sanguinis per os et per inferius, sine screatu saniei et eciam sine dolore in aliqua parte intrinseca et sic de aliis requisitis ad hoc vulnus si debet esse mortale penitus ymo in veritate mortuus fuit et est ex fluxu disinterico . . . sicut ad praesens multi homines perierunt simili morbo et continuo pereunt" (p. 213). On the development of forensic medicine at Bologna, see Münster, "La medicina legale in Bologna," and Edgardo Ortalli, "La perizia medica a Bologna nei secoli XIII e XIV. Normativa e practica di un istituto giudizario," *Deputazione di Storia Patria per le provincie di Romagna, Atti e Memorie,* n.s. 17-19 (1965-1968 in one):223-259.

[109] See note 35 to chapter four, above.

[110] Dino debated whether bloodletting should be considered part of medicine or of surgery; see *Dilucidatorium,* chap. 22, q. 9.

[111] On the assimilation of the treatment of wounds and ulcers in antiquity, see Majno, *The Healing Hand,* pp. 183-184.

cians of involvement in cases requiring surgical intervention. It may, however, owe a good deal to a desire to present their practice in the most scientifically interesting and intellectually respectable light. Although, as already noted n chapter four above, surgery came to form part of the university curriculum at Bologna and other Italian *studia*,[112] surgical methods were perhaps perceived as somewhat lacking in scientific interest by physicians v hose understanding of injury and illness was primarily in terms of alteration of complexion. Furthermore, as we have seen, Taddeo (at any rate when stressing the philosophical aspects of his scientific enterprise) expressed his disdain for *manualis operatio*, a disdain which those accustomed to later standards of medical propriety may find somewhat incongruous w th his willingness to devise recipes for cosmetics. It may well be that he and his colleagues delegated the actual performance of routine venesection, cautery, bonesetting, bandaging, and suturing to assistants wheneer possible. No doubt, too, these procedures were often carried out by practitioners who were not learned physicians, and with whom the latter would not have wished to be equated.

The *consilia* of Taddeo and his colleagues seldom or never give any indications of the outcome of a treatment, and provide only occasional glimpses of the level of expectation of physician or patient. Taddeo himself usually made no promise about the probable results of the treatment he recommended, although he would occasionally qualify a particular procedure or medicament as "remarkably effective," or "proven many times."[113] Mondino de' Liuzzi assured the readers of his *Practica de accidentibus* that a powder consisting of *terra sigillata* was "wonderful" (*mirabilis*) in its power to stop bleeding.[114] Both were more reticent than Guglielmo da Brescia, who confidently informed a physician who had consulted him by letter about a patient with a lump in a breast that the external application of local remedies to the lump would "quickly and easily dissolve it and perfectly heal it."[115] In one famous instance, however, Taddeo abandoned his usual reserve in order to endorse a medicinal

---

[112] For a summary of information concerning the position of surgery in the north Italian faculties of arts and medicine in the later Middle Ages, see Siraisi, *Arts and Sciences at Padua*, pp. 31, 165-166, and bibliography there cited.

[113] Taddeo, I "Consilia," no. 76, p. 138: "Pulvis mirabilis et expertus . . ."; ibid., no. 93, p. 141: "Pulvis probatissimus. . . ."

[114] Mondino, *Practica de accidentibus*, p. 22.

[115] "citius et facilius dissolvat eam et perfecte sanet," Guglielmo, *Consilia*, in E. Schmidt, *Die Bedeutung Wilhelms von Brescia*, p. 13.

substance in the warmest possible terms. As is well known, he devoted
no fewer than seven *consilia* to the manufacture and manifold virtues of
alcohol distilled from wine. Drawing upon the processes and techniques
of alchemy, he described distilling equipment and gave directions for its
use; he also noted with approval the capacity of distilled alcohol to absorb
the flavors of fruits, herbs, and spices steeped in it, and he gave his readers
several recipes for cordials.[116] As a medicine *aqua vitae* was, according to
Taddeo, "of inestimable glory, the mother and mistress of all medicine."[117] He remarked on its usefulness against melancholy (a little every
morning "makes one happy, jocund, and glad"),[118] as a toothache lini-
ment, and for cleansing wounds; he also claimed that it restored lost
memory, strengthened weak sight, and was an effective treatment in cases
of epilepsy, paralysis, and deafness—recommending its injection into the
ear in the latter instance.

The capacity to distill spirits was a relatively recent accomplishment in
western Europe in Taddeo's day;[119] so Taddeo's enthusiasm for *aqua
vitae* is no doubt partially explained by its novelty. His *consilia* on the
subject are striking but scarcely historically unique examples of the praise
of a new panacea that closer acquaintance would reveal as not without
drawbacks. Yet it is also clear from his encomium that he found alcohol
to be much more noticeable in its effects than most other medicinal substances known to him; the limited results produced by and expected of
most medieval herbal remedies is nowhere more clearly revealed than by
Taddeo's sense of the contrasting and much greater effectiveness of ardent
spirits.

If Taddeo generally hesitated to estimate the medical usefulness and
probable outcome of the treatments he advocated in particular cases, we
may be equally cautious in attempting to measure the overall impact of
his practice and that of other learned physicians of his day and of the
following generation on public health, on social conditions, and on intel-

---

[116] Taddeo, *I "Consilia,"* nos. 179-185, pp. 235-242; also edited in Edmund O. von
Lippmann, "Thaddäus Florentinus [Taddeo Alderotti] über den Weingeist," *Archiv für
Geschichte der Medizin* 7 (1913-1914):379-389.

[117] "Est igitur eius gloria inextimabilis, omnium medicinarum mater et domina," Taddeo, *I "Consilia,"* no. 180, p. 236.

[118] "quolibet mane dimidium coclear, ieiuno stomacho, cum parvo ciato vini odoriferi
sumptum, letificat, iucundum et ilarem facit," ibid., p. 237.

[119] See Multhauf, *Origins of Chemistry*, pp. 205-206 (cited in note 91, above).

lectual trends. Most of the patients treated by learned physicians were no doubt somewhat healthier than the rest of the population simply by dint of coming from a background that gave them access to the best that their society had to offer in the way of diet, housing conditions, and leisure. The attendance of a learned physician further provided them with sensible rules for health and hygiene, rational and perhaps therefore reassuring explanations of disease as a natural phenomenon, careful nursing along with helpful treatment for a good many minor complaints, and sympathetic concern. It also brought them into at least superficial contact with scientific learning. On the other hand, medical treatment is likely on occasion to have introduced infection where it was not already present; and the dietary regime usually recommended by the medical profession, with its strictures on fresh fruits, may have led to vitamin deficiencies if taken seriously.[120] Nonetheless, on balance it seems probable that the medical services of Taddeo and his colleagues improved the quality of life for those for whom they were available.

[120] A point made in Majno, *The Healing Hand*, p. 418. Fresh fruits may, however, have been regarded with suspicion by ancient physicians in the Mediterranean world (and hence by their medieval followers throughout Europe) because of an observed connection with intestinal illnesses.

CONCLUSION

The medicine with which we have been concerned in this study was a rigorous mental discipline requiring of its devotees a high degree of skill in handling abstract concepts and theoretical systems; simultaneously, it was a fairly simple technology or craft. The careers and writings of Taddeo Alderotti and his associates do not appear to substantiate the interpretation that the advent of "scholasticism" or "Aristotelianism" retarded the development of medicine. On the contrary, as has become apparent, it was the philosophizing learned physicians who, in the milieu of a faculty of arts and medicine, first developed and adopted such potentially fruitful innovations as the practice of writing *consilia* in individual cases and of carrying out dissections of human cadavers for purposes of study. This was neither coincidental nor wholly due to the partial survival of an earlier "practical" tradition. The *consilia* were Latin works based on theory, written by medical professors, and read, in all probability, by medical students; human dissection as a teaching tool (as opposed to the performance of occasional autopsies for legal purposes) appeared when the need for it was felt by an organized, and privileged, academic faculty and student university. Moreover, it was precisely the scholastic methods and the scholastic interest in ancient authorities that allowed problems such as the differences between Aristotelian and Galenic physiology to be exactly identified, and that encouraged rational discussion of differing theories to be carried on.

Nor can excessive reliance upon Hippocrates, Galen, and the Arabs as sources of medical teaching be regarded as limiting the medicine of the late thirteenth and early fourteenth centuries; rather, the attempts of Taddeo and his associates to extend and deepen the study of these authors were in themselves an important beginning of the expansion of medical learning. In medicine as in other disciplines, the ancient sources had to be recovered before they could be understood, and had to be understood before they could be criticized or rejected. The process that began in the twelfth century was not yet complete with Vesalius.

However, it is scarcely possible to sustain a claim that the association of technology with academic learning in the medicine studied, taught, and practiced by Taddeo Alderotti and his colleagues, and by other university-trained physicians in the Middle Ages, entitles one to think of their discipline as an applied science in anything like the modern sense of the term. Certainly, it is clear both that medical practice was influenced by theoretical concepts and that learned academic professors of medicine, trained also in arts and philosophy and noted for their pretensions to expertise in subtle speculation, spent a good deal of classroom time conveying mundane information about treatments and remedies. But the association of medicine as a craft with academic learning did not mean either that, as practitioners, learned physicians were required to adhere to a more rigorous methodology than members of other crafts, or that, as theoreticians, they carried out or were confronted with more frequent testing by experience than scholars in other learned disciplines. Indeed, no means were available to test much of current medical theory. In medicine, it was demanded of theoretical explanations merely that they not lead to actually harmful treatment. In some ways, moreover, the realities confronting physicians were less harsh than those facing other kinds of craftsmen; if a bridge or a cathedral tower fell down, human error was presumably responsible; but if a patient died, nature could be called upon to share the blame with the learned physician (even though the patient's family might not necessarily view the matter in that light).[1]

As philosophers and as scientists, too, Taddeo and his associates had their limitations. One cannot claim for them any major original contributions to philosophical thought or scientific discovery. Yet their contributions, along with those of other learned teaching physicians, in transmitting the philosophy and science of their day to large numbers of students and also in establishing a secular, professional faculty of medicine was surely of major significance. Taddeo and his associates played their part in shaping an enduring curriculum that gave certain of the Italian universities a scientific and secular cast evident throughout the later Middle Ages and Renaissance. The academic, professional, and scientific endeavors of these men merit lasting respect.

[1] Even the twelfth-century author Guibert of Nogent, who saw the hand of God or the devil in every possible (and impossible) occurrence, referred casually to the fall of a tower at Saint Denis as due to faulty construction by the masons; see his *De vita sua,* trans. in John F. Benton, ed., *Self and Society in Medieval France: The Memoirs of Abbot Guibert of Nogent* (New York, 1970), p. 228. For English examples of suits brought against physicians and surgeons in the later Middle Ages, see Madeleine Pelner Cosman, "Medieval Malpractice: The Dicta and the Dockets," *Bulletin of the New York Academy of Medicine,* 2d ser. 49 (1973):22-47. It is unlikely, however, that any of the practitioners involved were university trained.

REGISTER OF *QUESTIONES*

The following cumulative register of question titles contains a large majority, although not all, of the *questiones* examined by the members of Taddeo's circle in their medical works. Included are all the questions in eight major commentaries by these authors, all the questions in seven of their shorter commentaries or treatises, and a selection of questions from some of their other works, as well as questions surviving in independent form. Works covering the whole range of theoretical and practical medicine have been drawn upon, and each of the authors in the circle is represented. Questions by Taddeo and Dino preponderate, but this reflects their greater fecundity rather than any bias in selection. Even if every question in every commentary by Bartolomeo and Mondino were included, the total would come nowhere near that of Taddeo and Dino. The questions by Guglielmo and Turisanus that have been included apparently constitute almost the entire output of those authors in that form. Gentile da Cingoli wrote no medical commentaries, as far as is known, and appears to have left only one independently surviving question on a subject pertaining to medicine. For discussion of the uses made of the *questio* format in the circle of Taddeo, see chapter eight.

The question titles from the major commentaries have been drawn from the existing question registers (for full titles and details of publication of the cited editions of the major commentaries, the reader is referred to the list of abbreviations at the beginning of this volume):

Taddeo, *Aphor.*, question register on three unnumbered folios at the beginning of the volume;

Taddeo, *Pronost.*, question register on fols. 245v-246r;

Taddeo, *Reg. acut.*, question register on fol. 342v;

Taddeo, *Isagoge*, question register on fols. 400v-[402r];

Dino, *Dilucidatorium* and *Canon* 2, question registers on three unnumbered folios between the two works (printed together in the edition of Venice, 1514);

Dino, *Recollectiones reverendi artium et medicine doctoris magistri dini de Garbo de florentia super cirugiam avicene principis alboali,* Modena, Biblioteca Estense, MS Lat. 710 (alpha V.7.21), fols. 1r-102r (as noted in chapter eight, this question register is not found in the edition of Dino's *Chirurgia* printed at Ferrara in 1489 and several times cited earlier in this volume); this manuscript is hereafter cited as Dino, *Chirurgia* (Estense);

Turisanus, *Plusquam*, a register of questions, including *"digressiones,"* at fols. 137r-138r.

Each of the foregoing registers has been used in its entirety. The folio numbers or book and chapter citations that follow the question titles listed below indicate where the text of the question itself is to be found, according to the source register. In Dino's *Chirurgia*, however, the question titles listed in the manuscript register are simply enumerated at first, second, third, and so on, and this practice has been followed below (these numbered questions follow the alphabetized questions).

Where printed question registers exist, these have been used, even though in a few instances a register different from the printed version can be found in a single manuscript (compare, for example, the register found with Turisanus's *Plusquam commentum* in BAV, MS Vat. lat. 4472, fols. 19v-20v, and that found with Dino's *Dilucidatorium* in Vat. lat. 2484, fols. 182v-184v, with those in the editions of those works published in Venice in 1512 and 1514, respectively). The variations that I have seen between manuscript and printed versions of question registers for the same work appear to be relatively insignificant. A minute comparison of manuscript and printed registers would at this time serve little purpose, since the whole problem of possible interpolations, alterations, or omissions in manuscript and printed versions of the commentaries cannot be solved without the preparation of critical editions of the works themselves (a task far beyond the scope of this book). For the present, therefore, there seems to be no reason to shun the greater convenience offered by the printed registers.

The shorter treatises or commentaries from which all *questiones* have been included are the following (where the presence of a register is not indicated, question titles were drawn from the body of the work itself):

Bartolomeo, *De complexionibus* (BAV, MS Vat. lat. 4451, Bartholomaeus de Varignana, *Questiones super libro de complexionibus,* fols. 57r-87v);

Dino, *De natura fetus,* question register at fols. 89v-90r;

Guglielmo, *De tyriaca* (*Questiones de tyriaca*, ed. in McVaugh, "Theriac at Montpellier");

Guglielmo, *Canon* 1.4 (Padua, Biblioteca Universitaria, MS al numero provvisorio 202, *Questiones 4ᵉ fen libri primi avicenna recollecte sub provido viro . . . magistro Guilielmio de Brixia*, fols. 117v-124v), question register on fol. 29r;

Mondino, *De generatione* (BAV, MS Reg. lat. 2000, Mundinus de Bononia, *Expositio capituli de generatione embrionis* [*Canon* 3.21] fols. 1-23), question register on unnumbered folios at the beginning of the codex;

Taddeo, *Quod comeditur* (BAV, MS Palat. lat. 1246, *Dicta tadei de forma specifica in hoc capitulo primi canonis Quod comeditur et bibitur* [*Canon* 1.2.2.1.15], fols. 78v-79v;

Taddeo, *Practica de febribus* (Padua, Biblioteca Universitaria, MS al numero provvisorio 202, *Practica honorabilis doctoris medicine magistri thadei disputata*, fols. 107r-115r), question register on fol. 29r.

Other treatises or commentaries from which a few sample questions have been drawn, such as, for example, the commentaries on the *Prognostica* and *De regimine acutorum* (*reportationes super libro pronosticorum et primo, secundo et tertio libro regiminis acutorum morborum*), and on the *Tegni* by Mondino, which are contained in BAV, MS Vat. lat. 4466, are also indicated by abbreviated citations; for further information the reader is referred to the Bibliography.

In the case of *questiones* surviving independently in manuscript miscellanies, only one manuscript is cited below. Most of the few cases in which more than one manuscript or version of the same independent question is known are noted in the footnotes to the main text. In almost all instances only questions specifically attributed to a member of the group (by name) have been included, although in some cases anonymous questions found with the identified ones may belong to the same author. Thus, the set of six numbered miscellaneous questions by Dino del Garbo found in Munich, Bayerische Staatsbibliothek, CLM 13020, fols. 217r-222r (at fol. 220r: "Et in hoc terminatus determinacio veritatem questionum que fuerunt mote in palestris [?] nostris quam determinacio ego dinus de florencia posui") is immediately preceded by a much longer set that may also be his, but that in the absence of an attribution is not included here; it may be noted that several of the questions said to be by Dino in CLM

13020 are also to be found in a question miscellany in BAV, MS Vat. lat. 4454, fols. 99v-104v, where some of them occur anonymously.

The titles of *questiones* have been arranged under subject headings, in an effort to make the scope of discussion clearly apparent to the reader. Although the subject categories were deliberately kept very broad, some instances nonetheless turned up in which the same question could reasonably have been classified in more than one of the selected categories. The already considerable length of the register made it impractical to introduce cross-references from one category to another, or to repeat the same question in different categories. Thus, the final decision about the category to which certain questions should be assigned was on occasion somewhat arbitrary, a circumstance for which the reader's indulgence is sought. The spelling of the source registers has been retained; so some variants occur. Punctuation has been modernized and abbreviations have been expanded. A few obvious errors in the foliation given for some questions in the registers of Taddeo's commentaries have been silently corrected.

Fundamentals of Natural Philosophy
(scientific method, form and matter, the elements, the four causes, etc.)

An agens a forma specifica nutritur.   Taddeo, *Quod comeditur*, fol. 93v.
An attractio sit per identitatem.   Taddeo, *Quod comeditur*, fol. 91r.
An forma procedat ab extrinseco.   Taddeo, *Quod comeditur*, fol. 85v.
An forma specifica agat naturaliter.   Taddeo, *Quod comeditur*, fol. 90r.
An forma specifica sit.   Taddeo, *Quod comeditur*, fol. 83v.
An omnis res habeat formam specificam.
                    Taddeo, *Quod comeditur*, fol. 86r.
An operatio . . . sit per similitudinem.
                    Taddeo, *Quod comeditur*, fol. 91r.
An [forma specifica] participetur equaliter ab omnibus individuis.
                    Taddeo, *Quod comeditur*, fol. 85v.
An [forma specifica] sit accidens.   Taddeo, *Quod comeditur*, fol. 84r.
An unus possit habere plures formas specificas.
                    Taddeo, *Quod comeditur*, fol. 86v.
Qualis sit prima operatio, an alteracio an motus.
                    Taddeo, *Quod comeditur*, fol. 90v.
Utrum actio forme specifice sit per viam contrarii.
                    Taddeo, *Isagoge*, fol. 378v.

Utrum actio possit fieri a forma specifica.

Taddeo, *Isagoge*, fol. 378r.

Utrum aer inveniatur purus sine aliquis elementis.

Taddeo, *Isagoge*, fol. 346r.

Utrum aer sit humidior aqua. Taddeo, *Isagoge*, fol. 346r.

Utrum aqua inveniatur pura. Taddeo, *Isagoge*, fol. 346r.

Utrum attendende sint solum due conditiones, scilicet qualitatis et quantitatis; an tempus sit tertia conditio.

Turisanus, *Plusquam*, 3.7.

Utrum attractio possit esse a vacuo. Turisanus, *Plusquam*, 3.59.

Utrum caliditas et frigiditas elementorum sint cause gravitatis et levitatis elementorum. Taddeo, *Isagoge*, fol. 345r.

Utrum caliditas et frigiditas sint forme elementorum substantiales.

Taddeo, *Isagoge*, fol. 345r.

Utrum causa primitiva et antecedens dicantur materiales vel efficientes [*sic*].

Taddeo, *Isagoge*, fol. 393r.

Utrum causa primitiva sit res corporea.

Taddeo, *Isagoge*, fol. 393r.

Utrum diffinitio cause posita ab Avicenna sit bona.

Taddeo, *Isagoge*, fol. 391v.

Utrum diffinitio habeatur per viam divisionis vel demonstrationis.

Turisanus, *Plusquam*, 1.2.

Utrum diffinitio nature posita ab Avicenna sit bona.

Turisanus, *Plusquam*, 3.1.

Utrum doctrina resolutiva contineat omnia capitula huius libri.

Turisanus, *Plusquam*, 1.5.

Utrum doctrina resolutiva procedit ab effectu ad causam.

Mondino, *Tegni*, Vat. lat. 4466,
fol. 57v.

Utrum elementa remaneant similiter in mixto.

Turisanus, *Plusquam*, 1.15.

Utrum elementa sint in elementato potentia et non actu.

Taddeo, *Isagoge*, fol. 345r.

Utrum elementa sint res naturales. Taddeo, *Isagoge*, fol. 344r.

Utrum elementa sint tamen quattuor. Taddeo, *Isagoge*, fol. 345r.

Utrum elementum aliquid habeat duas qualitates in summo.

Taddeo, *Isagoge*, fol. 345r.

Utrum forma specifica causetur ex elementis.

Taddeo, *Isagoge*, fol. 378r.

Utrum futuri de fiente sit causa antecedens.

Turisanus, *Plusquam*, 3.34.

Utrum ignis elementaris veniat ad mixtionem.

Taddeo, *Isagoge*, fol. 345v.

Utrum inanimata sint consuetudinis receptiva.

Taddeo, *Aphor.*, fol. 68.

Utrum materia attrahat ad se. Turisanus, *Plusquam*, 3.59.

Utrum materia sit principium individuationis.

Turisanus, *Plusquam*, 2.44.

Utrum mulier sit de intentione natura.

Taddeo, *Isagoge*, fol. 370v.

Utrum mutatio cadat inter similia. Taddeo, *Aphor.*, fol. 69.

Utrum natura utatur previsione. Taddeo, *Aphor.*, fol. 22.

Utrum omnis res habeat formam specificam.

Taddeo, *Isagoge*, fol. 378v.

Utrum operatio possit totaliter mutari.

Taddeo, *Isagoge*, fol. 396v.

Utrum premise sint materia communis.

Turisanus, *Plusquam*, 1.6.

Utrum res mutans suum locum naturalem mutet etiam naturam.

Taddeo, *Aphor.*, fol. 174.

Utrum simpliciter talia sint que simpliciter tali corpori conveniunt.

Turisanus, *Plusquam*, 3.10.

Utrum species sensibilis vel intelligibilis habeat virtutem alterandi corpus.

Gentile da Cingoli, independent
question in Grabmann, "Gentile
da Cingoli."

Utrum terra et aqua magis dominent in nobis quam alia elementa.

Taddeo, *Isagoge*, fol. 345v.

Utrum tota materia possit effluere et tota renovari.

Turisanus, *Plusquam*, 2.44.

Utrum universale sit notius particulari.

Taddeo, *Reg. acut.*, fol. 256v.

The Heavenly Bodies
(astrology and the calendar)

Utrum aliqua stella possit immutare aerem.

Taddeo, *Isagoge*, fol. 374r.

Utrum aliquis aspectus celestis sit causa crisis.

Taddeo, *Aphor.*, fol. 49.

Utrum annus sit ter centum et sexaginta quinque dierum et quarta pars
ex centum partibus unius diei. Taddeo, *Pronost.*, fol. 237v.

Utrum aspectus lune sint tamen tres.   Taddeo, *Aphor.*, fol. 49.
Utrum aspectus lune et corporis supercelestis sit causa crisis.
                              Taddeo, *Pronost.*, fol. 236r.
Utrum corpus superceleste sit causa male crisis.
                              Taddeo, *Pronost.*, fol. 236v.
Utrum distinctio temporum sit eadem apud medicum et astrologum.
                              Taddeo, *Aphor.*, fol. 78.
Utrum inceptio temporum sit eadem apud omnes authores medicinales.
                              Taddeo, *Aphor.*, fol. 79.
Utrum motus celestis sit causa dierum creticorum intercidentium.
                              Taddeo, *Pronost.*, fol. 236v.
Utrum natura creticans recipiat adiutorium a constellatione.
                              Taddeo, *Pronost.*, fol. 236v.
Utrum propinquitas stellarum ad solem sit causa caliditatis aeris.
                              Taddeo, *Isagoge*, fol. 374r.
Utrum revolutiones periodorum sint tamen due.
                              Taddeo, *Pronost.*, fol. 237v.
Utrum sol sit causa crisis per motum proprium eius in circulo signorum vel
per solam aeris alterationem.   Taddeo, *Aphor.*, fol. 50.
Utrum sol sit causa efficiens venti.   Taddeo, *Isagoge*, fol. 364v.
Utrum sol sit ille que impellit vaporem elevatum ex quo sit ventus.
                              Taddeo, *Isagoge*, fol. 374v.
Utrum stelle fortunate et infortunate operantur ad bonam vel malam crisim.
                              Taddeo, *Aphor.*, fol. 50.
Utrum tempora anni sint equali inter se.
                              Taddeo, *Aphor.*, fol. 79.
Utrum tempora anni sint tamen duo.   Taddeo, *Isagoge*, fol. 373r.

Climate and the Seasons

Digressio de climatum habitatione.   Turisanus, *Plusquam*, 2.19.
Digressio de ventis.   Turisanus, *Plusquam*, 2.26.
Propter quid terra in estate interius est frigida econverso in hyeme.
                              Dino, *De natura fetus*, fol. 78r.
Utrum auster commoveat pluvias, et boreas eas destruat.
                              Taddeo, *Isagoge*, fol. 374v.
Utrum auster faciat malam auditum.   Taddeo, *Aphor.*, fol. 80.
Utrum autumnus debeat habere noctes hyemales et dies estivales.
                              Taddeo, *Isagoge*, fol. 373v.
Utrum boreas faciat corpora bene colorata.
                              Taddeo, *Aphor.*, fol. 80.

Utrum boreas faciat corpora bene nobilis.

Taddeo, *Aphor.*, fol. 80.

Utrum calor estatis remittatur in ortu canicule.

Taddeo, *Aphor.*, fol. 89.

Utrum frigiditas sit in media regione aeris.

Taddeo, *Isagoge*, fol. 345v.

Utrum hyems possit esse simul australis et pluviosa.

Taddeo, *Aphor.*, fol. 77.

Utrum hyems possit esse simul australis et tranquilla.

Taddeo, *Aphor.*, fol. 77.

Utrum mare debeat disponere terram a[d] frigidem et humidem.

Taddeo, *Isagoge*, fol. 375r.

Utrum omnis ventus sit frigidus et siccus.

Taddeo, *Isagoge*, fol. 374r.

Utrum plures et fortiores venti veniant a septentrione et a meridie quam ab oriente et occidente.   Taddeo, *Isagoge*, fol. 374v.

Utrum regiones vicine mari sunt frigide et humide.

Taddeo, *Aphor.*, fol. 78.

Utrum tempus possit facere aliquam mutationem in aere.

Taddeo, *Isagoge*, fol. 373r.

Utrum tempus siccum sit sanius pluviali.

Taddeo, *Aphor.*, fol. 79.

Utrum terra calida et humida sit causa longe vite.

Taddeo, *Isagoge*, fol. 375r.

Utrum terra elevata sit calidior quam depressa.

Taddeo, *Isagoge*, fol. 375r.

Utrum venti magis multiplicentur in vere et autumno quam in aliquo alio anni tempore.   Taddeo, *Isagoge*, fol. 374v.

Utrum ventus favonius sit frigidior borea.

Taddeo, *Isagoge*, fol. 374v.

Utrum ventus subsolanus sit calidior austro.

Taddeo, *Isagoge*, fol. 374r.

Utrum ver sit magis temperatum quam autumnus.

Taddeo, *Isagoge*, fol. 373r.

Utrum ver sit tempus calidum et humidum.

Taddeo, *Isagoge*, fol. 373v.

Utrum ver sit tempus temperatum.   Taddeo, *Aphor.*, fol. 74.

Miscellaneous Natural Phenomena
(properties of air and water, light and color, plants, wine, etc.)

Digressio de causis colorum.   Turisanus, *Plusquam*, 2.32.

Utrum acetum fortificet operationem vaporationis.

Taddeo, *Reg. acut.*, fol. 275v.

Utrum acuitas et caliditas augeantur in vino in processu temporis.

Taddeo, *Reg. acut.*, fol. 307v.

Utrum aqua calida intus exhibita possit redire ad frigiditatem naturalem.

Dino, *Canon*, 2, ch. 2, q. 1.

Utrum colores in tenebris sint actu colores.

Taddeo, *Isagoge*, fol. 369v.

Utrum dyaphana habeant colorem.   Taddeo, *Isagoge*, fol. 369v.

Utrum ex semine quando rumpitur primo oriantur frondes vel stipes.

Dino, *De natura fetus*, fol. 72r.

Utrum in ovo vitellum est sicut materia albumen sicut nutrimentum.

Dino, *De natura fetus*, fol. 86r.

Utrum Johannitius sufficienter posuerit species colorum.

Taddeo, *Isagoge*, fol. 369v.

Utrum lac sit facilis mutationis.   Taddeo, *Aphor.*, fol. 157.

Utrum lumen sit necessarium propter colorem vel diafanum.

Turisanus, *Plusquam*, 2.31.

Utrum nix et christallus sint frigidiores aqua.

Taddeo, *Aphor.*, fol. 134.

Utrum plante habeant actiones vel operationes.

Taddeo, *Isagoge*, fol. 344v.

Utrum plante habeant virtutem.   Taddeo, *Isagoge*, fol. 344v.

Utrum plante que generantur ex semine possint sine semine generari.

Dino, *De natura fetus*, fol. 74r.

Utrum propter multitudinem aqueitatis et aereitatis res rarificetur.

Dino, *Canon* 2, ch. 3, q. 4.

Utrum res grossiores velocius recipiant congelationem quam res subtiliores.

Dino, *Canon* 2, ch. 3, q. 3.

Utrum res rarificetur ex hoc quod partes aeree in aqueas convertuntur, vel condensetur quod partes aquee in aereas convertuntur.

Dino, *Canon* 2, ch. 3, q. 5.

Utrum semen ex quo generatur planta sic [*sic*] de essentia plante.

Dino, *De natura fetus*, fol. 73v.

Utrum virtus vitalis sit in plantis.   Taddeo, *Isagoge*, fol. 359r.

NATURE AND PURPOSE OF MEDICINE
(INCLUDING DEFINITIONS OF HEALTH AND SICKNESS
AND DISCUSSIONS OF THE PLACE OF MEDICINE AMONG THE SCIENCES)

Digressio de distinctione, subalternatione scientiarum.

Turisanus, *Plusquam*, 1.7.

Querabatur pridie de quadam questione in qua possunt tangi omnes
difficultates communes de corporibus. Et erat questio utrum corpus sanum
ut nunc habeat sanitatem adquisitam a rebus temporalibus sive a tempora . . . .
questio magistri mondini [*sic*].   Mondino, independent question,

CLM 244, fols. 135v-138r.

Queritur quia Avicenna non determinavit de parte practice que est resumtiam

Guglielmo, *Canon* 1.4, fol. 117v.

Queritur quia Galenus videtur continuari egritudinem nunc ad sanitatem
nunc, ut dicebam in loquendo literam, et nullam facit mentionem de
neutralitate nunc.   Bartolomeo, *De complexionibus*,

fol. 73r.

Utrum aliqua nota vulgo arti medicinali addenda sint.

Taddeo, *Reg. acut.*, fol. 247v.

Utrum aphorismus secundus sit theoria vel practica.

Taddeo, *Aphor.*, fol. 3.

Utrum ars conservativa possit conservare.

Turisanus, *Plusquam*, 3.2.

Utrum causa conservans sit alicuius generis cause.

Turisanus, *Plusquam*, 3.1.

Utrum causa conservans sit prior sanitate.

Turisanus, *Plusquam*, 3.1.

Utrum causa faciens sanitatem sit medicina.

Taddeo, *Isagoge*, fol. 392v.

Utrum cause que neutris nec conferunt nec nocent possint dici cause neutri.

Turisanus, *Plusquam*, 3.82.

Utrum corpus bone habitudinis possit manere in eodem quantum ad
medicum necne.   Taddeo, *Aphor.*, fol. 5.

Utrum corpus humanum sit subiectum in hoc libro.

Taddeo, *Isagoge*, fol. 343v.

Utrum corpus sanum in organicis et distemperatum in similibus
sit egrum.   Turisanus, *Plusquam*, 1.16.

Utrum corpus sanum sit plura vel unum.

Turisanus, *Plusquam*, 1.15.

Utrum corpus simpliciter sanum, infirmatum et sanitati restitutum, sit
simpliciter sanum.   Turisanus, *Plusquam*, 1.15.

Utrum corpus semper sanum sit in latitudine sanitatis.

Turisanus, *Plusquam*, 2.7.

Utrum corpus simpliciter sanum possit infirmari.

Turisanus, *Plusquam*, 1.15.

Utrum diffinitio medicina sit bona.   Turisanus, *Plusquam*, 1.7.

Utrum diffinitio neutri posita ab auctore sit bona.

Taddeo, *Isagoge*, fol. 391v.

Utrum diffinitiones sani et egri sint bone.

Turisanus, *Plusquam*, 1.16.

Utrum dispositio simpliciter talis sit congenita.

Turisanus, *Plusquam*, 1.15.

Utrum dispositiones corporis humani sint tamen due, sanitas et egritudo.

Taddeo, *Isagoge*, fol. 391v.

Utrum divisio qua medicina dividitur in theoricam et practicam sit divisio
generis in species.   Taddeo, *Isagoge*, fol. 344r.

Utrum divisio quam ponit author de morbo sit divisio generis in species.

Taddeo, *Isagoge*, fol. 390r.

Utrum doctrina huius libri sit ordinaria.

Taddeo, *Isagoge*, fol. 343v.

Utrum eadem possit esse causa sanitatis regiminis que et neutralitatis.

Turisanus, *Plusquam*, 3.82.

Utrum et qua sit significatio causarum conservantium ad corpus.

Turisanus, *Plusquam*, 3.21.

Utrum facere sanitatem in egro sit finis medicine vel potius eam conservare.

Taddeo, *Pronost.*, fol. 195v.

Utrum fortitudo virtutis sola significet salutem.

Taddeo, *Pronost.*, fol. 228v.

Utrum hec diffinitio [sc. medicine in *Tegni*] sit convenienter data.

Mondino, *Tegni*, fol. 58v.

Utrum idem aphorismus [1.2] sit de corpore, vel de causa, vel de signo.

Taddeo, *Aphor.*, fol. 3.

Utrum idem corpus sit egrum ut nunc, et sanum simpliciter.

Turisanus, *Plusquam*, 1.16.

Utrum inter sanum et egrum cadat medium.

Turisanus, *Plusquam*, 1.7.

Utrum ista sit diffinitio [sc. sanitatis in *Tegni*] conveniens.

Mondino, *Tegni*, fol. 59v.

Utrum ista divisio signorum sit conveniens.

Mondino, *Tegni*, fol. 63v.

Utrum iudicium vulgare sit verum.   Taddeo, *Reg. acut.*, fol. 250v.

Utrum medicatio sit finis medicine.   Taddeo, *Reg. acut.*, fol. 248v.

Utrum medici precedentes Hippocratem tradiderint pauca medicamina.
                              Taddeo, *Reg. acut.*, fol. 249v.
Utrum medicina sit composita ex theorica et practica.
                              Turisanus, *Plusquam*, 1.10.
Utrum medicina sit potius dicenda tota activa vel tota speculativa.
                              Turisanus, *Plusquam*, 1.10.
Utrum medicina sit scientia signorum.
                              Turisanus, *Plusquam*, 1.9.
Utrum medicina supponatur philosophie naturali.
                              Taddeo, *Isagoge*, fol. 343v.
Utrum modi doctrine ordinarie sint tamen tres.
                              Mondino, *Tegni*, fol. 57r.
Utrum omne indubitabile et manifestum sit inutile in arte.
                              Taddeo, *Aphor.*, fol. 127.
Utrum omne periculum a medico previsum ab eodem tolli possit.
                              Taddeo, *Pronost.*, fol. 196r.
Utrum optima sanitas sit in medio extremorum.
                              Turisanus, *Plusquam*, 2.9.
Utrum optima sanitas sit reperibilis.   Turisanus, *Plusquam*, 2.9.
Utrum philosophia [ph'ia] practica docet exerceri in pravis.
                              Turisanus, *Plusquam*, 2.43.
Utrum possit etiam aliquid corpus neutrum simpliciter neutri significati.
                              Turisanus, *Plusquam*, 1.18.
Utrum practica fuerit prior theorica vel econtra.
                              Taddeo, *Isagoge*, fol. 343v.
Utrum practica sit operatio vel non.   Taddeo, *Isagoge*, fol. 343v.
Utrum preservatio indigeat tribus generibus causarum salubrium.
                              Turisanus, *Plusquam*, 3.78.
Utrum recte procedat Galenus a corporibus ad signa, et non econtra.
                              Turisanus, *Plusquam*, 1.10.
Utrum sanum ut multum sit sanum ut nunc.
                              Turisanus, *Plusquam*, 1.15.
Utrum sanum ut nunc ponatur in genere corporum naturaliter dispositorum
vel preternaturaliter.   Turisanus, *Plusquam*, 1.15.
Utrum sanum ut nunc sit tale a generatione.
                              Turisanus, *Plusquam*, 1.15.
Utrum scientia medicine sit utilis.   Taddeo, *Pronost.*, fol. 214r.
Utrum scientia sit genus medici, an ars.
                              Turisanus, *Plusquam*, 1.7.
Utrum simpliciter neutrum ponatur medium inter sanum semper egrum
et nunc.   Turisanus, *Plusquam*, 2.9.

Utrum sit aliquod genus sub quo locetur corpus optime sanum.

Turisanus, *Plusquam*, 3.22.

Utrum sit aliquod neutrum non tactum a Galeno.

Turisanus, *Plusquam*, 1.18.

Utrum sit dabile corpus cuius quidam membra sunt sana quidam neutra.

Turisanus, *Plusquam*, 1.16.

Utrum sit possibile corpus conservare. Turisanus, *Plusquam*, 3.4.

Utrum sit reperibile corpus optime sanum.

Turisanus, *Plusquam*, 1.15.

Utrum subiectum medicine sit unum. Turisanus, *Plusquam*, 1.0.

Utrum sunt idem corpus egrotantem et egrum simpliciter.

Mondino, *Tegni*, BAV, Vat. lat. 4466,
fol. 51v.

Utrum theorica adiuvet nos in opere vel non.

Taddeo, *Isagoge*, fol. 343v.

Utrum theorica consideret res solo intellectu.

Taddeo, *Isagoge*, fol. 343v.

Utrum theorica et practica sint species medicine.

Turisanus, *Plusquam*, 1.10.

Utrum vulgus cognoscat tantum ea in quibus medicus bonus cum malo
communicat. Taddeo, *Reg. acut.*, fol. 250v.

70ª questio est utrum dictum sit verum cum dicit quod magis est
credendum experimentum quam rationi.

Dino, *Chirurgia* (Estense).

PSYCHOLOGY
(THE SOUL, COGNITION, THE EMOTIONS, SLEEP, MENTAL DISORDERS)

Digressio de mutatione corporis ex accidentibus anime.

Turisanus, *Plusquam*, 3.5.

Digressio de somno et causis eius. Turisanus, *Plusquam*, 2.21.

Dubitatio quare non fecit intentionem de frenese vera quia dicendum quod
dedit intelligere. Mondino, *Pronost.*, fol. 6r.

Utrum accidentia anime desiccent corpus nostrum.

Taddeo, *Isagoge*, fol. 380v.

Utrum accidentia anime possint corpus nostrum immutare.

Taddeo, *Isagoge*, fol. 380v.

Utrum aliquod universale possit memorari.

Taddeo, *Isagoge*, fol. 361v.

Utrum anima cum sit incorporea possit movere musculum qui est corporeus.

Taddeo, *Isagoge*, fol. 365v.

Utrum anima intellectiva sit una numero in omnibus hominibus.

Taddeo, *Isagoge*, fol. 360v.

Utrum anima sit actus corporis habentis vitam in potentiam.

Turisanus, *Plusquam*, 2.12.

Utrum contingat intelligere sine phantasmate.

Taddeo, *Isagoge*, fol. 360v.

Utrum essentia anime sit in corde.   Turisanus, *Plusquam*, 2.12.

Utrum ex ira possit quis citius mori quam ex aliquo alio anime accidenti.

Taddeo, *Isagoge*, fol. 381v.

Utrum frenesis sit passio mortifera propter nobilitatem membri in quo sit, non autem propter sui magnitudinem.

Taddeo, *Pronost.*, fol. 205r.

Utrum homo post mortem recordetur.

Taddeo, *Isagoge*, fol. 361v.

Utrum intellectus agens et materialis sint idem in substantia.

Taddeo, *Isagoge*, fol. 360v.

Utrum intellectus semper intelligat.   Taddeo, *Isagoge*, fol. 360v.

Utrum memoria sit in omnibus animalibus.

Taddeo, *Isagoge*, fol. 361v.

Utrum omne animal habeat phantasiam.

Taddeo, *Isagoge*, fol. 359v.

Utrum omne animal participet somno.

Taddeo, *Isagoge*, fol. 380v.

Utrum omnia anime accidentia corpus exiccent et contraria humectent.

Turisanus, *Plusquam*, 3.21.

Utrum omnis virtus animalis quiescat in somno.

Taddeo, *Isagoge*, fol. 380v.

Utrum phantasia componat.   Taddeo, *Isagoge*, fol. 360r.

Utrum phantasia semper operetur vel non.

Taddeo, *Isagoge*, fol. 360r.

Utrum ratio possit esse sana, imaginatione existent corrupta.

Taddeo, *Pronost.*, fol. 205r.

Utrum sit reperibile temperamentum in accidentibus anime quod faciat ad conservatione corporis optime sani.   Turisanus, *Plusquam*, 3.16.

Utrum somnus possit nocere.   Taddeo, *Aphor.*, fol. 28.

Utrum somnus sit res non naturalis.   Taddeo, *Isagoge*, fol. 380v.

Utrum somnus tollat sitim.   Taddeo, *Aphor.*, fol. 136.

Utrum timor et pusillanimitas sint causa manie.

Taddeo, *Aphor.*, fol. 175.

Utrum timor et pusillanimitas sint causa melancholie.

Taddeo, *Aphor.*, fol. 175.

Utrum virtus animalis sit in toto corpore.

Taddeo, Isagoge, fol. 359v.

Utrum virtus animalis sit semper in actu secundo in nobis.

Taddeo, Isagoge, fol. 359v.

Utrum virtus phantastica sit solum vera.

Taddeo, Isagoge, fol. 360r.

PHYSIOLOGY—GENERAL

An diastole in aliquam dispositionem possit esse maior sistole.

Dino in Tommaso del Garbo,
Digressiones, no. 36.

Digressio de causis dispositionum corporis.

Turisanus, Plusquam, 3.5.

Utrum corpus diffiniatur per oppositiones.

Turisanus, Plusquam, 2.2.

Utrum res annexe rebus naturalibus sint tamen quatuor.

Taddeo, Isagoge, fol. 344v.

Utrum res naturales sint tamen VII.   Taddeo, Isagoge, fol. 344r.

Utrum vita possit elongari ultra mensura sui primitivi calidi.

Turisanus, Plusquam, 3.87.

PHYSIOLOGY—COMPLEXION THEORY
(INCLUDING SOME QUESTIONS ON THE COMPLEXION OF SUBSTANCES OTHER THAN THE HUMAN BODY)

An ista forma precedat complexionem.

Taddeo, Quod comeditur, fol. 85v.

An sit materia, forma, a complexione.

Taddeo, Quod comeditur, fol. 84v.

Digressio de complexionibus et remanentia elementorum in mixtis.

Turisanus, Plusquam, 1.15.

Dubitatur quare cum proponat dicere signum complexionis dicat signorum compositionis.   Turisanus, Plusquam, 2.14.

Queritur que complexio sit longioris vite.

Dino, independent question, Vat. lat.
3144, fols. 12r-13v.

Quis stomachus melius digeret, an stomachus temperatus vel stomachus calidus.   Bartolomeo, De complexionibus, fol. 77r.

Utrum acetosum sit complexionis calide aut frigide.

Dino, *Canon* 2, ch. 3, q. 11.

Utrum acetosum sit complexionis humide aut sicce.

Dino, *Canon* 2, ch. 3, q. 12.

Utrum aer mutatis in complexione magis ledat quam mutatus in substantia.

Taddeo, *Isagoge*, fol. 375v.

Utrum aliqua etas temperata possit inveniri.

Taddeo, *Isagoge*, fol. 369r.

Utrum aliquam mulierem sit calidioris complexionis quem aliquis vir [*sic*].

Taddeo, *Isagoge*, fol. 370v.

Utrum aliqua terra sit calide et humide complexionis.

Taddeo, *Isagoge*, fol. 375r.

Utrum calida et sicca complexio sit conveniens ad generationem masculorum.

Turisanus, *Plusquam*, 2.53.

Utrum caliditas epatis possit contra operari frigiditati cordis.

Turisanus, *Plusquam*, 2.48.

Utrum caliditas innata quo ad subiectum sit maior in pueris quam in iuvenibus, quo vero ad qualitatem sit econverso.

Taddeo, *Aphor.*, fol. 17.

Utrum caliditas pectoris gaudeat similibus, sicut que ventris.

Turisanus, *Plusquam*, 2.71.

Utrum calidum conferat cerebro.   Taddeo, *Aphor.*, fol. 132.

Utrum calidum in ultimo rarificetur.   Taddeo, *Aphor.*, fol. 132.

Utrum calor attribuatur complexioni.   Taddeo, *Isagoge*, fol. 369v.

Utrum calor et spiritus sint mixti vel distincti.

Taddeo, *Isagoge*, fol. 368r.

Utrum calor innatus in hyeme multiplicetur.

Taddeo, *Aphor.*, fol. 19.

Utrum calor innatus sit magis in iuvene quo ad 4^m elementum quam in puero.

Taddeo, *Aphor.*, fol. 17.

Utrum calor iuvenis sit maior calore pueri.

Taddeo, *Aphor.*, fol. 16.

Utrum calor naturalis plus resolvat in hyeme quam in estate.

Taddeo, *Aphor.*, fol. 19.

Utrum calor naturalis sit temperate complexionis.

Taddeo, *Aphor.*, fol. 17.

Utrum calor sit calidior quam spiritus.

Taddeo, *Isagoge*, fol. 368r.

Utrum calor sit complexio.   Taddeo, *Isagoge*, fol. 369r.

Utrum cerebrum per eandem complexionem sit principium motive operationis et sensitive.   Turisanus, *Plusquam*, 2.18.

Utrum cerebrum sit calidum.   Taddeo, *Isagoge*, fol. 352v.
Utrum circa durum et molle cadat ista diversitas que cadit in macrem et
pinguedinem, sic ergo [?] non sequitur complexionem naturalem.
                                          Bartolomeo, *De complexionibus*,
                                          fol. 107v.
Utrum coitus infrigidet vel calefaciat.
                                          Taddeo, *Isagoge*, fol. 381r.
Utrum complexio antecedat formam specificam.
                                          Taddeo, *Isagoge*, fol. 378r.
Utrum complexio antecedat formam substantialem.
                                          Taddeo, *Isagoge*, fol. 346v.
Utrum complexio calida male se habeat ad tempus.
                                          Taddeo, *Aphor.*, fol. 72.
Utrum complexio equalis quo ad iustitiam non sit possibilis inveniri nisi in
solo homine.   Taddeo, *Isagoge*, fol. 347r.
Utrum complexio equalis quo ad iustitiam non sit possibilis inveniri nisi in
uno solo individuo.   Taddeo, *Isagoge*, fol. 347r.
Utrum complexio equalis quo ad iustitiam reperiatur.
                                          Taddeo, *Isagoge*, fol. 347r.
Utrum complexio equalis quo ad pondus sit possibilis.
                                          Taddeo, *Isagoge*, fol. 346v.
Utrum complexio et commixtio sint idem vel diversa.
                                          Taddeo, *Isagoge*, fol. 346r.
Utrum complexio et etas bene se habeant ad dietas contrarias male ad similes.
                                          Taddeo, *Aphor.*, fol. 72.
Utrum complexio frigida male se habeat ad hyemem.
                                          Taddeo, *Aphor.*, fol. 72.
Utrum complexio hominis sit magis propinqua complexioni temperate ad
pondus quam aliqua alia complexio.   Bartolomeo, *De complexionibus*,
                                          fol. 68r.
Utrum complexio innata possit permutari.
                                          Taddeo, independent question,
                                          BAV, Reg. lat. 2000, fols. 115v-116r.
Utrum complexio longioris vite cognoscatur.
                                          Turisanus, *Plusquam*, 2.65.
Utrum complexio naturalis possit permutari.
                                          [Dino], independent question, BAV,
                                          Vat. lat. 4454, fols. 101r-102r.
Utrum complexio sit causa forma specifica.
                                          Taddeo, *Isagoge*, fol. 378r.

Utrum complexio sit forma substantialis.

Taddeo, *Isagoge*, fol. 346r.

Utrum complexio sit genus numeri forme quantitatis et compositionis.

Taddeo, *Isagoge*, fol. 391r.

Utrum complexio temperata sit eque distans etc.

Turisanus, *Plusquam*, 1, 13.

Utrum cor sit frigide complexionis.   Taddeo, *Isagoge*, fol. 352r.

Utrum corpus calidum plus repugnat causis frigidis quam temperatum.

Turisanus, *Plusquam*, 2.6.

Utrum corpus humanum, remanente vita, possit labi ad frigus vel calorem.

Turisanus, *Plusquam*, 3.43.

Utrum crassi minus habeant de calore quam macri.

Taddeo, *Aphor.*, fol. 65.

Utrum cum malitia complexionis possit esse bonitas et temperantia
complexionis.   Bartolomeo, *De complexionibus*,
fol. 64r.

Utrum debuerit docuisse complexionem testium ab influxu, scilicet totum.

Turisanus, *Plusquam*, 2.52.

Utrum epar sit frigide complexionis.   Taddeo, *Isagoge*, fol. 353r.

Utrum epar temperatum reddat ventrem siccum.

Taddeo, *Aphor.*, fol. 43.

Utrum equalis sit caliditas in puero et iuvene.

Bartolomeo, *De complexionibus*,
fol. 70r-v.

Utrum etas iuventutis sit etas temperata.

Taddeo, *Aphor.*, fol. 72.

Utrum ex superficietate capitis debeat docere significare super complexione
cerebri.   Turisanus, *Plusquam*, 2.16.

Utrum forma specifica sit idem que complexio.

Taddeo, *Isagoge*, fol. 378r.

Utrum frigida conveniant nervis.   Turisanus, *Plusquam*, 3.55.

Utrum frigiditas ingrediatur opus nature per se.

Taddeo, *Isagoge*, fol. 366v.

Utrum frigiditas intret opus nature actu vel potentia.

Taddeo, *Isagoge*, fol. 367r.

Utrum frigiditas per se simplex intret opus nature.

Taddeo, *Isagoge*, fol. 366v.

Utrum frigidum sit bene appetere.   Turisanus, *Plusquam*, 2.71.

Utrum frigus possit calorem naturalem augere.

Taddeo, *Aphor.*, fol. 19.

Utrum genera signorum significantia super complexione cerebri sint tamen V.

Turisanus, *Plusquam*, 2.13.

Utrum habentes stomachum humidum faciliter famescant.

Turisanus, *Plusquam*, 2.70.

Utrum homo temperatus secundum se totus sit magis temperatus, vel minus,
vel equaliter, cum temperantia cutis.   Bartolomeo, *De complexionibus*,
fol. 65r.

Utrum humiditas possit recurrere ex mediis regionibus in venis.

Turisanus, *Plusquam*, 3.68.

Utrum in febre in qua est mala complexio diverse, complexio in omnibus
partibus tocius corporis . . . leditur.   Dino, *De malicia complexionis*,
BAV, Vat. lat. 2484, fol. 196v.

Utrum in humano corpore sit dari malam complexionem simpliciter.

Mondino, independent question, BAV,
Vat. lat. 3144, fol. 12r.

Utrum lac sit calide complexionis.   Taddeo, *Aphor.*, fol. 157.

Utrum lac sit frigidius sanguine.   Taddeo, *Aphor.*, fol. 141.

Utrum latus dextrum sit calidius sinistro.

Taddeo, *Aphor.*, fol. 140.

Utrum lenitas significet humiditatem.

Turisanus, *Plusquam*, 2.75.

Utrum maturatio non fiat nisi per calidum.

Taddeo, *Pronost.*, fol. 209r.

Utrum maxima pars aromatum sit calida et sicca.

Taddeo, *Aphor.*, fol. 136.

Utrum melancholia efficiatur a calore temperato.

Taddeo, *Isagoge*, fol. 350v.

Utrum melancholia sit frigidior quam flegma.

Taddeo, *Isagoge*, fol. 350v.

Utrum melancholia sit siccior quam cholera.

Taddeo, *Isagoge*, fol. 350v.

Utrum membrum possit corrumpi propter malam complexionem sine materia.

Dino, *Dilucidatorium*, 27.1.

Utrum modo determinandi complexionem in homine sit similis modo
determinandi complexionem in temporibus.

Bartolomeo, *De complexionibus*,
fol. 62r.

Utrum mulier possit esse temperate complexionis, sicut vir.

Taddeo, *Isagoge*, fol. 370v.

Utrum oculus sit calide et sicce complexionis.

Taddeo, *Isagoge*, fol. 370v.

Utrum omne amarum sit calidum.   Dino, *Canon* 2, ch. 3, q. 9.

Utrum omne aromaticum sit calidum et siccum.

Taddeo, *Isagoge*, fol. 364v.

Utrum omne mixtum habens complexionem secundam habeat complexionem
primam.   Dino, *Canon* 2, ch. 1, q. 4.

Utrum omne odorabile sit calidum a dominio.

Dino, *Canon* 2, ch. 3, q. 12.

Utrum omnes quatuor qualitates sint active.

Turisanus, *Plusquam*, 1.18.

Utrum omnis res mordicativa sit calida.

Taddeo, *Aphor.*, fol. 133.

Utrum parvitas occipitis est ita proprium signum prave complexionis
posterioris partis cerebri, sicut parvitas totius.

Turisanus, *Plusquam*, 2.15.

Utrum parvus recessus a temperamento sit causa morbi, et magnus recessus
sit morbus.   Taddeo, *Aphor.*, fol. 30.

Utrum per operationes sensitivas et motivas significetur super complexione
cerebri.   Turisanus, *Plusquam*, 2.13.

Utrum permutatio a complexione naturali sit possibile.

Turisanus, *Plusquam*, 3.22.

Utrum pinguedo fiat ex humiditate vicinis temperate, an ex humiditate calida.

Turisanus, *Plusquam*, 2.59.

Utrum pinguedo procedat a caliditate vel non.

Taddeo, *Isagoge*, fol. 371r.

Utrum pueri plus habeant de calore quam iuvenes.

Taddeo, *Isagoge*, fol. 368v.

Utrum qualitas mutata possit cognosci.

Taddeo, *Isagoge*, fol. 397r.

Utrum quot sunt operationes dependentes a caliditate, tot sint dependentes a
frigiditate.   Dino, *Canon* 2, ch. 4, q. 1.

Utrum sanguis sit temperate complexionis.

Taddeo, *Isagoge*, fol. 348v.

Utrum sanitas sit temperamentum.   Taddeo, *Isagoge*, fol. 391v.

Utrum sapor dulcis fundetur semper in substantia calida.

Dino, *Canon* 2, ch. 3, q. 6.

Utrum sapor dulcis sit calidior unctuoso vel econtra.

Dino, *Canon* 2, ch. 3, q. 10.

Utrum sensus tactus sit una competens in determinandi complexionem malam.

Bartolomeo, *De complexionibus*,
fol. 70r.

Utrum serum sit frigide et humide complexionis.

Taddeo, *Aphor.*, fol. 157.

Utrum siccitas acuta sit causa extractionis caloris naturalis.

Turisanus, *Plusquam*, 3.2.

Utrum sint plura corpora lapsa lapsu simili vel dissimili.

Bartolomeo, *De complexionibus*,
fol. 74v.

Utrum sit dare complexiones simplices inequales.

Bartolomeo, *De complexionibus*,
fol. 64v.

Utrum sit in natura aliquid corpus mixtum quod dicatur equata absolute.

Bartolomeo, *De complexionibus*,
fol. 64v.

Utrum sit possibile aliquam mulierem esse calidiorem viro.

Dino, *De natura fetus*, fol. 65v.

Utrum sperma sit calidum et humidum.

Taddeo, *Aphor.*, fol. 17.

Utrum spiritus sit calide et humide complexionis.

Taddeo, *Isagoge*, fol. 367v.

Utrum stomachus siccus sitiat et appetat similia.

Turisanus, *Plusquam*, 2.70.

Utrum tempus curationis male complexionis calide et frigide sit equali tempori curationis male complexionis humide et sicce.

Dino, *Dilucidatorium*, 2.1.

Utrum tempus humectationis sit longius tempore exiccationis.

Dino, *Dilucidatorium*, 2.3.

Utrum tempus infrigandi et calefaciendi sit equale.

Guglielmo, *Canon* 1.4, fol. 119r.

Utrum tempus infrigidationis sit equale tempori calefactionis.

Dino, *Dilucidatorium*, 2.2.

Utrum testes sint complexionis calide et humide.

Taddeo, *Isagoge*, fol. 353v.

Utrum venter siccus in iuventute propter caliditatem epatis fiat humidus in senectute.   Taddeo, *Aphor.*, fol. 43.

Utrum vinum calefaciat, infrigidet, humectet, et desiccet.

Taddeo, *Isagoge*, fol. 380r.

Utrum vinum sit frigide complexionis.

Taddeo, *Isagoge*, fol. 380r.

Utrum vinum sit humide complexionis.

Taddeo, *Isagoge*, fol. 380r.

Utrum vir sit humidior femina.   Taddeo, *Isagoge*, fol. 370v.

Physiology—The Humors

Digressio de sanguine an sit quartus humor.

> Turisanus, *Plusquam*, 2.44.

Utrum causa formalis melancholie sit sex hypostativa.

> Taddeo, *Isagoge*, fol. 350v.

Utrum cholera innaturalis habeat receptaculum.

> Taddeo, *Isagoge*, fol. 349v.

Utrum cholera inveniantur pura in corpore.

> Taddeo, *Isagoge*, fol. 349r.

Utrum cholera nigra rodat membra in quibus adunatur.

> Taddeo, *Pronost.*, fol. 225r.

Utrum cholera praxina generetur in stomacho totaliter.

> Taddeo, *Isagoge*, fol. 350r.

Utrum cholera que vadit ad stomacho possit iuvare digestionem.

> Taddeo, *Isagoge*, fol. 350r.

Utrum cholera sit calidissimus [humor] quod sit in corpore humano.

> Taddeo, *Isagoge*, fol. 350r.

Utrum cholera sit spuma sanguinis.   Taddeo, *Isagoge*, fol. 350r.

Utrum cholera sola possit nutrire.   Taddeo, *Isagoge*, fol. 349v.

Utrum cholera viridis fiat in venis.   Taddeo, *Pronost.*, fol. 223v.

Utrum cholera viridis generetur in stomacho ex oleribus.

> Taddeo, *Pronost.*, fol. 246r.

Utrum cholerici sint naturaliter pinguiores quam melancholici.

> Taddeo, *Isagoge*, fol. 371r.

Utrum descensus cholere ad intestina augeat solutionem ventris.

> Taddeo, *Reg. acut.*, fol. 293v.

Utrum diffinitio humoris posita a Joannitio sit bona.

> Taddeo, *Isagoge*, fol. 347v.

Utrum dulcedo in rebus sit causa conversionis earum ad choleram.

> Taddeo, *Reg. acut.*, fol. 318r.

Utrum ex rebus dulcibus aptius generetur cholera quam ex amaris.

> Taddeo, *Reg. acut.*, fol. 312r.

Utrum flegma dulce possit nutrire.   Taddeo, *Isagoge*, fol. 349r.

Utrum flegma habeat receptaculum.   Taddeo, *Isagoge*, fol. 349r.

Utrum flegma solum possit nutrire.   Taddeo, *Isagoge*, fol. 349r.

Utrum flegma vitreum fiat per congelationem.

> Taddeo, *Isagoge*, fol. 349r.

Utrum generatio humorum sit reciproca.

> Taddeo, *Isagoge*, fol. 348r.

Utrum generatio sanguinis compleatur in epate.

> Taddeo, *Isagoge*, fol. 348r.

Utrum gracilitas significet hominem esse cholericum.

Taddeo, *Pronost.*, fol. 89.

Utrum humor calidus et humidus magis debeat putrescere quam frigidus et siccus. Taddeo, *Isagoge*, fol. 385r.

Utrum humor generetur solum in epate.

Taddeo, *Isagoge*, fol. 347v.

Utrum humor melancholicus sit ineptus ad vomitum.

Dino, *Dilucidatorium*, 4.7.

Utrum humor temperatus inveniri possit.

Taddeo, *Isagoge*, fol. 348r.

Utrum humores evacuentur a locis extra venas vel a venis.

Guglielmo, *Canon* 1.4, fols. 121r-v.

Utrum humores generentur successive.

Taddeo, *Isagoge*, fol. 347v.

Utrum in corpore humano humor vere purus inveniatur.

Taddeo, *Pronost.*, fol. 223r.

Utrum in corpore humano sit plus de melancholia quam de sanguine.

Taddeo, *Isagoge*, fol. 350v.

Utrum in corpore possit inveniri humor purus.

Taddeo, *Isagoge*, fol. 348r.

Utrum in flegmate salso dominetur cholera vel flegma.

Taddeo, *Isagoge*, fol. 349r.

Utrum melancholia indigeat medicina fortiori quam alius humor.

Taddeo, *Aphor.*, fol. 90.

Utrum melancholia sit superfluitas sanguinis.

Taddeo, *Isagoge*, fol. 350v.

Utrum per evacutionem humorum qui sunt in venis fiat macies.

Taddeo, *Aphor.*, fol. 32.

Utrum quocumque humore in corpore habudante oporteat omnia signa ab Hippocrate posita considerare. Taddeo, *Aphor.*, fol. 4.

Utrum receptaculum cholere debeat esse in capite.

Taddeo, *Isagoge*, fol. 349v.

Utrum reperiatur cholera nigra que sit acetosa.

Taddeo, *Reg. acut.*, fol. 311v.

Utrum sanguine debeatur digestio. Dino, independent question, Padua 202, fols. 80v-82v.

Utrum sanguis existens in propria forma sanguinis possit putrescere.

Taddeo, *Isagoge*, fol. 348v.

Utrum sanguis in vena spumificetur que exit ad ex̄ (? exteriorem; or misprint for ad dextram) cordis.

Turisanus, *Plusquam*, 2.35.

Utrum sanguis possit putrescere. Taddeo, *Isagoge*, fol. 385r.

Utrum sanguis putrefiat extra venas.

Turisanus, *Plusquam*, 3.38.

Utrum sanguis sit minus putrescibile et utrum sit quartus humor.

Turisanus, *Plusquam*, 2.41.

Utrum sanguis spumosus veniat de pulmone.

Taddeo, *Aphor.*, fol. 131.

Utrum sanguis veniens de vena pulmonis sit spumosus.

Taddeo, *Aphor.*, fol. 131.

Utrum sola cholera inter humore digeri possit.

Taddeo, *Reg. acut.*, fol. 298v.

Utrum solus sanguis nutriat. Dino, independent question,

BAV, Vat. lat. 3144, fols. 13v-14v.

Utrum solus sanguis nutriat.

Taddeo, *Isagoge*, fol. 348v.

Utrum species detur humori a materia sua.

Taddeo, *Isagoge*, fol. 348r.

Physiology—Spiritus and the Virtues

A quod nutritur spiritus. Dino, *De natura fetus*, fol. 47v.

Ad solvendum dubitacionem, scilicet cuius virtutis risus sit passio.

Dino, *De risu*, CLM 7609, fol. 140r.

Digressio de virtutibus sensitivis. Turisanus, *Plusquam*, 2.17.

Utrum aliqua crasis sit differentia bonitatis et vitii cuiuscumque virtutum.

Turisanus, *Plusquam*, 2.76.

Utrum, corrupta una virtute in sua operatione, alie corrumpuntur.

Mondino, *Pronost.*, BAV, Vat. lat.
4466, fol. 12v.

Utrum destructio virtutum simul fiat.

Taddeo, *Pronost.*, fol. 215r.

Utrum diversitas que est inter virtutes procedat a diversitate membrorum.

Taddeo, *Isagoge*, fol. 355r.

Utrum genera lapsuum sint his que virtutem complent.

Turisanus, *Plusquam*, 2.4.

Utrum in statu virtus naturalis salvetur et animata laboret.

Taddeo, *Aphor.*, fol. 55.

Utrum multa bona materia semper sit cum forti virtute.

Taddeo, *Isagoge*, fol. 395r.

Utrum omne membrum habeat quatuor virtutes.

Taddeo, *Isagoge*, fol. 358v.

Utrum omnia que calefaciunt habeant spiritum.

Dino, *De natura fetus*, fol. 47v.

Utrum spiritus deferat virtutem per corpus vel non.

Taddeo, *Isagoge*, fol. 367v.

Utrum spiritus et sanguis vadent per eandem viam.

Taddeo, *Isagoge*, fol. 368r.

Utrum spiritus faciat ad digestionem.

Taddeo, *Isagoge*, fol. 367v.

Utrum spiritus frequens significet dolorem vel incensionem.

Taddeo, *Pronost.*, fol. 205r.

Utrum spiritus magnus cum intermissione significet alienationem.

Taddeo, *Pronost.*, fol. 205r.

Utrum spiritus possit putrescere.   Taddeo, *Isagoge*, fol. 385.

Utrum spiritus sit in rebus insensibilibus.

Taddeo, *Isagoge*, fol. 344v.

Utrum spiritus qui est vehiculum virtutis vitalis sit vehiculum virtutis animalis.   Taddeo, *Isagoge*, fol. 359v.

Utrum spiritus sit prior calore.   Taddeo, *Isagoge*, fol. 368r.

Utrum spiritus vitalis sit subtilior animali.

Taddeo, *Isagoge*, fol. 368v.

Utrum una virtute permanente fixa corpus in sua dispositione permaneat.

Taddeo, *Pronost.*, fol. 215r.

Utrum virtus appetitiva aliquando delectetur in malitia cibi.

Taddeo, *Aphor.*, fol. 62.

Utrum virtus appetitiva moveat omnes corporis iuncturas.

Turisanus, *Plusquam*, 2.17.

Utrum virtus attractiva sit creata ut nutrimentum iuvativum attrahat.

Taddeo, *Isagoge*, fol. 358v.

Utrum virtus augmentativa et nutritiva sint idem.

Taddeo, *Isagoge*, fol. 356v.

Utrum virtus augmentativa operetur continue in tempore adolescentie.

Taddeo, *Isagoge*, fol. 357r.

Utrum virtus augmentativa semper augeat corpus.

Taddeo, *Isagoge*, fol. 356v.

Utrum virtus digestiva operatur per villos.

Taddeo, *Isagoge*, fol. 358v.

Utrum virtus fortis sit causa distinctionis inter masculum et feminam.

Taddeo, *Isagoge*, fol. 372r.

Utrum virtus generativa que cum spermate descendit non possit operari.

Taddeo, *Isagoge*, fol. 358r.

Utrum virtus generativa sit non solum in masculis sed etiam in feminis.

> Taddeo, *Isagoge*, fol. 357v.

Utrum virtus immutativa prius operetur in fetu quam informativa.

> Dino, *De natura fetus*, fol. 56v.

Utrum virtus ministrans et ministrata sint idem.

> Taddeo, *Isagoge*, fol. 358v.

Utrum virtus naturalis sit illa que movet lacertos in apoplexia.

> Taddeo, *Aphor.*, fol. 64.

Utrum virtus nutritiva agat cum quiete.

> Taddeo, *Isagoge*, fol. 355v.

Utrum virtus nutritiva patiatur a cibo.

> Taddeo, *Isagoge*, fol. 356r.

Utrum virtus nutritiva sit fatigabilis, sicut sensitiva.

> Turisanus, *Plusquam*, 2.35.

Utrum virtus nutritive sit fixa in epate.

> Taddeo, *Isagoge*, fol. 356r.

Utrum virtus sensibilis vadat ad locum doloris.

> Taddeo, *Aphor.*, fol. 67.

Utrum virtus specialis det vitam.   Turisanus, *Plusquam*, 2.12.

Utrum virtus vitalis, animalis, et naturalis sint idem vel diverse.

> Taddeo, *Isagoge*, fol. 355r.

Utrum virtus vitalis possit comprehendi sub aliqua trium potentiarum anime.

> Taddeo, *Isagoge*, fol. 359r.

Utrum virtus vitalis precedat virtutem naturalem.

> Taddeo, *Isagoge*, fol. 359r.

Utrum virtutes ministrantes sint diverse adinvicem.

> Taddeo, *Isagoge*, fol. 358v.

Utrum virtutes nutritive recte dicantur naturales.

> Turisanus, *Plusquam*, 2.12.

Physiology—Growth, Aging, Nourishment, Excretion

Digressio circa evacuationem.   Turisanus, *Plusquam*, 3.81.

Digressio de causis grassitiei, macredinis, et medii.

> Turisanus, *Plusquam*, 2.59.

Digressio de digestione.   Turisanus, *Plusquam*, 3.39.

Digressio de digestione, perfectione, et quantitate et qualitate egestorum.

> Turisanus, *Plusquam*, 3.13.

Digressio de mutatione corporis ex cibis et potibus.

> Turisanus, *Plusquam*, 3.5.

Digressio de sudoris causis.   Turisanus, *Plusquam*, 3.11.

Digressio de virtutibus epatis circa nutrimentum.

Turisanus, *Plusquam*, 2.44.

Dubitatio de ypostasi [urine] utrum, scilicet, descendatur a membris 3[e]
digestionis aut 2[e].   Mondino, *Pronost.*, fol. 17r.

Questio de ypostasi urine. Quesivit a me vestra dilectio de ypostasi urine.

Turisanus, fol. 138r-141v.

Utrum aliquis cibus sit pure cibus.   Taddeo, *Isagoge*, fol. 378v.

Utrum aliquis cibus possit nutriri ea hora qua assumitur.

Taddeo, *Aphor.*, fol. 41.

Utrum aqua digeratur.   Taddeo, *Aphor.*, fol. 135.

Utrum aqua mixta cum cibo nutriat.   Taddeo, *Reg. acut.*, fol. 324r.

Utrum aqua possit digeri.   Taddeo, *Isagoge*, fol. 379v.

Utrum aqua possit nutrire.   Taddeo, *Isagoge*, fol. 379v.

Utrum aqua sit verus potus.   Taddeo, *Isagoge*, fol. 379v.

Utrum augmentum sit possibile.   Taddeo, *Isagoge*, fol. 356v.

Utrum bone habitudines sint ad ultimum evacuanda.

Taddeo, *Aphor.*, fol. 5.

Utrum bone habitudines sint evacuande.

Taddeo, *Aphor.*, fol. 4.

Utrum capilli nutriantur.   Taddeo, *Aphor.*, fol. 131.

Utrum cibaria dura minus nutriant quam mollia.

Taddeo, *Aphor.*, fol. 41.

Utrum cibus agat a forma specifica.   Taddeo, *Isagoge*, fol. 378v.

Utrum cibus humectet absolute.   Taddeo, *Aphor.*, fol. 92.

Utrum cibus immutet corpus.   Taddeo, *Isagoge*, fol. 378v.

Utrum cibus magis permutet corpora nostra quam aer.

Taddeo, *Isagoge*, fol. 375v.

Utrum cibus semper noceat ratione morbi.

Taddeo, *Reg. acut.*, fol. 269r.

Utrum color in urina generetur per alterationem an per permixtionem.

Mondino, *Pronost.*, BAV, MS
Vat. lat. 4466, fol. 16v.

Utrum color urine detur sibi a permixtione cholere cum ea, an ab actione
caloris naturalis in eam agentis.   Taddeo, *Pronost.*, fol. 221r.

Utrum cum res aliqua nutrit corpus et assimilatur ei possit ipsum alterare
et permutare.   Bartolomeo, *De complexionibus*,
fol. 85r.

Utrum digestio debeatur cause antecedenti vel coniuncte.

Taddeo, *Reg. acut.*, fol. 256v.

Utrum digestio debeatur sputo sanguineo puro.

Taddeo, *Pronost.*, fol. 226v.

Utrum digestio sequatur ad somnum.

                 Taddeo, *Reg. acut.*, fol. 299r.

Utrum dispositioni a cibis similibus sit proprium corporis optime sani.

                 Turisanus, *Plusquam*, 3.9.

Utrum etas sequatur virtutem.   Taddeo, *Isagoge*, fol. 369r.

Utrum etas sit spacium vite.   Taddeo, *Isagoge*, fol. 369r.

Utrum etates sint plures quam quattuor.

                 Taddeo, *Isagoge*, fol. 368v.

Utrum evacuatio naturalis et per consequens laudabilis possit fieri a membris superioribus per stomacho.   Mondino, *Pronost.*, BAV, MS

                 Vat. lat. 4466, fol. 13v.

Utrum evacuatio per urinam sit evacuatio propria alicui membro.

                 Taddeo, *Aphor.*, fol. 88.

Utrum in omni quod nutritur oportet cibum mole esse equale corpori, et esse quod augetur saltem augeri ad duplum continue.

                 Turisanus, *Plusquam*, 2.44.

Utrum lac det bonum nutrimentum.   Taddeo, *Aphor.*, fol. 158.

Utrum lac possit aliquo bene digeri.   Taddeo, *Aphor.*, fol. 158.

Utrum natura materiam aliquam evacuet per regionem inconvenientem.

                 Taddeo, *Aphor.*, fol. 24.

Utrum nos debeamus evacuare digesta.

                 Taddeo, *Aphor.*, fol. 24.

Utrum nutrimentum fiat a contrario vel a simili.

                 Taddeo, *Isagoge*, fol. 356r.

Utrum nutrimentum membrorum transeat per renes.

                 Taddeo, *Aphor.*, fol. 126.

Utrum nutritio sit generatio.   Turisanus, *Plusquam*, 2.44.

Utrum omnia membra nutriantur a substantia alba.

                 Taddeo, *Pronost.*, fol. 211r.

Utrum pueritia sit a 18 anno usque ad 25.

                 Taddeo, *Aphor.*, fol. 130.

Utrum secessus et urina simul multiplicari possint.

                 Taddeo, *Aphor.*, fol. 127.

Utrum sedimen in urina sit illud quod refugit operationem nature in conversione cibi in sanguinem.   Taddeo, *Pronost.*, fol. 211v.

Utrum simul et semel detur urine substantia et color an prius substantia et preterea color.   Mondino, *Pronost.*, BAV, MS

                 Vat. lat. 4466, fol. 16v.

Utrum sit aliqua etas media inter pubertatem et iuventutem.

                 Taddeo, *Aphor.*, fol. 85.

Utrum terminus adolescentia sit apud **XXX** annos.

Taddeo, *Isagoge*, fol. 368v.

Utrum ultima inanitio sit ita fallax sicut ultima repletio.

Taddeo, *Aphor.*, fol. 5.

Utrum urina causetur a solo potu.   Taddeo, *Pronost.*, fol. 221r.

Utrum urina et egestio sint accidentia.

Taddeo, *Isagoge*, fol. 396v.

Utrum urina habet formam ab epate, an a renibus.

Mondino, *Pronost.*, BAV, MS
Vat. lat. 4466, fol. 16v.

Utrum urina presit colorari.   Mondino, *Pronost.*, BAV, MS
Vat. lat. 4466, fol. 16v.

Utrum urina significet super fortitudinem et debilitatem virtutis expulsiva
an digestiva.   Mondino, *Pronost.*, BAV, MS
Vat. lat. 4466, fol. 17r.

Physiology—Pulsation

Digressio quomodo fiat pulsus et cuius virtutis.

Turisanus, *Plusquam*, 2.35.

Utrum dilatatio arterie sit per influxum spiritus repletivi a corde an per
ebulitionem sanguinis.   Turisanus, *Plusquam*, 2.35.

Utrum dilatatio chorde [*sic*] dilatentur simul omnes arterie.

Turisanus, *Plusquam*, 2.40.

Utrum pulsatio arterie sit a natura.   Turisanus, *Plusquam*, 2.35.

Utrum pulsus magnus possit esse velox et spissus.

Turisanus, *Plusquam*, 2.35.

Utrum recte fecit Galenus qui non dixit organum proprium cordis calidioris
temperato esse magnitudinem pulsus.

Turisanus, *Plusquam*, 2.35.

Physiology—Respiration

Digressio de respiratione.

Turisanus, *Plusquam*, 2.35.

Utrum in magna ascensione anhelitus sit magnus.

Taddeo, *Pronost.*, fol. 205v.

Utrum respiratio debet esse de necessitate tarda rara, sicut pulsus.

Turisanus, *Plusquam*, 2.37.

Physiology—Voice

Digressio de causis vocis et modo perventus eius.

Turisanus, *Plusquam*, 2.74.

Digressio de differentiis vocum.   Turisanus, *Plusquam*, 2.75.

Physiology—Exercise

Digressio de exercitio.   Turisanus, *Plusquam*, 3.2.

Digressio de speciebus lassitudinis.   Turisanus, *Plusquam*, 2.12.

Utrum excercitium calefaciat corpus nostrum vel non.

Taddeo, *Isagoge*, fol. 376r.

Utrum excercitium confortet digestionem.

Taddeo, *Reg. acut.*, fol. 280v.

Utrum excercitium debeat fieri ante cibum vel post.

Taddeo, *Isagoge*, fol. 376v.

Utrum exercitium magis confortet digestionem quam somnus.

Taddeo, *Reg. acut.*, fol. 285r.

Utrum excercitium sit res non naturalis vel non.

Taddeo, *Isagoge*, fol. 376r.

Utrum exercitium sit solum motus activus vel passivus.

Taddeo, *Isagoge*, fol. 376v.

Utrum exercitium sit solum motus localis.

Taddeo, *Isagoge*, fol. 376v.

Utrum motus que dicitur de exercitio sit comunis corpori et anime.

Taddeo, *Isagoge*, fol. 376v.

Utrum quies statim facta sit cura fatige cui supervenit.

Taddeo, *Aphor.*, fol. 67.

Physiology—Sensation

Digressio de bonitate et malitia [visus], quod sint et earum causis.

Turisanus, *Plusquam*, 2.32.

Digressio de visibili: quod sit videre, quod bonitas visus, et unde causetur.

Turisanus, *Plusquam*, 2.31.

Utrum alia membra nervo et chorda habeant sensum.

Turisanus, *Plusquam*, 3.55.

Utrum caro sentiat per se vel non.   Taddeo, *Isagoge*, fol. 365v.

Utrum caro sit medium sensus tactus.

Taddeo, *Isagoge*, fol. 365v.

Utrum cristallina sit membrum vel non.

Taddeo, *Isagoge*, fol. 370v.

Utrum cristallina sit particula principalis oculi.

Taddeo, *Isagoge*, fol. 370v.

Utrum gustus sit necessarius. Taddeo, *Isagoge*, fol. 365r.

Utrum homo habeat meliorem sensus odoratus quam cetera animalia.

Taddeo, *Isagoge*, fol. 364r.

Utrum homo possit dormiendo sentire.

Taddeo, *Isagoge*, fol. 362r.

Utrum homo possit videre rem que est in eius oculo.

Taddeo, *Pronost.*, fol. 205r.

Utrum humores constituentes oculum sint tamen tres.

Taddeo, *Isagoge*, fol. 371r.

Utrum id quod est intra oculum possit videri.

Mondino, *Pronost.*, BAV, MS
Vat. lat. 4466, fol. 6r.

Utrum idem nervus sit in lingua instrumentum gustus et tactus.

Taddeo, *Isagoge*, fol. 365r.

Utrum in oculo dominetur ignis. Taddeo, *Isagoge*, fol. 370v.

Utrum in omnibus membris sensibilibus sentiatur fames.

Turisanus, *Plusquam*, 2.70.

Utrum in quolibet sensu sit dolor. Turisanus, *Plusquam*, 2.88.

Utrum instrumentum sensus odoratus sit nervus.

Taddeo, *Isagoge*, fol. 364r.

Utrum instrumentum sensus tactus sit caro.

Taddeo, *Isagoge*, fol. 365r.

Utrum nervus sentiat per se vel non. Taddeo, *Isagoge*, fol. 365v.

Utrum odor fiat per resolutionem a corpore odorifero vel non.

Taddeo, *Isagoge*, fol. 364v.

Utrum sapor sit differentia propria vini.

Taddeo, *Reg. acut.*, fol. 307v.

Utrum sapor stipticus et dulcis sint contrarii.

Taddeo, *Reg. acut.*, fol. 307v.

Utrum sensibile positum, scilicet sensum, causet sensationem.

Turisanus, *Plusquam*, 3.55.

Utrum sensibilia communia sentiatur per accidens.

Turisanus, *Plusquam*, 2.16.

Utrum sensus communis, existens unus, movetur motibus diversis.

Turisanus, *Plusquam*, 2.17.

Utrum sensus per siccitatem fiant perfectiores.

Turisanus, *Plusquam*, 2.23.

Utrum sensus possit decipi. Taddeo, *Isagoge*, fol. 362r.

Utrum sensus sit in plus quam motus.

> Taddeo, *Isagoge*, fol. 362r.

Utrum sensus tactus et gustus in lingua sint idem in substantia [sb'a].

> Taddeo, *Isagoge*, fol. 365r.

Utrum sensus tactus sit plures sensus.

> Taddeo, *Isagoge*, fol. 365v.

Utrum sensus visus sit unus.   Turisanus, *Plusquam*, 2.31.

Utrum sentire sit pati vel agere.   Taddeo, *Isagoge*, fol. 362r.

Utrum tactus dicatur esse sensus alimenti.

> Taddeo, *Isagoge*, fol. 365r.

Utrum tactus sit in toto corpore.   Taddeo, *Isagoge*, fol. 365r.

Utrum videamus extramittendo.   Taddeo, *Pronost.*, fol. 205r.

Utrum videamus extramittentes vel intus suscipientes.

> Taddeo, *Isagoge*, fol. 362v.

Utrum visibile debet apparere duo.   Turisanus, *Plusquam*, 2.31.

Utrum visus fiat in tempore.   Taddeo, *Isagoge*, fol. 363r.

Physiology—Reproduction and Sex

Digressio an testiculi sint necessarii in generatione.

> Turisanus, *Plusquam*, 2.51.

Dubium quare in evacuatione spermatis sit maior delitia quam in evacuatione aliarum superfluitatem.   Turisanus, *Plusquam*, 3.17.

Propter quid in specie humana mammille sunt in pectore, in aliis animalibus inter coxas.   Dino, *De natura fetus*, fol. 66v.

Quare in quibusdam animalibus generatur lac, in quibusdam non.

> Dino, *De natura fetus*, fol. 66v.

Utrum aborsum sit egritudo vel accidens.

> Taddeo, *Aphor.*, fol. 148.

Utrum aliquis possit assimilari avo suo.

> Taddeo, *Isagoge*, fol. 372r.

Utrum animal ante generationem prius est animal quam in aliqua specie animalis.   Turisanus, *Plusquam*, 2.52.

Utrum animal generetur totum simul vel successive.

> Dino, *De natura fetus*, fol. 59v.

Utrum animalia generata ex putrefactione habeant virtutem generativam.

> Taddeo, *Isagoge*, fol. 357v.

Utrum coitus sit causa curativa egritudinis.

> Taddeo, *Isagoge*, fol. 381r.

Utrum coitus sit reponendus sub capitulo de inanitione vel de accidentibus anime.   Taddeo, *Isagoge*, fol. 380v.

Utrum conceptio possit fieri successive.

Taddeo, *Isagoge*, fol. 358v.

Utrum concipiens masculum sit coloratior concipiente feminam.

Taddeo, *Aphor.*, fol. 142.

Utrum cor generetur prius quam spiritus.

Dino, *De natura fetus*, fol. 48r.

Utrum cor sit primo generatum quam aliquid membrum corporis.

Taddeo, *Isagoge*, fol. 351.

Utrum cor sit principalius in actu generationis an testiculi.

Dino, *De natura fetus*, fol. 57v.

Utrum cortex generetur per putrefactionem.

Dino, *De natura fetus*, fol. 72v.

Utrum defectus nutrimenti sit causa quod fetus ante decem mensum oriatur.

Taddeo, *Aphor.*, fol. 139.

Utrum distinctio masculi a femina possit fieri ante formationem membrorum.

Taddeo, *Isagoge*, fol. 370v.

Utrum distinctio vel diversitas cellularum matricis possit esse causa
fetuum gemellorum vel plurimum.   Mondino, *De generatione*, fol. 20.

Utrum emissio spermatis faciat ad productionem pilorum.

Dino, *De natura fetus*, fol. 64r.

Utrum ex parte mulieris possit causari sexus masculinus.

Taddeo, *Aphor.*, fol. 145.

Utrum femina tardius formatur quam masculus, aut econtra.

Dino, *De natura fetus*, fol. 61r.

Utrum fetus in octavo mense vivat.   Dino, *De natura fetus*, fol. 84r.

Utrum fetus sanguine dulciori, et saporosiori, et subtiliori, et puriori nutriatur.

Taddeo, *Aphor.*, fol. 139.

Utrum fetus vel embrio debeat assimilari parentibus.

Mondino, *De generatione*, fol. 18r.

Utrum fluxus ventris faciat deficere nutrimentum fetui.

Taddeo, *Aphor.*, fol. 137.

Utrum frigiditas matricis sit causa sufficiens ad impediendum conceptionem.

Taddeo, *Aphor.*, fol. 152.

Utrum genitum semper debet assimilari generanti.

Dino, *De natura fetus*, fol. 76r.

Utrum gracilitas uberum sequatur necessario mulierum aborsuram.

Taddeo, *Aphor.*, fol. 147.

Utrum hora coytus veniat sperma a toto corpore vel a corde.

Dino, *De natura fetus*, fol. 80r.

Utrum in mammillis virorum sit possibilis generatio lactis.

Dino, *De natura fetus*, fol. 66v.

Utrum in partu debeat fieri dolor.   Dino, *De natura fetus*, fol. 58v.
Utrum in partu naturali mamille fiant graciles.
                              Taddeo, *Aphor.*, fol. 148.
Utrum in spermate mulieris sit aliqua virtus activa.
                              Dino, *De natura fetus*, fol. 49r.
Utrum lac fiat et dealbetur per digestionem.
                              Dino, *De natura fetus*, fol. 67v.
Utrum lac quod generatur tempore quo fetus incipit moveri sit melius an illud quod post generatur.   Dino, *De natura fetus*, fol. 67v.
Utrum ligamenta fetus sint fortiora in medio tempore quam in fine.
                              Taddeo, *Aphor.*, fol. 87.
Utrum maior fetus facilius pereat quam parvus.
                              Taddeo, *Aphor.*, fol. 136.
Utrum mamille nutriantur ex lacte.   Dino, *De natura fetus*, fol. 68r.
Utrum mamille nutriantur lacte.   Taddeo, *Aphor.*, fol. 139.
Utrum mamille pregnantium graciles subito fieri possit.
                              Taddeo, *Aphor.*, fol. 139.
Utrum masculus citius informetur in utero quam femella.
                              Mondino, *De generatione*, fol 7.
Utrum matrix ascendat usque ad diaphragma.
                              Taddeo, *Aphor.*, fol. 188.
Utrum matrix habeat aliquam virtutem activam in generatione.
                              Dino, *De natura fetus*, fol. 52v.
Utrum membra sint causa distinctionis inter masculum et feminam.
                              Taddeo, *Isagoge*, fol. 371v.
Utrum menses impregnationis sint medicinales vel solares.
                              Taddeo, *Aphor.*, fol. 49.
Utrum menstrua habeant colorem similem colori sanguinis per phlobothomiam aut per alium modum exeuntis.
                              Taddeo, *Aphor.*, fol. 138.
Utrum mulier habeat sperma.   Taddeo, *Isagoge*, fol. 357v.
Utrum mulier habeat sperma quod sit principium necessario requisitum ad generationem.   Dino, *De natura fetus*, fol. 46v.
Utrum nimia matricis pinguedo conceptionem prohibeat.
                              Taddeo, *Aphor.*, fol. 145.
Utrum omnia alia membra a corde generentur, a spiritu existente in spermate deciso a patre.   Dino, *De natura fetus*, fol. 79r.
Utrum omnis masculus debeat assimilari patri, et omnis femina matri.
                              Taddeo, *Isagoge*, fol. 372r.
Utrum oppilatio matricis sit causa sterilitatis.
                              Mondino, *De generatione*, fol. 23.

Utrum panniculus generetur a virtute generativa existente in spermate, an solum ex calefactione matricis. Dino, *De natura fetus*, fol. 49r.

Utrum partus in octavo mense sit naturalis.
Mondino, *De generatione*, fol. 9.

Utrum pharmacia faciat abortire. Taddeo, *Aphor.*, fol. 87.

Utrum phlobothomia faciat abortire pregnantes.
Taddeo, *Aphor.*, fol. 136.

Utrum pregnans macra prius abortiat quam crassescat.
Taddeo, *Aphor.*, fol. 143.

Utrum secundum medium spermatis fiat transitus spiritus ad intus, ad exteriora imo debuit dicere Hypocratis ad superiora.
Dino, *De natura fetus*, fol. 50r.

Utrum semen significet super totum corpus.
Taddeo, *Aphor.*, fol. 164.

Utrum semen virile proiectum in matricem digeratur in ea.
Taddeo, *Aphor.*, fol. 154.

Utrum sit possibile esse diversitatem et organizationem membrorum in fetu.
Dino, *De natura fetus*, fol. 56r.

Utrum sperma agat in virtute anima. Turisanus, *Plusquam*, 2.52.

Utrum sperma attrahit spiritum . . . a matrice.
Dino, *De natura fetus*, fol. 47v.

Utrum sperma augeatur a spermate mulieris descendente ad matricem.
Dino, *De natura fetus*, fol. 51v.

Utrum sperma decidatur a toto. Turisanus, *Plusquam*, 2.52.

Utrum sperma decidatur a toto vel a parte.
Dino, *De natura fetus*, fol. 69r.

Utrum sperma ex eo quod calefiat in matrice habeat spiritum.
Dino, *De natura fetus*, fol. 47v.

Utrum sperma generetur in testiculis.
Taddeo, *Isagoge*, fol. 353v.

Utrum sperma masculi cadat in substantiam fetus.
Dino, *De natura fetus*, fol. 50v.

Utrum sperma mulieris ingrediatur generationem.
Mondino, *De generatione*, fol. 3.

Utrum sperma mulieris sit necessarium ad generationem.
Taddeo, *Isagoge*, fol. 357v.

Utrum sperma possit calefieri a matrice.
Dino, *De natura fetus*, fol. 47v.

Utrum sperma viri sit animatum. Dino, *De natura fetus*, fol. 54v.

Utrum sperma viri sit pars concepti. Taddeo, *Isagoge*, fol. 358v.

Utrum spiritus existens in spermate sit instrumentum virtutis naturalis an alterius virtutis animate.　　　　　　Dino, *De natura fetus*, fol. 51r.

Utrum sternutatio expellat partum et materias a matrice.

　　　　　　　　　　Taddeo, *Aphor.*, fol. 137.

Utrum sternutatio prosit in suffocatione matricis.

　　　　　　　　　　Taddeo, *Aphor.*, fol. 137.

Utrum tam a mare quam a femina decidatur sperma.

　　　　　　　　　　Turisanus, *Plusquam*, 2.52.

Utrum tempus expulsionis post partum equiparetur tempori aggregationis earum.　　　　　　　Dino, *De natura fetus*, fol. 58v.

Utrum tempus motus masculi est usque ad tres menses, femine ad quatuor.

　　　　　　　　　　Dino, *De natura fetus*, fol. 65v.

Utrum testes sint de spermate.　　Taddeo, *Isagoge*, fol. 353v.

Utrum testiculi sint membra principalia in actu generationis.

　　　　　　　　　　Dino, *De natura fetus*, fol. 57r.

Utrum unicus fetus possit a venis utriusque lateris nutrimentum accipere.

　　　　　　　　　　Taddeo, *Aphor.*, fol. 140.

Utrum vir maxime delectetur ex coitu quam mulier.

　　　　　　　　　　Mondino, *De generatione*,
　　　　　　　　　　fols. 22v-23r.

Utrum vir plus delectetur in coitu quam mulier, an econverso.

　　　　　　　　　　Taddeo, *Isagoge*, fol. 380v.

PHYSIOLOGY AND ANATOMY—PARTS OF THE BODY

Digressio de generatione pillorum et causa colorum ipsius.

　　　　　　　　　　Turisanus, *Plusquam*, 2.18.

Digressio de nuche et cerebri quiditate et necessitate nervorum ortu.

　　　　　　　　　　Turisanus, *Plusquam*, 2.15.

Digressio de regeneratione membrorum spermaticorum.

　　　　　　　　　　Turisanus, *Plusquam*, 3.29.

Queritur in qua regione fiant capilli longiores et magis augmentates.

　　　　　　　　　　Bartolomeo, *De complexionibus*,
　　　　　　　　　　fol. 73v.

Utrum a natura possint capillari.　　Taddeo, *Aphor.*, fol. 183.

Utrum auctor debuerit determinare de colore capillorum illic ubi de eo determinavit vel alibi.　　　　　Taddeo, *Isagoge*, fol. 370r.

Utrum capilli nigri fiant ex abundantia humoris cholerici.

　　　　　　　　　　Taddeo, *Isagoge*, fol. 370r.

Utrum capitulum de capillis sit insufficiens nec ne.

　　　　　　　　　　Taddeo, *Isagoge*, fol. 370r.

Utrum caro corde sit de genere carnis lacti.

> Bartolomeo, *De complexionibus*, fols. 107r-v.

Utrum caro et ossa possint regere seipsa absque influentia ab alio.

> Taddeo, *Isagoge*, fol. 353v.

Utrum caro movetur ad carnem, et os ad os.

> Dino, *De natura fetus*, fol. 56v.

Utrum cerebrum sentiat. Taddeo, *Isagoge*, fol. 353r.

Utrum cerebrum sit ex sanguine. Taddeo, *Isagoge*, fol. 352v.

Utrum cerebrum sit generatum de sanguine menstruo.

> Taddeo, *Isagoge*, fol. 352r.

Utrum cerebrum sit nobilius corde. Taddeo, *Isagoge*, fol. 353r.

Utrum cor habeat iuvamentum. Taddeo, *Isagoge*, fol. 351r.

Utrum cor recipiat influentiam ab aliquo.

> Taddeo, *Isagoge*, fol. 351r.

Utrum cor sit dignius quam cerebrum et epar, vel econtra.

> Dino, *Dilucidatorium*, 1.26.

Utrum cor sit factum de spermate. Taddeo, *Isagoge*, fol. 352r.

Utrum cor sit nobilius membrum cerebro.

> Guglielmo, *Canon* 1.4, fol. 118r.

Utrum dentes incisi recrescant. Taddeo, *Aphor.*, fol. 174.

Utrum dentes sit membrum spermaticum.

> Turisanus, *Plusquam*, 3.29.

Utrum diffinitio membrorum posita a Joannitio sit bonus.

> Taddeo, *Isagoge*, fol. 351r.

Utrum divisio membrorum sit per opposita.

> Turisanus, *Plusquam*, 2.12.

Utrum epar possit attrahere cibum. Taddeo, *Isagoge*, fol. 353v.

Utrum epar sit membrum spermaticum.

> Taddeo, *Isagoge*, fol. 353r.

Utrum in corde sint nervi. Taddeo, *Isagoge*, fol. 352r.

Utrum intestinum subtile sit carnosum membrum.

> Taddeo, *Aphor.*, fol. 173.

Utrum iuncture sint membra nervosa.

> Taddeo, *Aphor.*, fol. 177.

Utrum medulla sit superfluitas ossium.

> Taddeo, *Aphor.*, fol. 141.

Utrum membra principalia habeant virtutem innatam et influentem.

> Taddeo, *Isagoge*, fol. 351v.

Utrum membra principalia sint consimilia.

> Taddeo, *Isagoge*, fol. 351v.

Utrum membra principalia sint tamen unum.

Taddeo, *Isagoge*, fol. 351v.

Utrum membrana suscipiat virtutem a cerebro.

Taddeo, *Isagoge*, fol. 353v.

Utrum membrum officiale patiatur perpetuam separationem.

Taddeo, *Isagoge*, fol. 391v.

Utrum membrum rarum citius veniat ad saniem quam spissum.

Taddeo, *Pronost.*, fol. 229r.

Utrum motus cordis sit continuus.   Taddeo, *Isagoge*, fol. 352r.

Utrum motus cordis sit motus animalis vel naturalis.

Taddeo, *Isagoge*, fol. 352r.

Utrum musculus ex carne et nervis componetur.

Turisanus, *Plusquam*, 2.57.

Utrum musculus habeat virtutem influentem.

Taddeo, *Isagoge*, fol. 353v.

Utrum nervi, vene, et arterie habeant virtutem innatam et influentem.

Taddeo, *Isagoge*, fol. 353v.

Utrum nucha sit continuata cum cerebro.

Taddeo, *Isagoge*, fol. 353r.

Utrum origo nervorum sit ex cerebro. Taddeo, *Isagoge*, fol. 353r.

Utrum orta a principali [membri] sibi invicem attestantur.

Turisanus, *Plusquam*, 2.16.

Utrum os et cartilago necessario recipiant influentiam ab epate et a corde.

Taddeo, *Isagoge*, fol. 351r.

Utrum ossa incisa in pueritia recrescant.

Taddeo, *Aphor.*, fol. 174.

Utrum pili a virtute informativa [formentur].

Dino, *De natura fetus*, fol. 63v.

Utrum pulmo habeat operationem.   Taddeo, *Isagoge*, fol. 351r.

Utrum quatuor membra sint equaliter principalia.

Turisanus, *Plusquam*, 2.12.

Utrum renes et vesica sint membra semper quiescencia.

Taddeo, *Aphor.*, fol. 167.

Utrum secundum quodlibet membrum consimile possunt operationes invenire
eque perfecte.   Turisanus, *Plusquam*, 2.3.

Utrum septem membra, scilicet cor, epar, etc., indigeant arteriis.

Turisanus, *Plusquam*, 2.12.

Utrum servientia servitute preparatoria sint comprehensa in divisione quadri
membri.   Turisanus, *Plusquam*, 2.12.

Utrum sicut caro crescit, ita os possit recrescere.

Turisanus, *Plusquam*, 3.56.

Utrum splena delectetur rebus dulcibus.

> Taddeo, *Reg. acut.*, fol. 320r.

Utrum stomachus delectetur rebus dulcibus.

> Taddeo, *Reg. acut.*, fol. 319r.

Utrum stomachus nutriatur chilo.   Taddeo, *Aphor.*, fol. 41.

Utrum stomachus sentiat sapores rerum quas assumit.

> Taddeo, *Reg. acut.*, fol. 319v.

Utrum ungues formentur a virtute informativa.

> Dino, *De natura fetus*, fol. 62v.

Utrum unitas quantitas, numerus, et virtus membri pertineant ad
naturam eius.   Dino, *Dilucidatorium*, 1.15.

Utrum unum membrum non possit habere nisi unam operationem.

> Taddeo, *Isagoge*, fol. 367v.

Utrum vena sit principalior pars epatis.

> Taddeo, *Isagoge*, fol. 353v.

Utrum vene et arterie habeant sensum.

> Taddeo, *Isagoge*, fol. 353v.

Utrum vene et arterie sentiant.   Taddeo, *Aphor.*, fol. 166.

Utrum vene oriantur a corde.   Taddeo, *Isagoge*, fol. 353v.

Utrum vene sint locus naturalis sanguinis.

> Taddeo, *Aphor.*, fol. 174.

Utrum venis debeatur aliqua operatio.

> Turisanus, *Plusquam*, 3.77.

Utrum venter grossus sit aptus purgationem inferiorem.

> Taddeo, *Aphor.*, fol. 61.

115ᵃ questio est numquid sit verum id quod dicit Avicenna, cum dicit quod
nervi sunt creati a materia humida quam frigiditas congelavit.

> Dino, *Chirurgia* (Estense).

Disease—Causes

An fortitudo alicuius virtutis possit esse causa morbi in illo membro.

> Dino in Tommaso del Garbo,
> *Digressiones*, no. 67.

An putredo in nobis causari possit cuius causa immediata non sit prohibitio
transpiratio.   Dino in Tommaso del Garbo,
> *Digressiones*, no. 13.

An sanguis possit facere febris putrida.

> Dino in Tommaso del Garbo,
> *Digressiones*, no. 60.

Que corpora plus vel minus ledantur ubi aere pestilentiali.
>   Dino in Tommaso del Garbo,
>   *Digressiones*, no. 20.

Utrum abundantia ciborum sit causa morbi frigidi.
>   Taddeo, *Isagoge*, fol. 394r.

Utrum apostema possit fieri a causa primitiva sola.
>   Taddeo, *Aphor.*, fol. 111.

Utrum author agat hic de causis morbi consimilis.
>   Taddeo, *Isagoge*, fol. 394.

Utrum autumnus faciat egritudines acutas.
>   Taddeo, *Aphor.*, fol. 75.

Utrum autumnus faciat multas egritudines.
>   Taddeo, *Aphor.*, fol. 75.

Utrum calor extraneus corruptivus naturalis sit ex aere.
>   Turisanus, *Plusquam*, 3.38.

Utrum causa apoplexie et epilepsie sit una et eadem.
>   Taddeo, *Aphor.*, fol. 66.

Utrum causa apoplexie sit in substantia cerebri vel in eius ventriculis.
>   Taddeo, *Aphor.*, fol. 64.

Utrum causa apoplexie sit solum humor frigidus.
>   Taddeo, *Aphor.*, fol. 64.

Utrum causa coniuncta sublata remaneat egritudo.
>   Taddeo, *Isagoge*, fol. 393r.

Utrum causa primitiva, antecedens, et coniuncta ita sint cause sanitatis
sicut egritudinis.   Taddeo, *Isagoge*, fol. 393r.

Utrum causa primitiva possit fieri mansiva.
>   Dino, *Dilucidatorium*, 30.7.

Utrum cause morbi frigidi sint tamen quinque.
>   Taddeo, *Isagoge*, fol. 394r.

Utrum cause morbi membri consimilis sint tamen V.
>   Taddeo, *Isagoge*, fol. 394v.

Utrum cause primitive possint esse causa doloris absque causa corporali
intrinseca.   Dino, *Dilucidatorium*, 30.5.

Utrum cibi calidi faciant morbum calidum.
>   Taddeo, *Isagoge*, fol. 394r.

Utrum clausio pororum faciat morbum frigidum.
>   Taddeo, *Isagoge*, fol. 394r.

Utrum coitus operetur ad podagrum.
>   Taddeo, *Aphor.*, fol. 177.

Utrum conversio visibilis et frigidatis faciat morbum frigidum.
>   Taddeo, *Isagoge*, fol. 394r.

Utrum debilitas morbi sit ex debilitate cause.

                         Turisanus, *Plusquam*, 3.32.

Utrum discrasia fiens habeat causam respectu facti de fiente, vel respectu
future fieri.   Turisanus, *Plusquam*, 3.32.

Utrum dispositio mansiva possit esse causa doloris.

                    Dino, *Dilucidatorium*, 30.6.

Utrum egritudo facta, si non habet causam efficientem, habeat conservantem.

                       Turisanus, *Plusquam*, 3.37.

Utrum ex sanguine manente in propria forma sanguinis possit fieri febris.

                  Dino, independent question, Paris
                  University 128, fols. 114v-115r.

Utrum ex sanguine possit fieri febris.   Taddeo, *Isagoge*, fol. 387r.

Utrum ex sanguine possit fieri febris putrida.

                  Dino, independent question, BAV, MS
                  Vat. lat. 4466, fol. 36v.

Utrum exercitium sit causa aliquarum egritudinum materialium.

                     Taddeo, *Aphor.*, fol. 82.

Utrum excercitium sit cause morbi calidi.

                     Taddeo, *Isagoge*, fol. 394r.

Utrum excercitium sit causa morbi calidi et frigidi.

                     Taddeo, *Isagoge*, fol. 394v.

Utrum exiens temperamentum proculdubio incidat in egritudinem.

                     Taddeo, *Aphor.*, fol. 30.

Utrum febris ephymera habeat causam antecedentem.

                     Taddeo, *Isagoge*, fol. 383v.

Utrum febris possit fieri de cholera pravissima.

                     Taddeo, *Isagoge*, fol. 386v.

Utrum fiat aggregatio egritudinis quando quatuor humore excrescunt.

                     Taddeo, *Isagoge*, fol. 344r.

Utrum fluxus sanguinis sit causa ventris sicci.

                     Taddeo, *Isagoge*, fol. 99.

Utrum frigiditas exterior sit causa bolismi.

                     Taddeo, *Aphor.*, fol. 44.

Utrum frigiditas faciat vomitum spissum.

                     Taddeo, *Pronost.*, fol. 223r.

Utrum frigidum faciat febrem.   Taddeo, *Aphor.*, fol. 132.

Utrum frigidum faciat spasmum.   Taddeo, *Aphor.*, fol. 132.

Utrum frigidum faciat spasmum de inanitione vel repletione.

                     Taddeo, *Aphor.*, fol. 132.

Utrum generatio saniei fiat a calore mixto ex naturali et preter naturam.

                     Taddeo, *Pronost.*, fol. 211r.

Utrum mala complexio sit causa morbi.

Taddeo, *Isagoge*, fol. 390r.

Utrum mala qualitas relicta in membris sit causa reversionis febris.

Taddeo, *Aphor.*, fol. 114.

Utrum materia frigida sit causa longe egritudinis.

Taddeo, *Aphor.*, fol. 107.

Utrum materia squinantie vadens ad pulmonem suffocationem aut empyma facere debeat.   Taddeo, *Aphor.*, fol. 131.

Utrum motus spiritus faciat morbum calidum.

Taddeo, *Isagoge*, fol. 394r.

Utrum nimium exercitium faciat morbum frigidum.

Taddeo, *Isagoge*, fol. 394v.

Utrum omnis exitus a natura compositionali faciat dolorem sicut exitus a natura complexionali.   Turisanus, *Plusquam*, 2.88.

Utrum omnis mala complexio causet dolorem.

Turisanus, *Plusquam*, 2.88.

Utrum ptisis possit fieri a causa sicca.

Taddeo, *Aphor.*, fol. 80.

Utrum ptisis possit fieri a frigiditate rumpente venam pulmonis.

Taddeo, *Aphor.*, fol. 80.

Utrum putredo sit causa coniuncta febris.

Taddeo, *Isagoge*, fol. 385r.

Utrum quelibet res naturalis debeat facere egritudines si propriam naturam amiserit.   Taddeo, *Isagoge*, fol. 389v.

Utrum quies faciat corpus facile ad vomitum.

Taddeo, *Aphor.*, fol. 92.

Utrum recte Galenus causas morborum ostendat.

Turisanus, *Plusquam*, 3.77.

Utrum rigor sit causa morbi.   Taddeo, *Isagoge*, fol. 381r.

Utrum siccitas aeris possit facere omnem morbum preter ptisim.

Taddeo, *Aphor.*, fol. 80.

Utrum sola frigiditas cum materia vel sine materia sit causa appetitus canini.

Taddeo, *Aphor.*, fol. 44.

Utrum sola quantitas sanguinis sine grossitie possit esse causa emorroidarum.

Taddeo, *Aphor.*, fol. 170.

Utrum solum flegma sit causa apoplexie.

Taddeo, *Aphor.*, fol. 64.

Utrum somnus in febre possit esse causa nocumenti mortalis.

Taddeo, *Aphor.*, fol. 28.

Utrum tempus siccum sit causa febris acute.

Taddeo, *Aphor.*, fol. 74.

Utrum timpania procedat a causa calida solum.

Taddeo, *Aphor.*, fol. 91.

Utrum ventositas generatur a caliditate et frigiditate.

Taddeo, *Pronost.*, fol. 218v.

Utrum ver faciat febres acutas. Taddeo, *Aphor.*, fol. 76.

3ª questio est quia dubitatur que causa apostematis sit dolor et quo modo.

Dino, *Chirurgia* (Estense).

4ª questio est quia videtur Avicennam fuisse diminutum in ponenda apostemata calida solum fieri ex sanguine et colera.

Dino, *Chirurgia* (Estense).

5ª questio est utrum apostemata fiat ex colera.

Dino, *Chirurgia* (Estense).

6ª questio est quia non videtur quod apostemata fiat ex sanguine laudabile.

Dino, *Chirurgia* (Estense).

9ª questio est quare Avicenna non posuit apostemata ita fieri a colera laudabili et alia a colera mala, sicut fecit de sanguine.

Dino, *Chirurgia* (Estense).

11ª questio est quare Avicenna posuit debilitatem membri inter causas primitivas, cum in superioribus posuisse ipsam inter causas antecedentes.

Dino, *Chirurgia* (Estense).

12ª questio est quare Avicenna posuit dolorem inter causas primitivas, et prius dixerat quod erat causa antecedens. Dino, *Chirurgia* (Estense).

13ª questio est quare Avicenna diversificat curam flegmonis facta a causa primitiva cum apostemata, cum apostematum non possit fieri sine causa.

Dino, *Chirurgia* (Estense).

31ª questio est quare Avicenna non fecit intentionem et causa primitiva et antecedenti in erisipila, sicut fecit de flegmone.

Dino, *Chirurgia* (Estense).

65ª questio est, ex qua causarum positarum ab Avicenna fiat sefricos [?].

Dino, *Chirurgia* (Estense).

121ª questio est utrum a causis primitivis summatur indicatio curativa.

Dino, *Chirurgia* (Estense).

DISEASE—NATURE AND COURSE, GENERAL

Digressio an egritudo membri iuvamentalis sit egritudo membri principalis.

Turisanus, *Plusquam*, 2.88.

Digressio de periodicatione. Turisanus, *Plusquam*, 3.38.

Digressio de temporibus particularibus morbi.

Turisanus, *Plusquam*, 3.32.

Digressio in quo genere morbi ponatur concavitas.

Turisanus, *Plusquam*, 3.56.

Questio mota fuit quid effectum periodicationis in egritudinibus que motum habent secundum periodos. Dino, independent question,

CLM 13020, fols. 221v-223r.

Utrum a temporibus morbi sit aliqua indicatio sumenda.

Turisanus, *Plusquam*, 3.68.

Utrum ad bonam crisim divisio requiratur.

Taddeo, *Aphor.*, fol. 98.

Utrum alii humores a sanguine egredientes venas in saniem convertantur.

Taddeo, *Aphor.*, fol. 174.

Utrum aliqua desipientia possit esse salubris.

Taddeo, *Aphor.*, fol. 192.

Utrum aliqua egritudo diversa potuerit esse tempore hyemis.

Taddeo, *Aphor.*, fol. 178.

Utrum aliquis dolor possit fieri antiquus.

Dino, *Dilucidatorium*, 20.57.

Utrum aliquis existens sanus possit fieri eger repente.

Taddeo, *Aphor.*, fol. 192.

Utrum aliquis morbus qui esset in patre posset hereditari in filio.

Dino, independent question, Paris University MS 128, fols. 113v-114v.

Utrum aliquis possit nasci eger. Taddeo, *Isagoge*, fol. 394v.

Utrum aliquis vomitus sit laudabilis aut naturalis.

Mondino, *Pronost.*, BAV, MS Vat. lat. 4466, fol. 20r.

Utrum aphorismus 12 doceat prescire consistentias cuiuslibet morbi.

Taddeo, *Aphor.*, fol. 14.

Utrum aphorismus primus habet locum in quolibet morbo.

Taddeo, *Aphor.*, fol. 28.

Utrum author debuerit ponere quinque morbos in forma.

Taddeo, *Isagoge*, fol. 391r.

Utrum bonus sudor debeat fieri in die cretica.

Taddeo, *Pronost.*, fol. 206r.

Utrum compassio que est condolentia sit possibilis.

Taddeo, *Aphor.*, fol. 172.

Utrum contingat egrum mori in declinatione universali.

Taddeo, *Aphor.*, fol. 29.

Utrum convalescentes possint habere fortem appetitum.

Taddeo, *Aphor.*, fol. 56.

Utrum corpus semper egrum sit aptum egrotare semper.

> Turisanus, *Plusquam*, 1.16.

Utrum crisis cadat in morbo compositionali.

> Taddeo, *Aphor.*, fol. 48.

Utrum crisis cadat in solutione continui.

> Taddeo, *Aphor.*, fol. 48.

Utrum crisis et dies cretici cadant in mala complexione sola.

> Taddeo, *Aphor.*, fol. 48.

Utrum crisis et dies cretici cadant in tempore conceptionis et partus.

> Taddeo, *Aphor.*, fol. 48.

Utrum crisis perfecta possit fieri a sola natura.

> Taddeo, *Aphor.*, fol. 22.

Utrum crisis quartane ventura post diem 15^m presciri possit.

> Taddeo, *Pronost.*, fol. 238v.

Utrum crisis sit motus localis.   Taddeo, *Aphor.*, fol. 37.

Utrum cum materia multa et mala stet fortitudo virtutis.

> Dino, *Dilucidatorium*, 3.20.

Utrum cutis scissa possit conglutineri.

> Turisanus, *Plusquam*, 3.57.

Utrum dies cretici intercidentes habeant dies indicativos.

> Taddeo, *Aphor.*, fol. 49.

Utrum dies creticus faciat aliquid ad bonitatem crisis.

> Taddeo, *Aphor.*, fol. 104.

Utrum dies nona indicet decimam septimam.

> Taddeo, *Aphor.*, fol. 119.

Utrum dies 4^r sit fortior 14°.   Taddeo, *Pronost.*, fol. 236v.

Utrum dies 4^r sit fortior 7°.   Taddeo, *Pronost.*, fol. 236v.

Utrum dies 14^s indicetur ab undecimo vel 7°.

> Taddeo, *Pronost.*, fol. 228v.

Utrum dies 7^s sit fortior 17°.   Taddeo, *Pronost.*, fol. 236v.

Utrum dies sexta sit ceteris pessima.   Taddeo, *Aphor.*, fol. 100.

Utrum dies 13 sit magis creticus quam 14.

> Taddeo, *Aphor.*, fol. 46.

Utrum dies 21 sit magis creticus quam 20.

> Taddeo, *Aphor.*, fol. 49.

Utrum duo tamen peccata humoribus contingant.

> Taddeo, *Aphor.*, fol. 190.

Utrum egritudines autumnales sint ut plurimum mortales.

> Taddeo, *Aphor.*, fol. 75.

Utrum egritudines magis in vere quam in estate per sudorem terminari
debeant.   Taddeo, *Aphor.*, fol. 74.

Utrum egritudines motu impari procedentes sint breves, contrarie vero longe.

Taddeo, *Aphor.*, fol. 104.

Utrum egritudo facta in tempore sicco sit mortalior facta in humido.

Taddeo, *Aphor.*, fol. 79.

Utrum egritudo facta per evacuationem curetur.

Taddeo, *Aphor.*, fol. 45.

Utrum egritudo in tempore simili sit minus periculosa quam in contrario.

Taddeo, *Aphor.*, fol. 60.

Utrum egritudo que ad saniem convertitur teneat medium inter salutiferam et insanibilem.   Taddeo, *Pronost.*, fol. 227r.

Utrum egritudo que est de grossis humoribus per apostemata terminetur.

Taddeo, *Pronost.*, fol. 222r.

Utrum egritudo sicca sit difficilioris curationis quam humida.

Taddeo, *Aphor.*, fol. 50.

Utrum erisipila in matrice pregnantis sit mortalis.

Taddeo, *Aphor.*, fol. 143.

Utrum evacuatio cretica per sudorem fieri possit.

Taddeo, *Aphor.*, fol. 103.

Utrum evaporatio in corpore pletorico plures attrahat quam resolvat.

Taddeo, *Reg. acut.*, fol. 273v.

Utrum ex aptitudine estate egrotandi corpus sit neutrum tertii significati.

Turisanus, *Plusquam*, 1.16.

Utrum ex forti dolore accidat primo frigiditas corporis et tremor.

Dino, *Dilucidatorium*, 30.2.

Utrum fluxus humoris sit morbus.   Turisanus, *Plusquam*, 3.58.

Utrum Galenus debuit dividere solutionem unitatis [*sic*: continuitatis] in fiente et factam.   Turisanus, *Plusquam*, 3.50.

Utrum generentur peiores morbi ab humoribus peccantibus in quantitate quam in qualitate.   Mondino, independent question at end of his comm. *Tegni*, BAV, MS Vat. lat. 4466, fol. 157v.

Utrum hec sit bona predicatio: malus numerus est morbus.

Taddeo, *Isagoge*, fol. 391r.

Utrum humiditas stomachi sequatur ad humiditatem lingue.

Taddeo, *Aphor.*, fol. 181.

Utrum Hypocratis in hoc libro super omnem egritudinem acutam pronosticari doceat.   Taddeo, *Pronost.*, fol. 198r.

Utrum Hypocratis in libris pronosticorum super egritudines acutas tamen pronosticari doceat.   Taddeo, *Pronost.*, fol. 198r.

Utrum impletio concavitatis sit generatio, vel nutritio, vel augmentatio.

Turisanus, *Plusquam*, 3.56.

Utrum in egritudinibus acutis status sit cum earum accidentia ultimantur.

Taddeo, *Aphor.*, fol. 8.

Utrum in principio morbi cronici et acuti possimus pronosticari super crisim bonam vel malam eorum. Taddeo, *Pronost.*, fol. 238r.

Utrum in principio morbi possit presciri an sit futurus salubris vel mortalis.

Taddeo, *Aphor.*, fol. 55.

Utrum in statu morbus sit maior. Turisanus, *Plusquam*, 3.32.

Utrum inanitio et repletio sint morbi vel causa morbi.

Turisanus, *Plusquam*, 3.55.

Utrum infirmitas sit intemperantia. Taddeo, *Isagoge*, fol. 391v.

Utrum iudicium possit esse circa morbos acutos et longos per considerationem quaternorum. Taddeo, *Pronost.*, fol. 246r.

Utrum lesio operationis impediat in consuetis exercitiis.

Turisanus, *Plusquam*, 2.97.

Utrum materia que cito colligitur in aliquo membro, cito etiam resolvatur ab eo. Taddeo, *Aphor.*, fol. 191.

Utrum membrum officiale sit infirmum quando solum eius principalis particula infirmatur. Taddeo, *Isagoge*, fol. 391r.

Utrum morbi acuantur in tempore sibi simili.

Taddeo, *Aphor.*, fol. 81.

Utrum morbus calidus simplex esse possit.

Taddeo, *Isagoge*, fol. 390v.

Utrum morbus calidus sit molestior quam frigidus.

Taddeo, *Isagoge*, fol. 394r.

Utrum morbus dependens a materia composita sit longior dependente a simplici. Taddeo, *Aphor.*, fol. 106.

Utrum morbus officialis et mala compositio sint equalia.

Taddeo, *Isagoge*, fol. 390v.

Utrum morbus officialis et mala compositio sint idem.

Taddeo, *Isagoge*, fol. 390v.

Utrum morbus officialis sit compositus.

Taddeo, *Isagoge*, fol. 391r.

Utrum morbus secundum se consideratus sit fortior in statu quam in principio

Taddeo, *Aphor.*, fol. 55.

Utrum morbus sit debilis in statu. Taddeo, *Aphor.*, fol. 55.

Utrum morbus sit in membro tanquam in subiecto.

Taddeo, *Isagoge*, fol. 390r.

Utrum natura possit facere egritudinem.

Taddeo, *Isagoge*, fol. 395r.

Utrum omnes morbi cronici sint frigidi.

Taddeo, *Aphor.*, fol. 63.

Utrum omnia accidentia sint fortiora in statu.

Taddeo, *Aphor.*, fol. 55.

Utrum omnis egritudo habeat contrarium.

Taddeo, *Aphor.*, fol. 44.

Utrum omnis egritudo que in pueris transit 40 dies debeat venire ad 7 menses.

Taddeo, *Aphor.*, fol. 85.

Utrum omnis humiditas possit putrescere.

Taddeo, *Isagoge*, fol. 385v.

Utrum omnis morbus sit longior in tempore frigido quam in calido.

Taddeo, *Aphor.*, fol. 50.

Utrum omnis morbus transiens pubertatem necessario ad senectutem
venire debeat.   Taddeo, *Aphor.*, fol. 85.

Utrum per sudorem factum in toto corpore fiat alleviatio.

Taddeo, *Pronost.*, fol. 206v.

Utrum periodus in febre interpollata idem faciat quod unus dies in continua
et econverso.   Taddeo, *Pronost.*, fol. 238v.

Utrum possit esse morbus in numero sine peccato materie.

Taddeo, *Isagoge*, fol. 395r.

Utrum post diem 20^m sit aliquis dies indicativus.

Taddeo, *Aphor.*, fol. 49.

Utrum presens consistentia possit conservari.

Turisanus, *Plusquam*, 3.3.

Utrum principalis et recidiva sit una egritudo vel plures.

Taddeo, *Aphor.*, fol. 35.

Utrum pronosticatio morbi acuti sit certior quam cretici.

Taddeo, *Aphor.*, fol. 42.

Utrum pronosticatio sit difficilior in egritudine acuta quam in longa.

Taddeo, *Pronost.*, fol. 238r.

Utrum purgatio facta a natura in principio morbi sit bona.

Taddeo, *Aphor.*, fol. 98.

Utrum purgato humore purgando purgatio conferat et purgate bene ferant.

Taddeo, *Aphor.*, fol. 3.

Utrum putredo possit fieri in corpore vivo.

Taddeo, *Isagoge*, fol. 385v.

Utrum putrefactio sit alteratio secundum substantiam.

Turisanus, *Plusquam*, 3.5.

Utrum putrefactio sit morbus.   Taddeo, *Isagoge*, fol. 385r.

Utrum putrefactio sit morbus.   Turisanus, *Plusquam*, 3.58.

Utrum putridum taliter possit alteri quod esset putredo.

Turisanus, *Plusquam*, 3.38.

Utrum quando egritudo est fortior virtute infirmus necessario moriatur.

Taddeo, *Pronost.*, fol. 214r.

Utrum quando medius digitus abscinditur, dicatur morbus in numero vel
in quantitate. Taddeo, *Isagoge*, fol. 391r.

Utrum quantitas virtutis et morbi a medico cognosci possit.

Taddeo, *Pronost.*, fol. 221v.

Utrum 4^8 dies sit creticus. Taddeo, *Pronost.*, fol. 236v.

Utrum repletio possit esse morbus. Taddeo, *Aphor.*, fol. 45.

Utrum sanguis exiens a venis in ventrem mutetur in qualitate sua.

Taddeo, *Aphor.*, fol. 174.

Utrum sanguis exiens venas necessario in saniem convertatur.

Taddeo, *Aphor.*, fol. 174.

Utrum senes plus egrotent quam iuvenes stante paritate regiminis in utrisque.

Taddeo, *Aphor.*, fol. 63.

Utrum septem periodi tertiane interpollate terminetur in 13 diebus.

Taddeo, *Aphor.*, fol. 113.

Utrum signa crisis possint apparere in principio universali.

Taddeo, *Aphor.*, fol. 14.

Utrum sit possibile accidens proprium alicuius egritudinis removere,
remanente vel non sanata egritudine.

Dino, *Dilucidatorium*, 31.3.

Utrum sit possibile egestionem naturalem sit in acutam egritudinem.

Mondino, *Pronost.*, BAV, MS Vat. lat.
4466, fol. 13v.

Utrum sit possibile medicum previdere omne accidens futurum in
quolibet morbo. Taddeo, *Pronost.*, fol. 195v.

Utrum sitis et fames [sint] naturales vel egritudinales, et utrum alicuius
virtutis. Turisanus, *Plusquam*, 2.70.

Utrum solutio continuitatis possit a natura contingere.

Turisanus, *Plusquam*, 3.31.

Utrum solutio continuitatis possit fieri in consimilibus membris quin fiat in
officialibus. Taddeo, *Isagoge*, fol. 391v.

Utrum solutio continuitatis possit fieri in officialibus quin fiat in consimilibus.

Taddeo, *Isagoge*, fol. 391v.

Utrum solutio continuitatis possit inducere dolorem.

Turisanus, *Plusquam*, 2.88.

Utrum solutio continuitatis sit immediata causa doloris.

Turisanus, *Plusquam*, 2.88.

Utrum solutio continuitatis sit morbus.

Taddeo, *Isagoge*, fol. 391v.

Utrum solutio continuitatis sit morbus compositus.

> Taddeo, *Isagoge*, fol. 391v.

Utrum species convalescentium sint tamen 4^r.

> Taddeo, *Aphor.*, fol. 57.

Utrum species crisis sint VI vel plures vel pauciores.

> Taddeo, *Pronost.*, fol. 236r.

Utrum subita mutatio que sit in crisi sit causa morbi vel morbus vel accidens morbi.   Taddeo, *Pronost.*, fol. 236r.

Utrum tamen in egritudinibus cronicis digestio expectetur.

> Dino, *Dilucidatorium*, 3.10.

Utrum tempora morborum presciri possint antequam veniant.

> Taddeo, *Aphor.*, fol. 15.

Utrum tempora morborum sint adinvicem proportionata.

> Taddeo, *Aphor.*, fol. 15.

Utrum tempus restaurationis debeat esse equale tempori resolutionis.

> Taddeo, *Aphor.*, fol. 32.

Utrum unus dolor destruat alterum.   Taddeo, *Aphor.*, fol. 66.

14^a questio est quare Avicenna non declarat principium flegmonis, sicut alia tempora.   Dino, *Chirurgia* (Estense).

15^a questio est utrum dictum Avicenna sit bonum dictum, cum dicit quod pulsatio incipit intensione et inflammatio incipit in sedationem.

> Dino, *Chirurgia* (Estense).

48^a questio est de illo verbo quod dicit Avicenna in capitulo de exituris, cum dicit "Nuncupatur ad interiorem et ventriculum continentem mirach."

> Dino, *Chirurgia* (Estense).

51^a questio est de eo quod dicit Avicenna in illo capitulo de signis exiturarum, cum dicit "Cum videris lenitatem quamdam et sedationem doloris, tunc exitura est in via maturationis."   Dino, *Chirurgia* (Estense).

52^a questio est quomodo fiant dolores vehementiores in principio quam in statu.   Dino, *Chirurgia* (Estense).

53^a questio est quare hic determinavit Avicenna de exituris interiore.

> Dino, *Chirurgia* (Estense).

59^a questio est quia videtur Avicennam dicere falsum de eo quod dicit in capitulo de undimia cum dicit "Quod non est in ellevatione."

> Dino, *Chirurgia* (Estense).

69^a questio est utrum solutionis continuitatis diffinitio communiter data sit bona.   Dino, *Chirurgia* (Estense).

87^a questio est quia queritur quis morbus sit putredo.

> Dino, *Chirurgia* (Estense).

104^a questio est quia dubitatur utrum quodam dictum Galieni allegatum a Dino applicetur omni solutioni continuitatis.

> Dino, *Chirurgia* (Estense).

DISEASE—NATURE AND COURSE, PARTICULAR AILMENTS NAMED

An complicata febris sit possibilis.   Dino in Tommaso del Garbo,
                                              Digressiones, no. 4.
An ethica possit fieri incipiendo non antecedente.
                                              Dino in Tommaso del Garbo,
                                              Digressiones, no. 40.
An febris effimera sit fiens vel facta.   Dino in Tommaso del Garbo,
                                              Digressiones, no. 34.
An febris pestilentialis sit febris putrida.
                                              Dino in Tommaso del Garbo,
                                              Digressiones, no. 23.
An omnis febris dicatur habere primum suum esse penes aliquam materiam
cordis.   Dino in Tommaso del Garbo,
                                              Digressiones, no. 2.
An sit tria genera febrium sed tres materias cordis et corporis distincta.
                                              Dino in Tommaso del Garbo,
                                              Digressiones, no. 3.
Digressio de canitie.   Turisanus, *Plusquam*, 2.27.
Digressio de febribus.   Turisanus, *Plusquam*, 3.38.
Digressio de fractura ossium attendis et in plasmatione ossis.
                                              Turisanus, *Plusquam*, 3.51.
Digressio de lesionibus operationum cerebri.
                                              Turisanus, *Plusquam*, 2.80.
Digressio de magnitudine febris.   Turisanus, *Plusquam*, 3.32.
Propter quid morsus a cane rabido ymaginatur viscera canum in aqua.
                                              Dino, independent question, BAV, MS
                                              Vat. lat. 4454, fols. 103r-v.
Que sint proprie et substantiales differentie febrium.
                                              Dino in Tommaso del Garbo,
                                              Digressiones, no. 1.
Utrum ad balbutiem sequatur diaria necessario.
                                              Taddeo, *Aphor.*, fol. 181.
Utrum ad longam dissinteriam spleneticorum hyrops aut lienteria sequatur.
                                              Taddeo, *Aphor.*, fol. 186.
Utrum ad vulnera principalium membrorum spasmus sequi possit.
                                              Taddeo, *Aphor.*, fol. 128.
Utrum aliqua febris possit esse composita.
                                              Taddeo, *Isagoge*, fol. 388r.
Utrum aliqua febris possit esse simplex.
                                              Taddeo, *Isagoge*, fol. 388r.
Utrum aliquis in ruptura apostematis pectoris suffocari possit.
                                              Taddeo, *Aphor.*, fol. 102.

Utrum aliquod corpus cuius calor est omnino extinctus vel vicinus extinctioni
febrire possit.   Taddeo, *Aphor.*, fol. 105.

Utrum anteriora et posteriora in tetano equaliter tendi possit.
                                             Taddeo, *Aphor.*, fol. 112.

Utrum apopletici apoplexia maiori in 7 diebus pereant.
                                             Taddeo, *Aphor.*, fol. 192.

Utrum apoplexia magna sit curabili.   Taddeo, *Aphor.*, fol. 64.

Utrum apoplexia possit esse sine anhelitu.
                                             Taddeo, *Aphor.*, fol. 64.

Utrum apoplexia sit accidens vel morbus.
                                             Taddeo, *Aphor.*, fol. 64.

Utrum apostema creticum contingat in egritudine, existentibus humoribus
eius digestis.   Taddeo, *Pronost.*, fol. 233v.

Utrum apostema quod magis approximat loco calidiori minus colligat de sanie.
                                             Taddeo, *Pronost.*, fol. 209v.

Utrum apostema sanguineum sit multe malitie.
                                             Taddeo, *Pronost.*, fol. 224v.

Utrum apostema saniosum possit transire de membro ad membrum.
                                             Taddeo, *Aphor.*, fol. 175.

Utrum apostema sit morbus.   Taddeo, *Isagoge*, fol. 389v.

Utrum apostema sit morbus membrorum consimilium vel officialium.
                                             Taddeo, *Isagoge*, fol. 389v.

Utrum apostema sit morbus simplex.
                                             Taddeo, *Isagoge*, fol. 389v.

Utrum apostema possit fieri in guttare subito et sine dolore.
                                             Taddeo, *Aphor.*, fol. 102.

Utrum apostemata [*sic*] cordis sit mortalius solutione continui eius.
                                             Taddeo, *Aphor.*, fol. 173.

Utrum aqua et sanies totaliter et subito ab hydropicis et empicis exeuntes
mortem inducant.   Taddeo, *Aphor.*, fol. 176.

Utrum aqua hydropicorum possit penetrare ad cannales pulmonis eorum.
                                             Taddeo, *Aphor.*, fol. 184.

Utrum autumnus noceat ptisicis.   Taddeo, *Aphor.*, fol. 75.

Utrum calor naturalis et febris sint idem.
                                             Taddeo, *Isagoge*, fol. 383r.

Utrum canities accidat flegmaticis.   Dino, *De natura fetus*, fol. 64v.

Utrum capitulum de febribus debeat precedere capitulum de morbis et causis.
                                             Taddeo, *Isagoge*, fol. 381v.

Utrum capitulum in quo author agit de morbo in generali debeat sequi
capitula in quibus agit de febribus et apostematis.
                                             Taddeo, *Isagoge*, fol. 389v.

Utrum collectio apostemosa possit transire de membro ad membrum.

Taddeo, *Aphor.*, fol. 175.

Utrum corpus fortiter febriens possit permanere in suo tumore.

Taddeo, *Aphor.*, fol. 53.

Utrum crisis cadat in apostematibus. Taddeo, *Aphor.*, fol. 48.

Utrum crisis contingat in febre ephymera.

Taddeo, *Isagoge*, fol. 384r.

Utrum diaria longa fiat in traulis. Taddeo, *Aphor.*, fol. 181.

Utrum diaria possit egritudo longa. Taddeo, *Aphor.*, fol. 181.

Utrum diffinitio febris sint bona. Taddeo, *Isagoge*, fol. 383r.

Utrum diffinitiones data ab auctore de apostemate sint bone.

Taddeo, *Isagoge*, fol. 389v.

Utrum dissinteria facte a felle nigro sit salubris.

Taddeo, *Aphor.*, fol. 99.

Utrum dissinteria sit curabilis. Taddeo, *Aphor.*, fol. 99.

Utrum dissinteria sit ex humoribus calidis tamen.

Taddeo, *Aphor.*, fol. 165.

Utrum dissuria sit defectus continendi urinam.

Taddeo, *Aphor.*, fol. 73.

Utrum diversitas situs humorum faciat diversam speciem febris.

Taddeo, *Isagoge*, fol. 386v.

Utrum divisio trimembris synochi possit competere synoche influente.

Taddeo, *Isagoge*, fol. 387r.

Utrum effimera et ethica sint discrasie fientes sicut putrida.

Turisanus, *Plusquam*, 3.32.

Utrum effimera sit febris fiens vel facta.

Turisanus, *Plusquam*, 3.38.

Utrum eger debeat prius mori antequam veniat ad ptisim per restrictionem emorroidarum. Taddeo, *Aphor.*, fol. 170.

Utrum egritudo de inanitione sit materialis.

Taddeo, *Aphor.*, fol. 45.

Utrum egritudo dependens a materia calida et subtile per apostema terminetur.

Taddeo, *Aphor.*, fol. 123.

Utrum emoroides sint res naturales. Taddeo, *Aphor.*, fol. 169.

Utrum empicus ex peripleumonia necessario sit simul ptisicus et empicus.

Taddeo, *Pronost.*, fol. 231v.

Utrum epilepsia aut apoplexia abortire faciat.

Taddeo, *Aphor.*, fol. 137.

Utrum epilepsia curetur in iuvenibus.

Taddeo, *Aphor.*, fol. 66.

Utrum epilepsia sit curabilis in 25 anno.

Taddeo, *Aphor.*, fol. 130.

Utrum epydimia tangat omnes universaliter.

Taddeo, *Isagoge*, fol. 375v.

Utrum error contingat in apostemate diu durante.

Taddeo, *Pronost.*, fol. 226v.

Utrum evacuatio in febre putrida secundum quod fiens est evacuatio putridi.

Turisanus, *Plusquam*, 3.40

Utrum evacuatio superflua secundum plurimum generet febres.

Dino, *Dilucidatorium*, 3.18.

Utrum ex sanguine manente in propria forma possit fieri febris.

Taddeo, *Isagoge*, fol. 387r.

Utrum ex sanguine manente in propria forma sanguinis possit fieri febris.

Dino, independent question, Paris
University MS 128, fol. 114v.

Utrum febricitans febre acuta possit esse abseque omni dolore.

Taddeo, *Pronost.*, fol. 239r.

Utrum febricitans febre interpollata febricitet in die interpollationis.

Taddeo, *Aphor.*, fol. 113.

Utrum febris acuta possit inducere spasmum.

Taddeo, *Aphor.*, fol. 50.

Utrum febris coniuncta buboni possit esse effimera.

Taddeo, *Aphor.*, fol. 111.

Utrum febris curet apoplexiam cui supervenit.

Taddeo, *Aphor.*, fol. 129.

Utrum febris de sanguine magis eveniat quam febris aliorum humorum.

Taddeo, *Isagoge*, fol. 387r.

Utrum febris de sanguine sit longior quam febris de cholera.

Taddeo, *Isagoge*, fol. 387r.

Utrum febris effimera in bubone sit bona.

Taddeo, *Aphor.*, fol. 111.

Utrum febris effimera per unicum diem duret.

Taddeo, *Aphor.*, fol. 111.

Utrum febris effimera sit mala complexio fiens.

[Dino?] independent question, BAV,
MS Vat. lat. 3144, fol. 13v.

Utrum febris ephimera possit supervenire alius febribus.

Taddeo, *Isagoge*, fol. 383v.

Utrum febris ephimera sit febris.　　Taddeo, *Isagoge*, fol. 383v.

Utrum febris ephimera sit solum in spiritu.

Taddeo, *Isagoge*, fol. 383v.

Utrum febris ephymera habeat paroxismos.

Taddeo, *Isagoge*, fol. 384r.

Utrum febris ephymera habeat quattuor tempora.

Taddeo, *Isagoge*, fol. 384r.

Utrum febris ephymera possit permutari in ethycam immediate.

Taddeo, *Isagoge*, fol. 384r.

Utrum febris ephymera pecipiat diversitatem in specie secundum diversos spiritus. Taddeo, *Isagoge*, fol. 384r.

Utrum febris ethica augeatur in tempore quo cibus digeritur aut dispergitur aut assumitur. Taddeo, *Pronost.*, fol. 230r.

Utrum febris ethica sit continua. Taddeo, *Pronost.*, fol. 230r.

Utrum febris hetica fiat subito. Taddeo, *Isagoge*, fol. 385r.

Utrum febris hetica habeat causam coniunctam.

Taddeo, *Isagoge*, fol. 384v.

Utrum febris hetica habeat quattuor tempora.

Taddeo, *Isagoge*, fol. 385r.

Utrum febris hetica possit fieri materia existente in venis.

Taddeo, *Isagoge*, fol. 385r.

Utrum febris hetica possit fieri sine alio morbo.

Taddeo, *Isagoge*, fol. 385r.

Utrum febris hetica sit mala complexio.

Taddeo, *Isagoge*, fol. 384v.

Utrum febris hetica sit mala complexio diversa.

Taddeo, *Isagoge*, fol. 384v.

Utrum febris hetica sit morbus. Taddeo, *Isagoge*, fol. 384v.

Utrum febris ideo anticipet quia eius materia ex grossa et subtili composita sit et grossa prius putrescat. Taddeo, *Aphor.*, fol. 13.

Utrum febris in generatione saniei augeatur.

Taddeo, *Aphor.*, fol. 67.

Utrum febris interpollata a principio usque ad finem omnium paroxismorum sit una et non plures. Taddeo, *Isagoge*, fol. 386v.

Utrum febris interpollata fiat in humide.

Taddeo, *Isagoge*, fol. 386v.

Utrum febris interpollata possit fieri ex sanguine.

Taddeo, *Isagoge*, fol. 386v.

Utrum febris interpollata sit una febris vel plures.

Taddeo, *Aphor.*, fol. 113.

Utrum febris interpollata possit fieri propter apostema intrinsecum.

Taddeo, *Aphor.*, fol. 107.

Utrum febris lipparia et empiala sint idem.

Taddeo, *Isagoge*, fol. 388v.

Utrum febris possit curare spasmum.   Taddeo, *Aphor.*, fol. 112.
Utrum febris putrida possit esse bonum signum cum bubone.
                              Taddeo, *Aphor.*, fol. 111.
Utrum febris sanguinis habeat quattuor tempora.
                              Taddeo, *Isagoge*, fol. 387r.
Utrum febris sanguinis sit febris acuta.
                              Taddeo, *Isagoge*, fol. 387r.
Utrum febris sanguinis sit febris ephymera.
                              Taddeo, *Isagoge*, fol. 387r.
Utrum febris sit calor naturalis mutatus in ignem.
                              Turisanus, *Plusquam*, 3.38.
Utrum febris sit calor naturalis mutatus in ignem.
                              Taddeo, *Aphor.*, fol. 20.
Utrum febris sit causa vel morbus vel accidens.
                              Taddeo, *Isagoge*, fol. 382v.
Utrum febris sit mala complexio equalis.
                              Taddeo, *Isagoge*, fol. 383r.
Utrum febris sit morbus compositus.   Taddeo, *Isagoge*, fol. 382v.
Utrum febris sit morbus officialis.   Taddeo, *Isagoge*, fol. 382v.
Utrum febris sit peior morbus que fiat in homine.
                              Taddeo, *Isagoge*, fol. 383r.
Utrum febris sit res naturalis, vel non naturalis, vel contra naturam.
                              Taddeo, *Isagoge*, fol. 382v.
Utrum febris superveniens alicui dolori auferat illum.
                              Taddeo, *Aphor.*, fol. 185.
Utrum febris synocha sit ex aliis humoribus a colera.
                              Turisanus, *Plusquam*, 3.38.
Utrum febris tertiana non vera plus duret quam vera, et quaterna econtra.
                              Taddeo, *Isagoge*, fol. 386v.
Utrum frenesis sit mortifera in suo genere necne.
                              Taddeo, *Aphor.*, fol. 120.
Utrum furfura possint venire de venis sine febre.
                              Taddeo, *Aphor.*, fol. 125.
Utrum gibbi ex asmate aut tussi moriantur ante iuventutem.
                              Taddeo, *Aphor.*, fol. 189.
Utrum gibbositas fiat ex asmate aut tussi.
                              Taddeo, *Aphor.*, fol. 189.
Utrum gibbositas pectoris spacium respirationis angustet.
                              Taddeo, *Aphor.*, fol. 189.
Utrum habens testiculos et abstinens a coitu podagrizare possit.
                              Taddeo, *Aphor.*, fol. 177.

Utrum humiditas faciat linguam ineptam literarum prolationi.

Taddeo, Aphor., fol. 181.

Utrum humiditas lingue sine humiditate cerebri possit facere bulbutiem [sic].

Taddeo, Aphor., fol. 181.

Utrum hydropicus tussiens evadere possit.

Taddeo, Aphor., fol. 183.

Utrum idropisis superveniens febri acute possit fieri vitio splenis.

Taddeo, Pronost., fol. 212r.

Utrum idropisis superveniens febri acute sit bonum signum et bona causa.

Taddeo, Pronost., fol. 212r.

Utrum in antrace competat sompnus.   Anon. independent question with questions of Dino, BAV, MS Vat. lat. 4454, fols. 104r-v.

Utrum in antrace competat sompnus.   Mondino, independent question, Bib. Marciana, fondo antico MS 534 (XIV.59), fols. 21-22.

Utrum in convalescentibus abstinentia consequens sit peior precedente.

Taddeo, Aphor., fol. 57.

Utrum in corporibus cacocimis possit esse vehemens appetitus.

Dino, Dilucidatorium, 1.10.

Utrum in die interpollationis homo patiens febrem sit eger.

Taddeo, Isagoge, fol. 386v.

Utrum in egritudine presente, scilicet cancri, competat [tyriaca].

Guglielmo, De tyriaca, pp. 130-133.

Utrum in epilepsia virtus motiva tota auferatur.

Taddeo, Aphor., fol. 66.

Utrum in febre acuta possit esse sudor frigidus.

Taddeo, Pronost., fol. 206v.

Utrum in febre ephymera attendatur signum digestionis.

Taddeo, Isagoge, fol. 384r.

Utrum in febre ephymera contingat mori ipsa existente in sua specie.

Taddeo, Isagoge, fol. 384r.

Utrum in febre putrida digestio debeatur cause antecedenti vel coniuncte.

Turisanus, Plusquam, 3.38.

Utrum in febris sanguis totus sanguis putrescat.

Taddeo, Isagoge, fol. 54.

Utrum in parva febre possit esse macies secundum rationem que significat debilitatem virtutis.   Taddeo, Aphor., fol. 54.

Utrum in passione iliaca exeat aliqua egestio.

Taddeo, Aphor., fol. 187.

Utrum in peripleumonia sanies adunetur in uno latere tamen.

Taddeo, *Pronost.*, fol. 229v.

Utrum in peripleumonia signa digestionis differant usque ad septimum diem.

Taddeo, *Pronost.*, fol. 226r.

Utrum in pleuresi sanies adunetur in uno latere tamen.

Taddeo, *Pronost.*, fol. 229v.

Utrum in podagricis fiant tumores in iuncturis.

Taddeo, *Aphor.*, fol. 191.

Utrum in principio lienterie semper sit oxiremia.

Taddeo, *Aphor.*, fol. 162.

Utrum in statu omnis pleuresis accidentia minorantur.

Turisanus, *Plusquam*, 3.32.

Utrum in tempore estivali omnes egritudines sint breves.

Taddeo, *Aphor.*, fol. 14.

Utrum in timpania sit aliqua aquositas.

Taddeo, *Aphor.*, fol. 91.

Utrum instabilitas accessionis febris significet brevitatem eius.

Taddeo, *Aphor.*, fol. 101.

Utrum lapide in renibus aut vesica existente sit necessarium arenam exire.

Taddeo, *Aphor.*, fol. 126.

Utrum lenitas rerum conferat in febribus acutis.

Taddeo, *Reg. acut.*, fol. 256r.

Utrum lumbrici permixti cum egestione sint boni.

Mondino, *Pronost.*, BAV, MS
Vat. lat. 4466, fol. 15r.

Utrum materia apostematis pleuretici debeat esse aut rubea aut nigra tantum.

Taddeo, *Aphor.*, fol. 182.

Utrum materia squinantie possit ire ad pulmonem.

Taddeo, *Aphor.*, fol. 131.

Utrum modus generationis apostematis positus a Galeno conveniat omnibus apostematibus.   Turisanus, *Plusquam*, 3.64.

Utrum motus auferatur in apoplexia.   Taddeo, *Aphor.*, fol. 64.

Utrum mulier podagrizare possit.   Taddeo, *Aphor.*, fol. 178.

Utrum mutatio etatis possit esse causa curativa epilepsie.

Taddeo, *Aphor.*, fol. 66.

Utrum natura possit removere superfluum de vulnera vel non.

Taddeo, *Isagoge*, fol. 398r.

Utrum nullus vulnus faciens saniem sit periculosum.

Taddeo, *Aphor.*, fol. 134.

Utrum omne membrum possit apostemari.

Taddeo, *Isagoge*, fol. 389v.

Utrum omnis febris durans per unicum diem sit effimera.

Taddeo, *Aphor.*, fol. 111.

Utrum omnis idropisis contingat propter peccatum epatis.

Taddeo, *Pronost.*, fol. 212r.

Utrum omnis peripleumonicus deductus ad saniem necessario moriatur.

Taddeo, *Pronost.*, fol. 234r.

Utrum opilationes nervorum sint peiores quam opilationes venarum et arteriarum.   Dino, *Dilucidatorium*, 24.7.

Utrum oporteat febrem lippariam super fieri de apostemate.

Taddeo, *Pronost.*, fol. 213v.

Urtum oxiremia appareat necessario in statu lienterie.

Taddeo, *Aphor.*, fol. 162.

Utrum passio artetica debeat magis venire in autumno quam in vere.

Taddeo, *Aphor.*, fol. 193.

Utrum passio iliaca fiat in solis intestinis.

Taddeo, *Aphor.*, fol. 188.

Utrum per exitum saniei ab empico ora venarum aperiantur.

Taddeo, *Aphor.*, fol. 176.

Utrum perforatio intestinorum grossorum sit curabilis.

Taddeo, *Aphor.*, fol. 176.

Utrum peripleumonia fiat equaliter ex omnibus humoribus.

Taddeo, *Aphor.*, fol. 182.

Utrum peripleumonia per apostema terminari possit.

Taddeo, *Pronost*, fol. 232v.

Utrum pestilentia possit contingere brutis et non hominus alicuius regionis.

Taddeo, *Isagoge*, fol. 375v.

Utrum pleuresi existente in dyaphramate dolor ascendat tamen ad furculam vel descendat tamen ad hypocundria.   Taddeo, *Reg. acut.*, fol. 280v.

Utrum, pleuresi existente in panniculo tegente quintam costam, dolor ascendat ad furculam vel descendat sub hypocundria.

Taddeo, *Reg. acut.*, fol. 280r.

Urtum pleuresis aliquod fiat sub diaphragmate.

Taddeo, *Reg. acut.*, fol. 280r.

Utrum pleuresis mundificabilis in 14 diebus mundificetur.

Taddeo, *Aphor.*, fol. 130.

Utrum pleuresis post 14 dies convertatur in empyma.

Taddeo, *Aphor.*, fol. 130.

Utrum pleuresis vera eveniat in solo panniculo tegente costas.

Taddeo, *Reg. acut.*, fol. 263v.

Utrum pleureticus possit transire diem 14^{m}.

Taddeo, *Aphor.*, fol. 14.

Utrum podagra sit morbus vel accidens.

> Taddeo, *Aphor.*, fol. 177.

Utrum possibile sit corpus febrire et non minui.

> Taddeo, *Aphor.*, fol. 53.

Utrum possit dari obtalmia in qua nihil egrediatur ab oculis.

> Taddeo, *Aphor.*, fol. 77.

Utrum possit fieri commixtio duarum febrium continuarum.

> Taddeo, *Isagoge*, fol. 388r.

Utrum possit fieri febris composita de flegma et cholera.

> Taddeo, *Isagoge*, fol. 388r.

Utrum ptisis facilius contingat in iuventute quam aliis etatibus.

> Taddeo, *Aphor.*, fol. 130.

Utrum pueri sint magis apti ad podagram quam eunuchi.

> Taddeo, *Aphor.*, fol. 178.

Utrum purgatio menstrualis defendat mulieres a podagra.

> Taddeo, *Aphor.*, fol. 178.

Utrum quelibet febris interpollata tantum faciat in uno periodo quantum facit continue in uno die.   Taddeo, *Aphor.*, fol. 113.

Utrum quies sit necessaria ad consolidationem ulcerum pulmonis.

> Taddeo, *Aphor.*, fol. 168.

Utrum rigor in febre quotidiana possit fieri a cholera rubea.

> Taddeo, *Aphor.*, fol. 114.

Utrum rigore superveniente febri crisis statim sequatur.

> Taddeo, *Aphor.*, fol. 100.

Utrum sanguis existens in apostemate pleuretico sit proportionalis sanguini totius corporis.   Taddeo, *Reg. acut.*, fol. 279r.

Utrum sanies existens in apostemate mirach possit intrare stomachum et intestina.   Taddeo, *Pronost.*, fol. 210v.

Utrum sanies sit a calore vehementi cum prevaluerit.

> Turisanus, *Plusquam*, 3.49.

Utrum sanies sit ab utroque calore.   Turisanus, *Plusquam*, 3.49.

Utrum senes evadentes a passionibus catarricis paralisim potius in latere dextro pati debeant quam in sinistro.   Taddeo, *Aphor.*, fol. 77.

Utrum senes magis pereant a collectionibus pectoris quam iuvenes et adolescentes.   Taddeo, *Pronost.*, fol. 234r.

Utrum sensus auferatur in apoplexia.   Taddeo, *Aphor.*, fol. 64.

Utrum siccitas possit facere suffocationem.

> Taddeo, *Aphor.*, fol. 102.

Utrum significandum sit super ptisicos.

> Taddeo, *Aphor.*, fol. 131.

Utrum sit possibile quod resolutum et resarcitum sint semper proportionata in quantitate in corpore nostro in quacumque eius etate.

Taddeo, *Aphor.*, fol. 19.

Utrum sola febris sit egritudo universalis totius corporis.

Taddeo, *Isagoge*, fol. 383r.

Utrum sola mala complexio possit esse causa apoplexie.

Taddeo, *Aphor.*, fol. 64.

Utrum solutio continui sit in omni apostemate.

Taddeo, *Isagoge*, fol. 389v.

Utrum somnus in declinatione contingens dolorem et apostemata augeat.

Taddeo, *Aphor.*, fol. 29.

Utrum somnus in declinatione contingens febrem augeat.

Taddeo, *Aphor.*, fol. 29.

Utrum species apoplexie sint solum due vel 3.

Taddeo, *Aphor.*, fol. 64.

Utrum species emitritrorum sint novem.

Taddeo, *Isagoge*, fol. 388v.

Utrum species febris ethice sint tantum quatuor, vel plures, sive pauciores.

Mondino, independent question, Paris University MS 128, fols. 128r-130r.

Utrum species febris hetice debeant esse quattuor.

Taddeo, *Isagoge*, fol. 385v.

Utrum stabilitas accessionis in febricus sit signum longitudinis earum.

Taddeo, *Aphor.*, fol. 100.

Utrum stomachus compatiatur intestinis in dissenteria.

Taddeo, *Aphor.*, fol. 165.

Utrum stranguiria possit esse causa ileos.

Taddeo, *Aphor.*, fol. 187.

Utrum surditas auferat cholericas egestiones.

Taddeo, *Aphor.*, fol. 100.

Utrum synochus possit dividi in tres species.

Taddeo, *Isagoge*, fol. 387r.

Utrum tertiana interpollata per fluxum ventris terminari possit.

Taddeo, *Aphor.*, fol. 113.

Utrum tertiana vera possit transire septem periodos.

Taddeo, *Aphor.*, fol. 113.

Utrum trauli longa diaria capi possint.

Taddeo, *Aphor.*, fol. 181.

Utrum tussis possit supervenire hydropisi.

Taddeo, *Aphor.*, fol. 183.

Utrum tympania generetur semper a calido.

> Mondino, *Pronost.*, BAV, MS
> Vat. lat. 4466, fol. 11v.

Utrum ultimus periodus tertiane sit creticus.

> Taddeo, *Aphor.*, fol. 113.

Utrum urina impediat consolidationem ulcerum vesice.

> Taddeo, *Aphor.*, fol. 168.

Utrum vapor calefactorii ingrediens per nares pleuretici noceat ei.

> Taddeo, *Reg. acut.*, fol. 275v.

Utrum ventositas timpanie sit inclusa in globoso intestino.

> Taddeo, *Aphor.*, fol. 91.

Utrum vulnera diafragmatis et pulmonis prohibeantur solidari propter motum.

> Taddeo, *Aphor.*, fol. 173.

Utrum vulnera difficilius sanentur in senibus quam in aliis etatibus.

> Taddeo, *Aphor.*, fol. 167.

Utrum vulnus frigidus sit morbus humidus sine humectatione.

> Taddeo, *Isagoge*, fol. 390v.

Utrum vulnus parvum epatis sit incurabili.

> Taddeo, *Aphor.*, fol. 173.

Prima questio est quia dubitatur quia videtur Avicennam male processisse, cum prius determinavit de apostematibus quam de solutione continuitatis.

> Dino, *Chirurgia* (Estense).

2ª questio est quia dubitatur utrum diffinitio apostematis communiter data sit bona.   Dino, *Chirurgia* (Estense).

8ª questio est quare Avicenna facit intentionem de erisipila in capitulo de flegmone.   Dino, *Chirurgia* (Estense).

16ª questio est quia videtur Avicennam fuisse superfluum et diminitum in ponendo solum tres terminationes apostematis.

> Dino, *Chirurgia* (Estense).

35ª questio est quia Avicenna nominat formicas ulceres cum sint pustule.

> Dino, *Chirurgia* (Estense).

37ª questio est quia Avicenna in fine capituli de pruria loquitur de formica cum dicit "Et quoniam sunt cum speciebus formice," etc.

> Dino, *Chirurgia* (Estense).

40ª questio est de eo quod dicit Avicenna in capitulo de althoin [?] que sensibiles carnes glandose sunt, sicut cancer mamillarum etc.

> Dino, *Chirurgia* (Estense).

41ª questio est quia dicit Avicenna quod cancer que est in subascellis et inguinibus et hiis similibus non habet sensum.

> Dino, *Chirurgia* (Estense).

42^a questio est in quo differt 4^m significatum althoin a tertio.

Dino, *Chirurgia* (Estense).

43^a questio est quia dicit Avicenna, loquendo de althoin, quod ex eo quidam ad nigredinem est declive, non evadit aliquis.

Dino, *Chirurgia* (Estense).

44^a questio est quia dicit Avicenna quod antrax vel althoin interficit eo quod introducit malam qualitatem ad cordem ex via arteriarum.

Dino, *Chirurgia* (Estense).

50^a questio est quia non videtur quod determinate de apostematibus glandosis specte ad hunc librum.   Dino, *Chirurgia* (Estense).

56^a questio est quare Avicenna posuit primo libro apostemata posuit apostematum aquosum, hic autem non.

Dino, *Chirurgia* (Estense).

57^a questio est quia dicit Avicenna quod scrofule et modi diversi sunt apostemata flegmatica, et in primo libro dixit ipsa esse melancolica.

Dino, *Chirurgia* (Estense).

58^a questio est sub qua specie apostematum ponantur glandulose, an sub specie apostematum melancolicorum an flegmaticorum.

Dino, *Chirurgia* (Estense).

71^a questio est que sint vulnera in quibus sit vehemens dolor et apostemata et quare in his fiant.   Dino, *Chirurgia* (Estense).

72^a questio est utrum in vulneribus apostemata accidere sit bona.

Dino, *Chirurgia* (Estense).

73^a questio est utrum dictum sit verum cum dicit in una rubrica "Sermo universalis de cirurgia vulnerum."   Dino, *Chirurgia* (Estense).

74^a questio est utrum quando apostematum supervenit vulneri possit vulnus curari preter quando curetur apostematum.

Dino, *Chirurgia* (Estense).

84^a questio est quare Avicenna non determinavit de vulneribus factis in concavitate membro spiritualium.   Dino, *Chirurgia* (Estense).

90^a questio est quare Avicenna magis in speciali tractavit in 4^a fen de cura vulnerum capitis quam aliorum membrorum.

Dino, *Chirurgia* (Estense).

100^a questio est unum problema, scilicet propter quid necesse est ex ablatione ossibus fieri cicatricem concavam.   Dino, *Chirurgia* (Estense).

101^a questio est utrum sit verum quod dicit Avicenna quod in capitulo de ulceribus dicit, quod ex fistula perveniente ad nervos ossa et ligamenta egreditur humiditas magis tenuis quam ex illa quod pervenit solum ad carnem.

Dino, *Chirurgia* (Estense).

102^{a} questio est quia queritur cum ulcerus fuerit in membro carnoso et caro
sit coloris rubei, utrum sanies ibi generata debeat esse coloris rubei.

Dino, *Chirurgia* (Estense).

111^{a} questio est quia queritur quis spasmus sit ille que consequitur ad vulnera
nervorum. Dino, *Chirurgia* (Estense).

112^{a} questio est propter quid potius consequitur spasmus ad vulnera nervorum
quam paralisis, et numquid aliquando possit consequitur paralisis.

Dino, *Chirurgia* (Estense).

113^{a} questio est quomodo est possibile quod in nervis sit apostematum
magnum et non sit cum dolore magno.

Dino, *Chirurgia* (Estense).

114^{a} questio est numquid adventus febris in vulnere nervorum sit bonus
et precipue quando ibi adest vel timetur adventus spasmi.

Dino, *Chirurgia* (Estense).

119^{a} questio est quia queritur super capitulo de fractura cranei quomodo est
possibile quod findatur craneum et non cutis nec caro cum tamen sint desuper.

Dino, *Chirurgia* (Estense).

INDICATIONS OF THE STATE OF HEALTH; REGIMEN

Dubitatur an in prandio conveniat plus de cibo quam in coena an econverso.

Questio famossissimi Dini de Florentia,
in *Opera Andreae Thurini Pisciensis*,
Rome, 1545, fols. 149r-153v.

Utrum a stomacho egrediatur aliquid sine vomitu vel fastidio.

Taddeo, *Aphor.*, fol. 65.

Utrum aer balnei infrigidet. Taddeo, *Isagoge*, fol. 377r.

Utrum aliqua signa possit dici neutra.

Turisanus, *Plusquam*, 2.100.

Utrum aliquod sedimen sit ventosum.

Taddeo, *Pronost.*, fol. 220v.

Utrum alteratio extrinseca reducatur ad aliquid genera signorum.

Turisanus, *Plusquam*, 2.13.

Utrum aqua balnei humectet membra subtilia.

Taddeo, *Isagoge*, fol. 377r.

Utrum aqua calida balnei possit calefacere.

Taddeo, *Isagoge*, fol. 377r.

Utrum aqua humectet membra substantialia.

Taddeo, *Aphor.*, fol. 92.

Utrum aqua magis tollat sitim quam vinum.

Taddeo, *Isagoge*, fol. 379v.

Utrum aqua mellis provocat urinam.   Taddeo, *Reg. acut.*, fol. 319v.

Utrum balneum adiuvet digestionem materie vel non.
Taddeo, *Isagoge*, fol. 377r.

Utrum balneum evacuet a toto corpore vel non.
Taddeo, *Isagoge*, fol. 377r.

Utrum balneum evacuet solum quod cuti vicinatur.
Taddeo, *Isagoge*, fol. 79.

Utrum balneum possit conferre ad digestionem cibi.
Taddeo, *Isagoge*, fol. 377r.

Utrum balneum purget equaliter de toto corpore.
Taddeo, *Aphor.*, fol. 89.

Utrum bonus appetitus adiuvet digestionem.
Taddeo, *Aphor.*, fol. 62.

Utrum bonus sudor debeat fieri in toto corpore.
Taddeo, *Pronost.*, fol. 206v.

Utrum caro bovina parum nutriat.   Taddeo, *Aphor.*, fol. 41.

Utrum color glaucus causetur a melancholia.
Taddeo, *Isagoge*, fol. 370r.

Utrum color hypostasis urine aliquam significandi habeat.
Taddeo, *Pronost.*, fol. 219v.

Utrum color puerorum debeat esse albus vel niger.
Taddeo, *Isagoge*, fol. 369v.

Utrum color rubeus clarus sanguinis sit medius inter rubeum et nigrum.
Taddeo, *Reg. acut.*, fol. 279r.

Utrum color rubeus fiat a sanguine adusto.
Taddeo, *Isagoge*, fol. 370r.

Utrum color rubeus urine sit melior colore albo.
Taddeo, *Pronost.*, fol. 218v.

Utrum color significans temperamentum debeat esse compositus ex albo
et rubeo.   Taddeo, *Isagoge*, fol. 369v.

Utrum color viridis causetur a melancholia.
Taddeo, *Pronost.*, fol. 204r.

Utrum color viridis significet super frigiditatem vel caliditatem.
Taddeo, *Pronost.*, fol. 199r.

Utrum consideratio etatis conferat in ordinatione diete.
Taddeo, *Aphor.*, fol. 15.

Utrum corpora senum sint neutra ut nunc.
Turisanus, *Plusquam*, 3.83.

Utrum corpus senis sit neutrum.   Turisanus, *Plusquam*, 2.94.

Utrum crassi minus vivant quam macri.
Taddeo, *Aphor.*, fol. 65.

Utrum delectatio cibi minuat eis maliciam et nocumentum.

Taddeo, *Aphor.*, fol. 62.

Utrum diffinitio rei naturalis et non naturalis posita ab autore sit bona.

Taddeo, *Isagoge*, fol. 372v.

Utrum divisio signorum sit bene posita.

Turisanus, *Plusquam*, 2.1.

Utrum etas calida magis possit ferre ieiunium quam frigida.

Taddeo, *Aphor.*, fol. 15.

Utrum etas humida melius ferat ieiunium quam sicca.

Taddeo, *Aphor.*, fol. 15.

Utrum experimentum de nutrientibus sit fiendum in corpore inanito.

Taddeo, *Aphor.*, fol. 41.

Utrum facies tornatilis facta in iuvene cholerico habenti humores subtiles existenti in regione calida et tempore calido sit deterius signum quam si facta sit in habenti conditiones oppositas.   Taddeo, *Pronost.*, fol. 200r.

Utrum facilius et velocius per potum quam per cibum nutriamur.

Taddeo, *Aphor.*, fol. 34.

Utrum Galenus recte requirit signa ex ortis.

Turisanus, *Plusquam*, 2.57.

Utrum homines quorum stomachus abundat flegma ferant ieiunium facile.

Taddeo, *Reg. acut.*, fol. 293v.

Utrum homines sani debeant mutare regimen in sua sanitate.

Taddeo, *Reg. acut.*, fol. 305v.

Utrum homines universali sint bono regimine tempore hyemis.

Taddeo, *Aphor.*, fol. 178.

Utrum hypostasis [urine] possit aliquid bonum significare.

Taddeo, *Pronost.*, fol. 219v.

Utrum hypostasis procedat a liquefactione adipsis.

Taddeo, *Pronost.,* fol. 220v.

Utrum hypostasis residens in fundo sit fidelis nuncia salutis.

Taddeo, *Pronost.*, fol. 219v.

Utrum hypostasis rubea contingat propter aquositatem sanguinea.

Taddeo, *Pronost.*, fol. 219v.

Utrum hypostasis sit maior in hyeme quam in estate.

Taddeo, *Aphor.*, fol. 19.

Utrum hypostasis stans in fundo bonum significet.

Taddeo, *Pronost.*, fol. 219v.

Utrum in hyeme venter sit calidus naturaliter vel violenter.

Taddeo, *Aphor.*, fol. 19.

Utrum in urina laudabilis debeat apparire ypostasis.

Mondino, *Pronost.*, BAV, MS Vat. lat. 4466, fol. 17r.

Utrum medicus debeat expectare aut deducere ad has significationes et ab eis
sumere significationem.   Dino, *Dilucidatorium*, 4.11.
Utrum medicus magis debeat considerare de vino quam de aqua.
                                           Taddeo, *Isagoge*, fol. 379v.
Utrum mulieres debeant regi in corpore dieta humida vel sicca.
                                           Dino, no. 1 in a set of six misc.
                                           questions, CLM 13020, fols. 217r-v.
Utrum mutatio urine ad spissitudinem significet digestionem.
                                           Taddeo, *Aphor.*, fol. 117.
Utrum mutatio urine ad subtilitatem significet digestionem.
                                           Taddeo, *Aphor.*, fol. 117.
Utrum mutatio urine de paucitate et grossitie ad multitudinem et subtilitatem
iuvet.   Taddeo, *Aphor.*, fol. 117.
Utrum ordinatio diete penes virtutem et statum simul necessario sit
attendenda.   Taddeo, *Aphor.*, fol. 8.
Utrum permixtio sputi cum saliva sit bonum signum.
                                           Taddeo, *Pronost.*, fol. 224v.
Utrum pinguedo urine possit in fundo residere.
                                           Taddeo, *Pronost.*, fol. 222v.
Utrum plenitudo sit semper mala.   Taddeo, *Aphor.*, fol. 30.
Utrum pueri bene se habeant in vere.
                                           Taddeo, *Aphor.*, fol. 81.
Utrum pulsus fortis post cibationem declaret corpus nutriri.
                                           Taddeo, *Aphor.*, fol. 41.
Utrum recte signa significantia modo sanitatem, modo mortem, dicantur
neutra.   Turisanus, *Plusquam*, 2.100.
Utrum res non naturales sint de substantia nostri corporis.
                                           Taddeo, *Isagoge*, fol. 372v.
Utrum res non naturales sint plures quam sex.
                                           Taddeo, *Isagoge*, fol. 372v.
Utrum res non naturales sint sex.   Turisanus, *Plusquam*, 3.5.
Utrum sal et milium ex quibus calefactorium est faciendum timeri debeat.
                                           Taddeo, *Reg. acut.*, fol. 276r.
Utrum sal sit mordicativum.   Taddeo, *Reg. acut.*, fol. 276r.
Utrum sani difficilius ferant peccantia quam egritudine.
                                           Taddeo, *Aphor.*, fol. 7.
Utrum sanitas et egritudo possint esse in signo.
                                           Taddeo, *Isagoge*, fol. 392v.
Utrum sedimen [urine] magnarum partium sit melius sedimine parvarum
partium.   Taddeo, *Pronost.*, fol. 220v.
Utrum senes bene se habeant in estate et in autumno.
                                           Taddeo, *Aphor.*, fol. 81.

Utrum senes multum cibum sustinere possint.

Taddeo, *Aphor.*, fol. 15.

Utrum signa sumpta a virtute animali sint fortiora in significando quam signa sumpta a virtute vitali.   Taddeo, *Pronost.*, fol. 214v.

Utrum signa sumpta a virtute naturali sint fortiora in significando quam sumpta ab animali et vitali.   Taddeo, *Pronost.*, fol. 214v.

Utrum signum et accidens convertantur.

Taddeo, *Isagoge*, fol. 395r.

Utrum signum possit esse verum cum significato.

Turisanus, *Plusquam*, 2.3.

Utrum signum sit in plus quam accidens.

Taddeo, *Isagoge*, fol. 396v.

Utrum sit aliqua ratio quare iste dicantur non naturales.

Turisanus, *Plusquam*, 3.5.

Utrum sit maius peccatum in dieta grossa quam in subtili.

Taddeo, *Aphor.*, fol. 7.

Utrum sit possibile sputum procedere sicut oportet, indigesta existente materia.

Taddeo, *Pronost.*, fol. 233v.

Utrum sputum album viscosum accidat a flegmate adusto.

Taddeo, *Isagoge*, fol. 224v.

Utrum sputum subrubeum clarum sit melius signum quam rubeum purum.

Taddeo, *Pronost.*, fol. 226v.

Utrum sputum subsanguineum clarum demonstret salutem si veniat in principio.   Taddeo, *Pronost.*, fol. 226r.

Utrum squinantia perfecte resoluta, pulsus equalis et ordinatus fiat.

Taddeo, *Aphor.*, fol. 131.

Utrum subita mutatio de nimia quiete ad motum et econtra sint nociva.

Taddeo, *Reg. acut.*, fol. 304v.

Utrum subita mutatio de nimia quiete ad motum sit magis nociva quam econtra.   Taddeo, *Reg. acut.*, fol. 304v.

Utrum sudor aptius fiat in somno quam in vigilia.

Taddeo, *Aphor.*, fol. 106.

Utrum tollerantia bona, mutatio humoris, somnus, et sitis sint bone significationes in evacuatione.   Dino, *Dilucidatorium*, 4.10.

Utrum urina aquosa magis contradicat nature puerorum quam nigra.

Taddeo, *Pronost.*, fol. 222r.

Utrum urina grossa, multa, et alba significet digestionem.

Taddeo, *Aphor.*, fol. 122.

Utrum urina in principio habeant hypostasim.

Taddeo, *Aphor.*, fol. 117.

Utrum urina in que est hypostasis multa sit grossior naturali.

Taddeo, *Pronost.*, fol. 232v.

Utrum urina pinguis possit esse bonum signum.

Taddeo, *Pronost.*, fol. 222v.

Utrum velocitas productionis sputi sit bonum signum.

Taddeo, *Pronost.*, fol. 224v.

Utrum vinum album dulce et hidromel sit pluris humectationis quam aqua ordei. Taddeo, *Reg. acut.*, fol. 260r.

Utrum vinum dulce et idromel equaliter ad choleram convertantur.

Taddeo, *Reg. acut.*, fol. 318r.

Utrum vinum dulce exopilet pulmonem et opilet epar.

Taddeo, *Reg. acut.*, fol. 310v.

Utrum vinum dulce noceat spleni. Taddeo, *Reg. acut.*, fol. 310r.

Utrum vinum dulce quando facit sitim adiuvet ad screandum.

Taddeo, *Reg. acut.*, fol. 313r.

Utrum vinum nigrum magis corporibus resumendis quam rubeum.

Taddeo, *Aphor.*, fol. 35.

Utrum vinum nisi dulce magis faciat permixtionem rationis quam viscosum.

Taddeo, *Reg. acut.*, fol. 309v.

Utrum vinum ponticum magis adiuvet ad screandum quam dulce.

Taddeo, *Reg. acut.*, fol. 313r.

Utrum vinum velocius nutria ceteris nutrientibus.

Taddeo, *Aphor.*, fol. 41.

Utrum vinum vicosum album magis provocet urinam quam ceteri potus.

Taddeo, *Reg. acut.*, fol. 314r.

Utrum vomitus ingrediatur conservationem corporis optimam compositionem habentis. Dino, *Dilucidatorium*, 13.1.

7ª questio est quia videtur Avicennam falsum dicere, cum dicit quod sanguis laudabilis aut est grossus aut est subtilis.

Dino, *Chirurgia* (Estense).

Symptoms of Disease

Digressio de generatione saniei.	Turisanus, *Plusquam*, 3.49.
Digressio de rigore et causis eius.	Turisanus, *Plusquam*, 3.11.
Digressio de spasmo et causa eius.	Turisanus, *Plusquam*, 3.55.
In quo sexu hec urina nigra sit peior.	Mondino, *Pronost.*, BAV, MS Vat. lat. 4466, fol. 19r.

Utrum accessiones plus solito morantes et anticipantes statum propinquum significent. Taddeo, *Aphor.*, fol. 13.

Utrum ad urinam tenuem cum fortitudine virtutis crisis cum apostemate necessario sequatur. Taddeo, *Pronost.*, fol. 222r.

Utrum alienatio et angustia in egritudine acuta mortem significent.

Taddeo, *Pronost.*, fol. 207v.

Utrum alienatio mentis sit signum mortis.

> Taddeo, *Pronost.*, fol. 204v.

Utrum aliquis eger possit habere bonum appetitum post egritudinem.

> Taddeo, *Aphor.*, fol. 56.

Utrum angustia sit signum pernitiosum in egrotantibus.

> Taddeo, *Pronost.*, fol. 203r.

Utrum anhelitus frigidus in egritudine acuta significet mortem.

> Taddeo, *Pronost.*, fol. 205r.

Utrum anhelitus spissus et parvus significet dolorem.

> Taddeo, *Pronost.*, fol. 205r.

Utrum appetitus sit bonum signum in principio convalescentie.

> Taddeo, *Aphor.*, fol. 57.

Utrum approprinquante crisi stercus condensari debeat.

> Taddeo, *Pronost.*, fol. 216v.

Utrum bene se habere ad oblationes in idropisi sit bonum signum.

> Taddeo, *Aphor.*, fol. 59.

Utrum bonitas anhelitus sit bonum signum in acutis egritudinibus tamen.

> Taddeo, *Aphor.*, fol. 59.

Utrum bonitas mentis significet bonum super quamlibet egritudinem.

> Taddeo, *Aphor.*, fol. 58.

Utrum calefactio stomachi et extremorum indicet nauseam.

> Dino, *Dilucidatorium*, 11.6.

Utrum color viridis et citrinus demonstrent parvum nocumentum.

> Taddeo, *Pronost.*, fol. 204r.

Utrum color viridis et lividus creticam evasionem significare possint.

> Taddeo, *Pronost.*, fol. 215r.

Utrum corpus febriens possit contabescere preter rationem.

> Taddeo, *Aphor.*, fol. 53.

Utrum debeat ponere signa aliorum lapsuum a cerebro sicut egri simpliciter.

> Turisanus, *Plusquam*, 2.26.

Utrum descensus doloris in pleuresi significet indigestionem farmacie.

> Taddeo, *Reg. acut.*, fol. 280v.

Utrum diaria sit bene posita esse signum malum in pleuresi.

> Taddeo, *Aphor.*, fol. 171.

Utrum diaria superveniens pleuresi et peripleumonie sit signum malum.

> Taddeo, *Aphor.*, fol. 171.

Utrum dolor et febris sint fortiores in generatione.

> Taddeo, *Aphor.*, fol. 67.

Utrum dolor secundum essentiam sentiatur.

> Taddeo, *Aphor.*, fol. 30.

Utrum dolor sit lesio operationis vel operatio corrupta.

Turisanus, *Plusquam*, 2.79.

Utrum dolorem non quiescere et febrem non desicere [*sic*] in pleuresi significet conversionem ad collectionem saniei.

Taddeo, *Pronost.*, fol. 208v.

Utrum duo dolores in eadem parte corporis esse possint.

Taddeo, *Aphor.*, fol. 67.

Utrum dura rigor incipit tunc sit febris.

Taddeo, *Isagoge*, fol. 389r.

Utrum egestio cholerica auferat surditatem.

Taddeo, *Aphor.*, fol. 100.

Utrum egestio fetida significet mortem.

Taddeo, *Pronost.*, fol. 217v.

Utrum egestio nigra sit signum mortis.

Taddeo, *Pronost.*, fol. 217v.

Utrum egestio pinguis significet mortem.

Taddeo, *Pronost.*, fol. 217v.

Utrum egestio que est sicut lotura [*sic*] intestinorum sit malum signum in acuta passione.   Taddeo, *Pronost.*, fol. 218r.

Utrum egestio viridis possit esse signum creticum.

Taddeo, *Pronost.*, fol. 217v.

Utrum egestio viscosa multa sit peior pauca.

Taddeo, *Pronost.*, fol. 217v.

Utrum egestiones melancholice sint peiores cholericis.

Taddeo, *Aphor.*, fol. 98.

Utrum egritudo de inanitione habeat paroxismos.

Taddeo, *Aphor.*, fol. 10.

Utrum eger habens egestionem cholericam in fine egritudinis sanetur.

Taddeo, *Aphor.*, fol. 98.

Utrum evasuri ab egritudine omnia signa bona, contrarii vero omnia signa mala, habere debeant.   Taddeo, *Pronost.*, fol. 239r.

Utrum ex poris uritidibus [*sic*] solutis sanguis egrediatur et doleant.

Taddeo, *Aphor.*, fol. 127.

Utrum exeuntia in lientaria significent peccatum in quantitate et non in qualitate.   Taddeo, *Aphor.*, fol. 163.

Utrum exitus sanguis emmorroidalis per intestina sit laudabilis.

Taddeo, *Aphor.*, fol. 170.

Utrum extenuatio irrationalis in corpore egrotante virtutis debilitatem significet.   Taddeo, *Aphor.*, fol. 54.

Utrum extenuatio irrationalis sequens quamlibet febrem sit signum malum.

Taddeo, *Aphor.*, fol. 54.

Utrum facies que assimilatur facie sane semper sit signum salutis, et utrum facies dissimilis faciei sane sit semper signum mortis.

> Mondino, *Pronost.*, BAV, MS Vat. lat. 4466, fol. 3v.

Utrum facilitas et bonitas et fortitudo motus in egris sint bonum signum necessario. Taddeo, *Pronost.*, fol. 214r.

Utrum facilitas productionis sputi sit bonum signum in omni egritudinis pulmonis. Taddeo, *Pronost.*, fol. 224v.

Utrum fetor sputi significet mortem in ptisis.

> Taddeo, *Aphor.*, fol. 131.

Utrum frigiditas extremitatum sit malum signum.

> Taddeo, *Pronost.*, fol. 213v.

Utrum frigiditas extremitatum sit signum mortale.

> Taddeo, *Pronost.*, fol. 213v.

Utrum generatio saniei sit digestio vel non.

> Taddeo, *Pronost.*, fol. 211r.

Utrum habens faciem tornatilem propter egritudinem evaderi possit.

> Taddeo, *Pronost.*, fol. 200v.

Utrum homo possit abstinere a tussi pro voluntate.

> Taddeo, *Pronost.*, fol. 213r.

Utrum Hypocratis ponat omnia mala signa a facie sumenda.

> Taddeo, *Pronost.*, fol. 199r.

Utrum hypostasis [urine] decidatur a materia morbi.

> Taddeo, *Pronost.*, fol. 219v.

Utrum hypostasis [urine] squamosa sit peior simulaginea.

> Taddeo, *Pronost.*, fol. 220v.

Utrum hypostasis [urine] squamosa sit pessima.

> Taddeo, *Pronost.*, fol. 220v.

Utrum icteritia ante septimum diem in febre acuta significet malum mortale.

> Taddeo, *Aphor.*, fol. 115.

Utrum icteritia contingens ante septimam diem in febre cholerica sit bonum signum. Taddeo, *Aphor.*, fol. 114.

Utrum icteritia in septima et ultra septimam possit esse mala.

> Taddeo, *Aphor.*, fol. 115.

Utrum icteritia possit esse crisis ad salutem in apostemate epatis.

> Taddeo, *Aphor.*, fol. 114.

Utrum icteritia possit esse determinatio cretice in febre continua.

> Taddeo, *Aphor.*, fol. 114.

Utrum in apostematibus calidis epatis et splenis fluxus sanguinis narium sit bonum signum simpliciter vel malum signum simpliciter.

> Taddeo, *Pronost.*, fol. 209r.

Utrum in corpore febriente calor possit esse in parte interiori et frigus
in exteriori. Taddeo, *Aphor.*, fol. 105.
Utrum in lienteria comestum et bibitum in eadem qualitate exeant.
Taddeo, *Aphor.*, fol. 91.
Utrum indigentia sit semper mala. Taddeo, *Aphor.*, fol. 30.
Utrum indigestio materia significetur per colorem citrinum urine, an per
substantiam tenuem eius, an per utrumque eorum simul.
Taddeo, *Pronost.*, fol. 221r.
Utrum irrationalis permanentia in corpore egro tante egritudinis longitudinem
necessario significet. Taddeo, *Aphor.*, fol. 54.
Utrum iste apparitiones sint signum mortis.
Mondino, *Pronost.*, BAV, MS Vat.
lat. 4466, fol. 6r.
Utrum labor spontaneus demonstret egritudinem vel eam pronosticet.
Taddeo, *Aphor.*, fol. 30.
Utrum labores spontanei pronosticent apostemata et solutiones continui.
Taddeo, *Aphor.*, fol. 30.
Utrum lacere corpore supino sit malum mediocre vel malum simpliciter.
Taddeo, *Pronost.*, fol. 202v.
Utrum lesio operationum semper ostendat membrum egrotans.
Turisanus, *Plusquam*, 2.79.
Utrum lienteria dicatur significare quantitative solum.
Taddeo, *Isagoge*, fol. 397r.
Utrum macies decrepitorum sit macies irrationabilis.
Taddeo, *Aphor.*, fol. 54.
Utrum multiplex color in egestione significet mortem.
Taddeo, *Pronost.*, fol. 218r.
Utrum multiplex color in egestione sit malum signum.
Taddeo, *Pronost.*, fol. 218r.
Utrum mutatio coloris menstruorum significet indigentiam purgationis.
Taddeo, *Aphor.*, fol. 138.
Utrum mutatio solius coloris urine in quarta significet crisim in septima.
Taddeo, *Aphor.*, fol. 119.
Utrum mutatio temporis menstruorum significet necessario indigentiam
purgationis. Taddeo, *Aphor.*, fol. 138.
Utrum mutatio urine de albedine in citrinitatem in quarta significet
crisim in septima. Taddeo, *Aphor.*, fol. 119.
Utrum nebula nigra [in urina] possit significare bonam crisim in acuta
passione. Taddeo, *Pronost.*, fol. 220v.
Utrum nebula [in urina] possit fieri ex flegmate et sanie.
Taddeo, *Pronost.*, fol. 220v.

Utrum nocumentum factum a somno necessario significet mortem.
                    Taddeo, *Aphor.*, fol. 28.
Utrum nocumentum factum a somno sit causa vel signum mortis.
                    Taddeo, *Aphor.*, fol. 28.
Utrum nocumentum somni in declinatione possit significare mortem.
                    Taddeo, *Aphor.*, fol. 29.
Utrum omne sputum perseverante dolore sit malum.
                    Taddeo, *Pronost.*, fol. 227r.
Utrum oxiremia in lienteria de phlegmate possit esse signum bonum vel
malum.   Taddeo, *Aphor.*, fol. 162.
Utrum oxiremia sit bonum signum in aliqua lienteria.
                    Taddeo, *Aphor.*, fol. 163.
Utrum paroxismi per incrementa significentur.
                    Taddeo, *Aphor.*, fol. 13.
Utrum per colorem unguium possimus pronosticari super mortem.
                    Taddeo, *Pronost.*, fol. 214v.
Utrum per exitum egestionum cholericarum possit cognosci mors diei
sequentis.   Taddeo, *Aphor.*, fol. 98.
Utrum per vomitum evacuetur solum illud quod est in stomacho.
                    Taddeo, *Aphor.*, fol. 91.
Utrum permanentia corporis febrientis in suo tumore sit signum malum.
                    Taddeo, *Aphor.*, fol. 54.
Utrum permanentia et macies irrationales in corpore febriente sint timende.
                    Taddeo, *Aphor.*, fol. 53.
Utrum possit apparere egro aves volare.
                    Taddeo, *Pronost.*, fol. 205r.
Utrum pulsus sit certius signum in significando super febres quam anhelitus.
                    Taddeo, *Pronost.*, fol. 205v.
Utrum putredo cholerica per sputum emissa mortem significet.
                    Taddeo, *Pronost.*, fol. 228r.
Utrum putredo cholerica significet super egritudinem pulmonis.
                    Taddeo, *Pronost.*, fol. 228r.
Utrum rigor debeat esse continuus in causone [*sic*].
                    Taddeo, *Aphor.*, fol. 112.
Utrum rigor multiplex cum virtute forti sit signum mortis.
                    Taddeo, *Aphor.*, fol. 107.
Utrum rigor necessario fiat cum icteritia.
                    Taddeo, *Aphor.*, fol. 114.
Utrum rigor sit impossibile continendi membra.
                    Taddeo, *Isagoge*, fol. 389r.

Utrum rigor sit res naturalis, vel non naturalis, vel contra naturam.

Taddeo, *Isagoge*, fol. 389r.

Utrum sedimen album leve [in urina] cuius causa est ventositas multa cum humore sit peius nebula. Taddeo, *Pronost.*, fol. 222v.

Utrum sedimen rubeus [in urina] egritudinis longitudinem significet.

Taddeo, *Pronost.*, fol. 219v.

Utrum signa a facie sumpta sint multe efficatie in significando.

Taddeo, *Pronost.*, fol. 199r.

Utrum signa indigestionis declarent consistentias futuras longas vel breves.

Taddeo, *Aphor.*, fol. 14.

Utrum signa mala irrationabilia sint magis timenda rationabilibus.

Taddeo, *Aphor.*, fol. 52.

Utrum signum sumptum a dolore in apopletico a medico inveniri possit.

Taddeo, *Aphor.*, fol. 192.

Utrum signum sumptum a testibus possit mortem vel salutem significare.

Taddeo, *Pronost.*, fol. 215v.

Utrum singultus posset fieri de inanitione.

Taddeo, *Aphor.*, fol. 185.

Utrum singultus sit motus fortior vomitu.

Taddeo, *Aphor.*, fol. 185.

Utrum sit aliquid genus accidentium ad quod reducatur tumor.

Turisanus, *Plusquam*, 2.79.

Utrum sit bonum diariam superveniri dolori oculorum.

Taddeo, *Aphor.*, 172.

Utrum sitis possit significare super multam vel paucam purgationem.

Taddeo, *Aphor.*, fol. 93.

Utrum sitis significet evacuationis complementum.

Taddeo, *Aphor.*, fol. 94.

Utrum spasmus de inanitione ex helleboro sit mortalis.

Taddeo, *Aphor.*, fol. 128.

Utrum spasmus de repletione accidat subito.

Taddeo, *Aphor.*, fol. 130.

Utrum spasmus de repletione curet febrem.

Taddeo, *Aphor.*, fol. 112.

Utrum spasmus de repletione superveniat solum corpori egro, spasmus vero de inanitione solum corpore sano, vel econtra.

Taddeo, *Aphor.*, fol. 50.

Utrum spasmus de repletione veniat citius quam spasmus de inanitione.

Taddeo, *Aphor.*, fol. 50.

Utrum spasmus possit esse motus naturalis.

Taddeo, *Aphor.*, fol. 185.

Utrum spasmus possit sequi ad fluxum sanguinis.

           Taddeo, *Aphor.*, fol. 128.

Utrum spasmus propter motum vomendi contingens sit de repletione.

           Taddeo, *Aphor.*, fol. 128.

Utrum spasmus sequens febrem sit de inanitione.

           Taddeo, *Aphor.*, fol. 112.

Utrum spasmus sequens febrem sit de inanitione et mortalis.

           Taddeo, *Aphor.*, fol. 50.

Utrum spasmus sit accidens.   Taddeo, *Aphor.*, fol. 128.

Utrum spuma sine motu fieri possit.   Taddeo, *Aphor.*, fol. 65.

Utrum sputum nigrum in pleuresi significet mortem.

           Taddeo, *Aphor.*, fol. 182.

Utrum sputum rubeum omnino sit malum signum.

           Taddeo, *Pronost.*, fol. 224v.

Utrum sputum sanguinis puri sit malum signum.

           Taddeo, *Pronost.*, fol. 225r.

Utrum sputum spumosum sit malum.

           Taddeo, *Pronost.*, fol. 225r.

Utrum sudor calidus existens solum in capite et cervice mortem demonstret.

           Taddeo, *Pronost.*, fol. 206v.

Utrum sudor existens in capite et cervice solum sit pessimus.

           Taddeo, *Pronost.*, fol. 206v.

Utrum sudor frigidus in egritudine lenta longitudinem eius vel potius mortem significet.   Taddeo, *Pronost.*, fol. 206v.

Utrum sudor frigidus in lenta egritudine significet mortem.

           Taddeo, *Aphor.*, fol. 105.

Utrum urina nigra sit pessima in pueris.

           Taddeo, *Pronost.*, fol. 222r.

Utrum sudor frigidus significet egritudinem frigidam.

           Taddeo, *Aphor.*, fol. 106.

Utrum sudor significet super febrem.   Taddeo, *Pronost.*, fol. 206v.

Utrum sudor sit evacuatio cretica febris continue.

           Taddeo, *Aphor.*, fol. 74.

Utrum tabescentia in febricitantibus in tempore et regione calidis sit rationalis, in frigidis vero econtra.   Taddeo, *Aphor.*, fol. 54.

Utrum tabescentia rationalis sit malum signum in febriente.

           Taddeo, *Aphor.*, fol. 54.

Utrum tussis sicca significet super privationem sitis.

           Taddeo, *Aphor.*, fol. 110.

Utrum tussis sit signum inseparabile ab hydropisi.

           Taddeo, *Aphor.*, fol. 183.

Utrum tussis tollat sitim.   Taddeo, *Aphor.*, fol. 110.

Utrum urina aquosa necessario mortem significet.
        Taddeo, *Pronost.*, fol. 221v.

Utrum urina fetida necessario mortem significet.
        Taddeo, *Pronost.*, fol. 221v.

Utrum urina grossa turbata significet necessario dolorem capitis.
        Taddeo, *Aphor.*, fol. 118.

Utrum urina grossior naturali significet crisim per apostemata.
        Taddeo, *Pronost.*, fol. 232v.

Utrum urina laudabiliter presit apparire in egritudinis acutis.
        Mondino, *Pronost.*, BAV, MS Vat.
        lat. 4466, fol. 17r.

Utrum urina nigra necessario mortem significet.
        Taddeo, *Pronost.*, fol. 221v.

Utrum urina nigra sit pessima in pueris.
        Taddeo, *Pronost.*, fol. 222r.

Utrum urina possit venire de venis sine febre cum furfureis resolutionibus.
        Taddeo, *Aphor.*, fol. 125.

Utrum venter tenuis in omni egritudine sit malus.
        Taddeo, *Aphor.*, fol. 61.

Utrum vomitus grossus sit malus.   Taddeo, *Pronost.*, fol. 223r.

Utrum vomitus niger significet malum mortale.
        Taddeo, *Pronost.*, fol. 223v.

Utrum vomitus significans multas egritudines significet mortem proximam.
        Taddeo, *Pronost.*, fol. 223v.

Utrum vomitus simplex sit malus.   Taddeo, *Pronost.*, fol. 223r.

10ª questio est quia videtur quod Avicenna fuerit superfluus in ponenda
signa flegmonis.   Dino, *Chirurgia* (Estense).

TREATMENT OF DISEASE

Digressio de dieta egrotantium.   Turisanus, *Plusquam*, 3.40.

Digressio de medicinis vulnerum.   Turisanus, *Plusquam*, 3.55.

Queritur de medicinis compositivis et labeficantis et exercitivis, utrum hii
faciant a proprietate aut a qualitate.
        Guglielmo, *Canon* 1.4, fol. 124v.

Questio generalis proposita fuit: utrum evacuatio sinchronatica sit utilis
et recipienda aut sit inutilis et constringenda.
        Dino, independent question, disputed
        at Siena, CLM 13020, fols. 223v-225v.

Utrum abstergentia removeant opilationem aperiendo.

         Dino, *Dilucidatorium*, 24.4.

Utrum abstersio conveniat in curatione ulcerum sicut exiccatio.

         Dino, *Dilucidatorium*, 28.4.

Utrum abstinentia sit bona corporibus cachochimis.

         Taddeo, *Aphor.*, fol. 58.

Utrum abundante humore flegmatico in sanguine prius debeat fieri flobothomia an solutio.   Dino, *Dilucidatorium*, 20.17.

Utrum abundante melancolia in sanguine prius debeat fieri flobothomia an solutio.   Dino, *Dilucidatorium*, 20.16.

Utrum abundante melancolia in sanguine sit potius flobothomandum quam abundante humore crudo.   Dino, *Dilucidatorium*, 20.15.

Utrum abundantibus humoribus malis cum sanguine pauco bono sit flobothomandus.   Dino, *Dilucidatorium*, 20.18.

Utrum accidenti debeatur curatio vel sanatio: et an cuilibet accidenti.

         Dino, *Dilucidatorium*, 31.2.

Utrum ad restorationem flobothomati melius sit exhibere assum vel elixum.

         Dino, *Dilucidatorium*, 20.43.

Utrum adeps egrediens ex vinere flobothomie debeat intromitti vel incidi.

         Dino, *Dilucidatorium*, 20.59.

Utrum albezaar et tyriace [*sic*] sint conservantia robur et sanitatem spiritus et caloris innati.   Dino, *Canon* 2, ch. 4, q.2.

Utrum aliqua medicina generet carnem.

         Taddeo, *Isagoge*, fol. 398r.

Utrum aliqua medicina sit temperata.

         Taddeo, *Isagoge*, fol. 379r.

Utrum aliquis potus reperiatur que sit potus, cibus, et medicina.

         Taddeo, *Isagoge*, fol. 380r.

Utrum alleviatio irrationalis possit fieri in egritudine.

         Taddeo, *Isagoge*, fol. 52.

Utrum apertio opilationis sit causa caliditatis.

         Dino, *Dilucidatorium*, 2.7.

Utrum apostemata ulcerosa sint infrigidanda et mollificanda.

         Dino, *Dilucidatorium*, 25.20.

Utrum apparentibus significationibus flobothomie melius sit preparare.

         Dino, *Dilucidatorium*, 20.29.

Utrum apparentibus signis repletionis semper fieri debeat flobothomia.

         Dino, *Dilucidatorium*, 20.14.

Utrum appositio ventosarum super partem anteriorem capitis noceat sensui et intellectui.   Dino, *Dilucidatorium*, 21.6.

Utrum aqua frigida competat febricitantibus putride febre.
Taddeo, independent question,
CLM 13020, fols. 81v-82r.

Utrum aqua frigida curet dolores articulorum.
Taddeo, *Aphor.*, fol. 135.

Utrum aqua frigida exhibita in febre vadat actu frigida ad membra.
Taddeo, *Reg. acut.*, fol. 268v.

Utrum aqua frigida iuvet apostemata.
Taddeo, *Aphor.*, fol. 134.

Utrum aqua frigida iuvet tumores et podagram.
Taddeo, *Aphor.*, fol. 135.

Utrum aqua frigida sola sit in pleuresi exhibenda.
Taddeo, *Reg. acut.*, fol. 268r.

Utrum ars melius et potentius evacuet quam natura.
Taddeo, *Aphor.*, fol. 88.

Utrum assa sint humidiora quam elixa vel econtra.
Dino, *Dilucidatorium*, 20.42.

Utrum augmentum humorum possit fieri secundum alium locum quam secundum venas.
Dino, *Dilucidatorium*, 20.1.

Utrum author ponat sufficienter omnes operationes medicine.
Taddeo, *Isagoge*, fol. 398r.

Utrum Avicenna fuerit diminutus cum non posuerit fen de conservatione.
Dino, *Dilucidatorium*, 1.1.

Utrum Avicenna ostendat rectum modum usus flobothomie in arteriis sicut facit in venis.
Dino, *Dilucidatorium*, 20.55.

Utrum Avicenna sit diminutus in ponendo canones curativos morbi in natura compositionali.
Dino, *Dilucidatorium*, 24.1.

Utrum Avicenna sufficienter ponat modos constrictionis evacuationis.
Dino, *Dilucidatorium*, 23.1.

Utrum balneum competat ante exhibitionem medicine.
Guglielmo, *Canon* 1.4, fols. 123r-v.

Utrum balneum competat immediate post exhibitionem medicinam.
Guglielmo, *Canon* 1.4, fol. 123v.

Utrum balneum competat post operationem medicine.
Dino, *Dilucidatorium*, 5.16.

Utrum balneum conveniat in dolore oculorum a quacumque materia facto.
Taddeo, *Aphor.*, fol. 179.

Utrum balneum conveniat in dolore oculorum cum multitudine humorum.
Taddeo, *Aphor.*, fol. 179.

Utrum calefactio educat menstrua.   Taddeo, *Aphor.*, fol. 136.

Utrum calefactorium appositum loco dolenti in pleuresi alleviet dolorem.
                                Taddeo, *Reg. acut.*, fol. 263v.

Utrum caro assa sit facilioris digestionis quam elixa an econtra.
                                Dino, *Dilucidatorium*, 20.41.

Utrum cauterium conveniat in omni mala complexione membri.
                                Dino, *Dilucidatorium*, 29.3.

Utrum cauterium conveniat quolibet tempore.
                                Dino, *Dilucidatorium*, 29.2.

Utrum cauterium convenienter fiat cum ferro vel cum auro.
                                Dino, *Dilucidatorium*, 29.4.

Utrum cauterizatio cum igne sit securior et melior quam cum medicina.
                                Dino, *Dilucidatorium*, 29.1.

Utrum cibaria insipida et sine sale sint preparantia ad vomitum.
                                Dino, *Dilucidatorium*, 11.3.

Utrum cibaria multe quantitatis et modici alimenti conveniant in corporibus
repletis humoribus crudis.   Dino, *Dilucidatorium*, 1.9.

Utrum cibus processu egritudinis sit augendus.
                                Taddeo, *Reg. acut.*, fol. 258v.

Utrum clistere sedet dolores renum et vesicce [*sic*].
                                Dino, *Dilucidatorium*, 17.1.

Utrum cogitatio qualitatis medicina abstracte possit haberi absque cogitatione
egritudinis.   Guglielmo, *Canon* 1.4, fol. 118r.

Utrum cognitio quantitatis medicine summatur ex complexione.
                                Dino, *Dilucidatorium*, 1.16.

Utrum colera et flegmate multiplicatis in stomacho melius sit in regimine
sanitatis uti vomitu an solutione.   Dino, *Dilucidatorium*, 13.4.

Utrum [medicina] commutatur ad humores ad quos habet aspectum.
                                Guglielmo, *Canon* 1.4, fol. 122v.

Utrum complexio calida et humida concedat evacuationem.
                                Dino, *Dilucidatorium*, 3.4.

Utrum complexio calida et humida prohibet evacuationem.
                                Dino, *Dilucidatorium*, 3.3.

Utrum complexio calida et sicca prohibeat evacuationem.
                                Dino, *Dilucidatorium*, 3.2.

Utrum compressio sit actio medicine.
                                Taddeo, *Isagoge*, fol. 398r.

Utrum confortantia debeant dari calida in fluxu a farmaco.
                                Dino, *Dilucidatorium*, 7.3.

Utrum consideratio signorum sequentium purgationem medico operanti prosit.
                                Taddeo, *Aphor.*, fol. 3.

Utrum consolidatio fieri debeat per medicamina exiccantia.

Dino, *Dilucidatorium*, 28.3.

Utrum consuetudo evacuandi indicet super evacuationem.

Dino, *Dilucidatorium*, 3.7.

Utrum contritio superflua faciat medicinam permutari ad aliam virtutem.

Dino, *Canon* 2, ch. 5, q. 2.

Utrum contritio superflua medicine auferat virtutem eius.

Dino, *Canon* 2, ch. 5, q. 1.

Utrum corpora cachochima a pharmaciis dissolvantur.

Taddeo, *Aphor.*, fol. 62.

Utrum corpora purganda sint prius fluida facienda.

Taddeo, *Aphor.*, fol. 33.

Utrum corpora similibus vel contrariis conserventur.

Turisanus, *Plusquam*, 3.20.

Utrum corporibus macris sit vomitus conveniens.

Dino, *Dilucidatorium*, 4.5.

Utrum cum senex indiget infrigidatione et humectatione debeat reduci ad temperamentum.   Dino, *Dilucidatorium*, 2.10.

Utrum cura fiat per contrarium.

Turisanus, *Plusquam*, 3.35.

Utrum cura morbi officialis fiat per contrarium.

Taddeo, *Isagoge*, fol. 397r.

Utrum curatio vulnerum fiat per exiccationem.

Taddeo, *Aphor.*, fol. 168.

Utrum, dato quod farmatia non evacuet, convertatur ad humores.

Guglielmo, *Canon* 1.4, fols. 122r-v.

Utrum, dato quod omne vulnus debeat desiccari, et desiccantia debeant esse sicca in tertio gradu.   Taddeo, *Isagoge*, fol. 398r.

Utrum debeamus ea uti [?] ex quo reperitur.

Guglielmo, *Canon* 1.3, fol. 124r.

Utrum debeamus medicinas permutare.

Guglielmo, *Canon* 1.4, fols. 118r-119r.

Utrum debeant dari simul, scilicet medicina fortis et medicina debilis.

Guglielmo, *Canon* 1.4, fols. 124r-v.

Utrum debentibus farmacum sumere sal et salsa danda sint.

Dino, *Dilucidatorium*, 5.15.

Utrum dieta, potio, et cyrugia convenienter ponantur instrumenta artis curative.   Dino, *Dilucidatorium*, 1.2.

Utrum dieta tenuissima competat in egritudine acuta.

Taddeo, *Aphor.*, fol. 6.

Utrum diete humide conferant omnibus febricantibus.

Taddeo, *Aphor.*, fol. 20.

Utrum digestio acutorum humorum prohibeat superfluitatem extinctionis.

Dino, *Dilucidatorium*, 2.8.

Utrum dignior hora evacuationis sit quando in corpore non est repletio.

Dino, *Dilucidatorium*, 3.13.

Utrum diversitas ciborum conveniat in morbis acutis.

Taddeo, *Reg. acut.*, fol. 257r.

Utrum dolor prius sedari debeat antequam fiat attractio.

Dino, *Dilucidatorium*, 1.24.

Utrum dosis tyriace debeat esse maior quam communitur detur.

Dino, *Dilucidatorium*, 30.11.

Utrum dum constringimus fluxum ventris vel vomitum per evacuationem debeat evacuatio fieri cum evacuantibus dissolvendo an comprimendo.

Dino, *Dilucidatorium*, 23.3.

Utrum ea [medicina] que sit frigida potentia permutetur a corpore nostro.

Bartolomeo, *De complexionibus*, fol. 83r.

Utrum eis competat ratio medii inter venenum et corpus, aut inter venenum et medicinas.   Guglielmo, *De tyriaca*, pp. 142-143.

Utrum egritudo mortalis sit a medico curanda.

Taddeo, *Aphor.*, fol. 55.

Utrum egritudo possit a medico ignorari.

Guglielmo, *Canon* 1.4, fol. 118v.

Utrum emanatio ultima sit fienda.   Dino, *Dilucidatorium*, 3.31.

Utrum emplastrum ex ordeo facto convenit in fluxu a farmaco facto.

Dino, *Dilucidatorium*, 7.2.

Utrum epithimata sit maioris virtutis quam embroce.

Dino, *Dilucidatorium*, 19.1.

Utrum epithimata ex stipticis conveniant in fluxu a farmaco facto.

Dino, *Dilucidatorium*, 7.1.

Utrum equalis sit timor in calefaciendo et infrigidando.

Dino, *Dilucidatorium*, 2.5.

Utrum etas que nondum venit ad complementum augeri prohibeat evacuationem.   Dino, *Dilucidatorium*, 3.5.

Utrum etates possint et debeant attribui tyriace.

Dino, *Dilucidatorium*, 30.12.

Utrum evacuandus per solutionem et vomitum debeat pluries comedere in die, etc.   Dino, *Dilucidatorium*, 4.1.

Utrum evacuantia removeant opilationem.

Dino, *Dilucidatorium*, 24.3.

Utrum evacuatio artificialis debeat assimilari naturali.

Taddeo, Aphor., fol. 3.

Utrum evacuatio debeat fieri per partem patientem vel per diversam.

Guglielmo, Canon 1.4, fols. 120r-v.

Utrum evacuatio debeatur corpori ratione magnitudinis morbi.

Dino, Dilucidatorium, 4.3.

Utrum evacuatio magna et subita fieri possit.

Taddeo, Aphor., fol. 70.

Utrum evacuatio possit fieri per partem longinquam sed duas dyametros.

Dino, Dilucidatorium, 3.14.

Utrum evaporatio sit dimittenda post evacuationem totius.

Taddeo, Reg. acut., fol. 276v.

Utrum evaporationem in pleuresi ex aqua calida factam conveniat.

Taddeo, Reg. acut., fol. 274v.

Utrum ex refrenatione evacuetur et recurrat materia in apostemate [sic] que iam exivit venas et iam pervenit ad spongiositates membrorum.

Dino, Dilucidatorium, 25.5.

Utrum ex siti semper summatur significatio super evacuationem sufficientem.

Dino, Dilucidatorium, 6.3.

Utrum ex temporibus morbi summatur aliqua indicatio super administrationem medicinarum.   Dino, Dilucidatorium, 1.30.

Utrum experientia ad indicium [sic] summendum de medicina debeat fieri in corpore egro vel in corpore temperato.

Dino, Canon 2, ch. 2, q. 2.

Utrum extractio sanguinis per sanguisugas sit profundior quam extractio per ventosas.   Dino, Dilucidatorium, 22.1.

Utrum farmacia competat.   Guglielmo, Canon 2.4, fol.121v.

Utrum farmaco ante solutionem conveniat panis solus aut vinum solum.

Dino, Dilucidatorium, 5.7.

Utrum farmacum debeat semper sumi ieiunio stomaco.

Dino, Dilucidatorium, 5.6.

Utrum farmacum post evacuationem proprii humoris evacuet alium humorem.

Dino, Dilucidatorium, 5.12.

Utrum farmacum solutivum superfluens in evacuatione cum pervenit ad evacuationem sanguinis evacuaverit alios humores.

Dino, Dilucidatorium, 5.13.

Utrum febricitantes in autumno multum et sepe cibandi sint.

Taddeo, Aphor., fol. 21.

Utrum febricitantes in hyeme multum et raro cibandi sint.

Taddeo, Aphor., fol. 21.

Utrum febricitantes in vere parvum et raro cibandi sint.

Taddeo, *Aphor.*, fol. 21.

Utrum flebotomia competat in omni febre.

Taddeo, *Practica de febribus*, fols.
110r-113r.

Utrum flobothomia arteriarum fieri debeat in manu vel brachio.

Dino, *Dilucidatorium*, 20.54.

Utrum flobothomia arteriarum manus conferat doloribus antiquis epatis
et diafragmatis.   Dino, *Dilucidatorium*, 20.56.

Utrum flobothomia basilice convenieat in pleuresi.

Taddeo, *Reg. acut.*, fol. 278v.

Utrum flobothomia basilice sufficiat in pleuresi.

Taddeo, *Reg. acut.*, fol. 278v.

Utrum flobothomia conveniat in pleuresi.

Taddeo, *Reg. acut.*, fol. 278r.

Utrum flobothomia et appositio ventosarum et sanguisugarum sint
intrumentum medicine vel cyrugie.   Dino, *Dilucidatorium*, 22.2.

Utrum flobothomia evacuet humores exeuntes extra venas.

Dino, *Dilucidatorium*, 20.2.

Utrum flobothomia ex basilica evacuet a partibus inferioribus.

Dino, *Dilucidatorium*, 20.53.

Utrum flobothomia, facta ubi non est necessaria, faciat ebullire coleram, etc.

Dino, *Dilucidatorium*, 20.45.

Utrum flobothomia fiat propter multitudinem, aut propter malitiam, aut
propter utrumque.   Dino, *Dilucidatorium*, 20.3.

Utrum flobothomia in pleuresi sit fienda in eodem latem vel in opposito.

Taddeo, *Reg. acut.*, fol. 278v.

Utrum flobothomia magis debeatur paratis ad egritudines sanguineas quare
dum actu inciderunt in eas.   Dino, *Dilucidatorium*, 20.6.

Utrum flobothomia pedis maxime conferat egritudinibus.

Dino, *Dilucidatorium*, 20.62.

Utrum flobothomia plus evacuet a profundo quam a superficie.

Dino, *Dilucidatorium*, 21.2.

Utrum flobothomia semper debeat precedere farmaciam.

Guglielmo, *Canon* 1.4, fols. 21v-122r.

Utrum flobothomia sit sufficiens in oppilatione facta ex multitudine humorum.

Dino, *Dilucidatorium*, 24.2.

Utrum flobothomia stricta sit magis conservativa virtutis quam lata.

Dino, *Dilucidatorium*, 20.22.

Utrum flobothomia venarum pedis plus debilitat quam venarum manus.

Dino, *Dilucidatorium*, 20.63.

Utrum flobothomia venarum post aures conferat capiti recipienti fumos
a stomacho.   Dino, *Dilucidatorium*, 20.65.
Utrum flobothomia ventrem constringat.
                                    Dino, *Dilucidatorium*, 20.13.
Utrum frigida et humida competant in omni febre.
                                    Taddeo, *Practica de febribus*, fols.
113r-115r.
Utrum graduatio medicinarum sit in ordine corpus temperatum.
                                    Turisanus, *Plusquam*, 3.36.
Utrum grossities calidarum medicinarum faciat distinctionem in canone
sicut caliditas.   Turisanus, *Plusquam*, 3.43.
Utrum habentes debilitatem in membris inferioribus cum mala complexione
calida debeant flobothomari.   Dino, *Dilucidatorium*, 20.4.
Utrum habentes stomachum debilem sint apti ad vomitum.
                                    Dino, *Dilucidatorium*, 11.1.
Utrum humectatio sit bona preparatio ad vomitum.
                                    Taddeo, *Aphor.*, fol. 92.
Utrum hyems prohibeat purgationem per superiora.
                                    Taddeo, *Aphor.*, fol. 90.
Utrum idromel conveniat habentibus choleram amaram et viscera magna.
                                    Taddeo, *Reg. acut.*, fol. 316v.
Utrum idromel conveniat habundantibus in cholera nigra.
                                    Taddeo, *Reg. acut.*, fol. 316v.
Utrum idromel conveniant habundantibus in sanguine.
                                    Taddeo, *Reg. acut.*, fol. 316v.
Utrum idromel conveniat in febribus peracutis.
                                    Taddeo, *Reg. acut.*, fol. 316r.
Utrum idromel faciat descendere sputum a superiori ad inferius.
                                    Taddeo, *Reg. acut.*, fol. 318v.
Utrum idromel faciat sputum viscosum.
                                    Taddeo, *Reg. acut.*, fol. 317v.
Utrum idromel magis permixtum magis provocet sputum quam parum
permixtum.   Taddeo, *Reg. acut.*, fol. 321v.
Utrum idromel possit ita sustentare virtutem sicut aqua ordei.
                                    Taddeo, *Reg. acut.*, fol. 323v.
Utrum idromel sedet tussim.   Taddeo, *Reg. acut.*, fol. 317v.
Utrum idromel sit humorum grossorum subtiliativum.
                                    Taddeo, *Reg. acut.*, fol. 311r.
Utrum idromel sit magis subtiliativum quam oximel.
                                    Taddeo, *Reg. acut.*, fol. 311r.

Utrum ille cuius sanguis malus est paucus declinans ad membrum sit
flobothomandus. Dino, *Dilucidatorium*, 20.19.
Utrum ille in quo est vomitus provocandus debeat assuefieri [*sic*] ad vomitum.
Dino, *Dilucidatorium*, 11.2.
Utrum ille post primam flobothomiam sit bono cibo cibandus, deinde
iterum flobothomandus. Dino, *Dilucidatorium*, 20.20.
Utrum illud quod faciliter calefiat et inflammatur ab igne, faciliter etiam
calefiat et inflammetur in corpore nostro.
Dino, *Canon* 2, ch. 3, q. 2.
Utrum immoderate repletioni debeatur immoderata evacuatio.
Turisanus, *Plusquam*, 3.59.
Utrum in acutis morbis minuendus sit cibus in quanto vel in quali.
Dino, *Dilucidatorium*, 1.11.
Utrum in aliqua egritudine debeat cibus augeri.
Dino, *Dilucidatorium*, 1.6.
Utrum in aliqua egritudine debeat cibus diminui.
Dino, *Dilucidatorium*, 1.4.
Utrum in aliqua egritudine debeat cibus equari.
Dino, *Dilucidatorium*, 1.5.
Utrum in aliqua egritudine debeat cibus omnino prohiberi.
Dino, *Dilucidatorium*, 1.3.
Utrum in aliquo casu sit licitum evacuare usque ad sincopim.
Dino, *Dilucidatorium*, 3.22.
Utrum in alleviatione paulative veniente et sine evacuatione confidendum sit.
Taddeo, *Aphor.*, fol. 52.
Utrum in apostemate [*sic*] a causa primitiva in corpore mundo in principio
debeant ap[p]licari resolutiva. Dino, *Dilucidatorium*, 25.11.
Utrum in apostemate a causa primitiva mundificat corpore debeant
applicari repercussiva. Dino, *Dilucidatorium*, 25.12.
Utrum in apostemate duro quod statum pertransivit debeat fieri mollificatio
cum habentibus siccitatem parvam. Dino, *Dilucidatorium*, 25.16.
Utrum in apostemate exeunte calore naturali debili glutinativa et opilativa
conveniant. Dino, *Dilucidatorium*, 25.15.
Utrum in apostemate facto propter flobothomia conveniat flobothomia ex
altero latere. Dino, *Dilucidatorium*, 20.52.
Utrum in apostemate non a causa primitiva, non existente repletione in toto
nec in aliquo membro quod transmittat, conveniat evacuatio.
Dino, *Dilucidatorium*, 25.3.
Utrum in apostemate stomaci debeamus plus uti stipticis quam in
apostemate epatis. Dino, *Dilucidatorium*, 25.24.

Utrum in apostematibus membrorum animatorum ut cerebri et miringarum debeant misceri stiptica cum resolutivis.

Dino, *Dilucidatorium*, 25.25.

Utrum in apostematibus post principium sit conveniens commixtio repercussivorum et resolutivorum super membrum.

Dino, *Dilucidatorium*, 20.8.

Utrum in attractione ad partem diversam consideranda sit societas.

Dino, *Dilucidatorium*, 1.22.

Utrum in contusione in principio debeant applicari resolutiva.

Dino, *Dilucidatorium*, 28.13.

Utrum in cura apostematis duri prius apponenda sint mollificativa deinde resolutiva.   Dino, *Dilucidatorium*, 25.19.

Utrum in cura apostematis per fluxum materie a toto vel a membro aliquo sufficiat evacuatio.   Dino, *Dilucidatorium*, 25.2.

Utrum in cura discrasie febrilis sit a causa inchoandum.

Taddeo, *Practica de febribus*, fols.

107r-v.

Utrum in curatione apostematis debeat considerari causa primitiva.

Dino, *Dilucidatorium*, 20.10.

Utrum in curatione ulceris debeat considerari complexio totius.

Dino, *Dilucidatorium*, 28.7.

Utrum in curatione ulcerum cavendum sit ne aliquid cadat inter labia eius.

Dino, *Dilucidatorium*, 28.5.

Utrum in die paroxismi sit provocandus somnus.

Dino, *Dilucidatorium*, 20.11.

Utrum in die paroxismi vel evacuationis sit facienda aliqua evacuatio.

Dino, *Dilucidatorium*, 20.10.

Utrum in egritudine cronica competat dieta grossa.

Taddeo, *Aphor.*, fol. 5.

Utrum in egritudine cronica competat dieta tenuis vel mediocris.

Taddeo, *Aphor.*, fol. 6.

Utrum in egritudinibus epatis flobothomanda sit vena communis et cephalica.

Dino, *Dilucidatorium*, 3.9.

Utrum in egritudinibus splenis conveniat flobothomia de basilica sinistra.

Dino, *Dilucidatorium*, 1.23.

Utrum in etate senectutis conveniat flobothomia.

Dino, *Dilucidatorium*, 20.36.

Utrum in evacuatione debeat fieri transitus super principale membrum.

Dino, *Dilucidatorium*, 1.25.

Utrum in evacuatione que debetur sanguini in egritudinibus factis ab eo debeat expectari digestio.   Dino, *Dilucidatorium*, 20.31.

Utrum in fastidito [*sic*] debeamus semper cavere a flobothomia.
                    Dino, *Dilucidatorium*, 20.39.
Utrum in febre aliquando fieri debeat flobothomia etiam si non sit necessaria.
                    Dino, *Dilucidatorium*, 20.30.
Utrum in febre que est sine putredine debeat minorari flobothomia.
                    Dino, *Dilucidatorium*, 20.26.
Utrum in febre que motu suo preparat conveniat flobothomia.
                    Dino, *Dilucidatorium*, 20.27.
Utrum in febre sanguinea post maturationem debeat fieri flobothomia
superflua.   Dino, *Dilucidatorium*, 20.32.
Utrum in febribus conclusis sit facienda flobothomia in die motus
egritudinis, etc.   Dino, *Dilucidatorium*, 20.12.
Utrum in febribus in quibus convenit flobothomia melior sit flobothomia
venarum quam arteriarum, vel econtra.
                    Dino, *Dilucidatorium*, 20.58.
Utrum in febribus vehementis inflammationis debeat caveri a flobothomia.
                    Dino, *Dilucidatorium*, 20.24.
Utrum in febricantibus conveniat simul exhiberi medicamenta digestivas
et expulsivas.   Dino, no. 2 in a set of six misc.
                    questions, CLM 13020, fols. 217v-218v.
Utrum in flobothomia diversiva debeat esse flobothomatus strictus.
                    Dino, *Dilucidatorium*, 20.44.
Utrum in flobothomia facta cibo exeunte in stomacho semper attrahatur
humor crudus sive materia cruda ad venas.
                    Dino, *Dilucidatorium*, 20.38.
Utrum in flobothomia fienda in paratis ad egritudines debeat expectari digestio.
                    Dino, *Dilucidatorium*, 20.7.
Utrum in forti dolore conveniat flobothomia.
                    Dino, *Dilucidatorium*, 20.34.
Utrum in habente stomachum fortis sensus ante flobothomiam debeant
dari acetosa.   Dino, *Dilucidatorium*, 20.40.
Utrum in habentibus apostemata [*sic*] in membris inferioribus competat
farmacum solutivum.   Dino, *Dilucidatorium*, 4.4.
Utrum in habentibus apostemata intrinseca conveniat balneum.
                    Dino, *Dilucidatorium*, 25.21.
Utrum in habentibus apostemata intrinseca conveniat vinum.
                    Dino, *Dilucidatorium*, 25.22.
Utrum in habentibus humores grossos mixtos sanguini ante flobothomiam
debeant administrari balneum, motus, et aperitiva, et subtiliativa, etc.
                    Dino, *Dilucidatorium*, 20.21.

Utrum in habentibus nauseam ante farmacum debeat provocari vomitus.
Dino, *Dilucidatorium*, 5.14.

Utrum in hora necessaria flobothomie attendat res prohibens eam.
Dino, *Dilucidatorium*, 20.67.

Utrum in hyeme sit fienda flobothomia ampla.
Dino, *Dilucidatorium*, 20.23.

Utrum in lepra purgatio cum sola pharmacia sit facienda.
Taddeo, *Aphor.*, fol. 190.

Utrum in lienteria conveniat vomitus.
Dino, *Dilucidatorium*, 4.8.

Utrum in istis medicaminibus [apostematum] debeat attendi virtus siccitatis et humiditatis, sicut attenditur virtus frigiditatis et caliditatis.
Dino, *Dilucidatorium*, 20.7.

Utrum in materia furiosa cum obstructione viarum debeamus vias aperire ante evacuationem humoris. Dino, *Dilucidatorium*, 4.6.

Utrum in materia grossa et spissa conveniat evacuatio ante maturationem.
Dino, *Dilucidatorium*, 3.12.

Utrum in materia magis grossa et magis compacta debeantur fortius subtilantia quam in minus grossa et compacta. Dino, *Dilucidatorium*, 24.6.

Utrum in medicinis generantibus carnem debeat esse fortior exiccatio quam in medicinis incarnantibus. Dino, *Dilucidatorium*, 28.9.

Utrum in omni apostemate [*sic*] calido medicamina que conveniunt in principio debeant esse equaliter frigida et equaliter stiptica.
Dino, *Dilucidatorium*, 25.6.

Utrum in omni tempore febris fieri possit flobothomia.
Dino, *Dilucidatorium*, 20.28.

Utrum in omnibus febribus non acutis in principio debeat caveri a flobothomia.
Dino, *Dilucidatorium*, 20.25.

Utrum in oppilatione epatis conveniat diuretica.
Dino, no. 4 in a set of six misc. questions, CLM 13020, fol. 219r.

Utrum in parato ad vomitum cum farmaco vomitivo debeat misceri solutivum, sicut in paratis ad colericum miscebatur.
Dino, *Dilucidatorium*, 5.3.

Utrum in passionibus liceat administrare contraria in maiori gradu quam sit distemperantia. Dino, *Dilucidatorium*, 1.32.

Utrum in passionibus membrorum principalium debeamus uti medicinis fortibus. Guglielmo, *Canon* 1.4, fol. 118r.

Utrum in pleuresi flegmatica conveniat flobothomia.
Dino, no. 3 in a set of six misc. questions, CLM 13020, fols. 218v-219r.

Utrum in preparatis colerice passioni debeant prohiberi ea que preparant vias et canales et humores purgandos contenutos in eis.

Dino, *Dilucidatorium*, 5.1.

Utrum in principio accessionis sit cibandum necne.

Taddeo, *Aphor.*, fol. 10.

Utrum in principio apostematis membrorum exteriorum competant repercussiva.   Dino, *Dilucidatorium*, 25.4.

Utrum in principio apostematis pectoris vel pulmonis conveniant repercussiva.   Dino, *Dilucidatorium*, 25.23.

Utrum in principio egritudinis per acute sit danda dieta tenuissima.

Taddeo, *Aphor.*, fol. 8.

Utrum in principio egritudinis sit evacuandum.

Taddeo, *Aphor.*, fol. 55.

Utrum in principio egritudinum ut podagre, epilepsie, conveniat flobothomia.

Dino, *Dilucidatorium*, 20.8.

Utrum in principio morbi sit uberius cibandum quam post.

Taddeo, *Aphor.*, fol. 9.

Utrum in purgationibus semper debeat deduci ad sitim.

Dino, *Dilucidatorium*, 6.4.

Utrum in qualibet discrasia digestio et evacuatio sit necessaria.

Turisanus, *Plusquam*, 3.38.

Utrum in regionibus vehementis frigiditatis debeat caveri a flobothomia.

Dino, *Dilucidatorium*, 20.33.

Utrum in sanguine grosso et nigro conveniat flobothomia et non in albo subtili.   Dino, *Dilucidatorium*, 20.37.

Utrum in sedatione doloris cum stupefactivis debeamus transcendere papaver.

Dino, *Dilucidatorium*, 1.35.

Utrum in statu apostematis resolutiva solum sint ponenda.

Dino, *Dilucidatorium*, 1.31.

Utrum in statu cuislibet morbi salvi dieta tenuissima sit exhibenda.

Taddeo, *Aphor.*, fol. 8.

Utrum in statu egritudinis sit evacuandum.

Taddeo, *Aphor.*, fol. 55.

Utrum in statu [apostematis] sit conveniens equatio ipsorum [repercussivorum et resolutivorum].   Dino, *Dilucidatorium*, 20.9.

Utrum in sudore multo ex repletione debeat fieri evacuatio.

Dino, *Dilucidatorium*, 20.68.

Utrum in superflua evacuatione quecumque sit universaliter debeant administrari stupefactiva.   Dino, *Dilucidatorium*, 23.4.

Utrum in talibus [apostematibus duris] debeat caliditas parva.

Dino, *Dilucidatorium*, 25.17.

Utrum in talibus [apostematibus duris] mollificatio debeat fieri per calida.
Dino, *Dilucidatorium*, 25.18.

Utrum in ulceribus intrinsecis medicine mundificante debeant misceri cum medicinis exiccantis et stipticis. Dino, *Dilucidatorium*, 28.11.

Utrum in ulceribus locorum urine debeant misceri diuretica cum eis.
Dino, *Dilucidatorium*, 28.12.

Utrum in vehementi causalitate membri debeamus uti nutrimentum grosso.
Dino, *Dilucidatorium*, 1.36.

Utrum in yctericia competat flobotomia.
Dino, no. 5 in a set of six misc.
questions, CLM 13020, fols. 219r-v.

Utrum incisio et subtiliatio sint diverse operationes.
Dino, *Dilucidatorium*, 24.5.

Utrum incisio venarum post aures faciat sterilitatem.
Dino, *Dilucidatorium*, 20.66.

Utrum indicatio sumpta a quantitate egritudinis sit necessaria in elligendo quantitatem medicine. Dino, *Dilucidatorium*, 1.27.

Utrum infra etatem 12 annorum conveniat flobothomia.
Dino, *Dilucidatorium*, 20.35.

Utrum instrumentum medicine sit triplex, dieta, potio, et chirurgia.
Guglielmo, *Canon* 1.4, fol. 117v.

Utrum intentio exhibendi clystera summatur ab etate.
Taddeo, *Reg. acut.*, fol. 272r.

Utrum intentio medicationis ab egritudine, cibationis vero a virtute summatur.
Taddeo, *Reg. acut.*, fol. 269r.

Utrum inter calefactorium et latus pleuretici aliquod medium liquidum poni debeat. Taddeo, *Reg. acut.*, fol. 275v.

Utrum inter flobothomiam et secundationem debeant cadere duo aut tres dies.
Dino, *Dilucidatorium*, 20.51.

Utrum investigatio prima quam facit Avicenna de rationem virtutis medicine sit sufficiens. Dino, *Canon* 2, ch. 3, q. 1.

Utrum lac competat siticulosis. Taddeo, *Aphor.*, fol. 156.

Utrum lac conferat febricantibus acute.
Taddeo, *Aphor.*, fol. 156.

Utrum lac conferat habentibus hypocundria suspensa et rugienta.
Taddeo, *Aphor.*, fol. 156.

Utrum lac sit malum dolentibus caput.
Taddeo, *Aphor.*, fol. 156.

Utrum lapso ad dissimile debeantur fortiores medicine quam lapso ad simile.
Dino, *Dilucidatorium*, 1.17.

Utrum liceat cum farmaco evacuare usque ad sincopim, sicut cum flobothomia.

Dino, *Dilucidatorium*, 3.23.

Utrum lubricitas faciat ptisanam digestibiliorem.

Taddeo, *Reg. acut.*, fol. 262r.

Utrum maior debeat esse intentio medici ad virtutem vel ad morbum.

Dino, *Dilucidatorium*, 1.8.

Utrum maius sit periculum in dieta grossiori quam in subtiliori.

Dino, *Dilucidatorium*, 1.7.

Utrum mala complexio calida indicet flobotomia fieri debeat.

Dino, *Dilucidatorium*, 20.5.

Utrum materia debeat evacuari per regionem unde reperit.

Dino, *Dilucidatorium*, 3.8.

Utrum materia in gibbo epatis debeat evacuari per diuretica et in concavo per secessum.

Dino, *Dilucidatorium*, 1.20.

Utrum materie contenute in venis sint facilioris evacuationis quam contenuta in membris.

Dino, *Dilucidatorium*, 3.16.

Utrum medicamen carnis generativum debeat esse ita exiccativum ut prohibeat materiam fluere ad ulcerem. Dino, *Dilucidatorium*, 28.10.

Utrum medicatio que sit cum medicinis habeat tres regulas tamen, secundum qualitatis, quantitatis, et temporis. Dino, *Dilucidatorium*, 13.1.

Utrum medicina attrahat humorem per convenientiam in substantia.

Dino, *Dilucidatorium*, 4.15.

Utrum medicina attrahat prius humorem grossum deinde subtillem.

Guglielmo, *Canon* 1.4, fol. 122v.

Utrum medicina calidior corpore nostro possit actuari ab illo.

Turisanus, *Plusquam*, 3.36.

Utrum medicina compressiva ex proprietate evacuet.

Dino, *Dilucidatorium*, 9.3.

Utrum medicina compressiva possit misceri cum lenitiva, et econtra.

Dino, *Canon* 2, ch. 5, q. 3.

Utrum medicina frigida in potentia actione corporis . . . permutetur.

Bartolomeo, *De complexionibus*, fols. 111v-112r.

Utrum medicina generativa carnis debeat esse in eodem gradum siccitatis an diversificari in gradibus. Turisanus, *Plusquam*, 3.57.

Utrum medicina generativa carnis debeat esse sicca in primo gradu.

Dino, *Dilucidatorium*, 28.6.

Utrum medicina laxativa attrahat cibi similia.

Taddeo, *Aphor.*, fol. 62.

Utrum medicina maturativa debeat esse calida.

Dino, *Dilucidatorium*, 25.13.

Utrum medicina maturativa debeat esse glutinantia et opilantia.

Dino, *Dilucidatorium*, 25.14.

Utrum medicina nutriat. Taddeo, *Isagoge*, fol. 279r.

Utrum medicina possit competere cause febre et accidentia.

Taddeo, *Practica de febribus*, fols. 107v-108r.

Utrum medicina possit reduci ad actum a calori nostri corporis.

Bartolomeo, *De complexionibus*, BAV, MS Vat. lat. 4454, fol. 112r; and in Puccinotti, *Storia della medicina*, vol. 2, pt. 1, pp. cxiii-cxxix.

Utrum medicina solutiva aut vomitiva possit convertit in humorem, et an in humorem ad quam habet aspectum.

Dino, *Dilucidatorium*, 4.13.

Utrum medicina solutiva convertatur potius ad humorem ad quem habet aspectum. Dino, *Dilucidatorium*, 4.14.

Utrum medicina solutiva evacuet per virtutem.

Dino, *Dilucidatorium*, 4.12.

Utrum medicina temperata possit inveniri.

Taddeo, *Isagoge*, fol. 347r.

Utrum medicina tyriacalis sit ponenda media inter corpus et venenum.

Guglielmo, *De tyriaca*, pp. 138-139.

Utrum medicina tyriacalis sit ponenda media inter venenum et medicinas.

Guglielmo, *De tyriaca*, pp. 139-142.

Utrum medicina vadat ad humorem substantialiter vel virtualiter.

Guglielmo, *Canon* 1.4, fols. 122v-123r.

Utrum medicina ventris solutiva moretur in stomaco vel in intestinis.

Dino, *Dilucidatorium*, 4.16.

Utrum medicinarum calidarum alique habeant principium calefactionis ex se, sicut hoc est in medicinis frigidis.

Dino, *Canon* 2, ch. 1, q. 3.

Utrum medicine compressive debeant misceri cum lenitivis.

Dino, *Dilucidatorium*, 9.4.

Utrum medicine cordiales sint aromatice, et econtra.

Dino, *Dilucidatorium*, 9.1.

Utrum medicine que faciunt labefacere sint commode.

Guglielmo, *Canon* 1.4, fol. 124v.

Utrum medicine sedantes dolorem vere debeant esse glutinative.

Dino, *Dilucidatorium*, 30.3.

Utrum medicine solutive debeant misceri cum provocativis urine.

Dino, *Canon* 2, ch. 4, q. 3.

Utrum medicine viscose acute sint magis opilantes orificia canalium quam
viscose tamen.   Dino, *Dilucidatorium*, 22.6.

Utrum medicinis solutivis in preparatis ad colericam passionem debeant
misceri medicine vomitiva.   Dino, *Dilucidatorium*, 5.2.

Utrum medicus cum ignorat esse egritudinem debeat aliquid agere.
                                    Dino, *Dilucidatorium*, 1.34.

Utrum medicus curaturus aliquam egritudinem debeat prius eam cognoscere.
                                   Taddeo, *Reg. acut.*, fol. 248v.

*Utrum medicus debeat adiuvare naturam creticantem.
                                    Taddeo, *Aphor.*, fol. 23.

Utrum medicus debeat interrogare infirmum de omnibus accidentibus et de
eis facere librum.   Taddeo, *Reg. acut.*, fol. 247v.

*Utrum medicus debeat naturam creticantem adiuvare.
                                    Taddeo, *Aphor.*, fol. 23.

Utrum medicus debeat temeri a superfluitate evacuationis.
                                   Dino, *Dilucidatorium*, 3.19.

Utrum medicus evacuans naturam imitari possit.
                                   Taddeo, *Aphor.*, fol. 3.

Utrum medicus evacuans naturam semper imitari debeat.
                                   Taddeo, *Aphor.*, fol. 3.

Utrum medicus evacuaturus materiam aliquam digestionem eius expectare
debeat.   Taddeo, *Aphor.*, fol. 24.

Utrum medicus possit imitari naturam evacuantem synthomatice.
                                   Taddeo, *Aphor.*, fol. 88.

Utrum medicus possit sequi naturam in bona evacuatione.
                                   Taddeo, *Aphor.*, fol. 88.

Utrum medicus possit supplere defectui nature que imperfecte creticaverit.
                                   Taddeo, *Aphor.*, fol. 24.

Utrum melancolici et epilentici flobothomari debeant cum flobothomo angusto.
                               Dino, *Dilucidatorium*, 20.49.

Utrum melius sit flobothomare et ventosare in prima quadra lune quam
in secunda, et in tertia quam in quarta.
                                   Dino, *Dilucidatorium*, 21.5.

Utrum melius sit flobothomare in die quam in nocte, vel contra.
                                   Dino, *Dilucidatorium*, 20.48.

Utrum melius sit provocare vomitum cum vino quam cum aqua.
                                   Dino, *Dilucidatorium*, 11.5.

Utrum membro raro debeatur medicina debilis, et spisso fortis.
                                   Dino, *Dilucidatorium*, 1.19.

* Repetition in original register.

Utrum methodus curativa morborum compositorum sit necessaria.

Dino, *Dilucidatorium*, 31.1.

Utrum minutio sit propria evacuatio humoribus equaliter augmentatis, et evacuatio alia a minutione sit propria uni humori augmentatio.

Dino, *Dilucidatorium*, 3.17.

Utrum miscere medicinas diversas solutivas sit conveniens.

Dino, *Dilucidatorium*, 4.9.

Utrum modus dietationis summi debeat a statu potius quam ab aliis temporibus morbi.   Dino, *Dilucidatorium*, 1.12.

Utrum morbus de inanitione curetur per medicinam.

Taddeo, *Aphor.*, fol. 46.

Utrum morbus de inanitione sit curabilior morbo de repletione.

Taddeo, *Aphor.*, fol. 45.

Utrum morituri sint dietandi.   Taddeo, *Aphor.*, fol. 8.

Utrum morituri sint dietandi.   Taddeo, *Reg. acut.*, fol. 306v.

Utrum motus augeat operationem medicine assumpte.

Taddeo, *Aphor.*, fol. 92.

Utrum multi humores per flobothomiam, unicus vero per pharmaciam, purgetur.   Taddeo, *Aphor.*, fol. 33.

Utrum multitudo exeuntium sit a medico consideranda.

Taddeo, *Aphor.*, fol. 25.

Utrum mutatio coloris sanguinis sit signum sufficiens complete flobothomie.

Taddeo, *Reg. acut.*, fol. 279r.

Utrum mutatio coloris sanguinis sit terminus generalis cuiuslibet flobothomie.

Taddeo, *Reg. acut.*, fol. 278v.

Utrum mutatio coloris sanguinis sit veridicum signum complementi cuiuslibet flobothomie.   Taddeo, *Reg. acut.*, fol. 278v.

Utrum nasturtium conveniat in fluxu, etc.

Dino, *Dilucidatorium*, 7.4.

Utrum natura possit iuvare in digestione materie a medicinis.

Taddeo, *Practica de febribus*, fols. 108r-110r.

Utrum nutrimentum debeat dari infrigidatum in fluxu a farmaco.

Dino, *Dilucidatorium*, 7.5.

Utrum oleum prohibeat consolidationem.

Dino, *Dilucidatorium*, 20.47.

Utrum omne vulnus debeat desiccari vel non.

Taddeo, *Isagoge*, fol. 398r.

Utrum omnes qui non indigent secundatione flobothomie debeant flobothomari cum flobothomo angusto.   Dino, *Dilucidatorium*, 20.50.

Utrum omnis curatio fiat per contrarium.

Dino, *Dilucidatorium*, 1.28.

Utrum omnis curatio fiat per contrarium equale in gradu.

Dino, *Dilucidatorium*, 1.29.

Utrum omnis egritudo de repletione curetur per evacuationem.

Taddeo, *Aphor.*, fol. 45.

Utrum omnis medicina sit venenosa.   Taddeo, *Isagoge*, fol. 379r.

Utrum omnis morbus curetur suo contrario.

Taddeo, *Aphor.*, fol. 45.

Utrum oportet causam prius abscindere.

Turisanus, *Plusquam*, 3.41.

Utrum orobum sit fortius in resolvendo quam ordeum.

Taddeo, *Reg. acut.*, fol. 275v.

Utrum ossa soluta possint continuari vera consolidatione.

Dino, *Dilucidatorium*, 28.1.

Utrum oximel assumptum digeratur.   Taddeo, *Reg. acut.*, fol. 268v.

Utrum oximel conveniat in pleuresi.   Taddeo, *Reg. acut.*, fol. 268r.

Utrum oximel sit administrandum in principio pleuresis.

Taddeo, *Reg. acut.*, fol. 268r.

Utrum pannus antiquus siccus sit ponendus inter calefactorium et corpus pleureticum.   Taddeo, *Reg. acut.*, fol. 275v.

Utrum penes accidentia debeant summi canones curativi.

Dino, *Dilucidatorium*, 30.1.

Utrum permutatio coloris sanguinis signum semper ostendens quantitatem sufficientem in evacuatione et horam ligationis vene.

Dino, *Dilucidatorium*, 20.60.

Utrum phlobothomia conveniat in fine veris.

Taddeo, *Aphor.*, fol. 190.

Utrum pillule dande sint cum apozimatibus, et quando.

Dino, *Dilucidatorium*, 5.9.

Utrum pillule dande sint cum apozimatibus homogeneis ipsis.

Dino, *Dilucidatorium*, 5.10.

Utrum pisces petrosi cum aneto porris sale et oleo preparati febricitantibus conveniant.   Taddeo, *Reg. acut.*, fol. 261v.

Utrum possimus uti aqua ordei convenienter in omnibus febribus acutis materialibus.   Taddeo, *Reg. acut.*, fol. 323v.

Utrum post flebotomiam statim competat sompnum.

Guglielmo, *Canon* 1.4, fol. 124r.

Utrum pleuresis possit stare sine cibo usque ad septimum diem.

Taddeo, *Reg. acut.*, fol. 269v.

Utrum pleuretico valde sitienti idromel sit exhibendum.

> Taddeo, *Reg. acut.*, fol. 268r.

Utrum ponticum sit subtilius et magis intrans quam stipticum.

> Dino, *Canon* 2, ch. 3, q. 8.

Utrum post medicinam lenitivam convenienter possit exhiberi compressiva et econtra. Dino, *Canon* 2, ch. 5, q. 4.

Utrum post operationem farmaci aqua ordei danda sit calida vel frigida.

> Dino, *Dilucidatorium*, 5.11.

Utrum post principium aut statum debeat fieri flobothomia in dictis egritudinibus [podagra, epilepsia]. Dino, *Dilucidatorium*, 20.9.

Utrum prava consuetudo evacuandi prohibeat evacuationem.

> Dino, *Dilucidatorium*, 3.6.

Utrum principales regule cognitionis medicinarum habeantur a membris quam ab egritudine. Guglielmo, *Canon* 1.4, fols. 118r-v.

Utrum principia in medicando solutionem continui in membris mollibus debeant esse tria, vel plura, aut pautiora [*sic*].

> Dino, *Dilucidatorium*, 28.2.

Utrum principium sit deterior hora cibandi quam status.

> Taddeo, *Aphor.*, fol. 11.

Utrum prius farmacum assumptum sit danda aqua calida per spacium.

> Dino, *Dilucidatorium*, 5.5.

Utrum prius tractandum sit de curatione apostematum quam de curatione solutionis continui. Dino, *Dilucidatorium*, 25.1.

Utrum ptisana conveniat in acutis morbis.

> Taddeo, *Reg. acut.*, fol. 256r.

Utrum ptisana conveniat in declinatone morborum acutarum.

> Taddeo, *Reg. acut.*, fol. 316v.

Utrum ptisana cum toto sit administranda in principio pleuresis.

> Taddeo, *Reg. acut.*, fol. 260v.

Utrum ptisana ordei fiat labilis per decoctionem.

> Taddeo, *Reg. acut.*, fol. 262r.

Utrum ptisana possit esse simul facilis digestionis et sitis excitativa.

> Taddeo, *Reg. acut.*, fol. 262r.

Utrum ptisana sit similium partium vel dissimilium.

> Taddeo, *Reg. acut.*, fol. 256v.

Utrum ptisana sit viscosa. Taddeo, *Reg. acut.*, fol. 256r.

Utrum pulmoni debeatur medicina debilis.

> Dino, *Dilucidatorium*, 1.18.

Utrum purgatio per partem inferiorem conveniat in omni tempore.

> Taddeo, *Aphor.*, fol. 89.

Utrum purgatio usqua ad sitim fienda sit.

Taddeo, *Aphor.*, fol. 94.

Utrum qualitas medicine solum elligatur ab essentia morbi.

Dino, *Dilucidatorium*, 1.14.

Utrum quando materia est in raptu ad membrum debeamus trahere ad partem diversam. Dino, *Dilucidatorium*, 1.21.

Utrum quantitas in medicina augeat contradum [?] omne.

Dino, independent question, BAV, MS
Vat. lat. 4454, fols. 102r-103r.

Utrum quelibet asperitas trachee sit removenda per humida glutinosa.

Turisanus, *Plusquam*, 3.62.

Utrum quelibet medicina que dicitur talis in potentia reducatur ad actum operationis a calore innato. Dino, *Canon* 2, ch. 1, q. 1.

Utrum quies in vulneribus conferat, motus vero noceat.

Taddeo, *Reg. acut.*, fol. 303r.

Utrum ratio et experimentum concordent in iuvamento vene saphene et vene sciatice. Dino, *Dilucidatorium*, 20.61.

Utrum reductio fiat paulatim. Turisanus, *Plusquam*, 3.29.

Utrum regimen decidentium et convalescentium ad eandem artis partem pertineat. Taddeo, *Reg. acut.*, fol. 298v.

Utrum res stiptice magis exasperet linguam secundum superficiem et profundum quam res stiptica, vel econverso [*sic*].

Dino, *Canon* 2, ch. 3, q. 7.

Utrum sal conveniat in cibis morborum acutorum.

Taddeo, *Reg. acut.*, fol. 257r.

Utrum secaniabim habeat solum virtutem medicine et non cibi.

Taddeo, *Reg. acut.*, fol. 269v.

Utrum secundum unam medicationem medicine sint permutande.

Dino, *Dilucidatorium*, 1.33.

Utrum seni febricanti febre acuta in eodem egritudinem cum iuvene competat [medicina] frigidiora quam iuveni. Guglielmo, *Canon* 1.4, fol. 120r.

Utrum servanda sit consuetudo in cibando egros quam habent tempora sanitatis. Taddeo, *Reg. acut.*, fol. 258v.

Utrum, si materia sit in dextra capiti, debeat trahi ad sinistram.

Dino, *Dilucidatorium*, 3.15.

Utrum, si medicina non solvat et mala non fiant accidentia, flobothomia fienda sit post duos aut tres dies. Dino, *Dilucidatorium*, 8.1.

Utrum siccitati lingue ex ebullitione colere debeat succuri cum zuccaro.

Dino, *Dilucidatorium*, 20.46.

Utrum sit aliqua medicina evacuativa carnis.
Taddeo, Aphor., fol. 62.

Utrum sit conveniens aliquid apozima cum vino construere.
Dino, Dilucidatorium, 5.8.

Utrum sit dare medicinam evacuativam sanguinem.
Guglielmo, Canon 1.4, fol. 124r.

Utrum sit invenire rem aliquam in qua natura cibi et natura medicine sit
ad equata.　　　　　　　　　　　Bartolomeo, De complexionibus,
fol. 85r.

Utrum sit magis periculosum uti medicina frigida an calida.
Guglielmo, Canon 1.4, fol. 119r.

Utrum sit maior timor in calefaciendo et infrigidando quam in humectando
et exiccando.　　　　　　　　　　Dino, Dilucidatorium, 2.4.

Utrum sit maior timor in humectando quam in exiccando.
Dino, Dilucidatorium, 2.6.

Utrum sit periculosior uti medicina sicca quam humida.
Guglielmo, Canon 1.4, fols. 110r-120r.

Utrum sit reperire medicinam temperatum.
Dino, Canon 2, ch. 1, q. 2.

Utrum sitis sit signum sufficientis evacuationis.
Dino, Dilucidatorium, 6.1.

Utrum sitis sit signum sufficientis evacuationis etiam in evacuatione per
vomitum.　　　　　　　　　　　　Dino, Dilucidatorium, 6.2.

Utrum solatrum habeat virtutem resolutivam.
Dino, Dilucidatorium, 26.26.

Utrum solutio ventris trahat a superioribus et eradicet ab inferioribus.
Dino, Dilucidatorium, 3.24.

Utrum solvere ventrem super solutionem ventris sit timorosum.
Dino, Dilucidatorium, 3.1.

Utrum somnus sistat [sic] operationem hellebori.
Taddeo, Aphor., fol. 92.

Utrum sompnus debeat fieri immediate post exhibitionem medicine.
Guglielmo, Canon 1.4, fols. 123v-124r.

Utrum, stante necessitate flobothomie et farmacie, flobothomia debeat premitti.
Dino, Dilucidatorium, 4.2.

Utrum stupefactio competat in spasmo.
Taddeo, Aphor., fol. 135.

Utrum subtilantia in egritudinibus cronicis debeant exhiberi ante
maturationem vel post maturationem.
Dino, Dilucidatorium, 3.11.

Utrum super medicinam debilem sit dormiendum.

Dino, *Dilucidatorium*, 5.4.

Utrum, supposito quod corpus frigidum, sive sit frigidum etate sicut est corpus sene vel ex complexione ut est flamaticum, equaliter febricatur cum corpore calido, sive sit calidum ex etate vel complexione, an cui in curatione hec febris debeant frigidiora.

Dino, independent question, BAV, MS Vat. lat. 2484, fols. 214r-217r.

Utrum sumpturi helleborum per multum nutrimentum et requiem sint preparandi.   Taddeo, *Aphor.*, fol. 92.

Utrum tradat curam solum opilationis ex humoribus viscosis, an etiam ex viscosis.   Turisanus, *Plusquam*, 3.60.

Utrum tyriaca fermentata operetur per unam virtutem in qua sunt confracte virtutes omnium simplicium componentium eam.

Dino, *Dilucidatorium*, 30.10.

Utrum tyriaca habeat solum complexionem secundam, an etiam primam, et habeat complexionem unam vel plures.

Dino, *Canon* 2, ch. 1, q. 5.

Utrum tyriaca nova sive recens debeat poni medicina narcotica.

Dino, *Dilucidatorium*, 30.8.

Utrum tyriaca recens sit pauci iuvamenti.

Dino, *Dilucidatorium*, 30.9.

Utrum ulcus in corpore et membro humidis indigeat ampliore exiccatione, et in corpore et membro siccis indigeat minori exiccatione.

Dino, *Dilucidatorium*, 28.8.

Utrum ultime egritudini competat ultima cura.

Taddeo, *Aphor.*, fol. 7.

Utrum una evacuatio possit esse cura duarum egritudinum contrarium.

Taddeo, *Aphor.*, fol. 169.

Utrum una medicina possit efficere in corpore humano operationes contrarias.

Dino, *Dilucidatorium*, 1.6.

Utrum unaquaque discrasia facile ledatur a simili et iuvetur a contraria.

Turisanus, *Plusquam*, 2.30.

Utrum universaliter in omni fluxu vel evacuatione superflua conveniat constrictio cum evacuatione per eandem partem vel per oppositam.

Dino, *Dilucidatorium*, 23.2.

Utrum universaliter in vulnere complexio servetur per exiccantia.

Turisanus, *Plusquam*, 3.49.

Utrum usus stipticorum universaliter conveniat in quolibet evacuatione superflua.   Dino, *Dilucidatorium*, 23.5.

Utrum vaporatio cum mileo sit conveniens in obthalmia ventosa.

Dino, *Dilucidatorium*, 30.13.

Utrum vena frontis flobothomari debeat secundum longum aut secundum latum.

Dino, *Dilucidatorium*, 20.64.

Utrum ventose apposite super nocram sint vicarie nigre et super alcheol basilice.

Dino, *Dilucidatorium*, 21.7.

Utrum ventose attrahat per naturam vacui.

Dino, *Dilucidatorium*, 21.1.

Utrum ventose evacuent ex profundo.

Dino, *Dilucidatorium*, 21.3.

Utrum ventose evacuent solum sanguinem subtilem et grossum.

Dino, *Dilucidatorium*, 21.4.

Utrum ventose posite super alchadam conferat tremori capitis.

Dino, *Dilucidatorium*, 21.8.

Utrum ventrem solventia et evacuantia sint de genere sedantium dolorem vere.

Dino, *Dilucidatorium*, 30.4.

Utrum ver sit tempus convenientius ad purgationem quam autumnus.

Taddeo, *Aphor.*, fol. 190.

Utrum videtur cerusa epithiata conveniat epatis calefactione.

Mondino, independent question, BAV, MS Vat. lat. 4455, fols. 41r-v.

Utrum vinum confortet virtutem acute febricitantium.

Taddeo, *Reg. acut.*, fol. 311r.

Utrum vinum conveniat in dolore oculorum pendenta a materia sanguinea.

Taddeo, *Aphor.*, fol. 179.

Utrum vinum curet appetitum caninum.

Taddeo, *Aphor.*, fol. 44.

Utrum vinum humectet an exiccet. Dino, *Dilucidatorium*, 2.9.

Utrum virtus curat morbum an medicina.

Turisanus, *Plusquam*, 3.35.

Utrum virtus expulsiva confortetur stipticis.

Turisanus, *Plusquam*, 3.67.

Utrum virtus solutiva in medicinis sit eadem cum forma specifica in eis.

Dino, *Dilucidatorium*, 9.2.

Utrum vomitivum leve debeat semper dari super cibum.

Dino, *Dilucidatorium*, 11.4.

Utrum vomitus attrahat ab inferioribus et eradicet a superioribus.

Dino, *Dilucidatorium*, 11.7.

Utrum vomitus competat in lienteria. Taddeo, *Aphor.*, fol. 91.

Utrum vomitus conferat asmati. Dino, *Dilucidatorium*, 13.5.

Utrum vomitus conferat epilepsie. Dino, *Dilucidatorium*, 11.9.

Utrum vomitus conferat lepre.   Dino, *Dilucidatorium*, 11.10.

Utrum vomitus fieri debeat duobus diebus continuis.

Dino, *Dilucidatorium*, 13.3.

Utrum vomitus fieri debeat unoquoque mense.

Dino, *Dilucidatorium*, 13.2.

Utrum vomitus maxime conferat egritudinibus cronicis.

Dino, *Dilucidatorium*, 11.8.

Utrum vomitus sit prohibendus in estate.

Dino, *Dilucidatorium*, 1.37.

Utrum vulnus debeat duci ad saniem.

Taddeo, *Isagoge*, fol. 398r.

17ª questio est quare Avicenna tractavit de cura apostematum interiorum, cum intentio sua sit hic loqui de apostematibus exterioribus.

Dino, *Chirurgia* (Estense).

18ª questio est quare Avicenna posuit diversitatem in cura flegmonis penes causam primitivam et antecedentem.   Dino, *Chirurgia* (Estense).

19ª questio est utrum sit verum quod dicit Avicenna, cum dicit quod quando causa primitiva obviat mundificationem non est necessaria nisi curatio apostematis in quantum est aperta.   Dino, *Chirurgia* (Estense).

20ª questio est utrum debeamus repercutere flegmonem a causa primitiva in principio post corporis purgationem.   Dino, *Chirurgia* (Estense).

22ª questio est quia dubitatur super capitulo de cura flegmonis de illo verbo quod dicit "ymo minus illa."   Dino, *Chirurgia* (Estense).

23ª questio est quomodo exponendo illum textum "ymo minus illa" secundum unam expositionem, scilicet, substantiam conveniat cura amborum illorum apostematum.   Dino, *Chirurgia* (Estense).

24ª questio est quia dicit Avicenna quod aliquando est necessaria evacuatio data quod corpus sit mundum.   Dino, *Chirurgia* (Estense).

25ª questio est utrum debeamus repercutere flegmonem in principio secundum quod ponunt Avicenna et Aliabas.   Dino, *Chirurgia* (Estense).

26ª questio est quare ponit Avicenna quod in augmento flegmonis debemus miscere mollitiva humectaria cum repercussivis; alii autem auctores quod debemus miscere resolutiva et non mollitiva.

Dino, *Chirurgia* (Estense).

27ª questio est cuius complexionis debeantur esse medicine repercussive flegmonis in principio quantum ad qualitatem earum, scilicet, utrum debeant esse frigidum, vel humidum, vel frigidum et siccum.

Dino, *Chirurgia* (Estense).

28ª questio est quia dicit Avicenna quod si volueris regere in principio cum sedatione doloris non aproximes ei aquam calidam.

Dino, *Chirurgia* (Estense).

29ª questio est quia dicit Avicenna quod cum apostemata calida indigent maturatione emplastretur caput eorum cum persilio, et similibus, etc.

Dino, *Chirurgia* (Estense).

30ª questio est quia dicit Avicenna quod in erisipila flobothomia non confert nisi quando materia est inter duas cutes, et si profundatur minoratus eius iuvamentum. Dino, *Chirurgia* (Estense).

32ª questio est quia videtur quod Rasis ponat quod in apostemate sanguineo competant magis frigida et stiptica quam in colerico frigida et humida.

Dino, *Chirurgia* (Estense).

33ª questio est quia videtur quod Avicenna dicit quod in statu erisipile medicina debeat esse magis frigida quam in principio.

Dino, *Chirurgia* (Estense).

34ª questio est quia Avicenna posuit curam erisipile solum quantum ad due tempora, scilicet quantum ad principium et statum, de augmento autem et statu nichil dixit. Dino, *Chirurgia* (Estense).

36ª questio est quia videtur quod exicatio quam ponit Avicenna non competat saltem in formica ambulativa. Dino, *Chirurgia* (Estense).

38ª questio est quia Avicenna videtur sibimet contradicere in capitulo de cura pruritis perfici, quia dicit ibi quod in ulceratio administrentur cura que fortiter exicant, et dicit postea quod non administrentur exicantia in quantum potes. Dino, *Chirurgia* (Estense).

39ª questio est quia videtur Avicennam non habuisse bonum ordinem in ponendo curam inflationum, etc., cum dixit "Et cum cadunt estate, etc."

Dino, *Chirurgia* (Estense).

45ª questio est utrum competat flobothomia in althoin.

46ª questio est quia non videtur quod in althoin competat aliqua evacuatio in principio. Dino, *Chirurgia* (Estense).

47ª questio est quia non videtur quod cibus huius morbi debeat esse infrigidativus ingrossans sanguinem. Dino, *Chirurgia* (Estense).

49ª questio est utrum debeamus curare althoin in principio cum hiis que infrigidant et repercutiunt, sicut dicit Avicenna.

Dino, *Chirurgia* (Estense).

54ª questio est quia dicit Avicenna quod si exitura rumpatur cum medicinis ruptoribus non debemus ipsam perforare cum ferro.

Dino, *Chirurgia* (Estense).

55ª questio est quid sit melius, an precipitare exitura cum medicinis an cum ferro. Dino, *Chirurgia* (Estense).

60ª questio est quia videtur quod Avicenna dicat in capitula de cura nodorum quod plumbum maturet; queritur quomodo.

Dino, *Chirurgia* (Estense).

61ᵃ questio est utrum in scrofulis competat vomitus.

Dino, *Chirurgia* (Estense).

62ᵃ questio est quomodo flobothomia iuvet in scrofulis cum ipse fiant ab humoribus flegmaticis grossis et viscosis.

Dino, *Chirurgia* (Estense).

63ᵃ questio est utrum ventosa competat in scrofulis.

Dino, *Chirurgia* (Estense).

64ᵃ questio est quia videtur quod Avicenna dicit quod in sefricos [?] non parvo sit aliqualis dolor et sensus; utrum sit verum.

Dino, *Chirurgia* (Estense).

66ᵃ questio est utrum sefricos possit sanari cum medicina ruptoriva et caustica. Dino, *Chirurgia* (Estense).

67ᵃ questio est quare Avicenna dixit materiam potius debere digeri in sephricos [?] quam in aliis apostematibus ante purgationem.

Dino, *Chirurgia* (Estense).

68ᵃ questio est quia dubitatur de eo quod dicit Avicenna quod medicus est audacior in administrando acetum in membro carnoso quam in nervoso.

Dino, *Chirurgia* (Estense).

75ᵃ questio est utrum sit verum id quod dicit aliquis, scilicet quod pulvis incarnativus non debet poni in orificio vulneris.

Dino, *Chirurgia* (Estense).

76ᵃ questio est utrum complexio sana conservetur per medicinas mediocriter exicantes. Dino, *Chirurgia* (Estense).

77ᵃ questio est quare Avicenna dixit in capitulo de cura vulneram quod medicamentum faciens nasci carnem facit nasci quandoque et non semper.

Dino, *Chirurgia* (Estense).

78ᵃ questio est utrum medicina generativa carnis debeat semper esse exicativa.

Dino, *Chirurgia* (Estense).

79ᵃ questio est utrum medicina exicativa debeat exicare usque ad terminum, sicut dicit Avicenna, et in quanto gradu debeat exicare.

Dino, *Chirurgia* (Estense).

80ᵃ questio est utrum medicina carnis generativa debeat exicativa in primo gradu, et utrum hoc intelligatur absolute vel respective.

Dino, *Chirurgia* (Estense).

81ᵃ questio est utrum dictum Avicenne sit verum cum dicit quod non oportet ut operentur ille medicine nisi in superficie vulneris.

Dino, *Chirurgia* (Estense).

82ᵃ questio est utrum medicina incarnativa debeat esse vehementis exicationis.

Dino, *Chirurgia* (Estense).

83ᵃ questio est in quo gradu debeat esse medicina generativa carnis in qualitatibus activis. Dino, *Chirurgia* (Estense).

85ᵃ questio est utrum dictum Avicenne sit verum, cum dicit quod medicinam consolidativam non debet administrari quando caro iam est adequata cum cute, quia ipse facit augeri carnem.

Dino, *Chirurgia* (Estense).

86ᵃ questio est utrum dictum Avicenne sit verum cum dicit quod medicina faciens nasci carnem non debet administrari nisi post perfectam mundificationem.   Dino, *Chirurgia* (Estense).

88ᵃ questio est utrum mixtio plurimum medicamentarum sit bona.

Dino, *Chirurgia* (Estense).

89ᵃ questio est utrum dictum Avicenne sit verum, cum dicit in capitulo de medicinis facientibus nasci carnem quod senes egent medicinis in quibus est caliditas et attractio fortior.   Dino, *Chirurgia* (Estense).

91ᵃ questio est utrum in vulnere prius debeamus sedare dolorem, cum dolor sit una causa apostematis que prohibet curam vulneris.

Dino, *Chirurgia* (Estense).

92ᵃ questio est utrum in cura attritionis et contusionis debeamus, sicut dicit Avicenna, flobothomare, dato quod corpus sit mundum.

Dino, *Chirurgia* (Estense).

93ᵃ questio est utrum sit verum quod dicit Avicenna, scilicet quod sedere dolor cum medicina faciet pus.   Dino, *Chirurgia* (Estense).

94ᵃ questio est utrum maior lesio accidat infantibus ex cautela et offensione quam iuvenibus.   Dino, *Chirurgia* (Estense).

95ᵃ questio est qualia debeant esse infrigidativa in cura combustionis ignis, scilicet an fortia an debilia.   Dino, *Chirurgia* (Estense).

96ᵃ questio est utrum dictum Avicenne contineat verum, cum dicit quod patiens fluxum sanguinis ex naribus flobothometur ex manu pertinenti nari patiente.   Dino, *Chirurgia* (Estense).

97ᵃ questio est utrum id quod videtur dicere Avicenna in capitulo de cura fluxus sanguinis sit verum. Cum videtur dicere quod si sit nimia propinquitas, sicut de una manu ad aliam, et fluxus sanguinis sit ex parte dextra, non debit fieri cum flobothomia diversio ad sinistram.

Dino, *Chirurgia* (Estense).

98ᵃ questio est utrum dictum Avicenne sit verum, cum dicit in capitulo de cura fluxus sanguinis "quod non expectet," ut hoc artificium sit adiuvans ad retentionem fluxus sanguinis.   Dino, *Chirurgia* (Estense).

99ᵃ questio est de uno dicto Avicenne; videtur enim dicere quod imponatur licinium in orificio arterie aperte et incarnabitur antequam solvantur ligature. Queritur nunc [?] quomodo existente ibi licinio fiet arterie incarnatio.   Dino, *Chirurgia* (Estense).

103ᵃ questio est quare Avicenna non dixit ita "Omnia ulcera indigent abstersionem," sicut dicit "exiccationem."

Dino, *Chirurgia* (Estense).

105ᵃ questio est quare dixit Avicenna in capitulo de cura ulcerum quod ulcera quandoque indigent dispositionibus aliis, scilicet mundificatione et abstersione, cum semper hiis indigeant.

Dino, *Chirurgia* (Estense).

106ᵃ questio est quia videtur Avicennam ponere curam ulcerum cum ligatura ac si essent vulnera simplicia.

Dino, *Chirurgia* (Estense).

107ᵃ questio est numquid observare debeamus suturam in cura ulcerum.

Dino, *Chirurgia* (Estense).

108ᵃ questio est utrum ulcus sub ratione qua vetustum est aut recens diversificent curam. Dino, *Chirurgia* (Estense).

109ᵃ questio est per quem modum caustica removeant ab ulcere id quod corruptum est. Dino, *Chirurgia* (Estense).

110ᵃ questio est propter quid est quod statim cum medicina caustica operata est in carnem, illa pars carnis causticate non decidit ab ulcere.

Dino, *Chirurgia* (Estense).

116ᵃ questio est utrum medicamentum vulnerum nervorum debeat esse calidum. Dino, *Chirurgia* (Estense).

117ᵃ questio est utrum in medicantibus vulnerum nervorum aliquando competat medicamentum fortis caliditatis.

Dino, *Chirurgia* (Estense).

118ᵃ questio est quare Avicenna docet administrare acetum in vulneribus nervorum cum ipse sit frigidus. Dino, *Chirurgia* (Estense).

120ᵃ questio est quia queritur si est possibile, vel quando est possibile, quod curetur fractura cranei absque incisione cutis et carnis et detectione ossis, et absque evitatione adventus alicuius accidentis mali, etc.

Dino, *Chirurgia* (Estense).

122ᵃ questio est numquid sit licitum in vulnere quod est cum fractura cranei in modo curationis procedere absque detectione et ellevatione ossis.

Dino, *Chirurgia* (Estense).

123ᵃ questio est utrum vulnus quod est cum fractura cranei convenienter possit curari alio modo quam cum incisione, et detectione, et ellevatione ossis.

Dino, *Chirurgia* (Estense).

124ᵃ questio est utrum post detectionem et ellevationem ossis sit conveniens super panniculos cerebri oleum rosatum apponere.

Dino, *Chirurgia* (Estense).

WORKS OF HIPPOCRATES AND GALEN LISTED BY MONDINO DE' LIUZZI AND BARTOLOMEO DA VARIGNANA

Spelling has been retained, but punctuation and capitalization have been modernized and abbreviations expanded. For discussion of these lists, see chapter four.

Mondino, commentary on Hippocrates, *Prognostica*, BAV, MS Vat. lat. 4466, fol 1ra, proem:

> Et ex hiis apparet ordo huius libri ad alios libros Ypocratis. Nam inter libros Ypocratis primus est liber *De lege*, post quem est liber *De natura humana*, post quem est liber *De natura puerorum*, post quem est liber iste, scilicet *Pronosticorum*, post quem est liber *Regiminis acutorum*, post quem est liber *Afforismorum*, qui secundum quidam alium modum perfectiorem omnes alios precedet preter librum *De lege*, post quem est liber *Epidimiarum*, post quem est liber de *Aere Aqua et Regionibus*, et hiis potest annexus liber *De farmaciis*.[1]

[Bartolomeo], commentary on Galen, *De interioribus* (De locis affectis), BAV, MS Vat. lat. 4452 (for the identification of this commentary as Bartolomeo's, see note 14 to chapter 5), proem, fols. 83vb-84ra:

> Si libri medicine distinguntur penes considerationem theoricam tunc habeant distingui per distinctionem subjecti de quo in ipsis determinatur. Modo cum subjectum habeat partes ymo passiones, et causas, aut libri medicine quantum ad considerationem theoricam erunt de partibus subjecti, vel de passionibus ipsius, vel de ipsius causis. Si sint de partibus subjecti, aut sunt de iuvamento parcium, et sic est liber *De iuvamentis membrorum*[2] qui

---

[1] Mondino incorporated the same list of Hippocratic works into the proem of his commentary on *De regimine acutorum*, BAV, MS Vat. lat. 4466, fol. 37r. For the medieval versions of the Hippocratic works named by him, and by Bartolomeo da Varignana in the passage that follows, see now Pearl Kibre, "Hippocrates Latinus: Repertorium of Hippocratic Writings in the Latin Middle Ages," pt. 1, *Traditio* 21 (1975):99-126, and continued in subsequent volumes (the concluding portion, pt. 8, is expected to appear in 1982).

[2] A compendium of *De usu partium*, the only Latin version of this work known before Niccolò da Reggio's complete translation; see Durling, "Corrigenda and Addenda," no.

in xi libros est divisus; aut sunt de compositione et substancia parcium et hoc dupliciter—aut enim in illis libris traditur determinatio de compositione et substancia parcium complete, et sic est liber *De medicatione per anothomiam*, aut incomplete, et hec diversificatur; quia aut hec est per conspectum sensibilem ad corpora viva, et sic est liber *De anothomia vivorum*, aut per conspectum sensibilem ad corpora mortua, et sic est liber *De anothomia mortuorum*. Et nullum horum trium habemus [in]permanentibus[?]; reffert tamen Galenus in fine *Tegni* se ipsos fecise.[3] Si autem ea que determina[n]tur in medicina sint de passionibus subjecti, cum tales sunt duplices, scilicet dispositiones et accidencia sive signa, aut erunt de dispositionibus aut de accidentibus sive signis. Si autem tractatio medicinalis sit de dispositionibus aut est de ipsis modo communi, et sic est liber *De accidenti et morbo*,[4] in quo eciam sub modo communi determinatur de causis peregrenianis [?], id est corruptibilibus, aut speciali et proprio, et tunc dupliciter: aut est de dispositionibus ut contracte sunt per essenciam vel ut contracte sunt per substanciam. Si sit de dispositionibus primo modo, sic sunt duo libri quos habemus, scilicet liber *De malicia complexionis diverse*[5] et liber *De febribus*.[6] Sed differunt isti libri adinvicem, quoniam in libro *De malicia complexionis diverse* solum determinatur essencia dispositionis ut est contracta per modos et doctrinas; in libro autem *De febribus* ut est contracta non solum per modos et doctrinas, sed eciam per accidentia et signa. Si autem sit tractatio medicinalis de dispositionibus ut contracte sunt per substanciam, et hoc dupliciter: aut tractat de illis modo communi, et sic est liber *De interioribus*,[7]

122a, p. 473. Bartolomeo's list may be compared with the list of works of Galen compiled by Guy de Chauliac (1363), the latter relying heavily upon the translations of Niccolò da Reggio. See Margaret S. Ogden, "The Galenic Works Cited in Guy de Chauliac's *Chirurgia Magna*," *Journal of the History of Medicine* 28 (1973):24-33.

[3] Several pseudo-Galenic works on anatomy circulated during the Middle Ages, including one entitled *Anatomia vivorum* and printed with works of Galen in early editions; according to George W. Corner this group of anatomical treatises all show dependence on medieval medical authorities and were composed between the late eleventh and the early thirteenth centuries. See Corner, *Anatomical Texts of the Earlier Middle Ages*, pp. 19, 27-32, 35-40.

[4] That is, Galen, *De morborum causis, De morborum differentiis, De symptomatum causis, De symptomatum differentiis*, in his *Omnia Opera*, ed. C. G. Kühn (Leipzig, 1821-33), 6:836-880, hereafter cited as Kühn; see Durling, "Corrigenda and Addenda," nos. 64a, 65a, 112a, 113a, pp. 467-468.

[5] Presumably Galen, *De inaequali intemperie*, in Kühn, 6:733-52; see Durling, "Corrigenda and Addenda," no. 55a, p. 466.

[6] Kühn, 7:273-332.

[7] That is, *De locis affectis*, Kühn, 7:1-452, see Durling, "Corrigenda and Addenda," no. 60a, pp. 466-467.

aut proprio, et sic est liber *De dislocatione*[8] et liber *De ptisi*[9] (del. et corr. in MS) *tipsi tipsi* [*sic*]. Si autem tractatio medicinalis sit de accidentibus et signis que eciam sunt passiones, aut est tractans de accidentibus et signis ut comparantur proprie dispositioni, scilicet passioni acute, et sic est liber *De crisi*[10] et *De creticis*.[11] In eis determinantur accidencia que acute

fol. 84ra:

passioni comparantur, secundum quod est de intentione Galeni, id est, et illa adhuc diversificantur secundum quod diversimode comparantur ad passionem acutam. Aut est de signis et accidentibus que non comparantur proprie dispositioni, et ista adhuc diversificatur, quia aut est tractans de accidentibus et signis que comparantur actionibus naturalibus, vel de hiis que comparantur actionibus vitalibus, vel de hiis que comparantur actionibus animalibus. Si tractat de accidentibus primo modo, sic est liber *De visitatione* Ypocratis qui sic intitulatur. Si autem tractat de illis secundo modo, sic est liber *De causis pulsus*,[12] vel liber que dicitur *Introductorius*;[13] si de illis tertio modo, sic est liber *De disnia*,[14] nam ipsa passio est hanelitus, modo hanelitus actio animalis est. Sed advertendum quod tractatio que est de accidentibus secundo modo diversificatur quia quedam est de ipsis per viam rationalem et quedam per viam experimentalem. In omnibus libris de pulsibus preter illum in quo traditur *De pronosticatione per pulsum*[15] est tractatio de illis accidentibus per viam rationalem, in illo autem solo per viam experimentalem. Si autem medicinalis scientia considerat causas subjecti, cum cause ipsius sint quatuor, scilicet materialis, efficiens, formalis, et finalis, tractatio de hiis aut erit de causis materialibus, aut formalibus, aut efficientibus, aut finalibus. Si est de causis materialibus aut est de illis sub modo considerationis proprie, et sic est liber *De chimis* sive *humoribus*,[16] aut sub modo communi, et hoc dupliciter, quia aut tractatur de illis sub brevitate et oscuritate, et sic est liber *De humana natura*, aut sub prolixitate et declaratione, et sic est liber *De ellementis secundum sentenciam Ypocratis*.[17] Si autem sit de causis formalibus, aut est de unitate aut de compositione, et de istis librum non habemus, aut de complexione; de hac

---

[8] I have not succeeded in identifying this title.

[9] Perhaps either *De ptisana*, Kühn, 6:816-831, or *De typis*, Kühn, 7:463-474.

[10] Kühn, 9:550-768; Durling, "Corrigenda and Addenda," no. 33a, p. 464.

[11] Kühn, 9:769-941; Durling, "Corrigenda and Addenda," no. 39a, p. 465.

[12] Kühn, 9:1-204.   [13] Perhaps the *Introductio, seu medicus*, Kühn, 14:674-797.

[14] Probably *De difficultate respirationis*, Kühn, 7:753-960.

[15] Presumably *De praesagitione ex pulsibus, Kühn*, 9:205-430.

[16] Kühn, 12:485-496.

[17] Kühn, 2:413-508; Durling, "Corrigenda and Addenda," no. 46a, pp. 465-466.

habemus librum unum, scilicet librum *De complexionibus*[18] qui dividitur in tres libros. In primo et secundo determinatur de complexione animalium, in tercio vero de complexione plantarum et omnium corporum non movencium. Si autem sit de causis efficientibus, aut est de causis efficientibus corruptibilibus, aut de causis efficientibus non corruptibilibus et primitivis. Si primo modo aut determinatur de illis sub modo communi, et sic determinatur de ipsis in libro *De accidenti et morbo,* aut sub modo proprio et sic est liber qui intitulatur *De plenitudine* sive *multitudine,*[19] et hunc se fecise fatetur Galenus VI *De regimine sanitatis.*[20] Si autem sit de causis efficientibus non corruptibilibus et primitivis, et hoc multipliciter: quia aut est de aere, et sic determinatur de ipsis in tertia particula *Afforismorum* et in libro *Epidimie* licet complecius et hoc quantum ad eorum duas particulas, aut est de cibo, et tunc de ipsis aut determinatur sub modo communi (del. et corr. in MS) communi et sic est liber Ypocratis *De dieta,* vel sub modo proprio, et sic est liber Galeni *De alimentis;*[21] aut est de medicina, et tunc tractat de medicinis simplicibus et compositis in universali, et sic est liber *De simplici medicina,*[22] aut modo particulari et tunc aut tractat de medicinis simplicibus, et sic est *Liber de virtutibus farmacorum,*[23] aut de compositis, et sic est liber *Experimentorum.*[24] Ad primum librum reduci potest tractatio *De medicinis simplicibus* quem fecit Serapio; ad secundum reduci potest *Antidotarius* Serapionis et Rasis, et *Antidotarius magnus* quem dicitur fecise in *Elementis* Galenus, et eciam *Antidotarius* iste Nicholay.[25] Nam in antidotariis determinatur de medicinis compositis. Si autem medicinalis scientia sit de causis finalibus, cum tales sunt virtutes et operationes, aut erit tractans de virtutibus et operationibus modo communi, et sic est liber qui intitulatur liber *De sentenciis pulmonis et ale* [?]

[18] That is, *De temperamentis.* The twelfth-century Latin version ascribed to Burgundio of Pisa is edited by R. J. Durling, *Galenus Latinus* 1 (Berlin-New York, 1976); Kühn, 1:509-694.

[19] Kühn, 7:513-583.

[20] Also known as *De ingenio sanitatis* and *De sanitate tuenda,* Kühn, 6:1-452; Burgundio of Pisa's translation of the sixth book sometimes circulated as a separate work. See Durling, "Addenda and Corrigenda," no. 103a, p. 470, and TK 87.

[21] Kühn, 6:453-748.

[22] Kühn, 11:379ff.; 12:377.

[23] Perhaps *De medicinis expertis,* attributed to Galen and printed with his works in Galen, *Opera* (Venice, 1490), 1:177r-181v; see Durling, "Addenda and Corrigenda," no. 62, p. 467, and TK, col. 658.

[24] No doubt one of the various collections of *experimenta* attributed to Galen in the Middle Ages; several are noted in TK 390, 420, 1093.

[25] Th *Antidotarii* of Rasis and Nicholas of Salerno and the various remedy collections attributed to Serapion were much relied upon by medieval physicians and survive in numerous manuscripts; see index entries in TK.

Ypocratis,[26] aut modo proprio—aut erit de virtutibus et operationibus naturalibus, aut vitalibus, aut animalibus. Si sit tractans de virtutibus et operationibus naturalibus, aut est tractans de ipsis sub modo speciali, et sic est liber *De natura puerorum* Ypocratis, vel sub modo communi, et sic est liber *De virtutibus naturalibus* Galeni.[27] Si sit tractans de virtutibus animalibus, non habemus nisi duos libros, scilicet librum *De voce* et librum *De hanelitu.*[28] Sed advertendum quod duplex est liber *De hanelitu.* Unus est qui est de motu hanelitus, alter qui est de motu pectoris et pulmonis. Et isti differunt ad invicem quoniam in uno determinatur de hanelitu in comparatione ad finem, in altero in comparatione ad virtutem que est causa motus. Si autem sit tractans de virtutibus et operationibus vitalibus, cum actio vitalis sit pulsus, aut erit tractans de pulsu modo communi, aut proprio; si proprio, aut tractat de utilitate ipsius, et sic est liber *De iuvamento pulsuum,*[29] aut tractat de eius speciebus, et sic est liber *De differentiis pulsuum,*[30] aut de causis specierum et sic est liber *De causis pulsus.* Si autem tractat de pulsu modo communi aut tractat de ipso sub brevitate et confuxione et sic est liber *De introductorio pulsus,*[31] aut sub prolixitate et declaratione, reprobando opinionem illorum qui male tractaverunt de pulsu; et iste est liber *De pulsibus Galeni contra Erasistratum.* Et sic apparet divisio Galeni secundum considerationem theoricam; alias si tractabimus de consideratione practica fiet distinctio librorum penes illam.

[26] I am unable to identify this title.

[27] That is, *De naturalibus facultatibus*, Kühn, 2:1-214.

[28] Perhaps equivalent to *De causis respirationis*, Kühn, 4:465-469, and TK 1455, or to pseudo-Galen, *De voce et anelitu*, in Galen, *Opera* (Venice, 1490).

[29] Presumably *De pulsuum usu*, Kühn, 5:149-180.

[30] Kühn, 8:493-765.

[31] Perhaps the short work on pulse ascribed to Theophilus that was usually included among the treatises of the *ars medicine.*

BIBLIOGRAPHY

In the Bibliography, the names Taddeo Alderotti, Guglielmo de' Corvi (Guglielmo da Brescia), Dino del Garbo, and Mondino de' Liuzzi are alphabetized under Alderotti, Corvi, Garbo, and Liuzzi, respectively, in order to conform to the style of the great majority of the other entries. However, the greater familiarity of the given names, and the general use of given names with places of origin (e.g., Thaddeus Florentinus) by the copyists of the manuscripts and by editors of the early editions of works by these authors, made it seem preferable to use first names for the abbreviated citations in the footnotes to this book and in the list of manuscripts in the Bibliography. Cross-references from the given name to the family name are supplied in part three of the Bibliography.

PART ONE: INCIPITS

Incipits of works by Taddeo Alderotti and his pupils (from the writings of Gentile da Cingoli, only his medical/natural philosophical question is included) are listed below. See the Abbreviations and Short Titles at the front of this volume, and part two of the Bibliography, below, for manuscripts, editions, and locations. Variants are indicated in brackets.

Alderotti, Taddeo

Amicorum copiam delectabilem et gloriosam permittit. . . .
                              Comm. Hippocrates, *Pronostica.*
Causa efficiens dicitur fuisse quidam mag. nomine Thadeus Florentinus
. . . sed secundum alios . . . quidam doctor parisiensis nomine Johannes. . . .
                              Comm. *De complexionibus* doubtfully
                              ascribed to Taddeo.
Cum nostra corpora diversis et occultis. . . .
                              Tabula de remediis.
Ecce tibi scribo et narro. . . .
                              Libellus medicinalis ad
                              conservationem sanitatis.
Finita prima fen in qua princeps Aboali tractavit de febribus. . . .
                              Comm. Avicenna, *Canon* 4.2.
Incipit expositio preclarissimi doctoris Al decrete medicorum telamen super

fen Primi Quarta. . . .

> Comm. Avicenna, *Canon* 1.4.1-5 and
> 20, doubtfully ascribed to Taddeo.

Inquit Ptolomeus. Qui scientiam vivificavit non est mortuus. . . .

> Comm. Hippocrates, *Aphorismi.*

Nostis enim quod neque hoc neque aliud aliquod opus. . . .

> Comm. Hippocrates, *De regimine
> acutorum.*

Optimus medicus est iste antecedens cum iudicio. . . .

> Comm. Galen, *De crisi.*

Quando incipit lepram etc. Ostendit quid sit lepra. . . .

> Comm. Avicenna, *Canon* 4.3.3
> (*de lepra*).

Quod comeditur et bibitur, etc. In hoc capitulo intendit. . . .

> Comm. Avicenna, *Canon* 1.2.2.1.15.

Quoniam compendiosa et lucida brevitate audientium. . . .

> Comm. Johannitius, *Isagoge.*

Quoniam mihi [nihil] ad veritatis indagationem. . . .

> *Practica* [*de febribus*].

Quoniam omne bonum desursum est a patre fluens. . . .

> Comm. Galen, *Tegni*, NLM 492,
> Naples, 1522.

Quoniam passibilis ac [et] mutabilis existit [extat] humani corporis
conditio. . . .

> *Libellus de sanitate* [*De conservanda
> sanitatis*];

and

Imperò che la chondizione del chorpo umano è passibile e mutevole. . . .

> *Libello per chonservare la sanità
> del corpo* (that is, regimen for Corso
> Donati—this is an Italian version of
> the preceding text).

Regimen eius consistit per sex res non naturales. . . .

> *Consilia* (various other incipits for
> Taddeo's *consilia* or *experimenta* are
> found, as some of the individual items
> circulated separately, and there are
> several manuscript collections of his
> *consilia* not all of which contain the
> same items in the same order).

Subiectum huius libri est corpus humanum sanabile operabile. . . .

> Comm. Galen, *Tegni*, BAV, MS Vat.
> lat. 4464.

Tu scis quod sanitas non est nisi equatio humorum. . . .

> *Introductorium ad practicam.*

Bartolomeo da Varignana

Medicina est philosophia corporis. . . .

> Comm. Galen, *De interioribus,*
> prologue;

with

Ex dictis apparet que sit causa materialis. . . .

> Comm. *De interioribus*, text.

Oportet qui curare naturam ut continuam cavet corpus. . . .

> Comm. Galen, *De complexionibus.*

Quem moralis imago. . . .

> Comm. pseudo-Aristotle, *Economica.*

Sicut apparet ex dictis Averrois in sua aggregatione. . . .

> Comm. Galen, *De accidenti et morbo.*

Subiectum [Causa materialis] in isto [huius] libro est corpus. . . .

> Comm. Galen, *Tegni.*

Vita brevis, etc. . . . ostensa quod sit causa materialis. . . .

> Comm. Hippocrates, *Aphorismi.*

Corvi, Guglielmo de' (Guglielmo da Brescia)

Dicemus quod res medicinalis. . . .

> Comm. Avicenna, *Canon* 1.4.

Illum [Oportet eum] qui vult esse magister et artifex. . . .

> *Practica [Aggregator]*, prologue;

with

De alopicia et tixia [tyria]. . . .

> *Practica*, text.

Impossibile est simile perficere. . . .

> Comm. Hippocrates, *Aphorismi*
> (partial).

Incipit cirurgia que distinguitur [dividitur] in tres. . . .

> *Practica in cyrurgia.*

Quia caro vippere cum in usu habetur conservat virtutem. . . .

> *Questiones de tyriaca.*

Quia regimen confortationis. . . .

De visu et oculo.

Quoniam ut mihi scripsistis in tumore [curatione] mammille. . . .

Consilia.

Garbo, Dino del

Ad solvendum dubitacionem scilicet cuius virtutis risus sit passio. . . .

questio or *tractatus De risu.*

Bonum ergo aliquid divitiarum et nostre vite. . . .

Comm. Galen, *Tegni.*

Circa istam [Cum primam] partem quarti libri Avicenne [quam]
intendimus exponere gratia operis cyrurgie. . . .

Comm. Avicenna, *Canon* 4.3, 4, 5
[*Chirurgia*], prologue;

with

De primo dico quod ad intelligendum quid sit cyrurgia. . . .

Comm. *Canon* 4.3, 4, 5, text.

Considerans verbum Galieni septimo Terapeutice Methodi. . . .

Comm. Avicenna, *Canon* 1.4
[*Dilucidatorium*], prologue;

with

Supra Avicenna determinavit de rebus que spectant ad partem. . . .

Comm. *Canon* 1.4, text.

Consuevit dubitari de titulo huius libri. . . .

Comm. *De malicia complexionis
diverse,* BAV, MS Vat. lat. 4464.

Distinctio mensurarum et ponderum diversificatur secundum
Avicennam et Serapion dupliciter. . . .

De ponderibus et mensuris (sometimes
also attributed to Mondino—variant
texts).

Excusati sumus ab hiis que in principio librorum. . . .

Comm. Avicenna, *Canon* 4.1.

Incipit scriptum super cantilena Guidonis de Cavalcantibus a magistro
Dino del Garbo egregio medicinae doctori editum. Ista cantilena
quae tractat de amoris passione. . . .

Comm. Cavalcanti, *Canzone d'amore.*

Postquam de [G. in] libro de accidenti et morbo determinavit. . . .

Comm. Galen, *De differentiis febrium.*

Quia intentio nostra est edere tractatum. . . .

> Comm. *De malicia complexionis
> diverse*, BAV, MS Vat. lat. 2484.

Rememoratio [Memoratio, Commemoratio] quarundum medicinarum que
sunt apte [de arte] cyrurgia. . . .

> *Compilatio emplastrorum et
> unguentorum* [*Receptarium in
> cyrurgia, unguenta*], sometimes also
> attributed to Mondino.

Serenissime princeps mundi rex Roberte. . . .

> Comm. Avicenna, *Canon* 2 [*De
> virtutibus medicamentorum*]
> prologue;

with

Horum librorum quos de medicina. . . .

> Comm. *Canon* 2, text.

Sicut scribitur a philosopho in principio quarti politicorum. . . .

> Comm. Hippocrates, *De natura fetus.*

Sunt quedam egritudines que semper procedunt. . . .

> Comm. Hippocrates, *Aphorismi* (on
> two aphorisms).

Ut videamus aliqualiter necessitatem eorum que in libro. . . .

> Comm. *De malicia complexionis
> diverse*, BAV, MS Vat. lat. 4452.

Gentile da Cingoli

Utrum species sensibilis. . . .

> *questio*, ed. Grabmann, "Gentile da
> Cingoli";

the same text as

Quia Galenus vult. . . .

> BAV MS palat. lat. 1246.

Liuzzi, Mondino de'

Cum accidentia que ad se vertunt [convertunt, pervertunt] curam. . . .

> *Practica* [*de accidentibus*], also
> attributed to Mondino of Forolivio
> and John of Paris.

Medicina est additio et subtractio scilicet a corpore. . . .

> Comm. Mesue, *Canones universales*
> [*Consolatio*].

Omnis qui medicine artis, etc. Quia in principio cuiuslibet libri. . . .

> Comm. Hippocrates, *Pronostica.*

Quamvis secundum Galienum VI de ingenio sanitatis. . . .

> *Consilia.*

Quia [Quare] [ut] ait [dixit] Galenus septimo [capitulo] therapeutice. . . .

> *Anatomia.*

Quoniam egritudinum causa querenti multoties. . . .

> *Compendium cirurgie.*

Sicut ponit Averroes primo sui Colliget. . . .

> Comm. Hippocrates, *De regimine*
> *acutorum.*

Tres sunt omnes docrine, etc. Ex his que fuerunt dicta in divisione. . . .

> Comm. Galen, *Tegni.*

Turisanus

Librum Galieni qui Microtegni intitulatur id est ars parva. . . .

> *Plusquam commentum in Microtegni*
> *Galieni.*

Quesivit a me vestra dilectio de hypostasi urine. . . .

> *De hypostasi urine,* prologue;

with

Dico ergo quod sicut dicit p. Abolai hypostasis apud medicos. . . .

> *De hypostasi urine,* text.

Part Two: Select List of Manuscripts

The following list consists principally of manuscripts consulted in the course of preparing this work. For some additional manuscripts of the medical works the reader is referred to TK and to Kibre, "Hippocrates Latinus," in part four of the Bibliography, below. Some additional manuscripts of works of Dino and Guglielmo are listed in Guy Beaujouan, "Manuscrits médicaux du Moyen Age conservés en Espagne," pp. 179-180, 186, 193, 198 (see Bibliography, part four). Manuscripts of Taddeo's supposed translation of the *Nicomachean Ethics* are listed in Marchesi, "Il compendio volgare dell'Etica," pp. 72-74 (Bibliography, part three), to which may be added no. 28 in W. H. Bond, ed., *Supplement to the Census of Medieval and Renaissance Manuscripts in the United States and Canada* (New York, 1962). I have also listed below a few manuscripts that I have not seen (drawing my information chiefly from the card index of medical manuscripts on microfilm at the National Library of Medicine), where these contain copies of works by Taddeo and his pupils not noted in TK. Manuscripts that I have not personally examined are marked with an asterisk; manuscripts that I have consulted only in microfilm or other photoreproduction are marked with a dagger.

As most of the codices are fourteenth- or fifteenth-century medical miscellanies in which various items may have been copied at different times, I have not normally indicated dating for each codex as a whole. The dates of composition and copying of individual works by Taddeo and his pupils are indicated, where possible, in the main text and notes of this study.

Aberystwyth, National Library of Wales

† 2050B, comm. *De complexionibus*, perhaps by Taddeo, fols. 126-135v.

Bethesda, Maryland, National Library of Medicine

492, Taddeo, comm. *Tegni, Isagoge, Pronost., Aphor., Reg. acut.*, 3 vols. This collection of Taddeo's major commentaries is contained in a set of three codices. They are very fully described in Dorothy M. Schullian and Francis E. Sommer, *A Catalogue of Incunabula and Manuscripts in the Army Medical Library* (New York, n.d.), pp. 216-218. Schullian and Sommer date the collection as a whole 14c, although vol. 3 includes the dates 1282 and 1283 at fols. 86 and 121.

Recent acquisitions, uncatalogued. Taddeo [?], comm. *Canon* 1.4.1-5 and 20, fols. 1-147; marginalia in Spanish.

Bologna, Biblioteca Universitaria

720(1418), Taddeo, *Consilia*, fols. 1r-30v.

Cesena, Biblioteca Malatestiana

* D Pluteo xxiv,3, Mondino, *Tractatus Mundini ad inveniendum dosim,* fols. 161v-162r.

* De Pluteo xxvi,1, Taddeo comm. *Pronost.*, fols. 65r-80v; Taddeo, comm. *Isagoge*, fols. 81r-108r; Dino, *De malicia complexionis diverse,* fols. 159r-165v; Dino, comm. *De diferentiis [sic] febrium*, fol. 165v-170v.

* D Pluteo xxvi,3, Mondino, *consilium*, fols. 35v-36v.

* S Pluteo xxvii,4, Dino, comm. *De natura fetus*, fols. 103r-140r; Mondino, *De speciebus febrium ethicorum* (questions), fols. 173v-174v.

* S Pluteo xxvii,5, Mondino, comm. *Pronost.*, fols. 53-114r; Mondino, comm. *Reg. acut.*, fols. 115r-140v; Mondino, comm. *Tegni*, fols. 141r-226r.

Florence, Biblioteca Medicea Laurenziana

Ashburnham 217 (149), Taddeo, *De lepra* (comm. *Canon* 4.3.3.), fols. 91v-93r;
Dino, *Unguenta*, fols. 115-132.

London, British Library

Harley 4087, Dino, *Chirurgia*, fols. 39r-108r.

Milan, Biblioteca Ambrosiana

C115 inf. (ex Q), Guglielmo, questions on *Canon* 1.4, fols. 60v-73v.

Modena, Biblioteca Estense

Lat. 14 (alpha F.1.27), Taddeo, *Libellus sanitatis*, fols. 61r-63r;
  Taddeo, *Consilium* (on aqua vita), fols. 63r-v.
Lat. 710 (alpha V.7.21), Dino, *Chirurgia*, fols. 1r-102r.
Lat. 959 (alpha K.6.2), Dino, comm. *De natura fetus*, fols. 1r-37v (explicit,
  bound out of order, at fol. 4r); Dino, comm. *Tegni*, fols. 42r-49r.

Munich, Bayerische Staatsbibliothek

† CLM 77, *Consilia Mundini* [*sic*], fols. 46r-59v.
† CLM 205, Dino, *Consilium*, fols. 246r-v.
† CLM 244, Mondino, question, fols. 135r-138r.
† CLM 7609, Dino, *De risu*, fol. 140r (139r).
† CLM 13020, Mondino, comm. *Pronost.*, fols. 1r-57; Mondino, comm. *Reg. acut.*,
  fols. 57-72v; Taddeo, *Practica* [*de febribus*], fols. 73r-82r; Mondino,
  Anatomia, fols. 82r-88v; Dino, *Dilucidatorium*, fols. 95r ff.; Dino, questions,
  fols. 187v-188v, 193r-194v, 217v-220r, 223v-225v.
† CLM 23912, *Consilia Mundini Bononiensis*, fols. 208r ff.; Bartolomeo,
  consilium for Henry VII, fols. 253r-254v.

Padua, Biblioteca Universitaria

Al numero provvisorio 202, Dino, question, fols. 80v-82v; Taddeo, *Practica
de febribus*, fols. 107v-115r; Guglielmo, comm. *Canon* 1.4, fols. 117v-124v.

Paris, Bibliothèque Nationale

Lat. 6860, *Anatomia Mundini*, fols. 71r-89r; Dino, comm. *Canon* 2, fols.
  99r-189r.
Lat. 6872, Dino, comm. *Tegni*, fols. 1r-58v; Bartolomeo da Varignana,
  comm. *Canon* 4.1, fols. 127v-133r; Guglielmo, questions on *Canon* 1.1,
  fols. 133r-v; Guglielmo, comm. *Aphor.*, fols. 134-224v; Bartolomeo da

Varignana, comm. *Aphor.*, fols. 227r-271v.

Lat. 6935, Dino, *Dilucidatorium*, fols. 1r-145v; Dino, comm. *Canon* 2, fols. 146r-199v.

Lat. 6935A, Dino, *Dilucidatorium*, fols. 1r-201r (entire codex).

Lat. 6964, Taddeo, *Experimenta*, fols. 100-117r; Taddeo, *Practica* [*de febribus*], fols. 117r-129v; Taddeo's verse epitaph, fol. 129v.

Lat. 6995, Dino, *Compilatio emplastrorum et unguentorum*, fols. 137r-156r (interpolation, fol. 154r).

Paris University, Bibliothèque de la Sorbonne

128, Dino, questions, fols. 113-115; Mondino (Mundinus de Leutiis Bononiensis), questions, fols. 128-130; Taddeo, *Experimenta*, fols. 147-155.

131, comm. Johannitius, fols. 61-88r; comm. Egidius on urines, fols. 88r-96v; comm. Egidius on pulse, fols. 96v-102r; comm. John Damascene, *Aphor.*, fols. 102r-108v. All attributed to "magistri Thaddei," fol. 108v, but doubtfully so.

Rome, Biblioteca Angelica

1489, *Cura crepatorum magni Thadei* (opening section of Brunus, *Practica*), fols. 152r-157v; Dino, *Compilatio emplastrorum et unguentorum*, fols. 170r-213r.

Vatican City, Biblioteca Apostolica Vaticana

Vat. lat. 2366, Taddeo, comm. *Isagoge*, fols. 48r-93r; Cecco d'Ascoli, *De principiis astrologie*, fols. 133r-142v.

Vat. lat. 2418, Taddeo, *Consilia*, fols. 93-114; Mondino (Mundinus de Lentiis), *Practica de accidentibus*, fols. 145r-148r; Dino, *De unguentis*, fols. 153r-163v.

Vat. lat. 2484, Dino, *Dilucidatorium*, fols. 1r-184v; Dino, *De malicia complexionis*, fols. 196v-210r; Dino, question, fols. 214r-217r.

Vat. lat. 3144, Dino, questions, fols. 12r-14v; Turisanus, *De hypostasi urine*, fols. 16v-19v.

Vat. lat. 4422, Taddeo, *Experimenta*, fols. 58r-88r.

Vat. lat. 4450, Dino, comm. *De differentiis febrium*, fols. 1r-21v.

Vat. lat. 4451, Taddeo, comm. *De crisi*, fols. 89r-101r; (Taddeo), comm. Avicenna, "Quod comeditur . . . ," fols. 87v-88v; Bartolomeo da Varignana, comm. *De complexionibus*, fols. 57r-87v.

Vat. lat. 4452, Bartolomeo da Varignana, comm. *De accidenti et morbo*, fols. 67r-82v; [Bartolomeo da Varignana], comm. *De interioribus*, fols. 83r-102r; [Dino?], *De malicia complexionis*, fols. 133r-142v.

Vat. lat. 4454, Dino, comm. *Aphor.*, fols. 52r-54r; Bartolomeo da Varignana, comm. *De interioribus*, fols. 55r-76v; Bartolomeo da Varignana, comm. *De complexionibus*, fols. 77r-85v; Dino and others, questions, fols. 99v-104r; Johannes Vath, questions on *De animalibus* reported by Gentile da Cingoli, fols. 87r-99v.

Vat. lat. 4455, Mondino, *De cerusa*, fols. 41r-v.

Vat. lat. 4464, Taddeo, comm. *Tegni*, fols. 1r-71r; Dino, *De malicia complexionis diverse*, fols. 74r-86v; Dino, comm. *De natura fetus*, fols. 88r-124r.

Vat. lat. 4465, Taddeo, comm. *Aphor.*, fols. 1-73 (entire codex).

Vat. lat. 4466, Mondino, comm. *Pronost.*, fols. 1r-36r; Mondino, comm. *Reg. acut.*, fols. 37r-55v; Mondino, comm. *Tegni*, fols. 57r-156v.

Vat. lat. 4472, Turisanus, *Plusquam commentum*, fols. 19v-105r.

Vat. lat. 5378, Dino, *De oleis, emplastris, unguentis*, fols. 161r-185r.

Palat. lat. 1240, Taddeo, *De lepra capitulum*, fols. 100v-102r.

Palat. lat. 1246, Taddeo, comm. Avicenna "Quod comeditur . . . ," fols. 78v-97v; Gentile, medical question, fols. 97v-112v.

Palat. lat. 1284, Taddeo, *Introductorium ad practicam*, fols. 143-153v.

Palat. lat. 1284, Taddeo, *Introductorium ad practicam*, fols. 143-153v.

Palat. lat. 1363, Taddeo, *Tabula de remediis*, fols. 167v-171r.

Reg. lat. 2000, Mondino, comm. *Canon* 3.21.1, *De generatione embrionis*, fols. 1r-23r; list of works of Galen "qui reperiuntur," fol. 73r; Taddeo, question, fols. 115v-116r.

Rossi 974, Dino, *Cirurgicalia* (i.e., emplastra, unguenta, etc.), fols. 73r-80r; Taddeo, *Consilia*, fols. 81r-150v.

Urb. lat. 244, Turisanus, *Plusquam commentum*, fols. 1-201.

Urb. lat. 247, Works of Galen (entire codex); *De interioribus*, "correptus" by Taddeo, fols. 254-281.

Venice, Biblioteca Marciana

Lat. vii,3 (2613), Taddeo, *Cura ad conceptum*, fols. 98v-99r.

Lat. vii,33 (2864) Dino, *Unguenta*, fols. 112r-147v.

Venice, Padri Redentoristi, Chiesa di Santa Maria della Fave

3 (445), Bartolomeo da Varignana, comm. *Economica*, fols. 33r-50r.

Part Three: Printed Works

The following general bibliography makes no claim to be comprehensive. In particular, editions of the works that constituted the sources of the philosophical and medical learning of Taddeo and his colleagues (for example, the writings of Aristotle, Hippocrates, Galen, and Avicenna) are not included. However, editions of such works that were used in preparing the present study are indicated when necessary in the notes. Furthermore, of the works cited in the notes, a few that pertain only indirectly to or touch only in passing on the circle of Taddeo have been omitted from the bibliography. Finally, considerations of space made it impossible to provide more than a very restricted listing of works pertaining to the earlier history of the various branches of knowledge studied by Taddeo and his colleagues.

Alderotti, Taddeo. *I "Consilia."* Ed. Giuseppe M. Nardi. Turin, 1937.

——. *Libello per conservare la sanità del corpo fatto per maestro Taddeo da Firenze, teste inedito del buon secolo della lingua toscana.* Ed. F. Z[ambrini]. Imola, 1852. For another edition, *see* Spina, G., and Sampalmieri, A., "La lettera di Taddeo Alderotti."

——. *Libellus de sanitate factus per Magistrum Thadeum de Florentia.* Printed with *Pulcherrimum et utilissimum opus ad sanitatis conservationem editum ab eximio artium professore magistro Benedicto de Nursia.* . . . Bologna, 1477. Despite assertions to the contrary in some secondary sources, this is a Latin version of the Italian regimen attributed to Taddeo.

——. *Thaddei Florentini Expositiones in arduum aphorismorum Ipocratis volumen, In divinum pronosticorum Ipocratis librum, In preclarum regiminis acutorum Ipocratis opus, In subtilissimum Joannitii Isagogarum libellum.* Venice, 1527.

——. *Thaddei Florentini medicorum sua tempestate principis in C. Gal. Micratechnen Commentarii.* . . . Naples, 1522.

For the commentary on part of Avicenna, *Canon,* Book 4, attributed to Taddeo, *see* Avicenna.

For the translation of the *Nicomachean Ethics* often attributed to Taddeo, *see* Marchesi, Concetto, "Il compendio volgare dell'Etica aristotelica."

Alston, Mary N. "The Attitude of the Church Toward Dissection Before 1500." *Bulletin of the History of Medicine* 16 (1944-1945):221-238.

Alverny, Marie Thérèse d'. "Pietro d'Abano et les 'naturalistes' à l'époque de Dante." In *Dante e la cultura veneta,* ed. Vittorio Branca and G. Padoan. Florence, 1966.

Amundsun, Darrel W. "Medieval Canon Law on Medical and Surgical Practice by the Clergy." *Bulletin of the History of Medicine* 52 (1978):22-44.

Arnald of Villanova. *Opera Medica Omnia.* Ed. L. Garcia-Ballester, J. A. Paniagua, and Michael R. McVaugh. Vol. 2, *Aphorismi de gradibus,* ed. Michael R. McVaugh. Granada-Barcelona, 1975.

Arnaldi, G. "Le origini dello studio di Padova. Dalla migrazione universitaria del 1222 alla fine del periodo ezzeliniano." *La cultura* 15 (1977):388-431.

——, ed. *Le origini dell'università.* Bologna, 1974.

Avicenna. *Presens maximus codex est totius scientie medicine principis Alboali Abinsene cum expositionibus omnium principalium et illustrium interpretum eius.* 5 vols. Venice, 1523. Includes Dino del Garbo's commentary on Book 2 (vol. 2) and Taddeo Alderotti's on 4.2 (vol. 5).

Beaujouan, Guy. "Fautes et obscurités dans les traductions médicales du moyen âge." *Revue de synthèse* 89 (1968):145-152.

————. *L'interdépendance entre la science scolastique et les techniques utili-taires.* Conférence faite au Palais de la Découverte. Université de Paris, January 15, 1957.

Beccaria, Augusto. "Sulle tracce di un antico canone latino di Ippocrate e di Galeno." *Italia medioevale e umanistica* 4 (1961):1-75; 14 (1971):1-23.

Bellomo, Manlio. *Aspetti dell'insegnamento giuridico nelle Università medi-evali. Le "quaestiones disputatae."* 1, *Saggi.* Reggio Calabria, 1974.

————. *Saggio sull'università nell'età del diritto comune.* Catania, 1979.

Belloni, L., and Vergnano, L. "Alderotti, Taddeo (Thaddaeus Florentinus)." In *Dizionario biografico degli italiani,* 2:85. Rome, 1960.

Bird, Otto. "The Canzone d'Amore of Cavalcanti According to the Com-mentary of Dino del Garbo: Text and Commentary." *Mediaeval Studies* 2 (1940):150-203; 3 (1941):117-160.

Birkenmajer, Aleksander. "Le rôle joué par les médecins et les naturalistes dans la réception d'Aristote au XIIᵉ et XIIIᵉ siècles." In *La Pologne au VIᵉ Congrès International des Sciences Historiques, Oslo, 1928,* pp. 1-15. Warsaw, 1930. Reprint, Aleksander Birkenmajer, *Etudes d'histoire des sciences et de la philosophie du Moyen Age. Studia Copernicana,* 1:73-87. Wroclaw-Warsaw-Cracow, 1970.

Bonora, Fausto, and Kern, George. "Does Anyone Really Know the Life of Gentile da Foligno?" *Medicina ne' secoli* 9 (1972):29-53.

Brody, Saul N. *The Disease of the Soul: Leprosy in Medieval Literature.* Ithaca, 1974.

Bullough, Vern L. *The Development of Medicine as a Profession: The Con-tribution of the Medieval University to Modern Medicine.* Basel and New York, 1966.

————. "Medieval Bologna and the Development of Medical Education." *Bulletin of the History of Medicine* 33 (1958):201-215.

————. "Medieval Medical and Scientific Views of Women." *Viator: Medieval and Renaissance Studies* 4 (1973):485-501.

————. "Mondino de' Luzzi." *DSB* 9 (1974):467-469.

————. "Taddeo Alderotti." *DSB* 1 (1970):107.

Busacchi, Vincenzo. "I primordi dell'insegnamento medico a Bologna." *Rivista di storia delle scienze mediche e naturali* 39 (1948):128-144.

Bylebyl, Jerome J. "Galen on the Non-Natural Causes of Variation of the Pulse." *Bulletin of the History of Medicine* 45 (1971):482-485.

Cadden, Joan. "The Medieval Philosophy and Biology of Growth: Albertus Magnus, Thomas Aquinas, Albert of Saxony, and Marsilius of Inghen on Book I, Chapter v, of Aristotle's *De generatione et corruptione.*" Ph.D. diss. Indiana Univ., 1971.

Calcaterra, G. *Alma mater studiorum.* Bologna, 1948.

Capparoni, P. *L'anatomia in Italia da Mondino a Mascagni.* Milan, 1938.

Cartulaire de l'Université de Montpellier, vol. 1, no. 25, pp. 219-221. Montpellier, 1890. Document pertaining to Guglielmo da Brescia.

Castelli, G. *La vita e le opere di Cecco d'Ascoli.* Bologna, 1892.

Cavazza, Francesco. "Le scuole dell'antico studio di Bologna." *Atti e memorie della R. Deputazione di storia patria per le provincie di Romagna.* 3d ser. 11 (1894):69-119, 242-302. Subsequently published as *Le scuole dell'antico Studio bolognese.* Milan, 1896.

Cecco d'Ascoli [Stabile, Francesco]. *L'Acerba.* Ed. Achille Crespi. Ascoli Piceno, 1927.

———. Il commento di Cecco d'Ascoli all'Alcabizzo. Ed. Giuseppe Boffito. Florence, 1905.

Cencetti, Giorgio. "Studium fuit Bononie." *Studi medievali* 7 (1966):781-833.

Ceva, Bianca. *Brunetto Latini, l'uomo e l'opera.* Milan-Naples, 1965.

Chartularium Studii Bononiensis: Documenti per la storia dell'università di Bologna dalle origine fino al secolo XV. Commissione per la Storia dell' Università di Bologna. 13 vols. to date. Bologna, 1909–.

Chartularium Studii Senensis. Ed. Giovanni Cecchini and Giulio Prunai. Vol. 1. Siena, 1942. Some documents pertaining to Dino del Garbo.

Ciasca, Raffaello. *L'arte dei medici e speziali nella storia nel commercio fiorentino dal secolo XII al XV.* Florence, 1927.

Cipolla, Carlo. *Public Health and the Medical Profession in the Renaissance.* Cambridge, 1976.

Clarke, Basil. *Mental Disorder in Earlier Britain.* Cardiff, 1975.

Cobban, A. B. *The Medieval Universities: Their Development and Organization.* London, 1975.

Colini-Baldeschi, Elia. "Per la biografia di Cecco d'Ascoli." *Rivista delle biblioteche e degli archivi* 22 (1921):65-72. Includes a document pertaining to the arts and medical faculty of Bologna.

Copelman, S. L., and Copelman-Fromant, L. "La contribution de la médecine toscana à la médecine médiévale." In XXI *Congresso internazionale di storia della medicina, Siena, 1968,* Atti, 1:229-231.

Corner, George W. *Anatomical Texts of the Earlier Middle Ages.* Washington, D.C., 1927.

Corsini, A. "Nuovo contributo di notizie intorno alla vita di maestro Tommaso del Garbo." *Rivista di storia delle scienze mediche e naturali* 16 (1925):268-278.

Corvi, Guglielmo de' [Guglielmo da Brescia]. *Excellentissimi medici Guielmi brixiensis dictorum illustrium medicorum ad unamquamque egritudinem a capite ad pedes practica. . . .* Venice, 1508.

———. *Questiones de tyriaca.* See McVaugh, Michael R., "Theriac at Montpellier."

For the *consilia* of Guglielmo da Brescia, see Schmidt, Erich Walter Georg.

Crombie, Alistair Cameron. *Robert Grosseteste and the Origins of Experimental Science.* 2nd ed. Oxford, 1961.

Dales, Richard C. "Marius 'On the Elements' and the Twelfth-Century Science of Matter." *Viator: Medieval and Renaissance Studies* 3 (1972):191-218.

Dallari, Umberto. "Due documenti inediti riguardanti Liuzzo e Mondino de' Liuzzi." *Rivista di storia delle scienze mediche e naturali* 14 (1932):1-7.

Dall'Osso, Eugenio. "Una questione dibattuta: quanti anatomici e medici di nome "Mondino" esistevano all'inizio del '300." *Bollettino dell'Accademia Medica Pistoiese Filippo Pacini* 26 (1955):245-255.

Dall'Osso, Eugenio, and Münster, Ladislao. "Una lezione inedita di Mondino de' Liuzzi sulla febbre autumnale." *Castalia: Rivista di storia della medicina* 14 (1958):151-159.

Davis, Charles T. "Education in Dante's Florence." *Speculum* 40 (1965):415-435.

Demaitre, Luke. "Nature and the Art of Medicine in the Middle Ages." *Medievalia* 2 (1976):23-47.

———. "Scholasticism in Compendia of Practical Medicine, 1250-1450." In *Science, Medicine, and the University, 1200-1550: Essays in Honor of Pearl Kibre,* ed. N. Siraisi and L. Demaitre. *Manuscripta* 20 (1976):81-95.

———. "Theory and Practice in Medical Education at the University of Montpellier in the Thirteenth and Fourteenth Centuries." *Journal of the History of Medicine and Allied Sciences* 30 (1975):103-123.

Denifle, H. *Die Entstehung der Universitäten des Mittelalters bis 1400.* Berlin, 1885.

Dino del Garbo. See Garbo, Dino del.

Ermatinger, Charles. "Averroism in Early Fourteenth-Century Bologna." *Mediaeval Studies* 16 (1954):35-56.

———. "The Missing Leaves of Codex Vaticanus Latinus 3066." *Manuscripta* 2 (1958):156-162.

———. "Some Unstudied Sources for the History of Philosophy in the Fourteenth Century." *Manuscripta* 14 (1970):3-23, 67-87.

Ermini, Giuseppe, *Storia dell'Università di Perugia.* 2 vols. Florence, 1971.

Fasoli, Gina. "Bologna e la Romagna durante la spedizione di Enrico VII." *Atti e memorie della Deputazione di storia patria per l'Emilia e la Romagna* 4 (1938-39):15-54.

———. *Per la storia dell' Università di Bologna nel Medio Evo.* Bologna, 1970.

Fasoli, G., and Sella, P., eds. *Statuti di Bologna dell'anno 1288.* 2 vols. Biblioteca Apostolica Vaticana, Studi e Testi 73 (1937) and 85 (1939).

Favaro, Antonio. "Nuovi documenti intorno all' emigrazione di professori e di scolari dallo Studio di Bologna avvenuta nel 1321." *Atti e memorie della R. Deputazione di storia patria per le provincie di Romagna*, 3d ser. 10 (1891-1892):313-323.

Favati, Guido. "Guido Cavalcanti, Dino del Garbo, e l'Averroismo di Bruno Nardi." *Filologia romanza* 2 (1955):67-83.

————, ed. *Il Novellino: testo critico, introduzione e note*. Genoa, 1970. No. 35 in this thirteenth-century collection of anecdotes is about Taddeo.

Filippini, F. "Cecco d'Ascoli a Bologna." *Studi e memorie per la storia dell'- Università di Bologna* 10 (1930):3-35.

Forni, G. G. *L'insegnamento della chirurgia nello studio di Bologna dalle origini a tutto il secolo XIX*. Bologna [1948].

Franchini, V. *Le arti di mestiere in Bologna nel secolo XIII*. Pubblicazione della Regia Università degli Studi Economici e Commerciale di Trieste. Vol. 1. Trieste, 1931.

Frati, L. "Per due antichi volgarizzamenti. II. L' 'Etica' volgarizzata da Taddeo di Alderotto." *Giornale storico della letteratura italiana* 48 (1916):- 192-195.

————. *La vita privata di Bologna dal secolo XIII al XVII*. Bologna, 1900.

Gabriel, A. L. "The College System in Medieval Universities." In *The For- ward Movement of the Fourteenth Century*, ed. Francis L. Utley, pp. 79- 124. Columbus, Ohio, 1961.

————. *Garlandia: Studies in the History of the Medieval University*. Frank- furt-am-Main, 1969.

————. "The Motivation of the Founders of Medieval Colleges." In *Beiträge zum Berufbewusstsein des mittelalterlichen Menschen, Miscellanea Mediae- valia*, 3:61-72. Berlin, 1964.

Garbo, Dino del. *Dyni florentini super quarta fen primi Avicenne preclarissima commentaria: que dilucidatorium totius practice generalis medicinalis scientie nuncupatur*. . . . Printed with *Expositio Dini super canones generales de virtutibus medicinarum simplicium secundi canonis Avicenne*. Venice, 1514.

————. *Expositio super III, IV et parte V Fen Avicennae*. Ferrara, 1489. Title from Hain *6166. There is no title page in the copy of this edition that I have consulted at the New York Academy of Medicine. On fol. a ii^r, how- ever, appears: *Clarissimi artium et medicine doctoris magistri Dini de Florentia expositio super 3^a et 4^a fen Avicenne et super parte quinte feliciter incipit*.

————. *Incipit compilatio emplastrorum et unguentorum Magistri Dini flo- rentini*. . . . Ferrara, 1489.

————. *De ponderibus et mensuris*. Printed with *Expositio Dini florentini super tertia et quarta et parte quinti canonis Avicenne*. . . . Venice, 1499.

————. "Quaestio famossissimi Dini de Florentia de coena et prandio." In *Opera Andreae Thurini Pisciensis* . . . , fols. 148-153v. Rome, 1545.

————. *Scriptum Dini super libro de natura fetus Hypocratis.* Printed with Jacopo [Giacomo] da Forli, *Expositio . . . supra capitulum Avicenne De generatione embrionis.* . . . Venice, 1502.

For Dino del Garbo's commentary on the Canzone d'Amore of Cavalcanti, see Bird, Otto.

Garbo, Tommaso del. *Liber de differentiis febrium a Galeno edito tres translationes videlicet antiquam Leoniceni et Laurentiani breviter ac faciliter exposite: et digressionibus scientificis Thadei: Dyni: et Thome de Garbo.* . . . Pavia, 1519. The *digressiones*, fols. 126v-224v, were compiled in 1345, apparently by Tommaso del Garbo. Taddeo is mentioned only once, but 12 of the 70 digressions expound the views of Dino.

Gaudenzi, A. "Gli antichi statuti del Comune di Bologna intorno allo studio." *Bullettino dell'Istituto Storico Italiano* 6 (1888):117-137.

Gentile da Cingoli. See Grabmann, Martin, "Gentile da Cingoli."

Gentile da Foligno. *Questiones et tractatus extravagantes clarissimi Domini Gentilis de Fulgineo.* . . . Venice, 1520. Question 46 records the views of Taddeo and his pupils on the reduction of medicine to act.

Ghirardacci, Cherubino. *Della historia di Bologna.* Vol. 1. Bologna, 1596.

Girolami, G. *Sopra Gentile da Fuligno, medico illustre del secolo XIV.* Naples, 1844.

Glorieux, Palémon. *La littérature quodlibétique de 1260 à 1320.* 2 vols. Bibliothèque Thomiste 5 (1925) and 21 (1935).

Goldbrunner, Hermann. "Durandus de Alvernia, Nicolaus von Oresme und Leonardo Bruni: Zu den Übersetzungen der pseudo-aristotelischen Ökonomik." *Archiv für Kulturgeschichte* 50 (1968):200-239.

Grabmann, Martin. "L'Aristotelismo italiano al tempo di Dante con particolare riguardo all'Università di Bologna." *Rivista di filosofia neo-scolastica* 38 (1946):260-277. Also appeared as "Das Aristotelesstudium in Italien zur zeit Dantes" in his *Mittelalterliches Geistesleben: Abhandlungen zur Geschichte der Scholastik und Mystik,* 3:197-212, Munich, 1956.

————. "Gentile da Cingoli, ein italienischer Aristoteleserklärer aus der Zeit Dantes." In *Sitzungsberichte der Bayerischen Akademie der Wissenschaften, Philosophisch-historische Abteilung,* vol. 9 (1940). Munich, 1941. Includes the text of Gentile's *questio "Utrum species sensibilis. . . ."*

————. *Die Geschichte der scholastischen Methode.* 2 vols. Freiburg-im-Breisgau, 1908-1911. Reprint. Graz, 1957.

Grant, Edward, ed. *A Source Book in Medieval Science.* Cambridge, Mass., 1974.

Guerrieri, Lorenzo. "Considerazioni sugli scolari bolognesi di Taddeo degli Alderotti in base ad una novella medioevale." In xxi *Congresso Internazionale di Storia della Medicina, Siena, 1968, Atti,* 1:126-129.

Guerrini, Paolo. "Guglielmo da Brescia e il Collegio Bresciano in Bologna." *Studi e memorie per la storia dell'Università di Bologna* 7 (1922):57-116. Prints Guglielmo's will and the foundation statute of his college.

Guglielmo de' Corvi [Guglielmo da Brescia]. See Corvi, Guglielmo de'.

Guido, Francesco. "Cenni biografici su Dino e Tommaso del Garbo." In xxi *Congresso Internazionale di Storia della Medicina, Siena, 1968, Atti,* 1:156-163.

Hall, Thomas S. "Life, Death, and the Radical Moisture: A Study of Thematic Patterns in Medical Theory." *Clio Medica* 6 (1971):3-23.

Harvey, E. Ruth. *The Inward Wits: Psychological Theory in the Middle Ages and Renaissance.* Warburg Institute Surveys, no. 6. London, 1975.

Haskins, Charles H. *Studies in Mediaeval Culture.* Oxford, 1929.

———. *Studies in the History of Mediaeval Science.* Reprint. New York, 1960.

Herrlinger, Robert, and Kudlien, Fridolf, eds. *Frühe Anatomie: Eine Anthologie.* Stuttgart, 1967.

Hewson, M. Anthony. *Giles of Rome and the Medieval Theory of Conception.* London, 1975.

Hyde, J. K. "Commune, University, and Society in Early Medieval Bologna." In *Universities in Politics: Case Studies from the Late Middle Ages and Early Modern Period,* ed. John W. Baldwin and Richard A. Goldthwaite, pp. 17-46. Baltimore and London, 1972.

Ijsewijn, J., and Paquet, Jacques, eds. *The Universities of the Late Middle Ages.* Louvain, 1978.

Jarcho, Saul. "Galen's Six Non-Naturals: A Bibliographic Note and Translation." *Bulletin of the History of Medicine* 44 (1970):370-377.

Kibre, Pearl. "Arts and Medicine in the Universities of the Later Middle Ages." In *The Universities in the Late Middle Ages,* ed. J. Ijsewijn and Jacques Paquet. Louvain, 1978.

———. "Hippocratic Writings in the Middle Ages." *Bulletin of the History of Medicine* 18 (1945):371-412.

———. *The Nations in the Mediaeval Universities.* Cambridge, Mass., 1948. Extensive bibliography of the medieval *studium* of Bologna on pp. 189-194.

———. *Scholarly Privileges in the Middle Ages.* Cambridge, Mass., 1962.

Klibansky, Raymond; Panofsky, Erwin; and Saxl, Fritz. *Saturn and Melancholy: Studies in the History of Philosophy, Religion, and Art.* New York, 1964.

Klubertanz, George P., S.J. *The Discursive Power: Sources and Doctrine of the Vis Cogitativa According to St. Thomas Aquinas.* St. Louis, Mo., 1952.

Kristeller, Paul Oskar. "Un 'ars dictaminis' di Giovanni del Virgilio." *Italia medioevale e umanistica* 4 (1961):181-200.

———. "Bartholomaeus, Musandinus, and Maurus of Salerno and Other Early Commentators on the 'Articella,' with a Tentative List of Texts and Manuscripts." *Italia medioevale e umanistica* 19 (1976):57-87.

———. "Matteo de' Libri, Bolognese Notary of the Thirteenth Century, and his *Artes Dictaminis*." In *Miscellanea Giovanni Galbiati*, 3 vols., 2:283-320. Milan, 1951.

———. "Il Petrarca, l'umanesimo e la scolastica a Venezia." In *La civiltà veneziana del Trecento*. Florence, n.d.

———. "Petrarch's 'Averroists': A Note on the History of Aristotelianism in Venice, Padua, and Bologna." *Mélanges A. Renaudet. Bibliothèque d'Humanisme et de Renaissance* 14 (1952):59-65.

———. "A Philosophical Treatise from Bologna Dedicated to Guido Cavalcanti: Magister Jacobus de Pistorio and his "Quaestio de felicitate.' " In *Medioevo e Rinascimento: Studi in onore di Bruno Nardi*, 2 vols., 1:425-463. Florence, 1955. Includes an edition of the text of the treatise.

———. "Philosophy and Medicine in Medieval and Renaissance Italy." In *Organism, Medicine, and Metaphysics*, ed. S. F. Spicker, pp. 29-40. Dordrecht, 1978.

———. *Renaissance Thought: The Classic, Scholastic and Humanist Strains*. New York, 1961.

———. "The School of Salerno: Its Development and Its Contribution to the History of Learning." In his *Studies in Renaissance Thought and Letters*, pp. 495-551. Rome, 1956.

———. "The University of Bologna and the Renaissance." *Studi e memorie per la storia dell'Università di Bologna*, n.s. 1 (1956):313-323.

Kuksewicz, Zdzislaw. *Averroisme bolonais au XIVᵉ siècle*. Wroclaw-Warsaw-Cracow, 1965.

———. *De Siger de Brabant à Jacques de Plaisance: La théorie de l'intellect chez les averroistes latins des XIIIᵉ et XIVᵉ siècles*. Wroclaw-Warsaw-Cracow, 1968.

Langlois, E., ed. *Les registres de Nicholas IV*. Fascicule 4, no. 2873, p. 474. Paris, 1890. Document pertaining to Taddeo.

Latini, Brunetto. *Li Livres dou tresor*. Ed. Francis J. Carmody. Berkeley, Calif., 1948.

Lawn, Brian. *The Salernitan Questions: An Introduction to the History of Medieval and Renaissance Problem Literature*. Oxford, 1963.

Lemay, Richard. "The Teaching of Astronomy in Medieval Universities, Principally at Paris in the Fourteenth Century." In *Science, Medicine, and the University, 1200-1550: Essays in Honor of Pearl Kibre. Manuscripta* 20 (1976):197-217.

Lindberg, David C. *Theories of Vision from Al-Kindi to Kepler.* Chicago, 1976.

Liuzzi, Mondino de'. *Anathomia Mundini.* In *The Fasciculo di Medicina, Venice, 1493,* ed. Charles Singer, 2 vols. Florence, 1925. Italian and English versions.

——. *Anatomia.* Ed. Lino Sighinolfi. Bologna, 1930. Edition of the fifteenth-century Italian translation, with facsimile of a Latin MS.

——. *Anatomies de Mondino de' Luzzi et de Guido da Vigevano.* Ed. Ernest Wickersheimer. Paris, 1926. Contains a facsimile of the edition of Mondino's *Anatomia* printed at Pavia in 1478.

——. *Mesue cum expositione Mondini super canones universales.* . . . Venice, 1508.

——. *Practica de accidentibus.* Ed. G. Caturegli. Pisa, 1966.

Lottin, O. *Psychologie et morale au XII* et XIII* siècles.* Vol. 1. *Problèmes de psychologie.* Louvain, 1942.

Lugano, P. "Gentilis Fulginas, Speculator, e le sue ultime volontà secondo un documento inedito del 2 agosto 1348." *Bollettino della Deputazione di storia patria per l'Umbria* 14 (1908):195-260.

McKeon, Richard P. "Medicine and Philosophy in the Eleventh and Twelfth Centuries: The Problem of the Elements." *The Thomist* 24 (1961):211-256.

McNeill, William H. *Plagues and Peoples.* Garden City, N.Y., 1976.

McVaugh, Michael R. "'Apud Antiquos' and Medieval Pharmacology." *Medizinhistorisches Journal* 1 (1966):16-23.

——. "An Early Discussion of Medicinal Degree at Montpellier by Henry of Winchester." *Bulletin of the History of Medicine* 49 (1975):57-71.

——. "The '*Humidum Radicale*' in Thirteenth-Century Medicine." *Traditio* 30 (1974):259-283.

——. "Theriac at Montpellier, 1285-1325 (with an Edition of the '*Questiones de tyriaca*' of William of Brescia)." *Sudhoffs Archiv für Geschichte der Medizin und der Naturwissenschaften* 56 (1972):113-143.

Maier, Anneliese. "Ein Beitrag zur Geschichte des italienischen Averroismus im 14. Jahrhundert." *Quellen und Forschungen aus italienischen Archiven und Bibliotheken* 33 (1944):136-157.

——. *An der Grenze von Scholastik und Naturwissenchaft: Die Struktur der materiellen Substanz, das Problem der Gravitation, die Mathematik der Formlatituden.* Rome, 1952.

——. *Die Vorläufer Galileis im 14. Jahrhundert: Studien zur Naturphilosophie der Spätscholastik.* Rome, 1966.

Majno, Guido. *The Healing Hand: Man and Wound in the Ancient World.* Cambridge, Mass., 1975.

Makdisi, George. "The Scholastic Method in Medieval Education: An Inquiry into Its Origins in Law and Theology." *Speculum* 49 (1974):640-661.

Malagola, Carlo. *Monografie storiche sullo Studio bolognese*. Bologna, 1888.

———, ed. *Statuti delle Università dei Collegi dello Studio bolognese*. Bologna, 1888.

Marangon, Paolo. *Alle origini dell'Aristotelismo Padovano*. Padua, 1977.

Marchesi, Concetto. "Il compendio volgare dell'Etica aristotelica e le fonti del vi libro del 'Tresor.'" *Giornale storico della letteratura italiana* 42 (1903):1-74. Prints excerpts from the translation attributed to Taddeo.

———. *L'Etica Nicomachea nella tradizione Medievale*. Messina, 1904.

Martinotti, Giovanni. "L'insegnamento dell'anatomia in Bologna prima del secolo xix." *Studi e memorie per la storia dell'Università di Bologna* 2 (1911):1-146.

Mazzoni-Toselli, Ottavio. *Racconti storici estratti dall'Archivio Criminale di Bologna*, 3:13-14, 351-352. Bologna, 1870. Documents pertaining to Bartolomeo da Varignana.

Medici, Michele. *Compendio storico della scuola anatomica di Bologna dal rinascimento delle scienze e delle lettere a tutto il secolo XVIII*. Bologna, 1857. Not always reliable.

Mondino de' Liuzzi. See Liuzzi, Mondino de'.

Monumenta Germaniae Historiae. Legum sectio IV: Constitutiones et acta publica imperatorum et regum. Ed. J. Schwalm. Vol. 4, pt. 1, no. 609, p. 572. Hanover and Leipzig, 1906. Document relating to Bartolomeo da Varignana.

Monumenti della Università di Padova (1222-1318). Ed. Andrea Gloria. Venice, 1884. Some documents pertaining to Dino del Garbo.

Morris, M. "Albertus de Zancariis." Leipzig, 1914.

Mundinus. See Liuzzi, Mondino de'.

Münster, Ladislao. "Alcuni considerazioni sul posto spettanto a Mondino de' Liuzzi nella storia dell'anatomia." In xx *Congresso Nazionale di Storia della Medicina, Rome, 1964, Atti*, pp. 601-608.

———. "Alcuni episodi sconosciuti o poco noti sulla vita e sull'attività di Bartolomeo da Varignana." *Castalia: Rivista di storia della medicina* 10 (1954):207-215. Includes documents.

———. "La medicina legale in Bologna dai suoi albori fino alla fine del secolo xiv." *Bollettino dell'Accademia Medica Pistoiese Filippo Pacini* 26 (1955):257-271.

———. "Taddeo degli Alderotti mancato medico condotto a Perugia (1287) e a Venezia (1293)." *Rivista di storia delle scienze mediche e naturali* 47 (1956):48-59.

———, and Dall'Osso, E. "Mondino de' Liuzzi lettore-clinico presso lo Studio di Bologna e le sue opera mediche ancora inedite." In xv *Congresso Italiano di Storia della Medicina, Torino, 1957, Atti*, pp. 212-220.

Mussato, Albertino. "Somnium in aegritudinem apud Florentiam." In *Thesaurus antiquitatum et historiarum Italiae*, ed. J. Graevius, 6:2. Leiden, 1722.

Nannini, Marco Cesare. "La cultura mistico-teologica Dantesca in Mondino de' Liucci." In xxi *Congresso Nazionale di Storia della Medicina, Perugia, 1965, Atti,* 1:209-215; 2:403-410.

Nardi, Bruno. "L'Averroismo bolognese nel secolo xiii e Taddeo Alderotto." *Rivista di storia di filosofia* 4 (1949):11-22.

———. "Noterella polemica sull'averroismo di Guido Cavalcanti." *Rassegna di filosofia* 3 (1954):47-71.

Nardi, Michele G. "Taddeo Alderotti." *Castalia: Rivista di storia della medicina* 19 (1963):25-26.

Neaman, Judith S. *Suggestion of the Devil: The Origins of Madness.* New York, 1975.

Needham, Joseph. *A History of Embryology.* 2nd ed. Cambridge, 1959.

Neuburger, Max. *History of Medicine.* Trans. E. R. Playfair. 2 vols. Oxford, 1925. Vol. 2, pt. 1, surveys medieval medicine.

Nicolini, Ugolino. "Documenti su Pietro Ispano (poi Giovanni XXI?) e Taddeo degli Alderotti nei loro rapporti con Perugia." In *Filosofia e cultura in Umbria tra Medioevo e Rinascimento. Atti del IV Convegno di Studi Umbri, Gubbio 22-26 maggio, 1966,* pp. 271-284. Gubbio-Perugia, 1967.

Niebyl, Peter H. "The Non-Naturals." *Bulletin of the History of Medicine* 45 (1971):486-492.

———. "Old Age, Fever, and the Lamp Metaphor." *Journal of the History of Medicine and Allied Sciences* 26 (1971):361-368.

Niedling, J. *Die mittelalterlichen und früneuzeitlichen Kommentare zur Techne Galenos.* Leipzig, 1924.

Ogden, Margaret S. "The Galenic Works Cited in Guy de Chauliac's *Chirurgia Magna.*" *Journal of the History of Medicine and Allied Sciences* 28 (1973):- 24-33.

O'Neill, Ynez Violé. "Michael Scot and Mary of Bologna: A Medieval Gynecological Puzzle." *Clio Medica* 8 (1973):87-111; 9 (1974):125-129.

Ongaro, Giuseppe. "Il metodo settorico di Mondino de' Liucci." In xxi *Congresso Internazionale di Storia della Medicina, Siena, 1968, Atti,* 1:68-82.

Orlandelli, G. *Il libro a Bologna dal 1300 al 1330.* Bologna, 1959.

Ortalli, Edgaro. "La perizia medica a Bologna nei secoli xiii e xiv. Normativa e practica di un istituto giudizario." *Atti e memorie della Deputazione di storia patria per le provincie di Romagna,* n.s. 17-19 (1965-1968 in one): 223-259.

Pansier, P. "Les maîtres de la faculté de médicine de Montpellier au Moyen Age." *Janus* 9 (1904):499-511.

———. "Les médecins des papes d'Avignon (1308-1403)." *Janus* 14 (1909):- 405-434.

Petella, J. B. "Les consultations oculistiques d'un maître italien du XIII^{éme} siècle." *Janus* 6 (1901):1-7, 61-67, 117-122, 173-178.

Peter of Abano. *Conciliator differentiarum philosophorum et precipue medicorum.* Venice, 1496.

Petracchi, Celestino. *Vita di Arrigo di Svevia, Re di Sardegna volgarmente Enzo chiamato.* Bologna, 1756. Prints Enzo's will, which refers to Taddeo.

Petrocchi, Giorgio. "Il Dolce stil nuovo." In *Storia della letteratura italiana,* ed. Emilio Cecchi and Natalino Sapegno, vol. 1, *Le origini e il Duecento,* pp. 729-774. Milan, 1965.

Pez, B. *Thesaurus Anecdotorum Novissimus.* Vol. 1, pt. 1, col. 430. Augsburg, 1721-29. Engelbert of Admont's letter about Guglielmo and Taddeo.

Piana, Celestino, O.F.M., ed. *Chartularium Studii Bononiensis S. Francisci (saec. XIII-XVI).* Analecta *Franciscana,* vol. 11. Florence, 1970.

———. *Nuove ricerche su le Università di Bologna e di Parma.* Spicilegium Bonaventurianum, vol. 2. Quaracchi, 1966.

Pinto, G. *Taddeo da Fiorenza e la medicina in Bologna nel secolo XIII. Discorso tenuto il giorno 14 giugno 1888 nell'Archiginnasio di Bologna ultimo della feste del VIII centenario.* Rome, 1888.

Pizzoni, Pietro. "I medici umbri lettori presso l'Università di Perugia." *Bollettino della Deputazione di storia patria per l'Umbria* 47 (1950):16-24.

Post, G. "Masters' Salaries and Students' Fees in the Medieval Universities." *Speculum* 7 (1932):181-198.

Premuda, L. "Pietro d'Abano." *DSB* 1 (1970):4-5.

Puccinotti, Francesco. *Storia della medicina.* 3 vols. Livorno, 1850-1866. Vol. 3 contains accounts of Bolognese physicians of the thirteenth and fourteenth centuries, with excerpts from their writings.

Randall, John Herman, Jr. *The School of Padua and the Emergence of Modern Science.* Padua, 1961.

Rashdall, F. Hastings. *The Universities of Europe in the Middle Ages.* 3 vols. 2nd ed. Ed. Maurice Powicke and A. B. Emden. Oxford, 1936.

Rather, L. J. "The 'Six Things Non-Natural': A Note on the Origins and Fate of a Doctrine and a Phrase." *Clio Medica* 3 (1968):337-347.

Renzi, Salvatore de. *Storia della medicina in Italia.* 5 vols. Naples, 1845-1848. Vol. 2 deals with the thirteenth and fourteenth centuries.

Riddle, John M. "Theory and Practice in Medieval Medicine." *Viator: Medieval and Renaissance Studies* 5 (1974):157-183.

Riesenberg, Peter. "The Consilia Literature: A Prospectus." *Manuscripta* 6 (1962):3-22.

Rodolico, N. *Dal comune alla signoria. Saggio sul governo di Taddeo Pepoli in Bologna.* Bologna, 1898.

Rosen, George. "The Historical Significance of Some Medical References in the *Defensor Pacis* of Marsilius of Padua." *Sudhoffs Archiv für Geschichte der Medizin und der Naturwissenschaften* 37 (1953):35-56.

Rossi, A., ed. "Documenti per la storia dell'Università di Perugia." *Giornale di erudizione artistica* 4 (1875). Nos. 47, 48, 50, pp. 323-325, pertain to Dino del Garbo.

Rossi, G. " 'Universitas scholarium' e comune." *Studi e memorie per la storia dell'Università di Bologna*, n.s. 1 (1956):173-266.

Saffron, Morris H., ed. and trans. *Maurus of Salerno Twelfth-Century "Optimus Physicus" with His Commentary on the Prognostics of Hippocrates.* Transactions of the American Philosophical Society, vol. 62, pt. 1, Philadelphia, 1972.

Sarti, Mauro, and Fattorini, Mauro. *De claris archigymnasii Bononiensis professoribus.* 2 vols. Ed. Carlo Albicini and Carlo Malagola. Bologna, 1888-1896.

Schipperges, Heinrich. *Die Assimilation der arabischen Medizin durch das lateinische Mittelalter. Sudhoffs Archiv für Geschichte der Medizin und der Naturwissenschaften.* Beinheft 3. Wiesbaden, 1964.

Schlam, Carl C. "Graduation Speeches of Gentile da Foligno." *Mediaeval Studies* 40 (1978):96-119.

Schmidt, Erich Walter Georg. *Die Bedeutung Wilhelms von Brescia als Verfasser von Konsilien.* Leipzig, 1922. Edits 21 *consilia.*

Schmitt, Charles B. "Philosophy and Science in Sixteenth-Century Universities: Some Preliminary Comments." In *The Cultural Context of Medieval Learning*, eds. John E. Murdoch and Edith D. Sylla, pp. 485-537. Dordrecht, 1975.
———. "Science in the Italian Universities in the Sixteenth and Early Seventeenth Centuries." In *The Emergence of Science in Western Europe*, ed. M. P. Crossland. London, 1975.

Segré, Cesare. *Lingua, stile e società.* Milan, 1963.

Segré, Cesare, and Marti, Mario, eds. *La prosa del Duecento.* Milan-Naples, n.d.

Seidler, E. "Die Spätzscholastik im Urteil der Medizingeschichte." *Sudhoffs Archiv für Geschichte der Medizin und der Naturwissenschaften* 48 (1964):-299-322.

Siegel, Rudolph E. *Galen on Sense Perception.* Basel and New York, 1970.
———. *Galen's System of Physiology and Medicine.* Basel and New York, 1968.

Silverstein, Theodore. "*Elementatum*: Its Appearance Among the Twelfth-Century Cosmogonists." *Mediaeval Studies* 16 (1954):156-162.

Simili, A. "Considerazioni storico critiche sui primordi dell' insegnamento medico in generale e di quello a Bologna in particolare." *Minerva medica* 65 (1974):2855-2868.

Singer, Charles. *The Evolution of Anatomy*. London, 1925.

Siraisi, Nancy G. *Arts and Sciences at Padua: The Studium of Padua Before 1350*. Toronto, 1973.

Smith, Edward G. "A Disagreement on the Need of a Sensible Species in the Writings of Some Medical Doctors in the Late Middle Ages." Ph.D. diss., St. Louis Univ., 1974.

Solmsen, Friedrich. "Greek Philosophy and the Discovery of the Nerves." *Museum Helveticum* 18 (1961):150-167, 169-197.

Sorbelli, Albano. *Storia della Università di Bologna*. Vol. 1. Bologna, 1940.

Soudek, Josef. "The Genesis and Tradition of Leonardo Bruni's Annotated Version of the (Pseudo-)Aristotelian *Economics*." *Scriptorium* 12 (1958):- 260-268.

Spina, G., and Sampalmieri, A. "La lettera di Taddeo Alderotti a Corso Donati e l'inizio della letteratura igienica medioevale." In xxi *Congresso Internazionale di Storia della Medicina, Siena, 1968, Atti*, 1:91-99. Prints text.

Stannard, Jerry. "Botanical Data in Medieval Medical Recipies." *Studies in History of Medicine* 1 (1977):80-87.

———. "Medieval Herbals and Their Development." *Clio Medica* 9 (1974):- 23-33.

———. "Medieval Italian Medical Botany." In xxi *Congresso Internazionale di Storia della Medicina, Siena, 1968, Atti*, 2:1554-1565.

Stapper, Richard. *Papste Johannes XXI*. Munster, 1898.

Steenberghen, Fernard Van. *Aristotle in the West*. Louvain, 1955.

Steneck, Nicholas H. "Albert the Great on the Classification and Localization of the Internal Senses." *Isis* 65 (1974):193-211.

Sudhoff, Karl. *Beiträge zur Geschichte der Chirurgie im Mittelalter*. 2 vols. Studien zur Geschichte der Medizin 11 and 12. Leipzig, 1918.

Tabanelli, Mario. *La chirurgia italiana nell-alto Medioevo*. 2 vols. Florence, 1965.

Taddeo Alderotti. See Alderotti, Taddeo.

Tarulli, L. "Documenti per la storia della medicina in Perugia." *Bollettino della Deputazione di Storia Patria per l'Umbria* 25 (1922):159-221. Includes documents pertaining to Taddeo.

Temkin, Owsei. *Galenism*. Ithaca, N.Y., 1973.

———. "Studies in Late Alexandrian Medicine. I. Alexandrian Commentaries on Galen's *De sectis ad introducendos*." *Bulletin of the History of Medicine* 3 (1935):405-430.

Theodoric of Lucca. *The Surgery of Theodoric*. 2 vols. Trans. C. Campbell and J. Colton. New York, 1955-1960.

Thompson, James Westfall. *The Literacy of the Laity in the Middle Ages*. Berkeley, Calif. 1939. Chap. 3 concerns Italy.

Thorndike, Lynn. "*De complexionibus.*" *Isis* 49 (1958):397-408.

———. *History of Magic and Experimental Science.* Vols. 1 and 2. New York, 1923.

———. *Michael Scot.* London, 1965.

———. "More Light on Cecco d'Ascoli." *The Romanic Review* (1946):293-306.

———, *The Sphere of Sacrobosco and Its Commentators.* Chicago, 1949. Includes the commentary by Cecco d'Ascoli.

———. "The Three Latin Translations of the Pseudo-Hippocratic Tract on Astrological Medicine." *Janus* 49 (1960):104-129.

Tiraboschi, G. *Storia della letteratura italiana.* 9 vols. Florence, 1805-1813. Vols. 4 and 5 contain detailed accounts of thirteenth- and fourteenth-century Bolognese physicians.

Torrigiano, Pietro, de' Torrigiani. See Turisanus.

Turisanus. *Turisani monaci plusquam commentum in Microtegni Galieni.* Venice, 1512.

Vaux, Roland de. "La première entrée d'Averroès chez les Latins." *Revue des sciences philosophiques et théologiques* 22 (1933):193-245.

Vecchi, G. *Il magistero delle "Artes" latine a Bologna nel Mediovo.* Pubblicazione della Facoltà di Magistro, Università di Bologna, no. 2. Bologna, 1958.

Verbeke, G. *L'évolution de la doctrine du Pneuma, du stoicisme à S. Augustin.* Paris and Louvain, 1945.

Villani, Filippo. *Liber de civitatis Florentia famosis civibus.* Ed. G. C. Galletti. Florence, 1848. Biographies of Taddeo, Dino, and Turisanus at pp. 26-29.

Villani, Giovanni. *Cronica.* In *Chroniche storiche di Giovanni, Matteo, e Filippo Villani* . . . , ed. F. G. Dragomanni. Milan, 1848.

Vitale, Vito. *Il dominio della Parte Guelfa in Bologna (1280-1321).* Biblioteca storica bolognese, no. 4. Bologna, 1902.

Wallace, William A. *Causality and Scientific Explanation.* 2 vols. Ann Arbor, Mich., 1972.

———. "Theodoric Borgognoni of Lucca." *DSB* 2 (1970):314-315.

Weisheipl, James A. "The Classification of the Sciences in Mediaeval Thought." *Mediaeval Studies* 27 (1965):54-90.

———. "Curriculum of the Faculty of Arts at Oxford in the Early Fourteenth Century." *Mediaeval Studies* 26 (1964):143-185.

———. "Developments in the Arts Curriculum at Oxford in the Early Fourteenth Century." *Mediaeval Studies* 28 (1966):151-175.

Weiss, Roberto. *Il primo secolo dell'umanesimo.* Rome, 1949.

Wellborn, Mary C. "Mondino de' Luzzi's Commentary on the *Canones Generales* of Mesue the Younger." *Isis* 22 (1934):8-11.

———. "Studies in Medieval Metrology: The *De ponderibus et Mensuribus* of Dino del Garbo." *Isis* 24 (1935-1936):15-16.

Wickersheimer, Ernest. "Une liste dressée au xve siècle des commentateurs du i^er livre du Canon d'Avicenne et du livre des Aphorismes d'Hippocrate." *Janus* 34 (1930):33-37.

Wieruszowski, Helene. *Politics and Culture in Medieval Spain and Italy.* Rome, 1971.

Wolfson, Harry A. "The Internal Senses in Latin, Arabic, and Hebrew Philosophical Texts." *Harvard Theological Review* 28 (1933):69-133.

Zaccagnini, Guido. *La vita dei maestri e degli scolari nello Studio bolognese nei secoli XIII e XIV.* Biblioteca dell "Archivum Romanicum," ser. 1, vol. 5. Geneva, 1926.

———. "Le scuole e la libreria del Convento di S. Domenico in Bologna dalle origini al secolo xvi." *Atti e memorie della R. Deputazione di storia patria per le provincie di Romagna,* 4th ser. 17 (1926-1927):228-327.

———. "L'insegnamento privato a Bologna e altrove nei secoli xiii e xiv." *Attie e memorie della R. Deputazione di storia patria per le provincie di Romagna,* 4th ser. 14 (1923-1924):254-301.

Part Four: Catalogues of Manuscripts, Bibliographical Tools, and Biographical Collections

Articles in the *Dictionary of Scientific Biography*, ed. C. G. Gillispie (New York, 1970-1978, are entered as items in part three, above.

Agrimi, J. *Tecnica e scienza nella cultura medievale: Inventario dei manoscritti relativi alla scienza e alla tecnica medievale (secc. XI-XV), Biblioteche di Lombardia.* Florence, 1976.

Aristoteles Latinus. Ed. G. Lacombe et al. Vol. 1. Rome, 1939. Vol. 2. Cambridge, 1955.

Beaujouan, Guy. "Manuscrits médicaux du Moyen Age conservés en Espagne." *Mélanges de la Casa de Velazquez* 8 (1972):161-221.

Beccaria, A. *I codici di medicina del periodo presalernitano.* Rome, 1956.

Biographisches Lexikon der hervorragenden Arzte aller Zeiten und Völker. Berlin, 1930.

Catalogo della Mostra tenutasi nella Regia Biblioteca Universitaria di Bologna in occasione del IIe Congresso della Società per la Storia delle Scienze Mediche e Naturali, Settembre, 1922. Istituto Nazionale Medio Farmacologico. Rome, 1924. Descriptions and photographic reproductions of some documents relating to Taddeo, Bartolomeo, and Dino.

Cencetti, Giorgio. *Gli archivi dello Studio bolognese.* Bologna, 1938.

Cosenza, Mario. *Biographical and Bibliographical Dictionary of the Italian Humanists (1300-1800).* 4 vols. Boston, 1962.

Cousturier, Pierre. *De vita cartusiana.* . . . Cologne, 1609. Biography of Turisanus included.

Diels, H. *Die Handschriften der antiken Ärzte.* 2 vols. Berlin, 1905-1906.

Durling, Richard J. *A Catalogue of Sixteenth-Century Printed Books in the National Library of Medicine.* Baltimore, 1967.

———. "Corrigenda and Addenda to Diels' Galenica." *Traditio* 23 (1967):463-476.

Fantuzzi, Giovanni. *Notizie degli scittori bolognesi.* 9 vols. Bologna, 1781-1794.

Fletcher, John M., ed. *The History of European Universities: Work in Progress and Publications, I, 1977.* Birmingham, 1978.

Frati, L., et al. "Indici dei codici latini conservati nella R. Biblioteca Universitaria di Bologna." *Studi italiani di filologia classica* 16 (1908):103-432; 17 (1909):1-171.

Gabriel, Astrik. *A Catalogue of Microfilms of One Thousand Manuscripts in the Ambrosiana.* Notre Dame, 1968.

———. *Summary Bibliography of the History of Universities of Great Britain and Ireland Up To 1800.* Notre Dame, 1974. Bibliography of the history of education in Europe at pp. 5-18.

Isis Cumulative Bibliography: A Bibliography of the History of Science formed from Isis Critical Bibliographies 1-90, 1913-65. 3 vols. Ed. Magda Witrow. London, 1971-1976.

Kibre, Pearl. "Hippocrates Latinus: Repertorium of Hippocratic Writings in the Latin Middle Ages." *Traditio* 31 (1975):99-126; 32 (1976):257-292; 33 (1977):253-295; 34 (1978):193-226. The series will comprise eight parts when completed.

Klebs, A. C. *Incunabula Scientifica et Medica: Short Title List.* Bruges, 1938.

Kristeller, Paul Oskar. *Iter Italicum.* 2 vols. London-Leiden, 1963, 1967.

———. *Latin Manuscript Books Before 1600.* 3d ed. New York, 1965.

Lohr, Charles H. "Medieval Latin Aristotle Commentaries." *Traditio* 23 (1967):313-413; 24 (1968):149-245; 26 (1970):135-216; 27 (1971):251-351; 28 (1972):281-396; 29 (1973):93-197; supplement in 30 (1974):119-144.

Marini, Gaetano. *Degli archiatri pontifici.* Rome, 1784.

Mazzetti, S. *Repertorio di tutti i professori antichi e moderni della famosa Università e del celebre Istituto delle scienze di Bologna.* Bologna, 1848.

Micheloni, Placido. *La medicina nei primi tremila codici del Fondo Vaticano.* Rome, 1950.

Negri, Giulio. *Istoria degli scrittori fiorentini.* Ferrara, 1722.

Pasquali Alidosi, G. N. *I dottori bolognesi di teologia, filosofia, medicina e d'arti liberali dall' anno 1000 per tutto marzo del 1623.* Bologna, 1623.

——. *Li dottori forestieri che in Bologna hanno letto. . . .* Bologna, 1623.

Petreius, Theodorus. *Bibliotheca Cartusiana, sive Illustrium sacri cartusiensis ordinis scriptorum catalogus.* Cologne, 1609. Includes biography of Turisanus.

Pocciantius, Michael. *Catalogus scriptorum florentinorum.* Florence, 1589.

Sarton, George. *Introduction to the History of Science.* 3 vols. in 5. Baltimore, 1927-1928.

Schullian, Dorothy M., and Sommer, Francis E. *Catalogue of Incunabula and Manuscripts in the Army Medical Library.* New York [1950].

Silverstein, Theodore. *Medieval Latin Scientific Writings in the Barberini Collection.* Chicago, 1957.

Thorndike, Lynn. "Some Medieval Medical Manuscripts at the Vatican." *Journal of the History of Medicine and Allied Sciences* 8 (1953):263-283.

——. "Vatican Latin Manuscripts in the History of Science and Medicine." *Isis* 13 (1929):53-102.

——, and Kibre, Pearl. *A Catalogue of Incipits of Mediaeval Scientific Writings in Latin.* 2nd ed. Cambridge, Mass., 1963.

Trithemius [Johannes de Tritterheim]. *De scriptoribus ecclesiasticis . . . collectanea.* Paris, 1512. Includes brief biographies of Taddeo, Dino, and Turisanus.

Wickersheimer, Ernest. *Dictionnaire biographique des médecins en France au moyen âge.* Paris, 1936. *Supplément*, ed. Danielle Jacquart. *Hautes études médiévales et modernes*, vol. 35. Geneva, 1979.

Wingate, Sybil D. *The Mediaeval Latin Versions of the Aristotelian Scientific Corpus, With Special Reference to the Biological Works.* London, 1931.

Zambrini, Francesco. *Le opere volgari a stampa del secoli XIII e XIV.* Bologna, 1866.

INDEX

All names of diseases are indexed under the main heading "diseases, injuries, and infirmities." The topics of *questiones* by Taddeo and his pupils are indexed under *"questiones."*

Library of Congress Cataloging in Publication Data

Siraisi, Nancy G
  Taddeo Alderotti and his pupils.

  Bibliography: p.
  Includes index.
    1. Medicine, Medieval—Italy—Bologna.   2. Thaddaeus
Florentinus, d. 1295.   3. Physicians—Italy—Bologna—
Biography.   4. Medical education—Italy—Bologna—
History.   5. Bologna.   Università.   Facoltà di
medicina e chirurgia—History.   6. Bologna—Intellectual
life.   I. Title.
R141.S55   610'.945'41   80-7554
ISBN 0-691-05313-8

Nancy G. Siraisi is Professor of History at
Hunter College of the City University of New York.